PHYSIOLOGY: MADE EASY

PHYSIOLOGY: MADE EASY

A K Basak PhD
Prof. & Head, Dept of Physiology
Haldia Institute of Dental Sciences & Research
Haldia, West Bengal

Formerly

Associate Professor and Head, Dept of Physiology
Institute of Dental Sciences, Bareilly, UP
Associate Professor and Head, Dept of Physiology
Avadh Institute of Dental Sciences, Lucknow, UP
Assistant Professor, Dept of Physiology
Universal College of Medical Sciences, Nepal
Assistant Professor, Dept of Physiology
Nepalgunj Medical College, Nepal

New Central Book Agency (P) Ltd

Co-Published by

Bijay Publications
E-mail : bijaypublications@gmail.com

Exclusively Distributed by

Bijay Pustak Bhandar (P) Ltd
90/6A M. G. Road, Bhawani Dutta Lane, Kolkata-700007
✆ : (033) 4605-7856, 8777898576, 8274916104
E-mail : bijaypustakbhandar@gmail.com

NCBA

REGD OFFICE
8/1 Chintamoni Das Lane, Kolkata 700 009, India
email: ncbakolkata@gmail.com

OVERSEAS
NCBA (UK) Ltd, 149 Park Avenue North, Northampton, NN3 2HY, UK
email: ncbauk@yahoo.com

CORPORATE OFFICE
212 Shahpur Jat, New Delhi 110 049
email: delhincba@gmail.com

BIJAY PUBLICATIONS
90/6A M. G. Road, Bhawani Dutta Lane, Kolkata-7
E-mail : bijaypublications@gmail.com

BIJAY PUSTAK BHANDAR (P) LTD
90/6A M. G. Road, Bhawani Dutta Lane, Kolkata-7
E-mail : bijaypustakbhandar@gmail.com

PHYSIOLOGY: MADE EASY • A K Basak

First Published: January 2012
Reprinted: April 2013, July 2014, August 2016, June 2019
Second Edition: January 2022
Reprinted: July 2024

PUBLISHER • TYPESETTER • PRINTER
New Central Book Agency (P) Ltd
8/1 Chintamoni Das Lane, Kolkata 700 009

CO-PUBLISHED BY
Bijay Publications
90/6A M G Road, Bhawani Dutta Lane, Kolkata 700007

TECHNICAL EDITOR : Dr Mita Sen

PROJECT SUPERVISOR : Nochiel Radhakrishnan

PROOF CHECKING : Sweeta Guha, Kakoli Banerjee and Pradip Biswas

ISBN: 978 81 7381 654 3

Price ₹ 750.00

CONTENTS

PREFACE TO SECOND EDITION

The author is glad to present the second edition of the book entitled "Physiology:Made Easy". It is also my great pleasure to have received numerous feedbacks from the students of different parts of the country. I am happy to know that this book on Physiology really helped them to excel in their examinations. It is due to their encouraging words and also the publisher's request, the author is hereby bringing the present edition of this book.

The present edition of this book has been thoroughly updated and revised as per the needs of the students. The unnecessary repetitions have been avoided with the incorporation of recent developments in the field of physiology. The explanations of the topics are supported with self-explanatory flow charts which will not only make the reading stress free but also help them to do better in the examinations especially in relation to time management during the examination.

This venture has been made possible only because of the blessings of my teachers, best wishes of my students and co-teachers to whom the author is indebted. The continuous encouragement from my wife Dhriti Basak and son Sohom is also greatly appreciated as without their support it would not have been possible to bring out this edition. The author is also grateful to Mr. Amitabha Sen, Director of New Central Book Aency, Kolkata and all his supportng staffs to make this venture successful.

I wish to have continuous feedback, valuable suggestions and opinions from one and all which will help me in making the book more student friendly and error free in the subsequent editions.

Dr. A. K. Basak

4th November, 2021

PREFACE TO FIRST EDITION

PHYSIOLOGY is the centre of the galaxy of all medical sciences. All other medical subjects revolve around Physiology.

After all, what is medical science for? To keep you and me well—our body healthy and free of diseases.

But how can you keep somebody physically fit and mentally fresh unless you know how his/her body works? So the primary need for any medical student is to know: What the body is? How does our 'SYSTEM ' work?

And you find all your answers here. In a student-friendly way—easy, concise, clear-cut, to the point.

The increasing demand of an examination-oriented (QUESTION-ANSWER) book from most of the medical and dental students, as also the vast syllabus which must be completed within a short duration, led me to author such a book—*Physiology: Made Easy*. The name itself implies that this book will make the difficult subject Physiology easier to the students—not only by building their concept within the short stipulated period but also helping them to excel in their examination.

The salient features of this book are:

- **As per the guidelines of new MCI and DCI regulations**
- **As per the pattern of University Examinations conducted by different Universities, i.e:**
  - **Easy-type long questions and answers**
  - **Short notes**
  - **Different ways of working of different 'Systems'**
  - **Brainstorming Short answer-type questions**
  - **MCQs**
- **Incorporation of *easy to present* type of diagrams and flow charts etc.**
- **Concise, point-wise and easy to understand**
- **Equally helpful for BSc (Physiology) and MSc (Medical Physiology) courses taught in different Universities—including all Universities in West Bengal.**

No venture of this kind is possible without the blessings of my teachers—especially Prof. B.N. Koley, Ex-Prof. in Physiology, CU; Dr. J. Koley, Ex-Reader in Physiology, CU: and my parents to whom I shall remain ever indebted. The generous help rendered by the faculty members of Nepalgunj Medical College, Universal College of Medical Sciences, Avadh Institute of Dental Sciences, Institute of Dental Sciences, Bareilley: and Haldia Institute of Dental Sciences is warmly acknowledged. I also wish to express my sincere thanks to my wife Dhriti Basak—who has helped me in each and every step of the preparation of this book, and also for editing the literary aspect of this book. I will be failing in my duty if I don't mention the name of my dear son, Sohom, who is always my inspiration for this type of venture.

The author is highly grateful to Mr. Amitabha Sen, Director, New Central Book Agency (P) Ltd., and his production staff, for publishing this book with due care and diligence.

I will be grateful if this book meets the umpteen demand of the students. The author is sorry for any typographical mistakes, human errors, inaccuracies or ambiguities. I will be very happy to receive any opinion, feedback and valuable suggestions from the teachers, senior and junior colleagues, and interested students for further improvement of this book. They will be beneficial both for me and the future students who will continue bearing the torch...to further heights.

Dr. A. K. Basak

1 Basic Concepts

A. Long type:

1. Define homeostasis. With suitable example justify how negative feedback mechanism helps in homeostasis.

Cellular function is entirely dependant on different constituents of ECF. In response to any change of even a single constituent in this ECF, the normal function of cell gets disturbed. So to maintain the normal function of cell it is essential to maintain this environment constant. *Homeostasis* is thus defined as the **maintenance of constancy of the internal environment i.e. ECF by the physiological mechanisms.**

Negative feedback mechanism:

- **Definition:** The homeostatic mechanism in which the final response is just opposite (negative) to initiating stimulus is called as ***negative feedback mechanism***.
- **Example with explanation:** An example of negative feedback mechanism is blood pressure control mechanism in which a high pressure causes a series of reactions that promote lowering of pressure. Similarly a low pressure initiates a series of reactions which results an elevated blood pressure. In these cases the response is negative to the initiating stimulus. The detail of this mechanism is illustrated by the following flow chart:

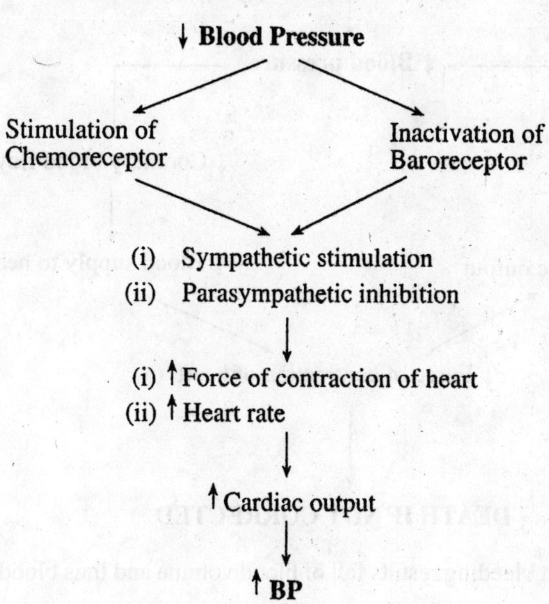

In this example the final response (i.e. ↑BP) is opposite to initiating stimulus (i.e. ↓BP). By this type of mechanism any type of change in the internal environment is counteracted and ultimately the internal environment is kept constant.

2. Define positive feedback mechanism. Is it beneficial to the body? Justify your answer with suitable example.

- **Definition:** The homeostatic mechanism in which the final response becomes similar to the initiating stimulus is known as *positive feedback mechanism.*
- **Example with explanation:**

If a person suddenly bled 2L of blood there is a drastic fall of BP and blood volume which is inadequate to fill the heart resulting initiation of positive feedback cycle instead of negative feedback as follows:

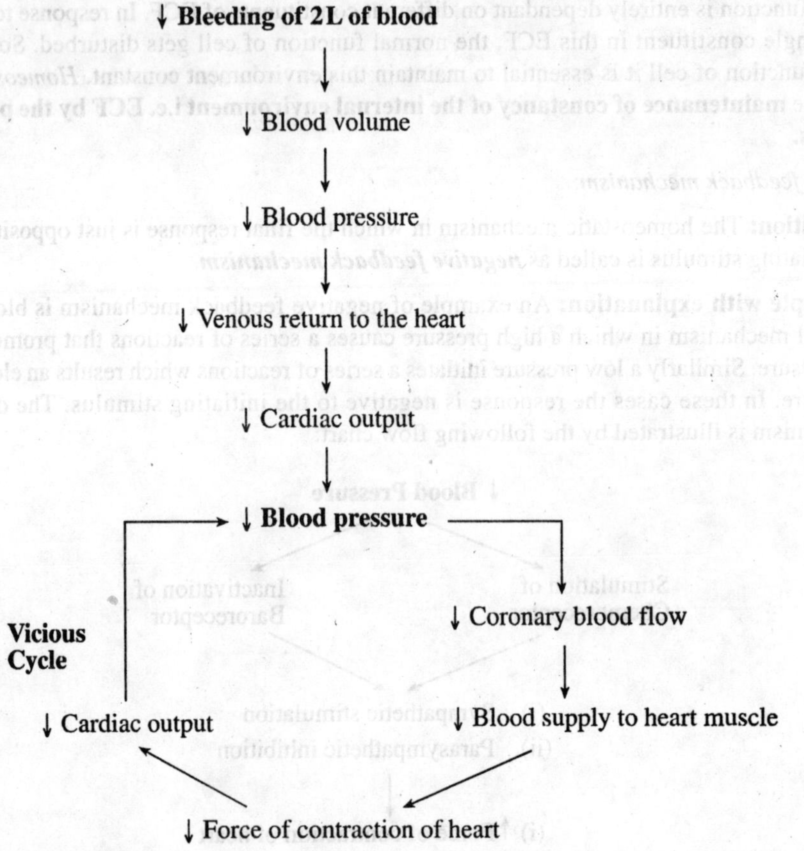

In this occasion sudden bleeding results fall of blood volume and thus blood pressure which initiates series of reactions those ultimately lead further fall of BP. As in this case the final response (i.e. ↓ BP) is similar to that of initiating stimulus (i.e. ↓BP) it is known as positive feedback mechanism.

From the above discussion it appears that positive feedback is harmful to the body as it leads a ***vicious cycle*** which ultimately leads to death. Though mild degree of positive feedback can be overcome by the negative control system which depends on the effectivity or ***Gain*** of the control system. If the gain of negative feedback is more than the positive feedback the vicious cycle can not continue, rather there is improvement of the situation and thus person survives. Whereas if the gain of negative feedback is less than that of positive feedback than negative feedback can not counteract that change and positive feedback continues to lead vicious cycle and thus death of that person occurs until not corrected by external therapy.

- **Examples where positive feedback is not harmful:** There are some instances where positive feedback is not harmful rather beneficial one. These are as follows:
  - (i) Birth of the child or parturition
  - (ii) Initiation of action potential
  - (iii) Blood clotting mechanisms

3. Enumerate the stages of Action Potential. What is the ionic basis of action potential?

- **Definition:** In response to a stimulus of threshold intensity there is *transient change* in potential difference across the cell membrane (to inside electropositive and outside electronegative). This change when reaches to a *critical level,* produces a electrical signal that can be *propagated* beyond it's site of origin. This transient change of membrane potential which is propagatory in nature is known as ***Action Potential*** (AP).

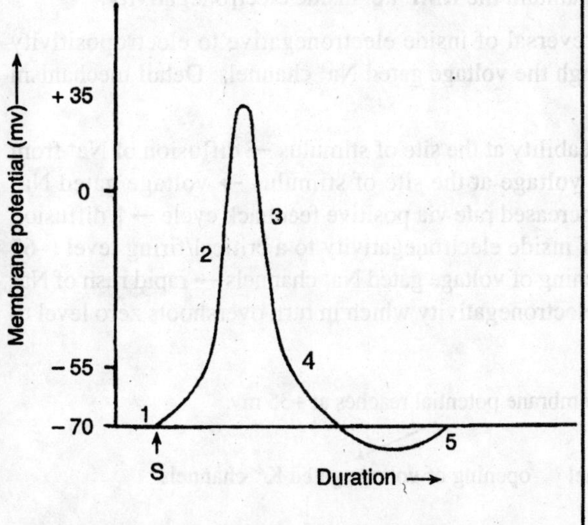

Fig. 1.1: Graphical representation of action potential (Monophasic). (1 = Polarised state; 2 = Depolarisation; 3 = Rapid Repolarisation; 4 = After depolarisation and 5 = Hyper polarisation) .

- **Phases and it's ionic basis:** Though the phases of the action potential vary from tissue to tissue, but the basic sequences of changes are almost similar. In case of nerve and some other tissues AP is mediated in following phases (Fig. 1.1).

1. **Polarized stage (Resting phase):** Under resting condition inside of the nerve fiber is electronegative in respect to the outside and the value of this potential difference (RMP) is –90 mv. This condition of the membrane is known as ***polarized stage***.

2. **Depolarization:** When a stimulus of threshold intensity is applied, after a brief time lag (latent period) inside electronegativity is decreased slowly at the initial half. When the inside electronegativity decreases to a value of approximately –65 to –70 mv (which is known as **firing level**) there is sudden and abrupt fall of electronegativity inside which ultimately reaches to **'zero'** and finally **overshoots** to reach electropositivity inside with the value of +35 mv. This reversal of electronegativity inside to electropositivity in response to stimulus of threshold intensity is known as ***depolarization.***

3. **Repolarisation:** Immediately after depolarization the electronegativity inside the membrane is reappeared initially in rapid rate followed by slow rate. This abrupt and steep rise of electropositivity inside followed by steep fall of electropositivity inside is known as ***Spike potential*** whereas the re-establishment of electronegativity inside is called as ***repolarisation*** which occurs in two phases – **initial rapid phase** followed by **slow phase**. The initial rapid phase is known as ***rapid repolarisation*** and late slow phase is known as ***after depolarization*** or ***negative after potential***.
4. **Hyperpolarisation** (after hyperpolarisation or positive after potential): At the end of repolarisation the re-establishment of inside electronegativity is not stopped at it's resting level, rather the electronegativity inside the membrane is further increased below its resting level (i.e. RMP) which finally regained after sometime. This phase in which electronegativity inside the membrane is further increased beyond RMP is known as ***Hyperpolarisation***.

- *Ionic basis*: The rise of electronegativity inside the membrane during action potential is basically due to the movement of Na^+ and K^+ through the **voltage gated Na^+ or voltage gated K^+ channels** present on the cell membrane. The detail of the ionic basis of AP in different phases is illustrated separately by the help of flow chart:

1. **Resting phase:** Under resting conditions when no stimulus is applied the voltage gated Na^+ and K^+ channels remain closed resulting no movement of Na^+ and K^+ through these channels. So the leak channels and Na^+ –K^+ pump maintain the RMP i.e. inside electronegativity.
2. **Depolarization:** Depolarization i.e. reversal of inside electronegative to electropositivity occurs due to entry of Na^+ inside through the voltage gated Na^+ channels. Detail mechanism is follows:

   Application of stimulus →↑ Na^+ permeability at the site of stimulus → diffusion of Na^+ from ECF to inside the fiber → change of voltage at the site of stimulus → voltage gated Na^+ channels ('m' gate) start to open at an increased rate via positive feedback cycle →↑ diffusion of Na^+ from outside to inside → fall of inside electronegativity to a critical/firing level (–65 to –70 mv) → sudden and complete opening of voltage gated Na^+ channels → rapid rush of Na^+ from outside to inside → rapid fall of electronegativity which in turn overshoots zero level to reach at +35 mv.

At the end of depolarisation when membrane potential reaches at +35 mv.

↙ ↘

Closure of 'h' gate of voltage gated Na^+ channel → No more Na^+ entry inside

opening of voltage gated K^+ channels → Exit of K^+ due to concentration gradient from inside of the membrane

↘ ↙

rapid fall of electropositivity inside
(RAPID REPOLARISATION)

↙ ↘

decreased K^+ gradient across the membrane

In the meantime voltage gated K^+ channels start closing

↘ ↙

slower rate of K^+ exit from inside to outside through the closing gate of K^+ channels

↓

slower fall of electropositivity or slower rise in electronegativity inside towards RMP which is known as after depolarisation

3. Repolarisation: At the end of depolarisation the inside electropositivity is reached to a value of +35 mv from –90 mv. At this phase voltage gated Na^+ channels start closing whereas voltage gated K^+ channels start opening. This results exit of K^+ out of the membrane leading fall of electropositivity inside and finally the inside of the membrane becomes electronegative again which is known as ***repolarisation.*** The detail mechanism is illustrated with the help of flow chart in **next page.**

4. Hyperpolarisation: When inside electronegativity is approached to the value of RMP voltage gated K^+ channels failed to close completely due to it's slowness in closing → exit of some extra K^+ outside → membrane potential goes negative side beyond the RMP which is known as hyperpolarisation.

4. Discuss in brief the mechanism of propagation of action potential along the nerve fiber. What do you mean by saltatory conduction of nerve impulse?

Mechanism of propagation of AP in unmyelinated nerve fiber: Once generated the action potential triggers a new action potential at the adjacent areas of the membrane by creating a **local circuit of current.** This new action potential in turn produces another local current of it's own that depolarizes the regions adjacent to it, producing action potential at the next site which is repeated cyclically (Fig. 1.2).

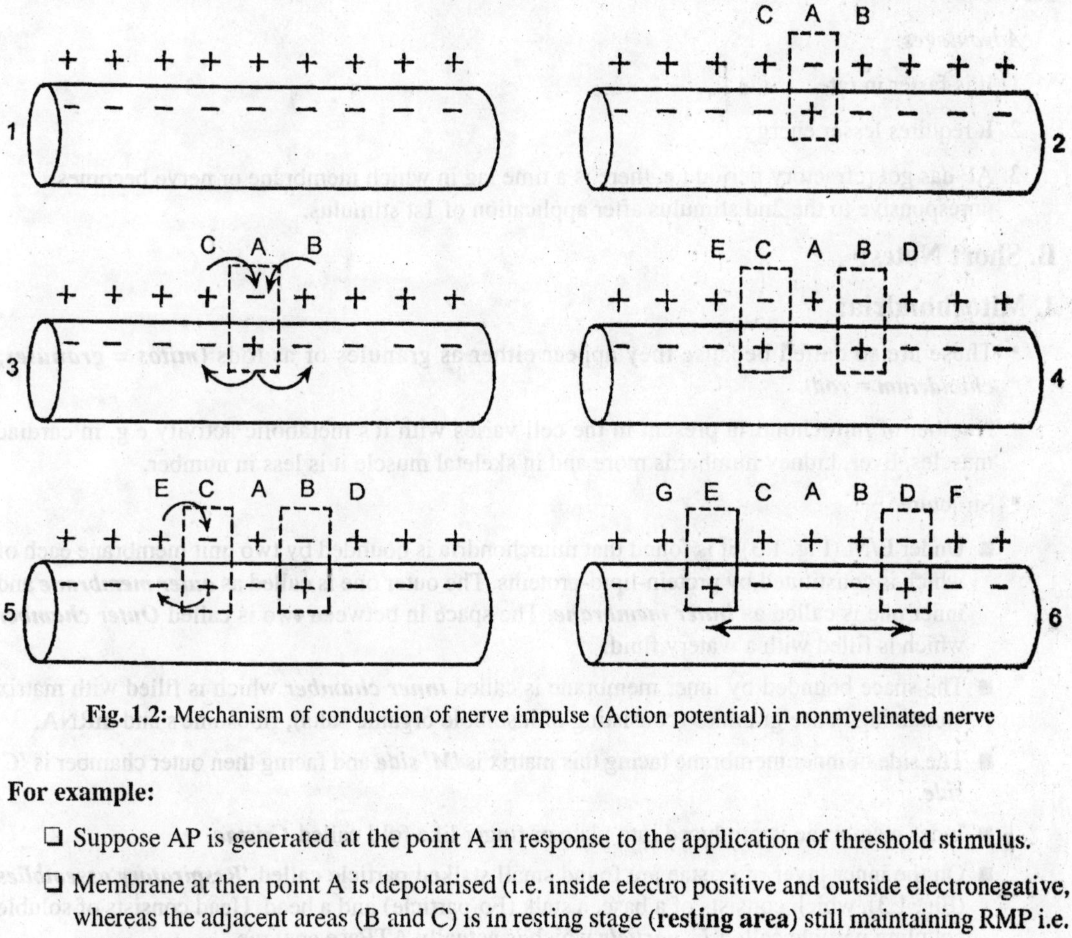

Fig. 1.2: Mechanism of conduction of nerve impulse (Action potential) in nonmyelinated nerve

For example:

- ❑ Suppose AP is generated at the point A in response to the application of threshold stimulus.
- ❑ Membrane at then point A is depolarised (i.e. inside electro positive and outside electronegative, whereas the adjacent areas (B and C) is in resting stage (**resting area**) still maintaining RMP i.e. **inside electronegativity.**

- ❑ This results flow of '+' ions from **depolarised area** (Point A) to **adjacent resting area** (Point B and C) in inside and flow of + ions from resting areas (B and C) to depolarised area (point A) in outside of the membrane thereby completing a local circuit.
- ❑ This local circuit of current flow alters the potential difference across the membrane at site B and C that leads sudden opening of voltage gated Na^+ channels at the site B and C.
- ❑ This results rapid entry of Na^+ inside at point B and C making these areas depolarized. In the meantime the previously depolarized area (i.e. point A) repolarised due to exit of K^+ through voltage gated K^+ channels.
- ❑ Thus depolarization wave is passed from point A to B and C which is continued resulting bilateral conduction of action potential.

Mechanism of propagation of AP in myelinated nerve (Saltatory conduction):

In case of myelinated nerve the myeline sheath acts as a insulator and does not allow the current flow. Therefore the flow of ions and local circuit of current flow occurs only through the **Nodes of Ranvier**. Thus current flows **from depolarised node of Ranvier** to nearby **resting node of Ranvier** which are placed apart resulting jumping of impulse from one node to another node. This type of propagation of action potential is known as ***Saltatory*** or ***Jumping conduction*** which is faster than in unmyelinated nerves.

Advantages:

1. It is faster in rate.
2. It requires lesser energy.
3. AP has got refractory period i.e. there is a time lag in which membrane or nerve becomes unresponsive to the 2nd stimulus after application of 1st stimulus.

B. Short Notes:

1. Mitochondria:

- These are so called because they appear either as granules or as rods (***mitos = granules; chondrium = rod).***
- Number of mitochondria present in the cell varies with it's metabolic activity e.g. in cardiac muscles, liver, kidney number is more and in skeletal muscle it is less in number.
- Structure:
  - ■ Under **E/M** (Fig. 1.3) it is found that mitochondria is bounded by two unit membrane each of which is constituted by protein-lipid-proteins. The outer one is called as ***outer membrane*** and inner one is called as ***inner membrane***. The space in between two is called ***Outer chamber*** which is filled with a watery fluid.
  - ■ The space bounded by inner membrane is called ***inner chamber*** which is filled with matrix containing dense granules (consisting of insoluble organic salts), ribosome's and mRNA.
  - ■ The side of inner membrane facing this matrix is ***'M' side*** and facing then outer chamber is ***'C' side.***
  - ■ Inner membrane is produced into plate or finger like fold called ***Cristae.***
  - ■ On the inner layer of cristae are found small stalked particle called ***'Respiratory assemblies*** (Fig. 1.3), which consists of a base, a stalk (Fo-particle) and a head. Head consists of soluble coupling particle called ***F_1 particle*** which is actually ATPase enzyme.

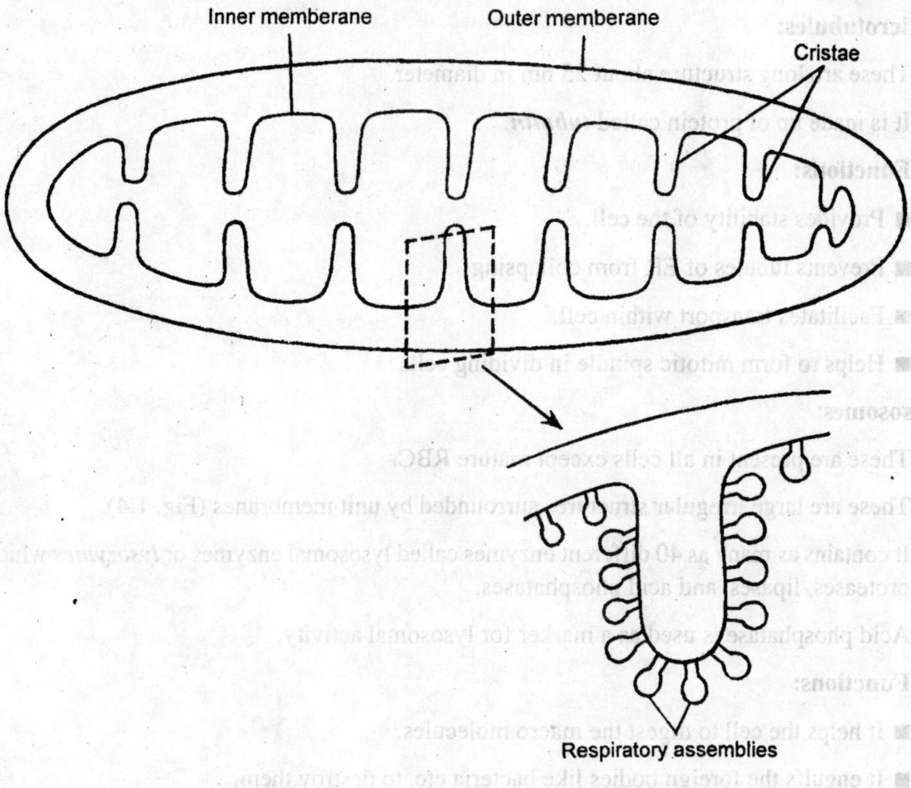

Fig. 1.3: Structure of mitochondria

- ■ The outer membrane of mitochondria is studded with enzymes concerned with biological oxidation. The enzymes of the TCA cycles are loaded in this matrix and the enzymes associated with the respiratory chain and ATP production (oxidative phosphorylation) are present on the inner mitochondrial membrane.

- **Functions:**
  - ■ It can generate the ATP and thus known as ***Power house*** of the cell.
  - ■ It can also synthesise some proteins.

2. Microtubules and Microfilaments:

Microfilaments:

- These are solid fibers of 4–6 nm in diameter.
- These are made up of protein **G-actin** which join together to form long chain called **F actin,** actin filaments or microfilaments.
- The actin filaments form a meshwork beneath the cell membrane called ***cell cortex*** which help to maintain the shape of the cell.
- **Functions:**
  - ■ Maintain shape of the cell.
  - ■ Involve in cell movement, chromosomal movement and movement of secretory granules.

Microtubules:

- These are long structure about 25 nm in diameter.
- It is made up of protein called ***tubulin***.
- **Functions:**
  - Provides stability of the cell.
  - Prevents tubules of ER from collapsing.
  - Facilitates transport within cell.
  - Helps to form mitotic spindle in dividing cells.

3. Lysosomes:

- These are present in all cells except mature RBC.
- These are large irregular structures surrounded by unit membranes (Fig. 1.4).
- It contains as many as 40 different enzymes called lysosomal enzymes or ***lysozymes*** which include proteases, lipases, and acid phosphatases.
- Acid phosphatase is used as a marker for lysosomal activity.
- **Functions:**
  - It helps the cell to digest the macro molecules.
  - It engulfs the foreign bodies like bacteria etc. to destroy them.
  - It helps to autolysis of the cell remnants and thus called as ***Suicidal bag***.

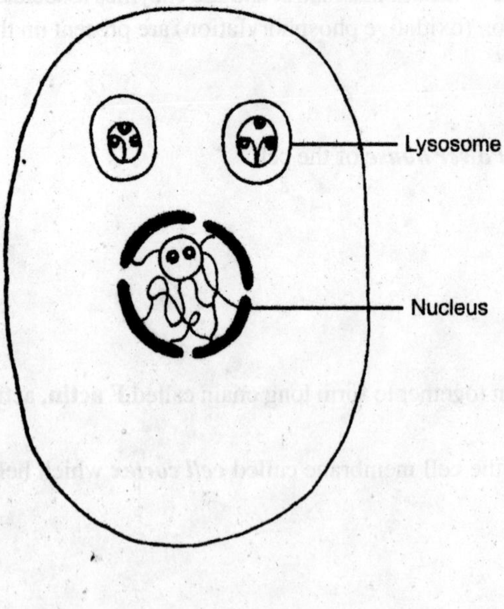

Fig. 1.4: Structure of Lysosome

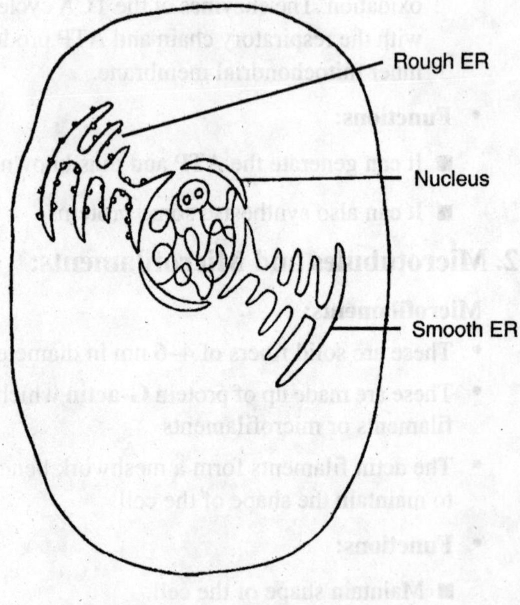

Fig. 1.5: Structure of Ribosome

4. Endoplasmic reticulum:

- It originates from nuclear envelope and connected to plasma membrane.
- It is a continuous network of tubular and flattened vesicular structure, wall of which is of unit membrane (Fig. 1.5).
- The most of the membrane surface of ER contains ribosome and thus called ***Rough Endoplasmic Reticulum*** (RER) which are responsible for protein synthesis. Whereas some membranes of ER are devoid of ribosomes called ***Smooth Endoplasmic Reticulum*** (SER) which are responsible for lipid synthesis (specially the membrane phospholipids for formation of membrane). It is also the site for the detoxification of hormones and toxins. The SER in muscle is known as sarcoplasmic reticulum.

5. Apoptosis:

- It is the natural process of coordinated and internally planned cell death that has genetic control.
- Examples:
  i. Degeneration of many tissues like web in the fingers during foetal development.
  ii. Death of neurones in CNS during brain development.
  iii. Normal shedding of intestinal epithelium.
  iv. Regression of lactating breast after cessation of breast feeding.
  v. Tumor cell death and degenerative diseases of CNS e.g. Alzheimer's disease. Parkinsons disease.

6. Tight junctions:

- These are formed through fusion of plasma membrane of two adjacent cells without leaving any intercellular space (Fig. 1.6).
- The junctions are made up of ridges half from one cell and half from other. The ridges are made up to proteins like ***Cingulin*** and ***ZO-1***.

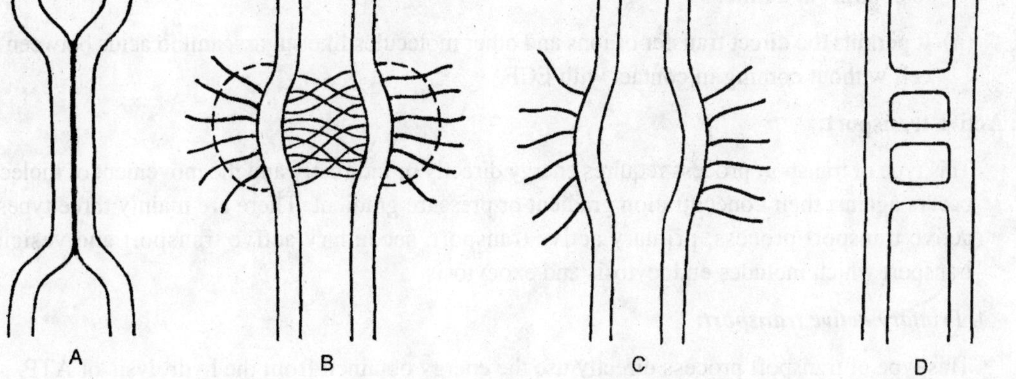

Fig. 1.6: Cell junction. (A = Tight junction; B = Desmosome; C = Zonula adherens; D = Gap junction)

- They are commonly located at the most apical part of the lateral surface of the cells in epithelium such as the intestinal epithelium, renal tubules, gall bladder, choroid plexus etc.
- **Functions:**

  (i) It forms a barrier to the movement of ions and other solute from one side of the epithelium to the other. However, in some tissues it is selectively permeable and allows the movement of NaCl.

  (ii) It maintains the cell polarity by preventing the movements of integral protein laterally.
- **Importance:**

  (i) Due to presence of tight junction within blood brain barrier (BBB) some toxic molecules can not pass through BBB from the blood to the brain tissue and thus protects the brain tissues from the hazardous effects of such substances.

  (ii) Due to presence of tight junctions, the lateral movement of protein like digestive enzymes through the intestinal mucosa is prevented allowing these to move into lumen of the tract.

  (iii) It does not allow the backflow of nutrients from the cell to lumen.

7. Gap junction:

- These are characterized by the presence of 3–4 channels in between two adjacent cells through which some molecules can pass from cytoplasm of one cell to another without coming in contact with ECF (Fig. 1.6).
- The channels are made by the fusion of cell membrane of two opposing cells which lie very close to each other (30 Å gap).
- The diameter of the channels are (normally 20 Å) regulated by intercellular Ca^{++} and also by pH and voltage around the membrane.
- The channels are formed by the collection of hexagonal arrays of protein units called ***Connexons***.
- These are present in heart muscles and also in smooth muscles.
- **Function/Importance:**

  (i) It allows rapid transmission of electrical impulse from one cell to another, thus helps the quick passage/conduction of impulse in the cardiac muscle and smooth muscle which enable them to contract at a time.

  (ii) It permits the direct transfer of ions and other molecules like sugars, amino acids between the cell without coming in contact with ECF.

8. Active transport:

This type of transport process requires energy directly or indirectly and the movement of molecule occurs against their concentration gradient or pressure gradient. There are mainly three types of active transport process, primary active transport, secondary active transport and vesicular transport which includes endocytosis and exocytosis.

A. Primary active transport:

- This type of transport process directly use the energy obtained from the hydrolysis of ATP.
- This process is mediated by the **'pump'** protein present in the cell membrane.

- **Examples:**

  (i) Na^+ K^+ pump (Fig. 1.7A) present in all cell membranes: This is actually a $Na^+ - K^+$ activated ATPase enzyme which catalyses the hydrolysis of ATP to convert ATP to ADP and energy.

  (ii) Ca_2^+ pump present in sarcoplasmic reticulum of muscles.

  (iii) $K^+ - H^+$ pump present in gastric mucosa and renal tubules.

B. Secondary active transport:

- This type of transport process does not require the energy directly but dependent on the primary active transport running simultaneously on other surface of the cell membrane. $Na^+ - K^+$ ATPase (i.e. ***primary active transport***) converts the chemical energy of ATP hydrolysis into an inward gradient for Na^+ and an outward gradient for K^+ (Fig. 1.7A) which ultimately determines the Na^+ or K^+ linked movement of other ions or substances in or out of the cell.
- This process is mediated by the ***Carrier*** protein present in the cell membrane.
- This carrier mediated process is mediated principally by two ways:

  (a) **Symport/Co-transport:** Here transport of two or more particles occur together in the same direction e.g. Na^+ – glucose transport in small intestine (Fig. 1.7B) and $Na^+ - HCO^{3-}$ transport in kidney.

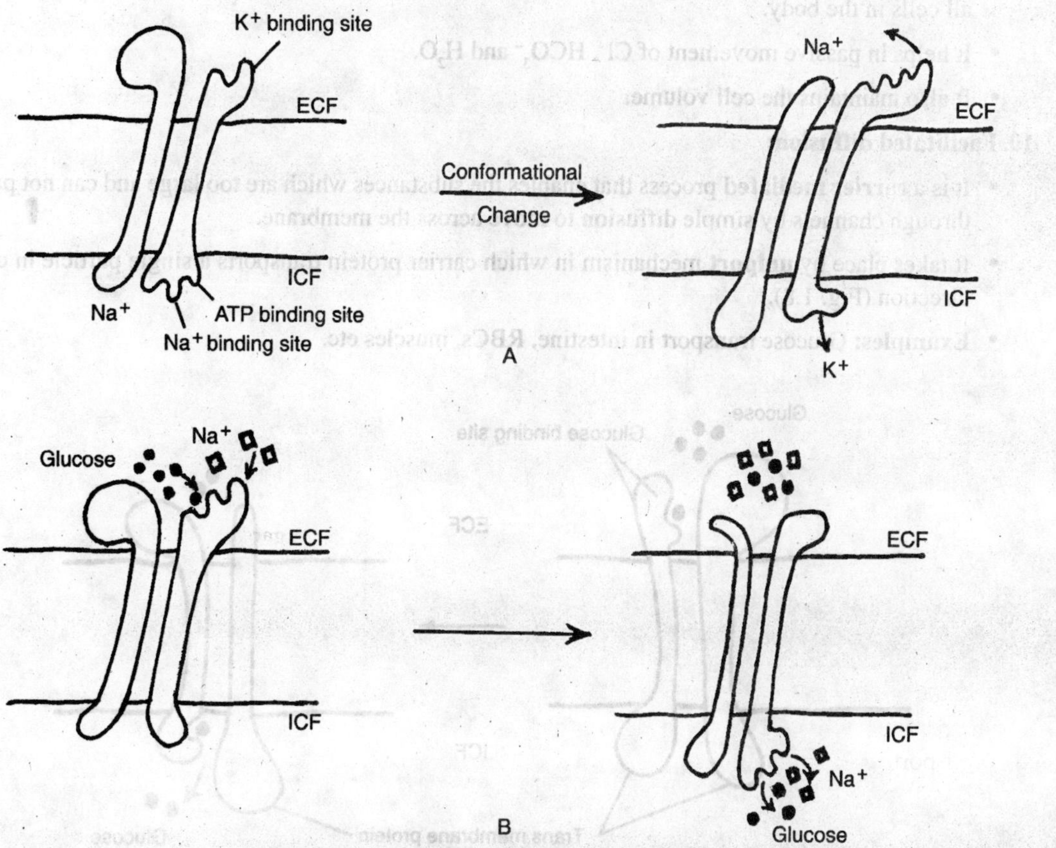

Fig.1.7: Diagrammatic representation of Primary active transport through $Na^+ - K^+$ pump (A) and Secondary active transport of glucose through carrier protein (B)

(b) **Antiport/Counter transport:** Here transportation of molecules take place in opposite directions, e.g. $Na^+ - Ca^{2+}$ transport in cardiac muscle.

9. $Na^+ - K^+$ pump:

Na^+ K^+ pumps (Fig. 1.7A) are present in all cell membranes. This is actually a $Na^+ - K^+$ activated ATPase enzyme which catalyses the hydrolysis of ATP to convert ATP to ADP and energy. The mechanism of operation of $Na^+ - K^+$ pump is illustrated in (Fig. 1.7). The $Na^+ - K^+$ pump actively and continuously pumps $3Na^+$ outside and 2 K^+ inside. Thus in single cycle there is deficit of single '+' ion inside. Continuous operation of this pump thus results the establishment of inside electronegativity (– 4 mv). The contribution of $Na^+ - K^+$ pump is far more important as this results the concentration gradient of Na^+ and K^+ across the cell membrane (i.e. More Na^+ outside and more K^+ inside) which in turn is responsible for diffusion of Na^+/K^+ across the membrane. Thus contribution of $Na^+ - K^+$ pump is the primary factor whereas K^+ diffusion and Na^+ diffusion potential are the secondary factors that determine the RMP.

Functions of Na^+ K^+ pump:

- It maintains the Na^+ and K^+ gradients by primary active transport across the cell membrane which helps to establish normal resting membrane potential.
- It directly helps in secondary active transport of amino acids and glucose through co-transport in all cells in the body.
- It helps in passive movement of Cl^-, HCO_3^- and H_2O.
- It also maintains the cell volume.

10. Facilitated diffusion:

- It is a **carrier mediated** process that enables the substances which are too large and can not pass through channels by simple diffusion to move across the membrane.
- It takes place by **uniport** mechanism in which carrier protein transports a single particle in one direction (Fig. 1.8).
- **Examples:** Glucose transport in intestine, RBCs, muscles etc.

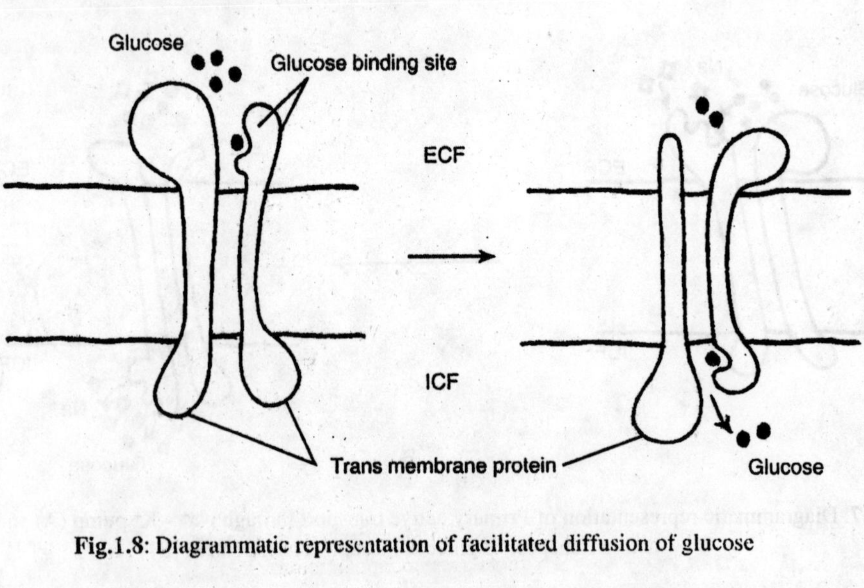

Fig.1.8: Diagrammatic representation of facilitated diffusion of glucose

- This is also assisted by hormones e.g. glucose transport from ECF to ICF by insulin.
- The factors affecting facilitated diffusion are concentration/electrical gradient, permeability of substances, molecular size of substances, temperature, number of carrier protein available, and hormones.

11. Intercellular communication:

Cell communicates each other via chemical messengers, the process of which is known as ***cell to cell communication*** or ***intercellular communication.*** There are 5 types of intercellular communication process as follows:

A. ***Neural communication***: In this process on stimulation the nerve cells release neurotransmitters which act on post synaptic cell to activate or inhibit it (Fig. 1.9).

B. ***Endocrine communication***: In this process the cells (erndocrine cells) release hormones which reaches target cell via circulating blood and thus communicate with other cells (Fig. 1.9).

C. ***Paracrine communication***: Depending on the requirement sometimes cell produces some substance which diffuses to ECF. While circulating through the ECF these substances control the activity of neighboring cells (Fig. 1.9).

D. ***Autocrine communication***: Sometimes some cells secrete chemical messengers which bind to receptors on the same cell to modify the activity of that cell (Fig. 1.9). This process is known as autocrine communication.

E. ***Juxtacrine communication***: In some situations some cells express multiple growth factors e.g. transforming growth factors alpha (***TGFα***) extracellularly on transmembrane proteins that provide an anchor to the cell. Other cells having TGFα receptors bind to those cells having TGFα on their membrane to communicate each other (Fig. 1.9).

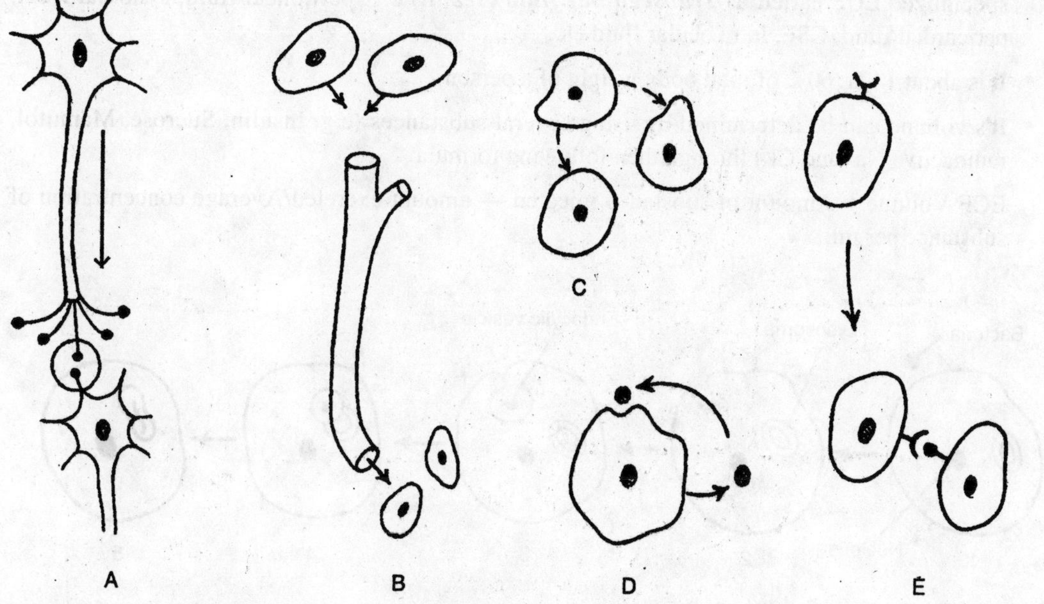

Fig.1.9: Intercellular communication (A = Neural; B = Endocrine; C = Paracrine; D = Autocrine and E = Juxtacrine communication)

12. Phagocytosis (cell eating):

In this process the extracellular (e.g. bacteria, dead tissue etc.) solid substances are engulfed by the cells. In this process when the bacterium or other foreign particles come in contact with phogocytic cell (Fig. 1.10) cell membrane invaginates the substance and forms ***digestive pouch or endocytic vesicle.*** This leads the fusion of endocytic vesicle with lysosome of the cell resulting degradation of the bacterium. The detail mechanism is illustrated as follows:

Step 1: Activation: This step of phagocytosis occurs when the phagocytic cell comes in close proximity to given objects/particles/foreign bodies. This step involves chemotaxis. Here, the cells are chemically stimulated to move towards the area with a high concentration of the foreign particles/cells or molecules.

Step 2: Binding: Surface receptors on the phagocyte then bind/adhere to the surface of the particle. Depending on the cell, there are different types of surface receptors that play an important role in this binding.

Step 3: Ingestion: The cell ingests the particle, and the particle is enclosed in a vesicle (a sphere of cell membrane with fluid in it) called a **phagosome**. The phagosome transports the particle into the cell.

Step 4: Digestion: A lysosome fuses with the phagosome called ***Phagolysosome*** and the particle is digested. Lysosomes are vesicles that contain hydrolytic enzymes that break down molecules.

Step 5: Egestion: The undigested debris of the foreign bodies are excreted out by the phagocytes by the help of exocytosis.

13. ECF:

- $\frac{1}{3}$of total body fluid (TBF) is extracellular fluid (ECF) which is comprised of 3 sub compartments known as ***Interstitial fluid*** ($\frac{3}{4}$th of ECF i.e. 10.5 lit), Plasma ($\frac{3}{4}$th of ECF i.e. 3.5 lit) and specialized ECF called as ***Transcellular fluid*** (1-2 lit) e.g. peritoneal fluid, synovial fluid, pericardial fluid, CSF, intra ocular fluid etc.
- It is about 14 L (60% of total body weight of a person).
- It's volume can be determined by using several substances (e.g. Insulin, Sucrose, Mannitol, radioactive Na^+ and Cl^-) through then following formula:

  ECF Volume = Amount of substance injected — amount excreted/Average concentration of substance per ml.

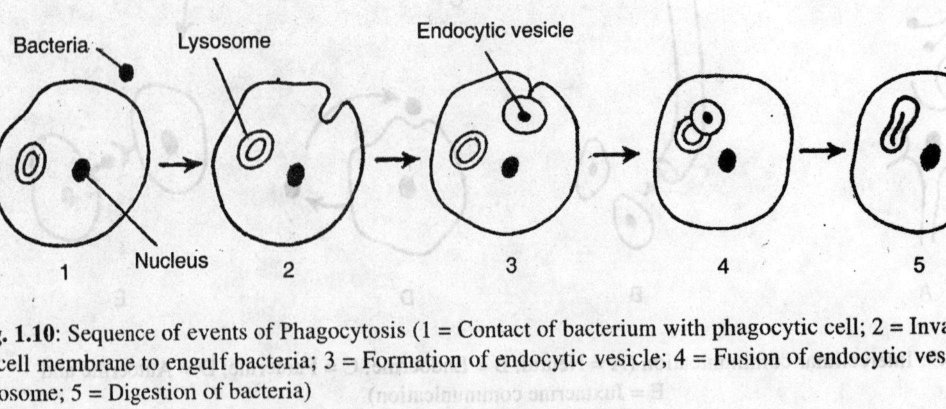

Fig. 1.10: Sequence of events of Phagocytosis (1 = Contact of bacterium with phagocytic cell; 2 = Invagination of cell membrane to engulf bacteria; 3 = Formation of endocytic vesicle; 4 = Fusion of endocytic vesicle with lysosome; 5 = Digestion of bacteria)

14. Dye dilution method:

Total body fluid or water can be measured by Dye (Indicator) dilution method based on the **conservation of mass law**. The general steps of measuring TBW is as follows:

Step 1: Known amount of indicator is dissolved in known amount of appropriate solution and injected in the compartment the volume of which is to be measured.

Step 2: Some time is allowed to distribute the indicator to that compartment.

Step 3: Then a known volume of sample from that particular compartment is collected.

Step 4: Concentration of the indicator is determined by appropriate biochemical method (Photometry or Colorimetry).

Step 5: Values are put in following formula:

$$\text{Volume of compartment} = \frac{\text{Amount of indicator injected}}{\text{Concentration of that indicator after dilution}}$$

$$= \frac{\text{Volume of solute} \times \text{concentration of indicator}}{\text{Concentration of that indicator after dilution}}$$

Characteristics of the Indicator substance:

- It must be nontoxic.
- It should neither be reabsorbed nor be secreted.
- It should not disturb the hemodynamics of blood flow.
- It's concentration can easily be measured.

15. Water intoxication:

- Excess of water intake or absence of ADH results water accumulation in the body → swelling of cells including neurone → convulsions and coma. This is known as water intoxication.
- In this case urine output increases upto 23-24 liters per day.

16. Graded potential (Electrotonic potential):

- Stimulation on specific region of cell membrane causes a transient change in membrane potential. If this change is so small (in case of application of stimulus of subthreshold intensity) that it can not pass to the adjacent area and die out within 1-2 mm of their site of origin then this small change of potential difference across the membrane is called as ***graded potential.***
- It is similar to receptor potential in case of receptor, End Plate Potential in case of N-M junction.
- It is of two types:
  - Catelectrotonic potential— the depolarising response that occurs in cathodal end of the stimulator.
  - Anelectrotonic potential—the hyperpolarising response that occurs in anodal end of the stimulator.

- It's properties are:
  - ■ It progressively decays with time and distance (decremental conduction).
  - ■ It can be summated.
  - ■ On the basis of type of stimulus it can occur either in depolarising or in hyperpolarising direction.
  - ■ It has no refractory period.
  - ■ It is non propagatory in nature.
  - ■ It does not obey all or none law.

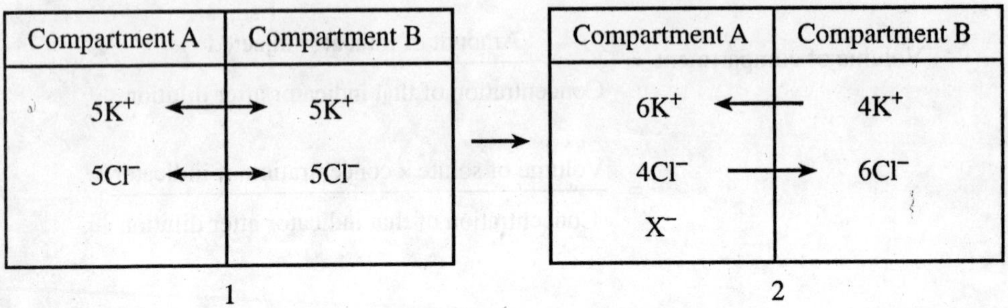

Fig. 1.11: Demonstration of Gibbs Donnan membrane Equation (1 = In presence of any non diffusible ion in compartment A; 2 = In presence of non diffusible ion i.e. X^- in compartment A there is more concentration of '+' i.e. K^+ in A and more '–' i.e. Cl^- in compartment B)

17. Gibb's Donnan membrane equilibrium:

The ionic difference across the cell membrane is established due to the asymmetric distribution of ions which is known as **Gibb's Donnan membrane equilibrium**. Suppose two compartments (separated by semi permeable membrane) contain some diffusible ions (e.g. K^+, Cl^-) and some non diffusion ions (e.g. X^-) as demonstrated in (Fig. 1.11). As in solution of compartment B no indiffusible ions are present so solution of compartment A will contain more positive ions (K^+) than the K^+ in compartment B because of attraction between X^- and K^+. Whereas in compartment B there will be more diffusible Cl^- than compartment A because of repulsion between X^- and Cl^-. Thus there is an asymmetric distribution of ions in between the compartment A and B. This asymmetric equilibrium of ions across the membrane is known as ***Gibbs's Donnan membrane equilibrium*** which is responsible for establishment of electrical difference across the cell membrane (i.e. **RMP**).

18. All or None law:

- As per the all or none law, once action potential (AP) is initiated it is initiated maximally or not at all. This means by application of subthreshold stimulus AP is not initiated, similarly any increase in the intensity stimulus beyond it's threshold level fails to further increase in the height of action potential (Fig. 1.12).
- It is applicable in single muscle cell or single nerve fiber and whole atria or whole ventricle.

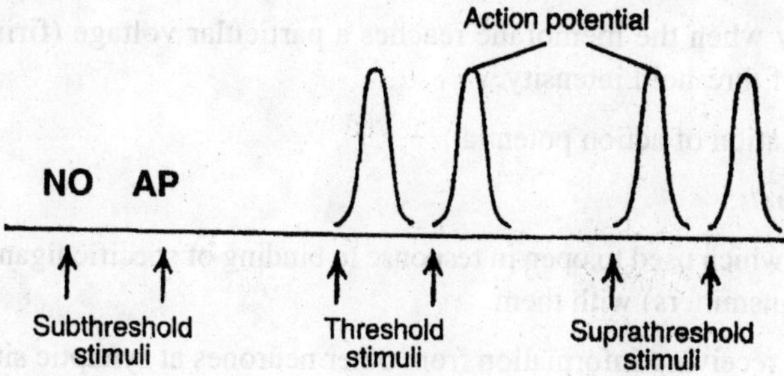

Fig. 1.12: Demonstration of all or none law

19. Na⁺ channels:

- **These are the channels (route) through which Na^+ diffuses from outisde to inside of the cell due to concentration gradient.**
- **These are of 2 types:**
  1. **Non gated or leaky Na^+ channels —responsible for establishment of RMP.**
  2. **Gated Na channels-responsible for origin of action potential in response to stimulus of threshold intensity. It is again of two types—**

(i) *Voltage gated Na channels*:

- **Present in all cell membrane though these are predominantly located in nodes of Ranvier and axon hillock of neuronal cell.**
- **These channels remain close during resting state due to closure of it's activation gate (Fig. 1.13).**

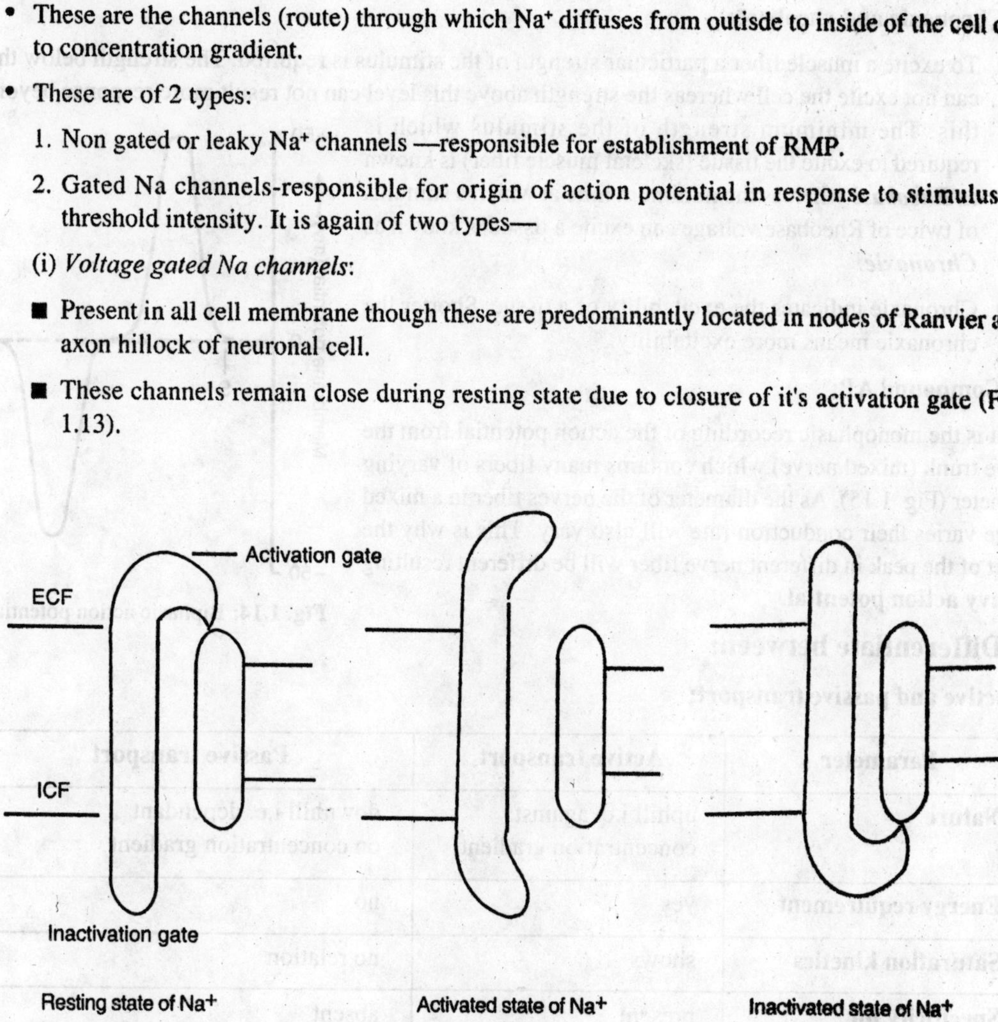

Fig.1.13: Diagrammatic representation of Na^+ channels

- They used to open only when the membrane reaches a particular voltage (firing level) in response to a stimulus of threshold intensity.
- It is responsible for initiation of action potential.

(ii) *Ligand gated Na channels*:

- These are like receptors which used to open in response to binding of specific ligand (chemical substances like neurotransmitters) with them.
- These are important for receiving information from other neurones at synaptic site.
- These are present predominantly on dendritic spine, dendrites and cell body of neurone.

• These are blocked either by using local anaesthetics like lidocaine, procain etc. or neurotoxins like tetrodotoxin, saxitoxin etc.

20. Chronaxie and rheobase:

• To excite a muscle fiber a particular strength of the stimulus is required. The strength below this can not excite the cell whereas the strength above this level can not result more response beyond this. The minimum strength of the stimulus which is required to excite the tissue (skeletal muscle fiber) is known as ***Rheobase*** whereas the minimum time at which a stimulus of twice of Rheobase voltage can excite a tissue is known as ***Chronaxie***.

• Chronaxie indicates the excitability of a tissue. Shorter the chronaxie means more excitability.

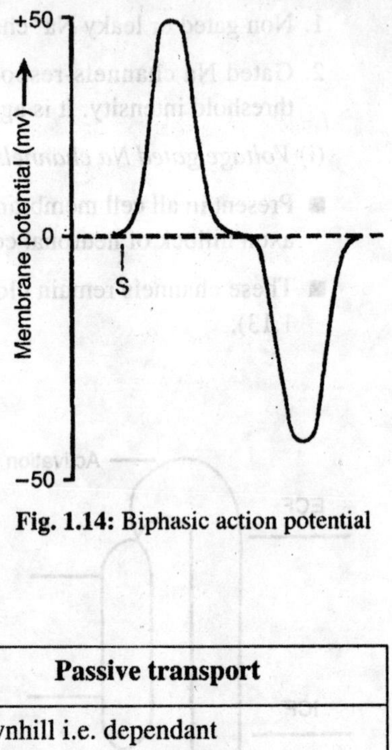

Fig. 1.14: Biphasic action potential

21. Compound AP:

It is the monophasic recording of the action potential from the nerve trunk (mixed nerve) which contains many fibers of varying diameter (Fig. 1.15). As the diameter of the nerves fiber in a mixed nerve varies their conduction rate will also vary. This is why the onset of the peak in different nerve fiber will be different resulting a **wavy action potential**.

C. Differentiate between:

1. Active and passive transport:

Parameter	Active transport	Passive transport
Nature	uphill i.e. against concentration gradient	downhill i.e. dependant on concentration gradient
Energy requirement	yes	no
Saturation kinetics	shows	no relation
Specificity for particular molecule	present	absent
Competitive inhibition	shows	no

2. Simple and facilitated diffusion:

Parameter	Simple diffusion	Facilitated diffusion
Rate of diffusion	directly related with concentration gradient and inversly related with permeability of the solute	dependant on kinetics of carrier mediated transport and can not exceed a certain maximum called V max
Example	diffusion of gases and solutes	Na^+-glucose co-transport and Cl^+ –HCO_3^-– antiport (in renal tubular and gastric pareital cell)
Route	through channels or pores	through carrier protein
Rate of transfer	slower	comparatively faster
Saturation kinetics	no saturation point	has saturation point i.e. all the available binding sites of carrier protein are occupied

3. Osmotic and oncotic pressure:

Osmotic: It is the minimum pressure applied to the solution with higher solute concentration to prevent osmosis.

Oncotic pressure: The colloidal osmotic pressure due to the plasma colloids is called as oncotic pressure.

4. Osmolarity and osmolality:

- Osmolarity is the number of .osmoles per liter of solution (e.g. plasma) whereas the osmolarity is the number of osmoles per kilogram of solvent.
- Osmolarity is affected by the volume of various solutes in the solution and temperature whereas the osmolality is not.

5. Endocytosis and exocytosis:

Endocytosis is the process of transport in which a substance is taken into the cells by means of vesicle formation whereas exocytosis is the process of discharge of particles from a cell.

6. Isotonic and isoosmotic solution:

The solution that has the same osmolality as plasma (e.g. 0.95 NaCl solution or 5% glucose solution) is known as isotonic whereas the solution that has the same osmolality as other regardless of it's composition is known as isoosmotic.

7. Primary and secondary active transport: Vide short note.

8. Graded and action potential:

Graded potential	Action potential
It is non prapagatory in nature	It is propagatory
It does not obey all or none law	It obeys all or none law
It has no threshold	It's threshold usually is 10-15 mv

Contd. next page

8. Graded and action potential (continued from previous page):

Graded potential	Action potential
It has no refractory period	It has refractory period
It is important in signalling over short distance	It is important in signalling over long distance
It can be summated	It can not be summated
It is either hyperpolarising or depolarising response	It is always depolarising response
It is the passive process	It is the active process

9. Monophasic and Biphasic action potential:

- The action potential initiated in response to the stimulus can be recorded through cathode ray oscilloscope by placing two electrodes in two separate site of the membrane (one electrode is placed outside the membrane and another is inserted inside the membrane or one electrode is placed externally on the surface of the healthy site of the membrane and another at the damaged/ injured/sectioned site). In both the cases the recorded action potential (AP) will be ***monophasic*** (Fig. 1.1).
- Whereas if both the electrodes are placed at the outside of the membrane the AP is recorded as an upward deflection followed by short isoelectric period and then a downward deflection (Fig. 1.14) which is known as ***biphasic action potential.***
- Monophasic AP is intracellular recording whereas biphasic AP is extracellular recordings.
- Biphasic AP is clinically more important e.g. ECG, EEG, EMG are all biphasic type (extra-cellular) of AP.

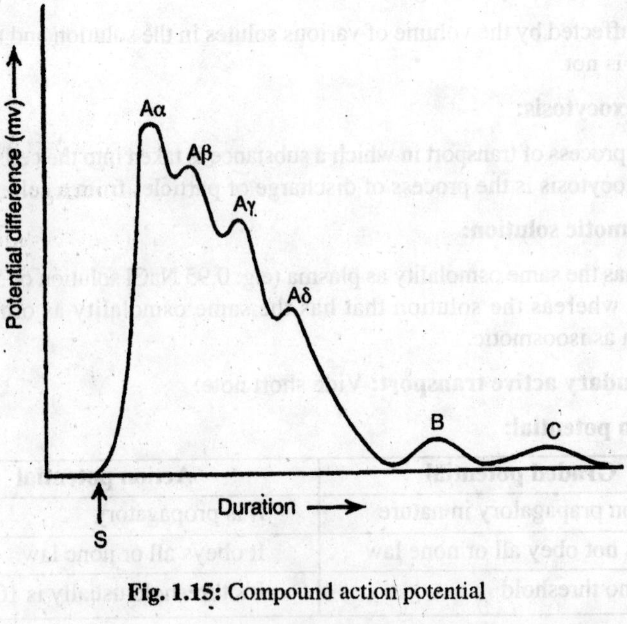

Fig. 1.15: Compound action potential

10. RMP and action potential:

RMP	Action potential
The potential difference across the membrane during resting conditions (without application of stimulus) is known as resting membrane potential (RMP)	The potential difference in response to stimulation of threshold intensity is called as action potential
During this condition the inside of the membrane is electronegative	During this condition the inside of the membrane is electropositive
It is maintained and established by the involvement of leak ion channels and also $Na^+ - K^+$ pump	It is due to action of gated ion channels
It is not propagatory	It is propagatory
It does not obey all or none law	It obeys all or none law

D. Brainstorming short answer type:

1. Enumerate the functions of membrane proteins and lipids.

(a) Function of proteins:

i. It is the structural component of membrane.

ii. It acts as pump, carriers and ion channels.

iii. It also acts as receptors and enzymes.

iv. It (glycoprotein) acts as antigens on the surface of the cell (blood group antigens)

(b) *Function of lipids*: Lipid layer of the membrane is responsible for fluidity of the membrane because of which membrane becomes flexible and allows cells to undergo considerable changes in shape without disruptions of their structural integrity.

2. What are the factors affecting membrane fluidity?

These are: lipid composition of the membrane, density of the integral proteins and temperature.

3. Give an account of "*Ping Pong model*" of carrier mediated transport.

The carrier mediated transport carriers do not move the substances through the thickness of the membrane to carry it but by Ping Pong mechanism. As per this model carrier protein exits in two

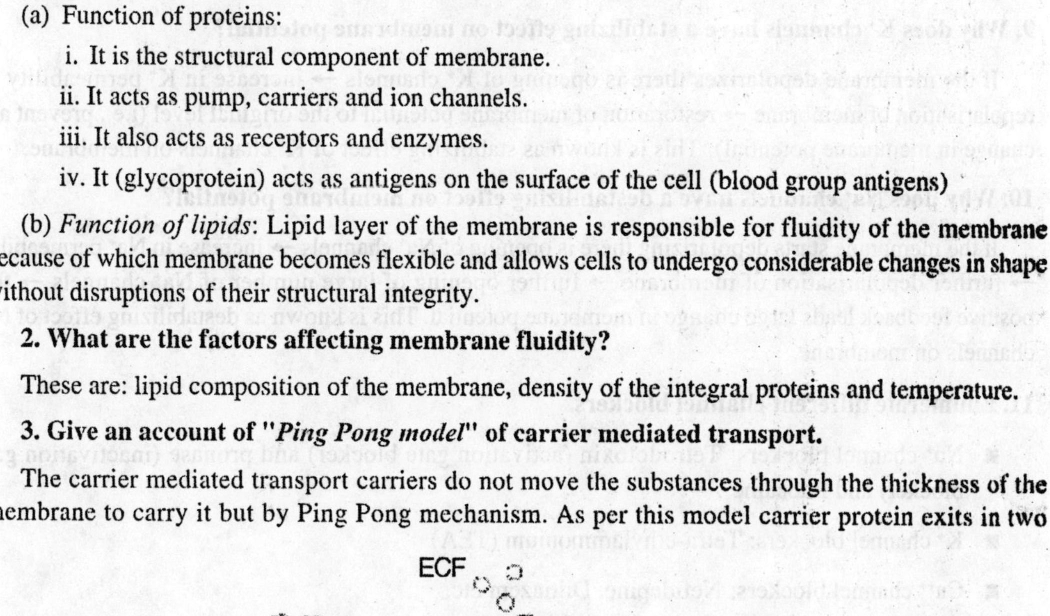

Fig. 1.16: Ping Pong model of carrier mediated transport

principal configurations: ***Ping*** and ***Pong*** state. In ***Pong state*** the carrier proteins bind the molecules of the solute when it is exposed to high concentration of solutes. Transport occurs when the conformation changes to ***Ping state*** exposing the carrier to a lower concentration of solute (Fig. 1.16).

4. How NO produces vascular smooth muscle relaxation?

NO diffuses to vascular smooth muscle → binds guanylate cyclase → converts GTP to cGMP → relaxation of smooth muscle.

5. Explain why dehydration develops rapidly and is more often in children.

It is because of low absolute volume of ECF in children and infants.

6. What is the normal pH of blood? What blood pH is compatible with life? Why it is important to maintain the normal range of blood pH?

Normal pH is 7.4 ± 0.02, whereas the blood pH that is compatible with life is 7.7 to 6.9.

It is important because most of the enzyme functions optimally at this particular range of blood pH.

7. What are the buffer system present in our body?

These are: bicarbonate, biphosphate, ammonia and proteins.

8. What is the effect of addition of KCl in the bathing fluid?

It may depolarize the membrane.

9. Why does K^+ channels have a stabilizing effect on membrane potential?

If the membrane depolarizes there is opening of K^+ channels → increase in K^+ permeability → repolarisation of membrane → restoration of membrane potential to the original level (i.e., prevent any change in membrane potential). This is known as stabilizing effect of K^+ channels on membrane.

10. Why does Na^+ channels have a destabilizing effect on membrane potential?

If the membrane starts depolarizing there is opening of Na^+ channels → increase in Na^+ permeability → further depolarisation of membrane → further opening of large number of Na^+ channels → this positive feedback leads large change in membrane potential. This is known as destabilizing effect of Na^+ channels on membrane.

11. Enumerate different channel blockers.

- Na^+ channel blockers: Tetrodotoxin (activation gate blocker) and pronase (inactivation gate blocker) and lidocaine
- K^+ channel blockers: Tetra-ethylammonium (TEA)
- Ca^{++} channel blockers: Nefidepine, Diltiazem etc.

12. What do you mean by catelectrotonic and anelectrotonic potential?

If a cathode is brought near the external surface of the membrane, the internal surface of the membrane becomes electropositive. This depolarization induced by cathode is Catelectronic potential whereas, if a anode is brought near the external surface of the membrane, the internal surface of the membrane becomes electronegative (hyperpolarisation) which is known as anelectrotonic potential.

E. MCQ:

1. The intrinsic proteins present in the cell membrane mainly functions as (i) enzyme (ii) carrier (iii) pump (iv) channels. (i)
2. Following are the membrane bound cell organelles except (i) endoplasmic reticulum (ii) lysosome (iii) ribosomes (iv) peroxisome. (iii)
3. The site of lipid synthesis in the cell is (i) RER (ii) SER (iii) golgibodies (iv) secretory vesicles. (ii)
4. F_0 particle present in (i) ribosome (ii) peroxisomes (iii) golgibodies (iv) mitochondria. (iv)
5. The normal ECF volume is (i) 10 L (ii) 28 L (iii) 14 L (iv) 20 L. (ii)
6. The osmolality of isotonic fluid is (i) 250 mosm/L (ii) 300 mosm/L (iii) 350 mosm/L (iv) 400 mosm/L. (ii)
7. Reduction in colloidal osmotic pressure results (i) edema (ii) acidosis (iii) alkalosis (iv) dehydration. (i)
8. Oral rehydration therapy utilizes following mechanism (i) diffusion (ii) filtration (iii) cotransport (iv) primary active transport. (iii)
9. RBC will swell up and burst if it is kept (i) 0.9% saline (ii) 10% saline (iii) distilled water (iv) 9% saline. (i)
10. The largest compartment of intracellular fluid is (i) plasma (ii) interstitial fluid (iii) transcellular fluid (iv) Synovial fluid. (ii)
11. All are the examples of transcellular fluid except (i) peritoneal fluid (ii) CSF (iii) intraocular fluid (iv) interstitial fluid. (iv)
12. The resting membrane potential of nerve fiber is (i) – 70 mv (ii) + 70 mv (iii) – 35 mv (iv) 0 mv. (i)
13. The resting membrane potential is mainly due to (i) Na^+ diffusion potential (ii) K^+ diffusion potential (iii) $Na^+ – K^+$ pump (iv) Cl^- diffusion potential. (ii)
14. The contribution of $Na^+ – K^+$ pump towards establishment RMP is about (i) – 70 mv (ii) – 90 mv (iii) – 86 mv (iv) – 4 mv. (iv)
15. A decrease in K^+ concentration in ECF will result (i) depolarization (ii) hyperpolarisation (iii) repolarisation (iv) none of the above. (ii)
16. Depolarisation occurs due to (i) Na^+ influx (ii) K^+ efflux (iii) CL^- i influx (iv) Ca^{++} influx. (i)
17. The part of action potential that coincides with absolute refractory period is (i) depolarization (ii) repolarisation (iii) hyperpolarisation (iv) depolarisation and 1/3 of repolarisation. (iv)
18. All the potentials do not follow the all or none law except (i) EPSP (ii) action potential (iii) IPSP (iv) MEPP. (ii)
19. Depolarisation in smooth muscle occurs due to — (i) Na^+ influx (ii) K^+ efflux (iii) Cl^- influx (iv) Ca^{++} influx. (iv)

20. Action potential develops in a neurone at (i) node (ii) internode (iii) dendrite (iv) axon hillock. (iv)

21. The plateue phase of AP in cardiac muscle is caused by (i) Na^+ influx (ii) K^+ efflux (iii) Cl^- influx (iv) Ca^{++} influx. (iv)

22. The potential of cardiac SA nodal cells is caused by (i) decreased Na^+ influx and K^+ efflux (ii) K^+ efflux (iii) decreased K^+ efflux and Ca^{++} influx (iv) increased K^+ efflux and Ca^{++} influx. (iii)

23. RMP is more in (i) small neurone (ii) larger neurone (iii) both (iv) none of the above. (i)

24. Following are the types of biphasic AP except (i) ECG (ii) EMG (iii) EEG (iv) all of the above. (iv)

25. Saltatory conduction takes place in (i) myelinated nerves (ii) non myelinated nerves (iii) single neurone (iv) cardiac muscle. (i)

26. Following are the examples of graded potential except (i) receptor potential (ii) action potential (iii) EPP (iv) MEPP.

■ SPACE FOR NOTES

Blood and Reticuloendothelial System

2

A. Long type:

1. Define Erythropoiesis. Where does it occur? Describe the stages of erythropoiesis. Enumerate the factors affecting erythropoiesis.

Definition: The process of RBC formation from the stem cells of bone marrow is known as erythropoiesis.

Site of erythropoiesis:

a. In foetal life:

- Upto 3 month of foetal life **(Mesoblastic stage)**—It is formed from mesoderm of yolk sac. As it occurs within the blood vessels it is known as **intravascular erythropoiesis.**
- From 3 months to about 6 months **(Hepatic stage)**—Liver and spleen.
- During last 3 months **(Myeloid stage)**—Red bone marrow mainly.

Erythropoiesis during hepatic and myeloid stage is known as extra vascular erythropoiesis.

b. In postnatal life and adults:

- **Up to the age of 5-6 years:** red bone marrow of all bones.
- **From 6-20 years:** red bone marrow of long and membranous bones.
- **Beyond 20 years:** red bone marrow of ends of long and membranous bones like vertebra, sternum, ribs etc.

***Stage and process of erythropoiesis*:** Erythropoiesis takes place in different stages as diagrammatically represented by (Fig. 2.1). The stages are: Proerythroblast, Early normoblast, Intermediate normoblast, Late normoblast, Reticulocyte and Mature erythrocyte. The details of the differentiation of mature erythrocytes are described in following steps:

(i) Differentiation of multipotent stem cell to committed stem cell: The most primitive totipotent stem cell in the marrow is capable of reproducing itself indefinitely to be differentiated into uncommitted stem cells which further divide mitotically to produce different committed stem cells.

(ii) Differentiation of committed stem cell to erythrocytes progenitor cell: These committed stem cells divide mitotically and differentiate into progenitor cells. The progenitor cell from which erythrocytes are developed is known as **Erythroid progenitor cell** which are of two types-***Blast***

Forming Unit **(BFU-E)** and ***Colony Forming Unit*** **(CFU-E)** of E series. However, CFU-E represents the most differentiated erythroid progenitors.

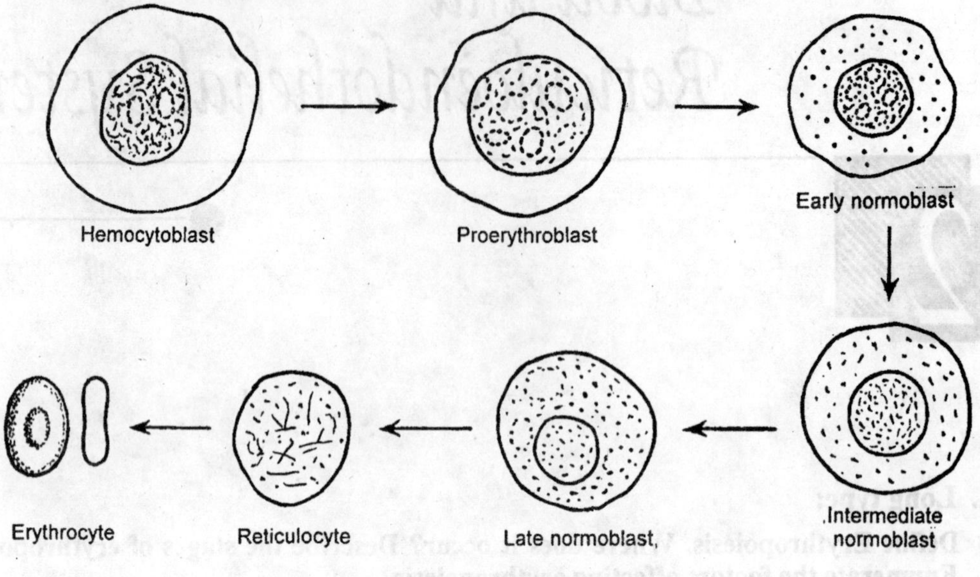

Fig. 2.1: Diagrammatic representation of erythropoiesis

(iii) Differentiation of erythrocyte progenitor cell to normoblast and thence to reticulocyte: The erythroid progenitor cells mitotically differentiate to first ***Proerythroblast*** which further differentiate to most mature nucleated cells. Eventually the nucleoli disappears, hemoglobin starts appearing and the cell is called then a ***Normoblast (early)***. Subsequently the size of normoblast diminishes progressively, the nucleus shrinks and finally extruded. In the ***Late normoblast*** the cell division stops and the cells are released through the capillaries of the marrow into the blood stream as ***Reticulocyte***.

(iv) Maturation of reticulocyte to form erythrocytes: In early stage the reticulocytes still possess some cytoplasmic RNA, mitochondria and surface transferring receptors i.e. the synthetic machinery required to continue hemoglobin synthesis. It also contains ribosomes in the reticular network form for which it is named as reticulocyte. A reticulocyte normally matures for 1-2 days in the marrow before entering the circulation as mature erythrocytes.

Factors affecting erythropoiesis (Regulation):

Regulators

- General factors
  - Hypoxia
  - Diet
- Maturation factor
  - Vit B_{12}
  - Folic acid
  - Extrinsic factors
  - Castle's intrinsic factor
- Growth factors (CSF)
- Chemical messenger

1. Hypoxia

It is the main regulatory factors influencing erythropoiesis. Hypoxia due to haemorrhage, high altitude, cardio-pulmonary disturbances or methemoglobin excess or renal hypoxia causes release of erythropoietic factors **(REF) or** *erythrogenin* from JG cells to kidney which acts on plasma substrate, erythropoietinogen (α-globin) to form ***erythropoietin.*** Hypoxia also increases this specific globulin formation from the liver. This erythropoietin inturn causes —

- Early differentiation of erythropoietin sensitive stem cells into proerythroblast and thence to mature RBC within 2-3 days.
- Increased release of reticulocytes from the bone marrow.
- Increases synthesis of RNA, DNA, globin and ferritin which increases ***'heme'*** synthesis and thus increasing hemoglobin synthesis in already existing normoblast.

The whole mode of action is represented by following schematic diagram.

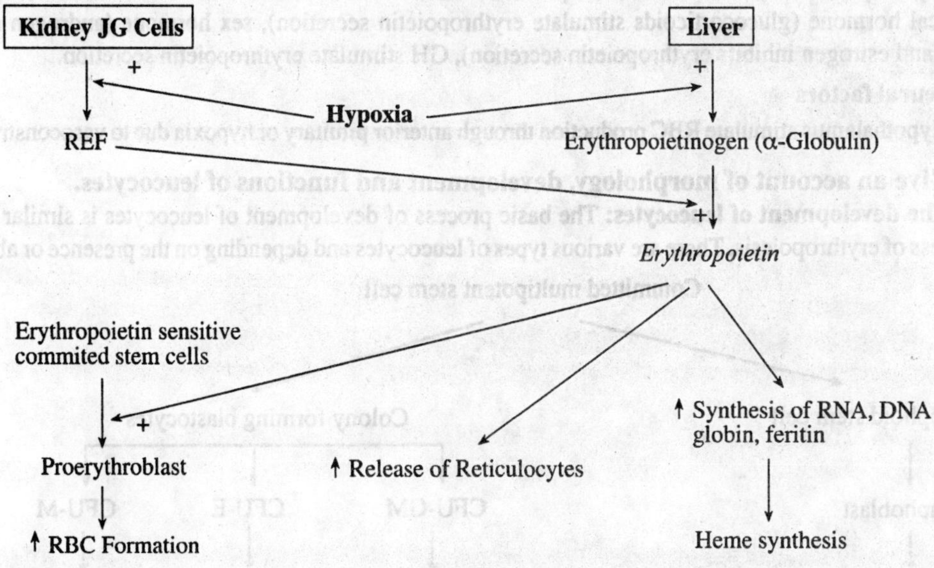

2. Interleukins (Il)

IL-1, 3, 6 causes differentiation of multipotent uncommitted stem cells to committed stem cells and also increases secretion of colony stimulating factors.

3. Colony stimulating factor (CSF)

These are growth factors or hormones which cause differentiation of committed stem cell to matured stem cell with then help of erythropoietin.

4. Maturation factors:

(i) *Vit B_{12}* and *Folic acid* — These are required for the final maturation of RBC by helping the synthesis of DNA. Therefore lack of either vitamin B_{12} or folic acid causes diminished DNA and consequently failure of nuclear maturation and division. Therefore it is said that vitamin B_{12} and folic acid deficiency causes maturation failure in the process of erythropoiesis.

(ii) *Castle's intrinsic factor*—Absorption of vitamin B_{12} and folic acid through GI tract is aided by glycoprotein secreted from parietal cells of stomach called ***Castle's intrinsic factor.*** This intrinsic factor combines with vitamin B_{12} of the food and protects it from being digested and thus makes available for absorption through mainly ileum. Thus lack of this factor because of atrophy of gastric mucosa causes loss of vit. B_{12} from the body and thereby develops **maturation failure** or ***pernicious anemia.***

5. Diet:

- Carbohydrates—required for energy supply
- Proteins—help in formation of globin
- Fats—required for cell membrane
- Vitamins—Vitamin C,D are essential for Hb synthesis besides vit B_{12} and folic acid
- Iron—helps in formation of 'Haem'
- Copper—helps in absorption of iron from GIT
- Cobalt and Nickel—enhance utilization of iron for Hb synthesis.

6. Hormonal factors:

Erythropoietin, thyroid hormones (required for maintenance of metabolism and maturation), adreno-cortical hormone (glucocorticoids stimulate erythropoietin secretion), sex hormone (androgen stimulates and estrogen inhibits erythropoietin secretion), GH stimulate erythropoietin secretion.

7. Neural factors

Hypothalamus stimulate RBC production through anterior pituitary or hypoxia due to vasoconstriction.

2. Give an account of morphology, development and functions of leucocytes.

The development of leucocytes: The basic process of development of leucocytes is similar to the process of erythropoiesis. There are various types of leucocytes and depending on the presence or absence

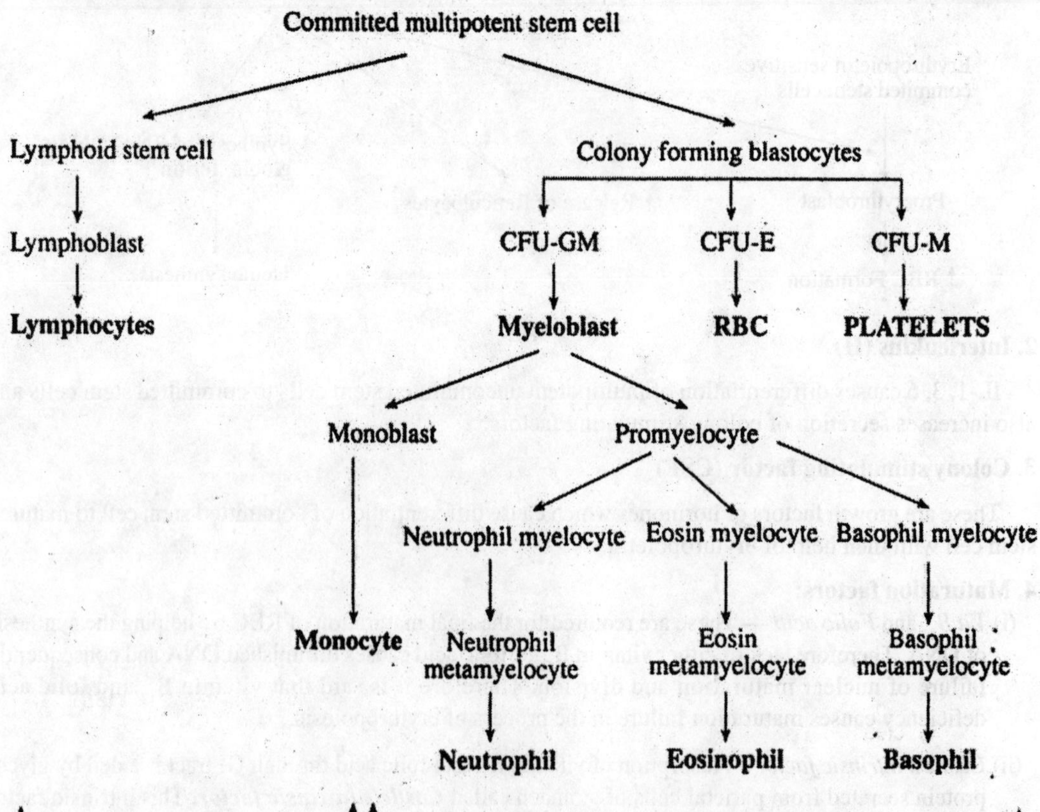

of granules in their cytoplasm they are classified as granulocytes that include Neutrophil, Eosinophil and Basophil and agranulocytes which include Lymphocyte and Monocyte. The development of each type of leucocytes are represented by the help of previous flow chart:

The structure and functions of different leucocytes are:

A. Neutrophil:

(a) Structure of Neutrophil (Fig. 2.2):

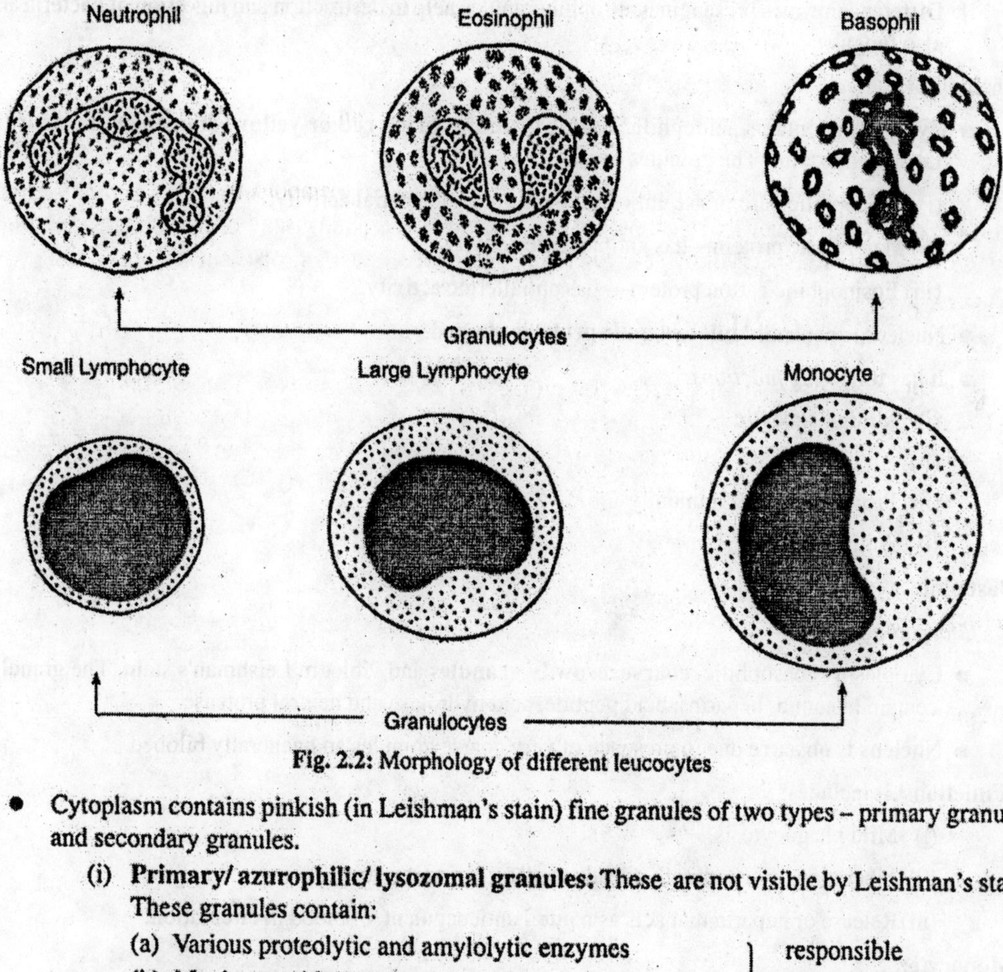

Fig. 2.2: Morphology of different leucocytes

- Cytoplasm contains pinkish (in Leishman's stain) fine granules of two types – primary granules and secondary granules.
  - (i) **Primary/ azurophilic/ lysozomal granules:** These are not visible by Leishman's stain. These granules contain:
    - (a) Various proteolytic and amylolytic enzymes
    - (b) Myeloperoxidase enzyme granules
    - (c) Lysozyme enzyme granules

    } responsible for destruction and digestion of bacteria
  - (ii) **Secondary granules:** These contain—
    - (a) Lactoferin: inhibits bacterial growth
    - (b) Alkaline phosphatase
    - (c) Vitamin B_{12} binding protein

    } indirectly help in bacterial killing
- Nucleus is: **2 to 6 lobed** (polymorphonuclear)
  - ■ Young cell has got single horse shoe shaped nucleus
  - ■ Lobes signify the maturity of cell as follows:
    - ❑ $N_1 - N_2$: Immature and inactive

- ❑ N_3: Fully mature and most active
- ❑ N_4: Mature and less active than N_3
- ❑ N_5-N_6: Over matured and fragile.

(b) Important function of neutrophils are as follows:

I. Phagocytosis—It is the body's Ist line of defence against invading bacteria.

II. Different enzymes present in neutrophil granules help in destruction and digestion of bacteria and also fungus.

B. Eosinophil:

- Cytoplasm contains acidophilic **coarse granules brick red or yellowish orange** in colour (in Leishman's stain). The granules contain :
  - (i) Eosinophilic peroxidase enzymes—has got antibacterial activity.
  - (ii) Major basic protein—has antiparasitic activity.
  - (iii) Eosinophilic cation protein— has antiallergic activity.
- Nucleus is generally **bilobed and spectacle shaped.**
- It has following *functions:*
  - (i) Mild phagocytic
  - (ii) Anti allergic
  - (iii) Provide mucosal immunity
  - (iv) Anti parasitic

C. Basophil:

Morphology:

- Cytoplasm is basophilic, **coarse, crowdy granules** and violet in Leishman's stain. The granules contain histamin, heparins, acid peptide, acid hydrolase and neutral protease.
- **Nucleus is obscure** due to presence of very coarse granules and generally bilobed.

Functions: It includes:

(i) Mild phagocytosis.

(ii) Liberation of histamin that leads to allergic manifestation.

(iii) Release of heparin that acts as natural anticoagulant of blood in circulation.

D. Monocyte:

Morphology:

- Cytoplasm is clear and pale blue in Leishman's stain.
- Nucleus is **single, kidney shaped or indented, eccentric** in position.
- The overall size is 10–18 μ with irregular cell outline.
- It is the **largest WBC** in peripheral blood.

Functions: It includes:

(i) **Formation of tissue macrophage**—Some monocytes leave the circulation and enter into the extra vascular system liver like lung and etc. where they are called as macrophages (monocytic macrophage). In these organs these monocytic macrophases kill bacteria by active phagocytosis.

(ii) **2nd line of defense in acute infection**— It acts as a body's 2nd line of defence against invading bacteria by liberation of H_2O_2 and also by digesting the bacteria.

(iii) **Play role in chronic infection**—It acts as monocytic macrophage system in case of chronic infection to eliminate the foreign bodies e.g. bacteria.

(iv) **Play role in lymphocyte mediated immunity**—It has role in both cell mediated and humoral immunity by releasing monokines.

E. Lymphocytes:

Morphology of Lymphocytes:

- Overall size is 10-14 μm in larger one (large lymphocytes) and 7-10 μm in smaller one (small lymphocytes).
- Cytoplasm is clear, pale blue and **scanty**.
- Nucleus is single, big, purple in colour in Leishman's stain, round or oval or even indented, central in position.
- **Small lymphocyte is most matured.**

Functions: T-lymphocytes help in cell mediated immunity and B-lymphocytes helps in humoral immunity.

3. **Define hemostasis. What Are it's stages? Describe the mechanism of coagulation with special; reference to clot retraction. List the factors involved in coagulation.**

Spontaneous stoppage of bleeding, in response to any injury of blood vessels, by physiological process is called ***Hemostasis***.

Stages and mechanism of hemostasis: Hemostasis takes place in 3 stages—

(A) Vasoconstriction

(B) Formation of primary platelet plug

(C) Formation of secondary platelet plug (Clot formation).

The whole process of hemostasis that occurs in these 3 stages are sequentially represented by schematic diagram (Fig. 2.3).

A. Vasoconstriction: Immediately after injury the traumatized vessels initiate contraction of vessel wall to reduce the loss of blood from the ruptured vessels. This contraction is due to—

(a) Nervous reflexes—initiated by pain or other impulses from injured vessels or tissue.

(b) Local myogenic spasm—that is initiated by direct damage of vessel wall.

(c) Local humoral factors—initiated by vasoconstrictor substances like 5HT, thromboxane A_2 from injured vessel wall and platelets.

This local vasoconstriction lasts for minutes to hours during which the platelet plugging and blood coagulation can occur.

B. Formation of primary platelet plug: When platelets come in contact with the collagen fibers or damaged endothelial cells of the damaged vessel wall they immediately change their characteristics drastically as follows:

(a) They begin to swell and assume irregular forms.

(b) Numerous processes irradiate from their surfaces.

(c) Their contractile proteins contract forcefully and release granules containing active factors.

(d) They become sticky and get stick to the collagen fibers of the injured vessel.

(e) They secrete ADP and thromboxane A_2 which activate nearby platelets which then adhere to originally activated platelets at injury site.

The vicious cycle of activation of increasing number of platelets form the platelet plug which is initially loose but successful in blocking the blood loss if the vascular opening is small. This type of loose platelet plug is known as ***temporary*** or ***primary hemostatic platelet plug*** which later on form a tight plug by the process of blood coagulation or clot formation.

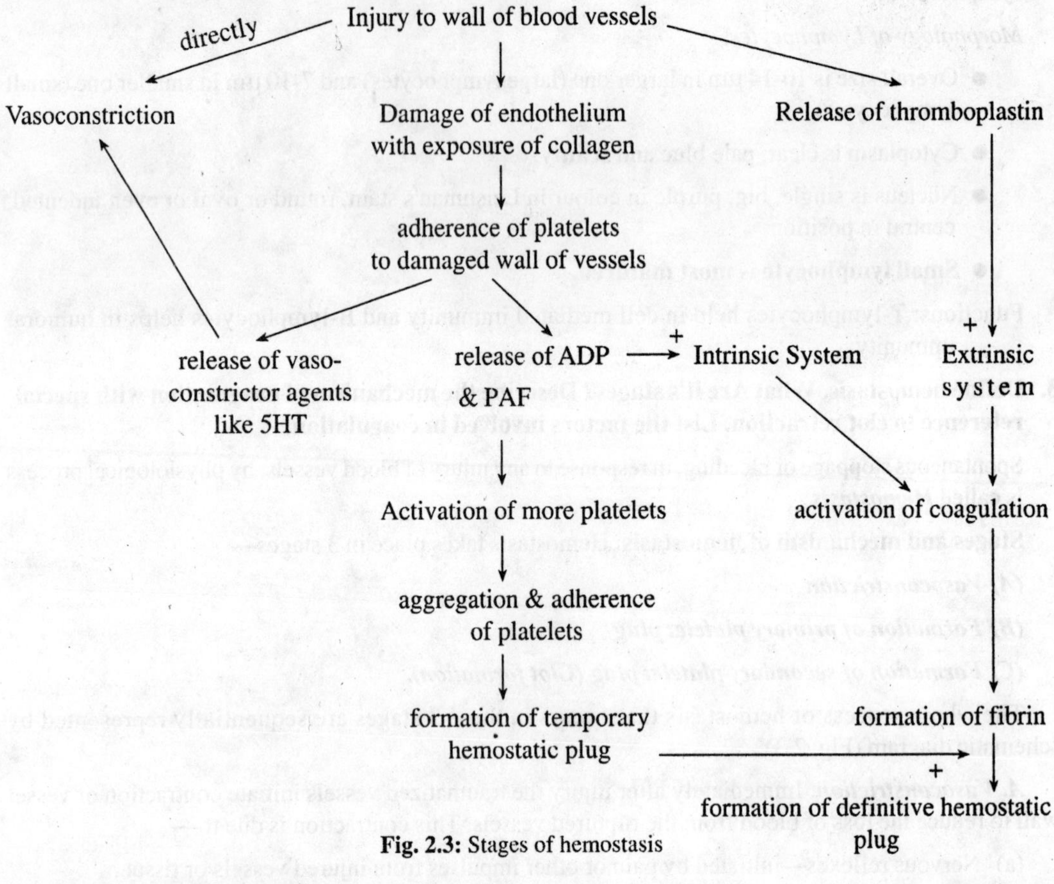

Fig. 2.3: Stages of hemostasis

C. Formation of blood clot (Blood coagulation):

(a) *Definition*: Blood coagulation is defined as the process by which the blood, sheded out or collected in a container, looses it's fluidity and becomes a jelly like mass due to the formation of meshwork of fibrin threads entangling the blood cells.

(b) *Mechanism of blood coagulation*: Over 50 substances that affect the blood coagulation are present in blood and tissue. Some of them promote coagulation (Vide Table 2.a) called ***Procoagulants*** or ***clotting factors***, others inhibiting coagulation called ***Anticoagulants.*** The degree of balance between them determines whether the clot will formed or not. Normally the anticoagulants predominant and procoagulants remain inactivated, so the blood does not coagulate in the vessels but when a vessel is damaged, the procoagulants become active in the area of damage and clot develops. The detail of the procedure is as follows: With the help of different factors enlisted in (Table -2.a) the clotting takes place in 3 essential steps:

Step I : Formation of **Prothrombin Activator** simultaneously by the—

(a) Extrinsic pathway (Fig. 2.4) (b) Intrinsic pathway (Fig. 2.4)

1. Formation of Prothrombin activator (PA): Blood clotting starts with the formation of prothrombin activator which is a complex of clotting factors like activated factor X, factor V, Phospholipid & Ca^{2+}. This complex is formed by both Intrinsic and Extrinsic pathway as shown by Fig. 2.4.

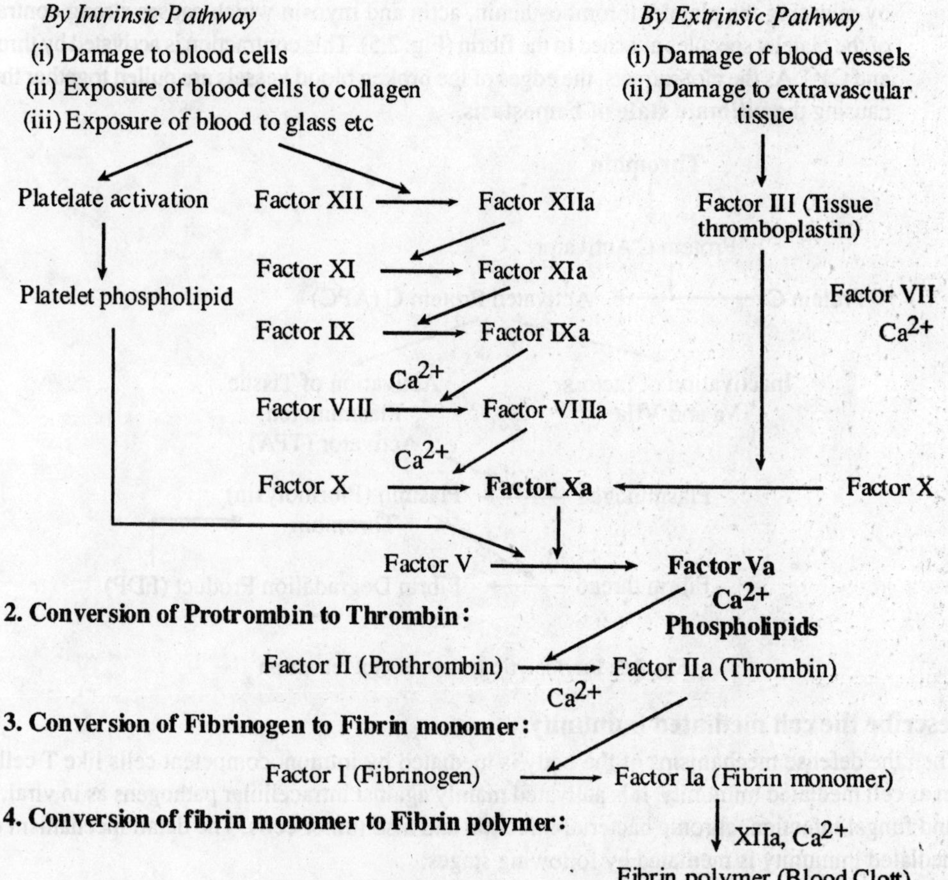

Fig. 2.4: Mechanism of blood coagulation

Step II: Conversion of prothrombin to **thrombin** in presence of Ca^{2+}

Step III: Conversion of fibrinogen to **fibrin** and thence polymerization of fibrin to form **fibrin thread** in presence of fibrin stabilizing factor (Factor III) and Ca_2^{++}

Table 2.a : List of clotting factors

Factor I	:	Fibrinogen	Factor VIII	:	Antihemophilic factor
Factor II	:	Prothrombin	Factor IX	:	Christmas factor
Factor III	:	Thromboplastin	Factor X	:	Stuart Prower factor
Factor IV	:	Calcium	Factor XI	:	Plasma thromboplastin antecedent
Factor V	:	Labile factor or proaccelerin	Factor XII	:	Hegeman's factor
Factor VI	:	Not known	Factor XIII	:	Fibrin stabilizing factor
Factor VII	:	Stable factor or proconvertin			

(c) *Role of Ca^{2+} in blood coagulation*: Except for the first 2 steps in the intrinsic pathway Ca^{2+} are required for the promotion of all reactions involved in both intrinsic and extrinsic pathway. Therefore in the absence of Ca^{2+} blood clotting will not occur.

(d) *Clot retraction*: After the formation of clot, it starts contracting and after about 30-45 min, a straw coloured fluid called ***serum*** oozes out. The process of contraction of clot and oozing of serum out of clot is called ***clot retraction***. The platelet contributes directly to clot retraction by releasing the platelet thrombosthenin, actin and myosin which causes strong contraction of the platelet specules attached to the fibrin (Fig. 2.5). This contraction is activated by thrombin and Ca^{2+}. As the clot retracts, the edges of the broken blood vessels are pulled together thereby causing the ultimate state of hemostasis.

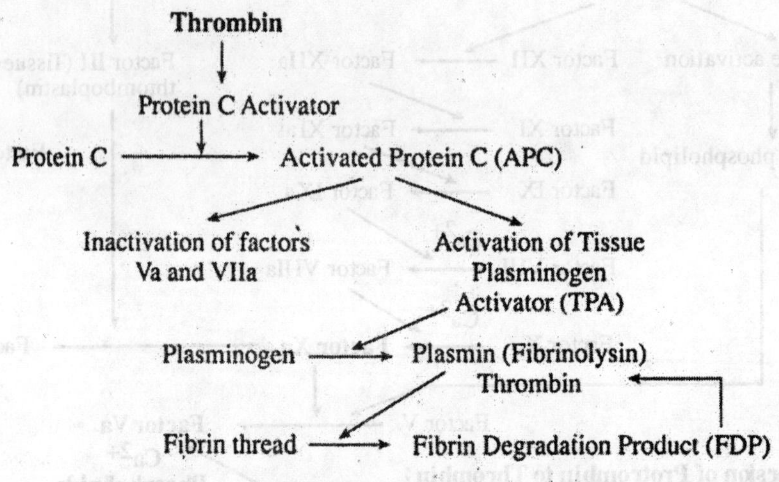

Fig. 2.5: Fibrinolytic system of clot retraction

4. Describe the cell mediated immunity.

When the defense mechanisms of the body is mediated by immunocompetent cells like T cells it is known as cell mediated immunity. It is activated mainly against intracellular pathogens as in viral, parasitic and fungal infection, chronic bacterial infection and also tumor cells. The detail mechanism of the cell mediated immunity is mediated by following stages:

- Stage-I : **Antigen processing and presentation**
- Stage-II : **Recognization of antigen by lymphocytes**
- Stage-III : **Activation of T-lymphocytes**
- Stage-IV : **Release of differentiated T cells**
- Stage-V : **Defensive role of differentiated T cell**

The detail of these phages is illustrated by flow chart FC. 2.A from next page.

5. Describe the humoral immunity.

The humoral immunity is the defense mechanisms of the body and is mediated by antibodies produced from plasma cell which are formed B cells on specific antigenic stimulation. The humoral response of acquired immunity is mediated by following stages:

- Stage-I : **Antigen processing and presentation**
- Stage-II : **Recognisation of antigen**

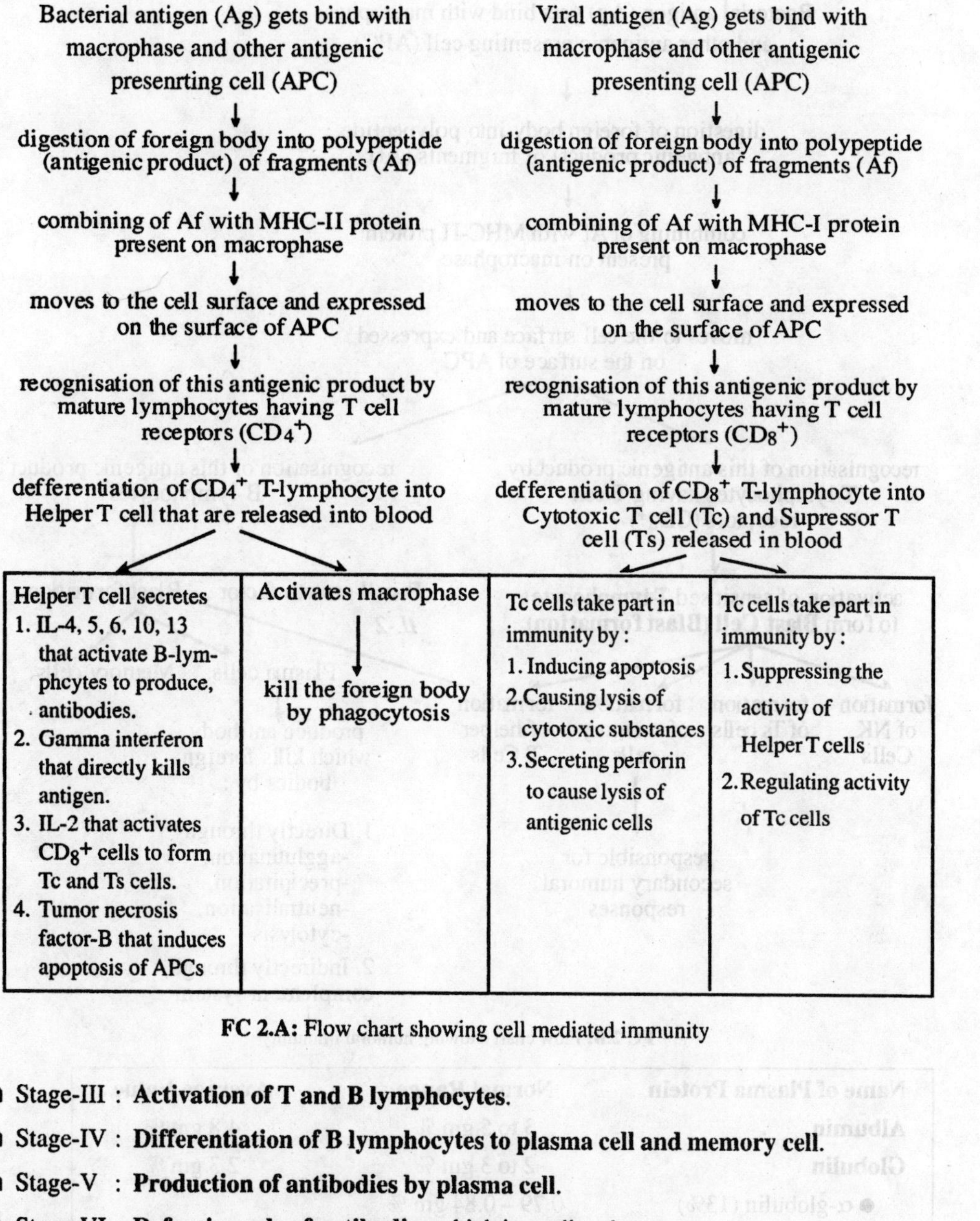

FC 2.A: Flow chart showing cell mediated immunity

- Stage-III : **Activation of T and B lymphocytes.**
- Stage-IV : **Differentiation of B lymphocytes to plasma cell and memory cell.**
- Stage-V : **Production of antibodies by plasma cell.**
- Stage-VI : **Defensive role of antibodies** which is mediated.
  - directly by agglutination, precipitation, neutralization, lysis etc.
  - indirectly through the complement system.

The detail of these stages is illustrated by flow chart FC 2.B from next page.

6. Name the plasma proteins. Describe it's functions. What is edema ?

Plasma proteins are mainly constituted by 55% albumin, 38% globulin, 7% fibrinogen and traces of prothrombin. The normal level of this components are illustrated in the table of next page.

Bacterial antigen (Ag) gets bind with macrophase and other antigenic presenting cell (APC)

↓

digestion of foreign body into polypeptide (antigenic product) of fragments (Af)

↓

combining of Af with MHC-II protein present on macrophase

↓

moves to the cell surface and expressed on the surface of APC

↙ ↘

recognisation of this antigenic product by T-lymphocytes having T cell receptors (CD_4^+)

↓

activation of sensitised T-lymphocytes to form **Blast Cell (Blast formation)**

- formation of NK Cells
- formation of Ts cells
- formation of memory cells → responsible for secondary humoral responses
- formation of helper T Cells → B-cell growth factor *IL-2*

recognisation of this antigenic product by B-lymphocytes

↓

Blast formation

- Plasma cells → produce antibody which kills foreign bodies by :
  1. Directly through
     - -agglutination,
     - -precipitation,
     - -neutralisation,
     - -cytolysis
  2. Indirectly through complement system
- Memory cells

FC 2.B: Flow chart showing humoral immunity

Name of Plasma Protein	Normal Range	Average Value
Albumin	3 to 5 gm %	4.8 gm %
Globulin	2 to 3 gm %	2.3 gm %
● α-globulin (13%)	0.79 – 0.84 gm %	
● β-globulin (14%)	0.78 – 0.81 gm %	
● γ-globulin (11%)	0.66 – 0.70 gm %	
Fibrinogen	150-300 mg %	0.3 mg%
Prothrombin	30-50 mg %	40 mg %

Function:

A. Coagulation of blood—Fibrinogen, prothrombin and other coagulation factors help in coagulation of blood.

B. ***Maintenance of colloidal osmotic pressure***—The plasma proteins (specially albumin) do not pass through capillary membrane easily during normal state. So it remains in the blood and exerts osmotic pressure. This helps to maintain the exchange of fluid at tissue level.

C. ***Maintenance of viscosity of blood and Blood pressure***—It (especially albumin) regulates viscosity of the blood and as resistance of blood flow is directly proportional to viscosity of blood, it also maintains the systemic arterial blood pressure.

D. ***Maintenance of acid base balance***—The plasma proteins, particularly albumin, play an important role in maintaining the acid base balance in the blood. This is due to the fact that in physiological pH plasma proteins exist as an ***'ionised'*** form and in this form it's C terminal end (i.e. COO^-–) can buffer the change due to the addition of an acid and N terminal end (i.e. –NH_3^+) can buffer the change that follow addition of an alkali.

E. ***Regulation of ESR***—Globulin and fibrinogen increase the rate of rouleaux formation and thus increase ESR.

F. ***Providing of suspension stability of RBC***—During circulation, the RBCs remain suspended uniformly in the blood without rouleaux formation. This property of RBC is known as **suspension stability of RBC**, which is provided mainly by globulin and fibrinogen.

G. ***Act as a reservoir***—Plasma proteins act as a reservoir during the conditions like fasting, starvation etc.

H. ***Production of trephone***—Leukocytes produces ***Trephones*** from plasma proteins which are required for nourishment of tissue cells in culture.

I. ***Immune function***—Globulin produces antibodies and thus provides immunity to the body.

J. ***Transportation***—It combines loosely with hormones, metal, drugs etc. and transports to appropriate site for their release as an active components.

K. ***Fibrinolysis***—Intravascular clot (thrombus) is digested by the enzymes of fibrinolytic system present in plasma which saves from disastrous effects of thrombus.

In case of hypoproteinaemia (decrease in plasma protein level) colloidal osmotic pressure is decreased resulting increased filtration in arterial end and increased absorption in venous end. Thus there is an abnormal fluid collection in interstitial spaces called as ***Edema***.

7. What is Landsteiner's law? Enumerate the basic rules of blood transfusion. What are the indications of blood transfusion? Mention the hazards of mismatched blood transfusion.

Landsteiner's law: It states that—

i. If an agglutinogen is present in the RBC of a person, the corresponding agglutinin must be absent in his plasma.

ii. If an agglutinogen is absent in the RBC of a person, the corresponding agglutinin must be present in his plasma.

Basic rules observed during blood transfusion:

A. Group A blood does not contain any antibody against A antigen. So it can receive A type of blood and also O group (as it does not contain any antigen).

B. Group B blood does not contain any antibody for antigen B in their plasma. So it can only receive B types of blood and also O group.

C. Group AB blood does not contain antibody in their plasma so it can take any of the blood group i.e. A, B, AB and also O. That is why this AB group of blood is called as **Universal recipient group.** Though AB^+ blood groups are known as **'True universal recipient'** as AB negative individuals can not accept AB^+ blood but AB positive persons can receive blood from all type of blood groups.

D. Group O blood contains both antibody in their plasma. So it cannot receive other blood except group O. On the other hand as it has no antigen in their RBC, so it can be given to any other blood group. This is why it is known as **Universal donor.** Whereas O⁻ is considered as **'True Universal donor'**.

Indication of blood transfusion: In some occasions there are the need to transfuse the store blood to the persons who suffer from the followings:

- **Blood loss**—Due to accidents and surgical operation.
- **Blood disorders**—Like hemophilia, purpura, clotting defects.
- **Blood diseases**—Like severe anemia, leukaemia, thalassemia etc.
- **Blood poisoning**—CO poisoning.
- **Acute infections or fever.**
- **Shock.**
- **Pre** and **post operations** to build up and make up the loss due to operation.
- **Burns**—plasma rich in protein is lost from the burn surface which is corrected by transfusing plasma and colloids. If it is associated with severe anemia packed RBCs are also transfused.

Transfusion hazards due to mismatching of blood: As per the onset of complications it is of two types:

A. Early reaction: It includes:

a. *Hemolytic reaction*—This is the collection of reaction like restlessness, anxiety, fever basically due to the hemolysis of RBCs.

b. *Allergic reactions*

c. *Pyrogenic reactions*—Pyrogen may come from bottle, tube or blood itself and produces fever and etc.

d. *Circulatory overload*

e. *Air embolism*

f. *Hyperkalemia*

g. *Citrate toxicity*

h. *Clotting abnormalities in case of massive transfusion.*

i. *Acute renal* failure due to blockade and damage of renal tubules by Hb casts and vasoconstriction by toxic substances from them lysed RBCs.

B. Late reaction: This includes:

a. *Disease transmission*-like hepatitis, AIDS, syphilis, malaria etc.

b. *Iron overload.* c. *Immune sensitization.*

B. Short Notes:

1. Varieties of hemoglobin:

A. Normal adult hemoglobin: 97% of hemoglobin in normal adult persons is of **HbA** type which consists of 2α and 2β chains ($\alpha_2\beta_2$). Rest 3% of adult hemoglobin is HbA_2 type which consists of two α chains and two delta (δ) chains instead of β chain. Each delta chain possesses the same number (i.e. 146) amino acids that of β chain but differs from the latter in the nature of 10 amino acids.

B. Normal fetal hemoglobin: Embryonic hemoglobin occurs in human erythrocytes in the 1st three months of embryonic life and has **Gower I** and **Gower II hemoglobin** which are replaced by fetal Hb (HbF) later in fetal life containing a globin with $\alpha_2\gamma_2$. Each γ chain consists of 146 amino acids, like that of β chain but differs from the later in 37 amino acids.

*C. **Abnormal Hb in sickle cell anemia*** (HbS): Here Hb consists of α_2 β_2 but the glutamic acid in position of 6 of β chain of normal Hb is replaced by valine. When exposed to hypoxic condition this abnormal hemoglobin tends to produce crystals called '*Tactoids*' within RBC, resulting in increased fragility of the RBC and changing it into sickle shaped. The resulting clinical condition is known as **Sickle Cell Anemia** which is characterized by hemolysis, hemolytic jaundice and susceptibility to infection.

*D. **Abnormal Hb in thalassemia***: In this case the synthesis of either the α chain or β chain is not sufficient in amount, though the chains once synthesized are normal. In some thalassemia synthesis of β chain is insufficient (β Thalassemia) which is more common. In other cases synthesis of α chain is insufficient known as α—Thalassemia which is very rare. β thalassemia may be of two types—Major and Minor (more common). In case of major one total absence of β chain synthesis is present where as in case of minor β—Thalassemia there is a partial synthesis of β chain.

2. Hematinic principle:

- Absorption of vitamin B_{12} and folic acid through GI tract is aided by glycoprotein secreted from parietal cells of stomach called ***Castle's intrinsic factor***. This intrinsic factor combines with vitamin B_{12} of the food and protects it from being digested and thus makes available for absorption through mainly ileum. These vitamins inturn help to form the mature the RBCs. Thus the vit B_{12} and folic acid along with intrinsic factor are collectively known as hematinic principle.
- Thus the deficiency of these vitamins and also lack of this factor because of atrophy of gastric mucosa which causes loss of vit. B_{12} from the body develops **maturation failure** or ***pernicious anemia***

3. Reticulocyte response:

While treating pernicious anemia and iron deficiency anemia when vit-B_{12} or iron is administered initially there is increase in reticulocyte count which indicates that the pateint is responding well to that treatment. This risc in reticulocyte count is known as reticulocyte response.

4. Interleukins:

- These are a group of cytokinins (a group of hormone like substances) which act in a paracrine manner to control immunological responses.
- There are different types of interleukins (IL) however the physiologically important ILs are IL-1 to IL-13.
- These are produced by macrophages, activated T cells, Antigen presenting cells (APCs), NK cells, Mast cells etc.
- They help in proliferation of B and T cells, activation of leucocytes, and hemopoiesis.
- The functions of specific ILs are as follows:
  - IL-1 : activation of cellular immunity, inflammation, hemopoiesis.
  - IL-2 : stimulation of cellular immunity, NK cells and macrophages.
  - IL-3 : activates hemopoiesis.
  - IL-4 : stimulates humoral immunity.
  - IL-5 : stimulates eosinophil development.

5. Van den Berg Test:

- This test helps to detect whether bilirubin is conjugated or not.
- In this test excess of water soluble bilirubin glucoronide is treated with diazo reagent. If the reddish violet colour appears immediately after the reaction it is considered as **direct positive** whereas if the colour appears late or only after addition of alkali it is considered as **indirect positive**.

- In hemolytic jaundice this test is indirect positive and in obstructive jaundice it is direct positive. In hepatic jaundice it may be biphasic.

6. Neonatal jaundice (Physiological jaundice):

- In some newborns the plasma bilirubin is high (5 mg%-12 mg%) which declines after a week. This condition is known as neonatal jaundice.
- It is common in premature babies and neonates having low birth weight.
- It occurs due to subnormal activity of glucoronyl transferase enzyme that impairs conjugation of bilirubin in hepatocytes.
- It is unlikely to be due to hemolysis.
- It is usually treated by 1) phototherapy which converts bilirubin to lumirubin which has shorter life span 2) injection of phenobarbitone which increases glucoronyl transferase enzyme.

7. Prothrombin activator:

- The complex consisting of activated factor X (Stuart–Prower factor), activated factor V (Proaccelerin), factor IV (Calcium) and phospholipids that helps to convert inactive form of thrombin i.e. prothrombin to thrombin is known as prothrombin activator.
- This is formed in both intrinsic and extrinsic system of blood coagulation i.e. this is a common pathway of both the system.
- This helps to form thrombin which inturn helps in clot formation as follows:

Prothrombin activator
↓
Prothrombin ⟶ Thrombin
↓
Fibrinogen ⟶ Fibrin monomer ⟶ Fibrin polymer (Clot formation)

8. Iron deficiency anemia:

- It is the commonest form of anemia in the developing countries.
- It is due to:
  - Increased physiological demand for iron as seen during pregnancy, lactation and growing children.
  - Decreased iron intake due to deficiency of iron in diet.
  - Blood loss due to peptic ulcer, piles, worm infestations etc.
- It is microcytic hypochromic type.

9. Aplastic anemia:

- It is due to impaired RBC production due to absence of hemopoietic precursor cells.
- The common causes are:
  - Acquired condition like chemical exposure (DDT, Benzene), drug therapy (anticancer, chloramphenicol, diuretics) X ray radiations, viral infections (hepatitis).
  - Hereditory defects.
  - Idiopathic.

10. Clot retraction:

After the formation of clot, it starts contracting and after about 30-45 min, a straw coloured fluid called *serum* oozes out. The process of contraction of clot and oozing of serum out of clot is called ***clot***

retraction. The platelet contributes directly to clot retraction by releasing the platelet thrombosthenin, actin and myosin which causes strong contraction of the platelet specules attached to the fibrin. This contraction is activated by thrombin and Ca^{2+}. As the clot retracts, the edges of the broken blood vessels are pulled together thereby causing the **ultimate state of hemostasis**.

11. Heparin:

- It is a powerful anticoagulant effective both in vivo and vitro.
- In the body it is produced by mast cells and also basophils.
- Chemically it is a sulphate containing mucopolysaccharides.
- It facilitates antithrombin III which inhibits activated factors II, IX, X, XI, XII and Kallikrein and thus prevents coagulation.
- It is used in acute conditions like open heart surgeries, dialysis, acute MI and also in acute animal experiments.
- Activity of heparin can be neutralized by Protamin and Toludine blue which are the basic substances.

12. Fibrinolytic system:

In certain organs specially in the heart and brain, the blood clot may obstruct the minute blood vessels leading to myocardial infarction and cerebral damage respectively. The lysis of the blood clot or fibrinolysis allows reopening of affected blood vessels and prevents the development of infarction and cell necrosis. Thus it is defined as the lysis of blood clot inside the blood vessels to establish the normal blood flow through the affected blood vessels after few days of injury. The mechanism of fibrinolysis is as follows:

After few days damaged tissues and endothelium releases lysosomal enzymes and tissue plasminogen activator which converts plasminogen to plasmin that digests the fibrin into soluble fragments (Fig. 2.5).

13. Procoagulants:

Over 50 substances that affect the blood coagulation are present in blood and tissue. Some of them promote coagulation called ***Procoagulants*** or ***clotting factors***, others inhibiting coagulation called ***anticoagulants.*** The degree of balance between them determines whether the clot will formed or not. Normally the anticoagulants predominant and procoagulants remain inactivated, so the blood does not coagulate in the vessels but when a vessel is damaged, the procoagulants become active in the area of damage and clot develops. The most important procoagulants present normally in the blood are tabulated in Table 2.a.

14. Anticoagulants:

There are 4 types of anticoagulants as follows:

A. Natural anticoagulants which includes:

(a) Heparin: Naturally occuring, produced by mast cells. It prevents blood clotting by:

(i) Suppressing thrombin activity

(ii) Removal of thrombin from circulation

(iii) Activation of active clotting factors like factor IX, X, XI

(iv) Activation of antithrombin

(b) Protein C: It prevents factor Va and VIIa and also plasminogen activator resulting lysis of blood clot. Congenital absence of protein C leads to uncontrolled intravascular coagulation and thus cause death in infancy. Vit-K is required for the production of protein C in the liver.

(c) Fibrinolytic system as described in detail under Question No. 12.

(d) Smoothness of endothelium prevents activation of factor XII and produces a plasminogen activator that helps in fibrinolysis. Prostacyclin produced by endothelial cells.prevents platelet activation and thus coagulation.

(e) Antithrombin

B. Anticoagulants for blood bank:

(a) Acid citrate dextrose (ACD)—it forms a complex with Ca^{++} and thus decrease Ca^{++} level

(b) Citrate phosphate dextrose (CPD)—has similar mechanism.

C. Laboratory anticoagulants:

(a) EDTA:

- It is strong anticoagulant used in vitro.
- Prevent blood clotting by removing Ca^{2+}.

(b) Oxalate and citrate: precipitates Ca^{++} and thus prevents coagulation.

(c) Na_2SO_4 forms weak compound with Ca^{++}.

D. Therapeutic anticoagulant: Heparin and Dicoumarol which prevent the synthesis of factor II, VII, IX, X and Protein C.

15. Rh factor:

- Rh factor is an **antigen** present in RBC membrane whereas there is no natural corresponding antibody (anti-D) present for the Rh antigen (D antigen). However in Rh negative (Rh^-) persons having absence of any D antigens anti-D antibodies can be produced if.
  - (i) Rh positive blood is transfused to him.
  - (ii) Rh positive RBCs from Rh^+ fetus gets enter into the maternal circulation.
- *Classification*: Depending on the presence of D antigen blood group is again classified as follows:

D Antigen	Anti-D antibody	Blood group	Distribution
Present	Absent naturally	Rh^+	55%
Absent	Present naturally	Rh^-	15%

- *Inheritance*: Rh factor is an inherited dominant factor inherited as per Mendelian's law. The main antigenic antigen D is responsible for it's inheritance. The person will be Rh positive if homozygous (DD) or heterozygous (Dd) is present in allele. In case of Rh negative the allele is dd.
- *Rh factor and hemolytic disease*: Incompatibility of Rh factor results mainly two hemolytic disease known as hemolytic disease of new born which is associated with—
  - *Hemolytic anemia*
  - Erythroblastosis fetalis
  - Kernicterus
  - Hydrops fetalis.

16. Erythroblastosis fetalis:

- If a Rh negative mother conceives a Rh positive fetus, at the time of delivery the Rh antigen containing fetal RBC enters into mother's blood. In response of this Rh antigen in mother's blood now anti-D antibody is formed within few days and thus there is no complications of 1st child. However in successive pregnancies if that Rh negative mother again carry Rh^+ fetus then those anti-D antibody can cross the placenta to enter into fetal blood and causes agglutination of fetal RBC resulting hemolysis. This in turn increases rate of RBC formation. This results appearance of large sized RBC (immature) in blood. This condition of the fetus is known as erythroblastosis fetalis.

- *Prevention of erythroblastosis details*:
  - If mother is Rh negative and fetus is found Rh positive, anti-D should be administered to the mother at 28th and 34th week of gestation as prophylactic measure.
  - If the mother is Rh negative and delivers Rh^+ baby then within 48 hours of delivery anti-D should be injected to mother to avoid complications during later pregnancies.
- Treatment: In severe cases following treatment is required.
  - Exchange transfusion immediately after birth.
  - Phototherapy to reduce bilirubin level.

17. Hemolytic disease of newborn:

- This is due to incompatibility of Rh factor in women. If a Rh negative mother conceives a Rh positive fetus, at the time of delivery the Rh antigen containing fetal RBC enters into mother's blood. In response of this Rh antigen in mother's blood now anti-D antibody is formed within few days and thus there is no complications of 1st child. However in successive pregnancies if that Rh negative mother again carry Rh^+ fetus then those anti-D antibody can cross the placenta to enter into fetal blood and causes agglutination of fetal RBC resulting hemolysis. This may lead to death of the fetus or if survived may suffer from hemolytic disease which is characterised by:
  - *Hemolytic anaemia*
  - Erythroblastosis fetalis—due to rapid hemolysis RBC formation is increased resulting release of large sized immature RBCs (Erythroblast) in the circulation which is known as erythroblastosis fetalis.
  - Kernicterus—due to rapid hemolysis excess bilirubin is formed resulting jaundice. The excess bilirubin enters then brain specially basal ganglia causing it's permanent damage which results deafness, choreo-atheotosis, spasticity which is known as Kernicterus.
  - Hydrops fetalis—Fetus may develop edema in all the organs leading to intrauterine death.

18. Bombay blood groups:

- It is a rare blood group in which no antigen H, A and B are present on red cells. H antigen is the sugar moiety present on RBC membrane of all the individuals which differentiates into A or B antigens.
- But the plasma contains anti-A, anti-B and anti-H antibodies as a result such a person can receive blood only from the person having Bombay blood group.

19. Storage of blood:

Different blood bank used to store the blood for ready-made use during acute emergency. The collected blood (420 ml) is mixed with simple 2% citrate solution in which 20 ml of 15% glucose is added. This glucose helps in two ways:

(i) It liberates lactic acid thereby decreases pH which increases the survival capacity of RBC.
(ii) It also helps RBC to maintain it's metabolic activity.

Blood is stored at 4°C up to 14 days in siliconised bottles. Of course this stored blood is not suitable for WBC and platelets for the recipients.

20. Functions of spleen:

Spleen is the largest lymphoid organ which has following functions:

- Macrophages in spleen play an important role in immunity by initiating phagocytosis.
- It helps in the development of lymphocytes.
- It is the site of production of antibodies.
- It removes old and abnormal RBCs, WBCs and platelets.
- During intrauterine life and also some pathological conditions it also helps in RBC production.

- It acts as reservoir of blood.
- It also helps in iron recycling for reutilisation of iron to synthesise Hb.

21. Tissue macrophage system:

- These are basically monocytes which after releasing from bone marrow are circulated through blood and ultimately enter into different tissues like liver (Kupffer cells), spleen, lymph nodes, lungs, bones (osteoclast), CNS (microglial cells), connective tissue etc. In these tissues they attain maturity and phagocyting capacity which are now known as ***macrophages.***
- Some of the macrophages travel tissues and perform scavenger functions of eliminating micro-organisms and other foreign particles that invade the tissues. These type of macrophages are known as ***mobile macrophages.***
- Whereas some of these macrophages become attached to certain tissues in the body and remain their for several month which are known as ***fixed macrophages***. These fixed macrophages present in the tissues are known as ***tissue macrophage system*** or ***mononuclear phagocytic system*** (MPS).
- *Functions*:
  - It provides defense against the bacteria invading the body tissue by phagocytosis or by releasing some bacteriocidal agents.
  - It also helps to ingest cell debis, broken bacteria etc. from the inflammed area and facilitate healing process.
  - Macrophages after engulfing the bacteria by phagocytosis, liberate antigenic products that activate B lymphocytes and helper T cells (i.e. induces cell mediated and humoral immunity).
  - Macrophages secrete some hormonal substances (Interleukin-I), which activates the maturation and proliferation of B-lymphocytes and T-lymphocytes.
  - The senile RBCs are destroyed with consequent release of hemoglobin by the cells of MPS in different organs like spleen, liver etc.
  - They are also responsible for conversion of hemoglobin to bile pigments.

22. Lymph:

- It is the clear, watery fluid present in the lymphatic vessels.
- It is composed of water – 94% and solid – 6% which includes lymphocytes, plasma cells, electrolytes, clotting factors, antibodies, plasma enzymes, urea, amino acids and creatinine.
- The rate of formation is 1-1.5 ml/min.
- The factors which favours the lymph formation are increase in hydrostatic pressure, capillary surface area, capillary permeability, functional activity etc.
- The functions are:
  - It helps in body defense by it's lymphocytes and antibodies.
  - It supplies nutrients and O_2 to those part of the body where blood is not reached e.g. cornea and cartilage etc.
  - It helps in redistribution of body fluids from one to another compartment whenever required.
  - It maintains interstitial fluid level.
  - It helps in fat absorption in the intestine.
  - It removes the particulate matter and bacteria in lymph node.

23. Interferons:

- Interferons are types of cytokinins produced by virally infected cells and help in protecting the uninfected cell and thus limit the spread of infection.
- There are 3 types of interferons–IFN-α, IFN-β, IFN-γ of which IFN-α and β are produced by macrophages, neutrophils and other somatic cells and IFN-γ by activated type-I helper cells and NK cells.

24. Complement system:

- There is a group of plasma proteins designated as complement system as they complement the effects of antibodies in killing antigen like virus, bacteria and etc.
- This includes more than 30 proteins out of which 11 are important and named as C1 to C9.
- These are system of plasma enzymes which remain inactivated form normally and once activated they exert the humoral immunity mainly by causing lysis of the foreign invaders by opsonization, phagocytosis, osmotic lysis of cell membrane by inserting pore forming protein ***'Perforins'*** and inflammation.
- This system is activated by two pathway:
  - Classical pathway: In this pathway antigen antibody complex activate C1 which then activate C2 and C4 and then C5 which then others.
  - Alternative or Properdin pathway: In this pathway a circulatory protein called factor–I recognises the polysaccharide unit present on the surface of microorganism which activates C3 and C5 and thus other proteins.

25. Non T-non B lymphocytes:

- These are 3rd category of lymphocytes also known as natural killer cells or NK cells which are the 1st line of defence specially against viral infection.
- They constitute 15% of total lymphocytes in the body and present in spleen, lymph nodes, bone marrow, and blood.
- They do not mature in thymus and lack surface antigen receptors.
- They do not require prior sensitization to fill microorganisms.
- They kill microbes by:
  - Incorporating ***perforin*** into cell membrane of microbes → osmotic lysis.
  - Release interferons which activate phagocytosis.
  - They also kill the antibody coated viruses.

26. Plasma cells:

- These are formed from B cells on specific antegenic stimulation which takes party in humoral immunity by producing antibodies.
- It has larger cytoplasm containing numerous RER.
- A specific antigen stimulates a specific B cells that undergo proliferations of a selective clone of plasma cell which is known as ***Clonal selection of plasma cell***. Specific clone of plasma cells produce specific antibodies which attack antigen and kill them by neutralisation, activating complement systems, precipitation of antigens, activating phagocytosis etc.

27. Polycythemia:

A. Definition: Increase in RBC above the normal range is defined as polycythemia.

B. Types:2 types

*a. Primary polycythemia (**polycythemia vera**)*

- It is the condition in which RBC count increases as high as 8-9 (ocassionally as high as 11) million/cubic mm of blood.
- In this condition erythropoietin production is either normal or less.

b. Secondary polycythemia: Increase in RBC count (6-8 million per cu mm of blood) due to hypoxia or any other known factors is known as secondary polycythemia. It may be due to:

- Physiological — in high altitude
- Pathological—in lung disease, congenital heart disease and cardiac failure.

C. Effect of polycythemia on circulation:

- Decrease in cardiac output due to decreased blood flow rate resulted from rise of viscosity of blood.
- Blood pressure remains normal in most cases due to homeostatic mechanism. However, in some cases rise of BP is due to increase in peripheral resistance resulted from rise of viscosity.
- Cyanosis due to stagnation of blood in the capillaries of skin causing greater deoxygenation of blood.

28. Pernicious anemia:

- This is an autoimmune disorder in which the gastric mucosa is atrophic with loss of pareital cells causing intrinsic factor deficiency. In the absence of intrinsic factor less than 1% of dietary vit-B_{12} is absorbed.
- This results the similar signs and symptoms as observed in vit-B_{12} deficiency i.e. megaloblastic anemia, which includes altered skin pigmentation, smooth tongue, poor memory, depression, pyrexia and neurological problems like subacute combined degeneration of spinal cord, upper motor neurone signs, optic atrophy etc. which results paresthesia, weakness, unsteady gait, decreased vibration and position sense and Rhomberg's sign. In severe cases spasticity with hyper-reflexia, clonus and positive Babinski sign may also be observed.
- It is more common in individuals with other autoimmune diseases like Grave's disease. Hashimoto's thyroiditis, Addision's disorder.

29. ESR

A. Definition: It is the rate at which the red cells settle down when blood mixed with proper anti-coagulant is made to stand vertically for an hour.

B. Determination: It can be determined by two methods named as Westergren's Method and Wintrobe's method.

C. Normal; Values:

(a) Wintrobe's method:

In male : 2-8 mm in first hour
In female : 4-10 mm in first hour (due to low PCV).

(b) Westergren's method:

In male : 3-7 mm in first hour
In female : 5-9 mm in first hour.

D. Variations of ESR

(a) Physiological:

- Age: Low in infants and high in elderly people
- Sex: Higher in females
- High altitude: High in high altitude
- Pregnancy: Increase in pregnancy

(b) Pathological increase:

- All acute infections
- Acute episodes of chronic infection
- Bone diseases
- Tuberculosis of lungs
- Malignant and collagen diseases
- Anaemia

(c) Pathological decrease: Polycythemia and disease related with decreased fibrinogen level.

E. Factor affecting ESR: Following factors affect the ESR:

(a) Increase in **rate of rouleaux** formation increases ESR

(b) Increase in **viscosity of blood** decreases ESR

(c) Increase in **RBC count** of blood decreases ESR

(d) Increase in specific gravity of RBC increases ESR

F. Clinical significance

- It is **not** a diagnostic test as it increases in large number of pathological conditions.
- It is used as **prognostic test** (i.e. to judge the progress of the diseases in patients under treatment especially in TB and Rheumatic fever).
- It is also used to rule out the presence of any organic diseases.

30. Packed cell volume:

***(a) Definition*:** It is defined as the volume of red blood cells packed at the bottom of hematocrit tube when the anticoagulant mixed blood is centrifuged.

***(b) Determination*:** To determine the PCV, blood is mixed with suitable anticoagulant (EDTA, heparin etc.) and filled in Wintrobe's tube upto 100 mark. It is then centrifuged at 3000 rpm for 30 minutes. The RBCs are packed up in the bottom and occupy a volume leaving a clear supernatant (plasma). Volume of these packed formed elements is determined from the gradation of the tube. It is commonly expressed as vol per 100 ml of blood.

***(c) Normal value*:**

- In male—40-45 ml/100 ml of blood
- In female—38-42 ml/100 ml of blood

31. Autoimmuno diseases:

- ***Definition*:** It is defined as the immune response to self antigen i.e. production of antibodies or T cells against self antigen (own cells or tissues).
- ***Causes*:** It may be due to—
  - Deficiency of suppressor T cells
  - Unbalanced activity of helper T cells and suppressor T cells.

- ■ Alteration of certain cells of the body due to mutation or exposure to irradiations, drugs etc. which behaves like foreign antigen.

- *Examples*: Myasthenia gravis, Grave's disease, Hashimoto's thyroiditis, Rheumatoid arthritis, Insulin dependant (Type-I) Diabetes mellitus.

32. Bleeding disorder:

These are grossly classified into two types:

A. Bleeding caused by a **defects in primary hemostasis** (purpura) that includes vessel wall abnormalities which are of two types:

i. *Thrombocytopenic purpura* which may be due to decreased production of platelets or increased destruction of platelets or excessive pooling that occurs in splenomegaly. The characteristics features of purpura are:

- Spontaneous hemorrhagic spots beneath the skin, mucous membrane etc.
- BT increases and CT remains normal in this condition.

ii. *Non thrombocytopenic purpura* which include Von Willebrand disease and vessel wall abnormality etc.

iii. *Thromboaesthenic purpura*: This is due to presence of abnormal platelets through it's count in normal.

B. **Coagulation disorder** which involve deficiency of only clotting factor. These are basically due to either deficiency of clotting factors like Factor VIII and IX (hemophilia) or Vitamin K.

i. ***Hemophilia***:

- It is an sex linked inherited disease due to abnormal gene on X chromosome.
- Mostly male is affected whereas female being the carriers.
- It occurs due to deficiency of either antihemophilic factor (factor VIII) or christmas factor (Factor IX) and thereby lack of formation of prothrombin activator.
- CT is prolonged in this case keeping the BT and prothrombin time normal.
- It is of 2 types—Classical hemophilia (Hemophilia–A): due to deficiency of Factor VIII and Hemophilia-B (Christmas disease) due to deficiency of factor IX.

ii. ***Vitamine K deficiency*** which occurs in the new born or in patients with intestinal malabsorption or biliary obstruction.

33. Edema:

- The accumulation of free fluid in excess in the interstitial tissue space is called as edema.
- It can occur either due to increased filtration of fluid into the interstitial tissue space or decrease removal of fluid from the interstitial spaces or both.
- Increased hydrostatic pressure of capillaries, decreased oncotic pressure, increased capillary permeability and decreased lymphatic drainage causes edema formation.
- It is of two types:
  - ■ *Pitting edema*:
    - ❑ Normally very little water is present in the interstitial space that too bound to proteoglycan meshwork. When more water accumulates in the interstitial space most of the water remains free in interstitial space, so when pressed with a finger water is displaced causing a *pit formation* which takes few minutes to disappear.
    - ❑ It is usually influenced by the effect of gravity on venous hydrostatic pressure and so accumulation of fluids in ankles during the day and improves overnight.
  - ■ *Non pitting edema*:
    - ❑ It is usually due to decreased lymphatic drainage.

- It is treated generally by diuretics and salt restriction (in case of generalised edema as occurs in heart failure) and anti inflammatory drugs (in case of localised edema) or steroids (in case of pulmonary edema).

34. Von-Willebrand factors:

- It is bleeding disorder due to deficiency of Von-Willebrand factors which is a protein synthesised by endothelial cells and megakaryocytes which—

  (a) Acts as a carrier protein for factor VIII and thus deficiency of this factor results secondary reduction in plasma factor VIII.

  (b) Form bridges between platelets and sub endothelial component (collagen) of blood vessels allowing platelets to adhere to damaged vessel wall.

- Factor VIII is a complex made up of VIII-C and VIII-R. Deficiency of factor VIII-R results Von-Willebrand disease.
- In this case the BT is prolonged but CT remains normal.

C. Differentiate between:

Plasma	Serum
❑ It is a cell free clear liquidic portion of blood which forms 55% of whole blood.	❑ It is the straw coloured fluidic portion of plasma remained after clotting.
❑ It contains fibrinogen and other clotting factors.	❑ It does not contain fibrinogen and other clotting factors.

Adult hemoglobin	Foetal hemoglobin
❑ The globin chain of this type of hemoglobin consists of 2α and 2β chains.	❑ The globin chain of this type of hemoglobin consists of 2α and 2γ chains.
❑ It has less affinity to O_2.	❑ It has more affinity to O_2.
❑ It has more affinity to 2-3-DPG.	❑ It has less affinity to 2-3-DPG.
❑ Life span more (120 days).	❑ Life span less (80 days).

Major thalassaemia	Minor thalassaemia
❑ It is a less common type of β-thalassaemia.	❑ It is a more common type of β-thalassaemia.
❑ There is total absence of β chain synthesis.	❑ There is partial synthesis of β chain.
❑ Mode of transmission is homozygous.	❑ Mode of transmission is heterozygous.
❑ Moderate to severe type of anemia is seen.	❑ Mild type of anemia is seen.
❑ HbF level is very high.	❑ HbF level is moderate.
❑ Life span of the sufferer is shorter (17th year).	❑ Life span of the sufferer is longer.

Red bone marrow	Yellow bone marrow
❑ It is the active marrow which participates in hemopoeisis.	❑ It does not participate in hemopoeisis.
❑ It contains more blood vessels.	❑ It contains less blood vessels and more fat cells and fibro-fatty tissue.

Red bone marrow	Yellow bone marrow
❑ Present in almost all bones of the body at birth. However with advancement of age it is replaced by yellow bone marrow and red marrow is limited to the membranous bones i.e. skull, vertebrae, ribs, sternum etc.	❑ Present in bones at older age.

Lymphokinins	Cytokinis
❑ These are chemical messengers (e.g. interleukins, interferons) secreted by the lymphocytes.	❑ These are the small proteins like chemical messengers secreted by WBCs and some other cells like macrophages, fibroblasts, glial cells.

Intravascular erythropoiesis	Extravascular erythropoiesis
❑ Erythropoiesis in blood vessels is known as intravascular erythropoiesis. ❑ It occurs in upto 3 months of foetal life (mesoblastic stage).	❑ Erythropoiesis outside the blood vessels (e.g. liver, spleen) is known as extra-vascular erythropoiesis. ❑ It occurs after 3 months of foetal life (Hepatic and Myeloid stage) and also on post natal and adult life.

Leucocytosis	Leukaemia
❑ Increased in TLC above 11,000/cu mm of blood is termed as leucocytosis. ❑ Mature WBCs are predominant. ❑ It occurs during some physiological and some pathological conditions.	❑ It is the cancerous condition in which TLC becomes more than 50,000/cu mm. ❑ Immature WBCs are predominant. ❑ It occurs during malignancy of bone marrow.

Temporary hemostatic plug	Definitive hemostatic plug
❑ It is the stage two of hemostasis process in which a loose temporary platelet plug is formed by aggregation of platelets to close the vessels. ❑ It is unstable in nature.	❑ It is the ultimate stage of hemostasis in which bleeding is stopped permanently by forming fibrin thread on the injured site of blood vessels. ❑ It is stable.

Warm antibodies	Cold antibodies
❑ The antibodies act best in the normal body temperature is known as warm antibodies. ❑ Example: Rh antibodies. ❑ These are IgG types of immunoglobin. ❑ It can cross the placenta.	❑ The antibodies the action of which is not affected by temperature is known as cold antibodies. ❑ Example: ABO antibodies. ❑ These are IgM type. ❑ It can not cross the placenta.

Natural immunity	Acquired immunity
❑ It is the inborn capacity of the body to resist the entry of microorganisms into the body.	❑ It is acquired by the subject during his lifetime.
❑ It protects the body from any pathogens and thus is called as nonspecific immunity.	❑ It is the resistance developed in the body against any specific foreign body like virus, bacteria etc. So this is known as specific immunity.
❑ It is not dependant on any invading organisms i.e. prior contact is not essential.	❑ It is developed only when the body is exposed to the specific antigen i.e., prior contact is essential.
❑ Ability to recognise the antigen and respond against it is quick.	❑ Ability to recognise is complex and more time is required.

Humoral immunity	Cellular immunity
❑ When the immunity is provided by the synthesis of antibodies it is known as humoral immunity.	❑ When the immunity is provided by the production of immuno competent cells like lymphocytes (cytotoxic cells, natural killer cells), it is known as cellular immunity.
❑ It is mediated by B-lymphocytes.	❑ It is mediated by T-lymphocytes.
❑ It is effective against intracellular organisms like viruses, parasites, fungi, cancer cell, tumor cells and etc.	❑ It is effective against extra cellular organisms e.g. bacteria, etc.

B-lymphocyte	T-lymphocyte
❑ It is responsible for humoral immunity.	❑ It is responsible for cellular immunity.
❑ It is originated from bone marrow and processed in bone marrow and liver.	❑ It is originated from bone marrow and processed in thymus gland under the influence of thymopoietin hormone.
❑ It is of two types; plasma cell and memory B cell.	❑ It is of three types; Helper T cell (T4 cells), Cytotoxic (T8, killer cells) cells and Memory T cell.
❑ Population-20-30%.	❑ Population-60-80%.
❑ Life span is few days to week.	❑ Life span is 2-4 years.

Active immunisation	Passive immunisation
❑ It is acquired by activating immuno systems of the body.	❑ It is produced without challenging the immuno system.
❑ It is produced following exposure to antigens.	❑ It is produced by administration of serum/ gamma globulin from a person who is already immunised to a non-immuno persons.

Primary immuno response	Secondary immuno response
❑ When antigen enters the body for the 1st time there is slow rise of antibody formation which is known as primary response.	❑ When the same antigen enters the body for the 2nd time there is speedy and intense rise of antibody formation which is known as secondary response.
❑ The response is smaller and slow.	❑ It is faster and intense.
❑ Antibody produced in this case are mainly IgM types.	❑ Antibody produced in this case are mainly IgG types.
❑ Antibody titer becomes normal within few days to weeks.	❑ Antibody titer falls very slowly and never returns to normal.
❑ Plasma antibody level is low.	❑ Plasma antibody level is high.
❑ Latent period is 5-10 days.	❑ Latent period is 1-3 days.
❑ Response is given by unsensitised B cells.	❑ Response is given by memory B cells.

Vascular bleeding disorder	Coagulation disorder
❑ It is due to capillary abnormality.	❑ It is due to deficiency or absence of clotting factors like VIII or IX.
❑ Bleeding is usually restricted to skin.	❑ Bleeding is usually restricted to deeper tissue.
❑ Spontaneous bleeding is common.	❑ Spontaneous bleeding is uncommon.
❑ Wound healing is excessive and lasts for < 48 hours.	❑ Wound healing is less profuse and lasts for > 48 hours.
❑ Stops quickly by applying local pressure.	❑ Does not stop quickly by applying local pressure.

Thrombocytopenia	Thromboasthenia
❑ Low platelet count is known as thrombocytopenia.	❑ The functional deficiency of platelets is known as thromboasthenia.
❑ Platelet count is decreased below 1.5 lakh/cumm.	❑ Platelet count remains normal.

Unconjugated hyperbilirubinemia	Conjugated hyperbilirubinemia
❑ It occurs in case of excess breakdown of RBCs.	❑ It occurs in case of obstruction of bile ducts.
❑ Urinary excretion of urobillinogen is increased.	❑ Urinary excretion of urobillinogen is decreased.
❑ Van-den-Bergh's test indirect positive.	❑ Van-den-Bergh's test direct positive.
❑ Liver functions are normal.	❑ Liver functions are exaggerated.
❑ Hemorrhagic tendency is absent.	❑ Hemorrhagic tendency is present due to lack of vit-K.
❑ Jaundice is acholuric.	❑ Jaundice is choluric.
❑ Kernicterus can occur.	❑ Kernicterus can never occur.
❑ Stool is never clay colour.	❑ Stool is clay coloured.
❑ Mostly due to prehepatic causes.	❑ Mostly due to posthepatic causes.

Iron deficiency anemia	Folic acid deficiency anemia	Vit-B_{12} deficiency anemia
❑ Inadequate intake is a common cause.	❑ Inadequate intake is a common cause.	❑ Inadequate intake is a rare cause.
❑ RBCs are microcytic and hypochromic.	❑ RBCs are macrocytic.	❑ RBCs are macrocytic.
❑ Nuclear maturity of RBC is normal.	❑ Nuclear maturity of RBC is impaired.	❑ Nuclear maturity of RBC is impaired.
❑ WBCs are unaffected.	❑ Decrease in Neutrophil count.	❑ Decrease in Neutrophil count.
❑ It is not associated with any neurological problem.	❑ It is commonly associated with neurological problems.	❑ It is commonly associated with neurological problems.
❑ Hyperplasia of RBC precursor cells is seen.	❑ Megaloblastic changes of RBC precursor cells is seen.	❑ Megaloblastic changes of RBC precursor cells is seen.

D. Brainstorming short answer type:

1. What will happen if plasma protein concentration decreases?

(a) less than 2 gm%

(b) to 4 gm%

(a) It results in shock and even death.

(b) It results in exhaustion of protein reserves in the body.

2. How hypoproteinemia produces edema?

Hypoproteinemia → decrease in capillary oncotic pressure → decrease in filtration at arterial end → decrease in absorption of fluid at venous end → abnormal collection of fluid in interstitial spaces → edema.

3. What is A/G ratio?

It is the ratio of albumin to globulin. Normally it is 1.7: 1.

4. Name three conditions when there is a physiological decrease of albumin.

In infancy, newborns and early pregnancy.

5. Can any of the plasma proteins pass through capillary endothelium?

Capillary endothelium normally is impermeable to plasma proteins though in some diseases like glomerulonephritis, nephrotic syndrome albumin can pass through the capillary membranes.

6. What are the advantages of biconcave shape of RBC?

These are:

- ❑ It can withstand considerable changes of osmotic pressure by altering its cell volume and thereby prevent hemolysis.
- ❑ Allows easy passage of RBC through narrow capillaries by folding itself.
- ❑ Facilitates quick and optimal exchange of gases in and out of hemoglobin.

7. What are the advantages of having no nucleus, no mitochondria and no ribosome in RBC?

It is to accommodate more amount of hemoglobin and also to decrease the use of O_2 by its own structure and thereby increases the availability of O_2 to the other cells.

8. What are the disadvantages of non-nucleated RBC?

- It can not multiply.
- It can not synthesise necessary enzymes so has less life span.

9. How does RBC survive for 120 days though it has no nucleus, mitochondria and ribosomes?

For energy supply RBCs depend on glucose metabolism only, which comes through facilitated diffusion. These glucoses are oxidised by cytoplasmic enzymes already present inside the cells to get the energy for their activity. When these cytoplasmic enzymes are exhausted, i.e. after 120 days, it dies.

10. Why RBC is stained pink by Leishman's stain though it has no ribosomes in their cytoplasm?

It is because of presence of hemoglobin.

11. Why hemoglobin is present within RBC not in plasma?

There are several reasons like:

- To prevent rise of viscosity of plasma that may lead to increase in blood pressure.
- To prevent the increase in osmotic pressure of plasma and thereby prevent the disturbances of fluid exchange mechanism due to rise in osmotic pressure.
- To prevent breakdown of Hb by tissue macrophage system.
- To prevent loss of Hb through urine.

12. What is the site of production of heme of Hb?

It is in mitochondria.

13. Mention the average daily production of Hb in the body.

It is about 7-8 gms/day.

14. In which form iron is stored in reticuloendothelial cells?

Ferritin and hemosiderin form.

15. Mention the varieties of haemoglobin with special reference to difference of each.

These are as follows:

- Adult Hb (HbA) — Contains 2 α and 2 β globin chain.
- Adult Hb (HbA_2) — Contains 2 α and 2 δ chain.
- Foetal Hb (HbF) — Contains 2 α and 2 γ chain.
- HbS — Contains 2 α and 2 β chain but in β chain glutamate of 6th position is replaced by a valine residue.

16. Why does Hb level lower in female?

This is due to the:

- Presence of estrogen which inhibits erythropoietin secretion resulting less RBC formation.
- Absence of testicular androgens which stimulate erythropoietin secretion in male and thereby increases RBC count.

17. Why does Hb level high in the newborn?

The newborns are generally in a state of mild hypoxia which in turn stimulate erythropoietin secretion and thereby increase in RBC count and thus Hb concentration.

18. What is the etiology of pernicious anemia?

It is due to deficiency of hematinic principle, i.e. lack of Castle's intrinsic factor, resulting failure of absorption of vitamin B_{12} from diet through ileum.

19. What will happen?

a. If iron in heme is present in ferric form

b. If HBF persists during adult life

(a) Ferric form of iron will bind O_2 tightly resulting no removal of O_2 from iron atom and then O_2 can not be used by the body.

(b) If HBF is present in adult blood there is shifting of O_2 dissociation curve to the left because of less affinity of HbF for 2-3-DPG resulting more uptake of O_2 in lungs and less release of O_2 in tissues.

20. What will happen if folic acid is given to pernicious anemic patient?

The administration of folic acid to pernicious anemic patient will improve the blood picture but it can not protect against neuropathy which is due to deficiency of vit-B_{12}.

21. What is the blood and bone marrow picture in iron deficiency anemia?

The RBCs are microcytic, hypochromic and MCH, MCHC and total RBC count is reduced, whereas the bone marrow shows proliferation of the precursor cells with a larger proportion of the mature forms. Some of the precursor cells may show scanty, polychromatic cytoplasm with a pyknotic necleus i.e. the cytoplasmic maturity is less than nuclear maturity.

22. What is the blood and bone marrow picture in megaloblastic anemia?

The blood picture is characterised by macrocytosis, anisocytosis, poikilocytosis, neutropenia with over matured neutrophils and also thrombocytopenia. Whereas in bone marrow all the RBC precursors show megaloblastic changes that includes:

1. Larger cell with larger nucleus
2. More reticular chromatin
3. Normal hemoglobinisation of cytoplasm

23. What is the dietary, active and therapeutic form of folic acid?

- ***Dietary form***: polyglutamates
- ***Active form***: tetrahydropholate
- ***Therapeutic form***: pteroylglutamic acid

24. What are the effects of foliate deficiency?

This results defective erythropoiesis resulting megaloblastic anemia.

25. Compare and contrast the folic acid, vit-B_{12} and iron deficiency anemia.

See answer in page 53.

26. Give characteristics features of (i) iron deficiency anemia (ii) pernicious anemia.

i. *Characteristics feature of iron deficiency anemia* is as follows:

- Microcytic hypochromic RBC
- MCV, MCH, MCHC and CI decreases

- RBC count decreases or remains normal
- Normoblastic hyperplasia of bone marrow
- Normal WBC and platelet count
- Soft, brittle and spoon shaped nail
- Angry red tongue and dysphagia
- Irritability, loss of concentration, headache, impotence
- Early breathlessness, palpitation.

ii. Characteristics feature of pernicious anemia is as follows:

- Microcytic normochromic RBC
- Marked decrease in RBC count and Hb concentration
- Lemon yellow coloured skin due to anemic paleness and mild jaundice
- MCV, MCH increases and MCHC remains normal
- Increase in reticulocyte count
- Low grade hemolytic jaundice
- Increase in serum iron concentration
- Paresthesia i.e. numbness, tingling, burning sensation ataxia etc.

27. What is ESR? How it differs from PCV?

ESR is the rate of settling of red cells in a special tube fixed vertically. To determine PCV the tube containing anticoagulant mixed blood is required to be centrifuged whereas in ESR centrifugation is not required.

28. What is importance of ESR?

It helps to diagnose broader aspect of some disease though it has got more prognostic value. It helps in assessing the progress of patients treated for chronic diseases like pulmonary tuberculosis and rheumatoid arthritis.

29. What happens if the RBC is kept in hypotonic and hypertonic saline?

- In hypotonic solution, water moves inside the RBC cell due to concentration gradient → swelling up of RBC → increase of RBC volume → rupture (hemolysis) of RBC takes place.
- In hypertonic solution, water moves out of the cell → shrinkage of the cell (crenated).

30. At what serum bilirubin level clinical jaundice occurs in adults and infants?

- *In adult:* If serum bilirubin increases beyond 2 mg% it results jaundice
- *In infants*: If serum bilirubin increases beyond 5 mg% it results jaundice

31. Why jaundice is first detected in the eyes?

It is because of whiteness of sclera. Sclera has a protein known as elastin which has high affinity to bind bilirubin. So even in low grade of jaundice bilirubin can get bind with sclera.

32. What is the clinical importance of glycosylated hemoglobin?

The blood level of glycosylated hemoglobin (HbA_{1C}) reflects the average blood glucose level over the period of preceding 5-8 weeks and thus serves as an index of long term control of diabetes mellitus. Thus a pateint if becomes careless about controlling his hyperglycemia and takes an insulin injection only before visiting his doctor would have normal blood glucose but his HbA_{1C} will be raised.

33. Why does stool darken on standing in air?

It is due to the conversion of residual urobilinogen (colourless) to coloured urobillin.

34. What is prehepatic jaundice? Why it does result in unconjugated hyperbilirubinemia?

When jaundice occurs due to increased formation of bilirubin it is called as prehepatic or hemolytic jaundice. In this case the liver is unable to conjugate the large amounts of bilirubin produced resulting in unconjugated hyperbilirubinemia.

35. What is post hepatic jaundice? Why it does result in conjugated hyperbilirubinemia?

If the jaundice occurs due to biliary obstruction it is known as post hepatic jaundice. In this case the conjugated bilirubin produced in the liver regurgitates back into blood instead of flowing out into the duodenum. This is why it results in conjugated hyperbilirubinemia.

36. What is hepatic jaundice? Why it does usually result in conjugated hyperbilirubinemia?

The jaundice due to the impairment of all steps of bilirubin metabolism in liver is known as hepatic jaundice. The commenest cause is infective hepatitis. In this case the excretion of bilirubin is worstly affected that results in conjugated hyperbilirubinemia.

37. What is the average period for normal development of neutrophils?

12 days.

38. What is respiratory burst?

Within seconds of stimulation neutrophils sharply increase their oxygen uptake which is known as respiratory burst.

39. Why blood do not clot in the body?

This is because of following reasons:

- Smoothness of endothelial lining which prevents platelet adhesion.
- Negativity of endothelial lining that repels the negatively charged plasma clotting factors.
- High blood pressure that increases velocity of blood.
- Presence of natural anticoagulants like heparin and protein C in the blood.
- Simultaneous activation of fibrinolytic system along with clotting mechanism. This causes lysis of fibrin molecules.

40. What is the mode of action of heparin as an anticoagulant?

It inhibits the reaction between thrombin and fibrinogen and also interferes in formation of thromboplastin.

41. Which one is the principal plasma protein associated with rate of sedimentation of RBCs.?

It is fibrinogen.

42. Mention the conditions when BT and CT is prolonged.

BT is increased during thrombocytopenic purpura, allergic and also senile purpura, infection like typhus, bacterial endocarditis, deficiency of vitamin C, etc.

CT is prolonged in hemophilia, afibrinogenemia, vitamin-K deficiency, liver disease, etc.

43. What is the basic difference between intrinsic and extrinsic system of blood clotting?

In the intrinsic system, injury to blood cells like platelets, releases phospholipid that activate different clotting factors to induce clotting. Whereas in the extrinsic system injury to blood vessels or nearby tissues releases tissue thromboplastin which induces clotting mechanism by activating different clotting factors by cascade mechanism.

44. What is prothrombin time? What is its significance?

Prothrombin time is the test for prothrombin activity and thereby it is a test for testing the extrinsic system of blood coagulation. Normal value of prothrombin time is 11-16 sec. and it is increased in liver failure and deficiency of vitamin-K. It is generally used to monitor patients with anticoagulants therapy to adjust its dose.

45. Mention the role of Ca^{++} in clotting mechanism.

Except for the first 2 steps in the intrinsic pathway calcium ions are required for the promotion of all reactions involved in both intrinsic and extrinsic pathway.

46. Why Ca^{++} deficiency does not produce coagulation defects?

Only traces of calcium ions are required for coagulation of blood which are normally available in the body.

47. Why clot does not spread in the injured vessel after blood coagulation?

The reasons are:

- Removal of some activated clotting factors specially IX, X, and XII from the circulation by anti-thrombin III secreted by the liver.
- Reduction in the supply of clotting factors.
- Balancing activity of thromboxane A_2 and prostacyclin that prevent excessive extension of clot and maintaining blood flow around it.

48. Why does blood become incoagulable following violent death?

In case of violent death, the blood remains in fluidic and incoagulable in nature due to fibrinolysis resulted due to adrenaline induced rapid release of plasminogen activators from endothelial cells.

49. What is the difference between rouleaux formation and agglutination?

Rouleaux formation is simply stacking of RBCs without any hemolysis whereas in agglutination there is antigen-antibody reaction on the red cells resulting hemolysis of RBC.

50. In 'O' blood group no antigens are there, still both antibodies are present in plasma. How these antibodies are formed?

Any of the specific blood group antibodies are absent at birth but in childhood while taking some foods like seed and plants or from intestinal bacteria these nonself-antigens are absorbed from GI tract to blood and thereby induces to develop the antibodies against that particular antigen or antigens.

51. What changes RBCs undergo during cold storage?

Cold storage results following changes:

- Appearance of spherocytic RBC due to net increase in volume of cell.
- Increase in tendency of hemolysis.

52. At what age after birth a child's blood group is set in it's true ABO type?

During adolescence i.e. upto 10 years.

53. How hemolytic disease in a newborn can be prevented?

It is by removing small quantities of infant's blood successively from IVC and replacing an equal amount of compatible Rh^- blood.

54. What is the management of hemolytic transfusion reactions?

In case of hemolytic transfusion reactions transfusion must be stopped immediately and the patient is to be given intravenous injection of rapid acting corticoids.

55. What do you mean by secretors and non-secretors?

The A and B antigens are also present in other tissues like liver, pancreas, kidney, etc. and also in body fluids like saliva, semen, etc. The individuals who have high concentration of these antigens in their body fluids are called secretors and those having low concentration of these antigens in their body fluid are known as non-secretors.

56. What are human leucocyte antigens (HLA) and what is their importance?

HLA are the antigens present on the surface of WBCs. HLA typing is done before tissue or bone marrow transplant since they are responsible for early rejection of transplant.

57. Why spleen is not essential for life?

The function of spleen can also be maintained by some other organs and tissues like Kupffer cells in liver, lymph nodes, sub cutaneous tissue, osteoclasts, microglia in brain, lymphocytes, thymus gland etc. This is why it is not essential in life, however in absence of spleen bacterial infections are more common and severe.

58. Why incidences of tumours are more with advancing age?

It is because of the gradual declining of cellular immune mechanism.

59. Why we do not make an immunological response of our own body proteins?

Body has got the capacity to identify it's own 'self' protein against of which no immunological response is evoked.

60. Has phototherapy any role in patients suffering from hemolytic jaundice?

Phototherapy has some role in treating any form of jaundice in infants because it converts bilirubin to lumirubin which has a shorter life than bilirubin.

61. Enumerate the role of aspirin in prevention of a stroke.

Aspirin by inhibiting Thromboxane A_2 formation prevents platelet aggregation. Therefore it has got immense value in preventing MI and Stroke.

62. Name two well known vascular causes of bleeding.

These are: Scurvy and Cushing Syndrome.

E. MCQ:

1. Normal pH of the blood is (i) 7.30 (ii) 7.40 (iii) 6.32 (iv) 8.20 (ii)
2. All are the NPN substances except (i) urea (ii) creatinin (iii) xanthine (iv) cholesterol. (iv)
3. Following are the blood buffers except (i) hemoglobin (ii) phosphate (iii) plasma proteins (iv) bicarbonate. (ii)
4. ESR is high in the following conditions except (i) female (ii) pregnancy (iii) high altitude (iv) infants. (iv)
5. Within a normal RBC following biochemical pathway operates (i) Kreb's cycle (ii) EMP (iii) both (iv) none. (ii)
6. In an young adult red bone marrow is seen in (i) shaft of femur (ii) cranial bones (iii) both (iv) none of the above. (ii)
7. Erythropoietin is produced by (i) loop of henlee (ii) liver (iii) peritubular capillaries of renal cortex (iv) none of the above. (iii)
8. Microcytic anemia develops in (i) Vit B_{12} deficiency (ii) folic acid deficiency (iii) both (iv) none of the above. (iii)

9. Iron absorption occurs mostly in (i) initial half of the small intestine (ii) ileum (iii) stomach (iv) all of the above. (i)
10. Free bilirubin refers to (i) bilirubin not complexed with protein or glucoronic acid (ii) bilirubin albumin complex (iii) bilirubin glucoronic complex. (ii)
11. Lymph in the blood predominantly are (i) T lymphocytes (ii) B lymphocytes (iii) both. (i)
12. Neutrophils are maximally present in (i) bone marrow (ii) tissue (iii) blood. (i)
13. Antigen presenting cell is a (i) T lymphocytes (ii) B lymphocytes (iii) Macrophage (iv) all of the above. (iii)
14. Imunoglobulins are produced by (i) plasma cell (ii) macrophage (iii) T lymphocytes (iv) N K cells. (i)
15. Following immunoglobulin can cross the placental barrier (i) IgG (ii) IgM (iii) IgA (iv) all of them. (i)
16. In healthy young persons the following serum lipoproteins are present (i) HDL (ii) LDL (iii) VLDL (iv) only i and ii. (iv)
17. Serum albumin concentration is low in (i) Kwashiorkor (ii) Malnutrition edema (iii) gross liver failure. (iv) all. (iv)
18. Plasma protein that exert maximum colloidal osmotic pressure is (i) prothrombin (ii) albumin (iii) fibrinogen (iv) globulin. (ii)
19. Prothrombin time is normal in (i) factor VIII deficiency (ii) factor VII deficiency (iii) both (iv) none of the above. (i)
20. Extrinsic system of blood clotting is initiated by (i) factor –III (ii) factor –VIII (iii) factor –II (iv) factor-I. (i)
21. Hemophilia A is caused by the deficiency of (i) factor-II (ii) factor-X (iii) factor-VIII (iv) factor-XII. (ii)
22. Von Willebrand factor helps in (i) platelet adhesion (ii) activation of clotting factors (iii) clotting lysis (iv) vasoconstriction. (i)
23. Which test is the test for extrinsic system of blood clotting (i) Platelet count (ii) Bleeding time (iii) Prothrombin count (iv)Thromboplastin generation time. (ii)
24. One of the following is not an anticoagulant (i) heparin (ii) protein C (iii) antithrombin-III (iv) thrombin. (iv)
25. The type of immunoglobulin present in human milk is (i) IgG (ii) IgE (iii) IgD (iv) IgA. (iv)
26. The normal stored form of iron in liver and spleen is (i) transferrin (ii) apoferritin (iii) ferritin (iv) hemosiderin. (iii)
27. The daily requirement of iron in adult male is (i) 5mg (ii) 50 mg (iii) 25 mg (iv) 30 mg. (iii)
28. The antibody takes part in allergic reaction is (i) IgA (ii) IgM (iii) IgG (iv) IgE. (iv)
29. All the plasma proteins except one increase ESR (i) fibrinogen (ii) albumin (iii) globulin (iv) prothrombin. (ii)
30. All the indices are increased in macrocytic anemia except (i) MCV (ii) PCV (iii) MCHC (iv) MCH. (iii)
31. Complements has all the following function except (i) chemotaxis (ii) phagocytosis (iii) cytolysis (iv) opsonization. (ii)
32. The cell that acts 1st line of defence in acute infection is (i) lymphocytes (ii) monocytes (iii) basophils (iv) neutrophils. (iv)
33. The stage of erythropoiesis at which Hb starts to appear is (i) reticulocyte (ii) mature stage (iii) proerythroblast (iv) intermediate normoblast. (iv)

Neuro-Muscular System

3

A. Long type:

1. Describe the NM junction with suitable diagram. Add a note on NM transmission.

The junction between the terminal branch of the motor nerve fiber and the muscle fiber is known as *Neuromuscular junction* or *Myo-Neural Junction*.

Structure: Both the light and E/M structure is represented by (Fig. 3.1).

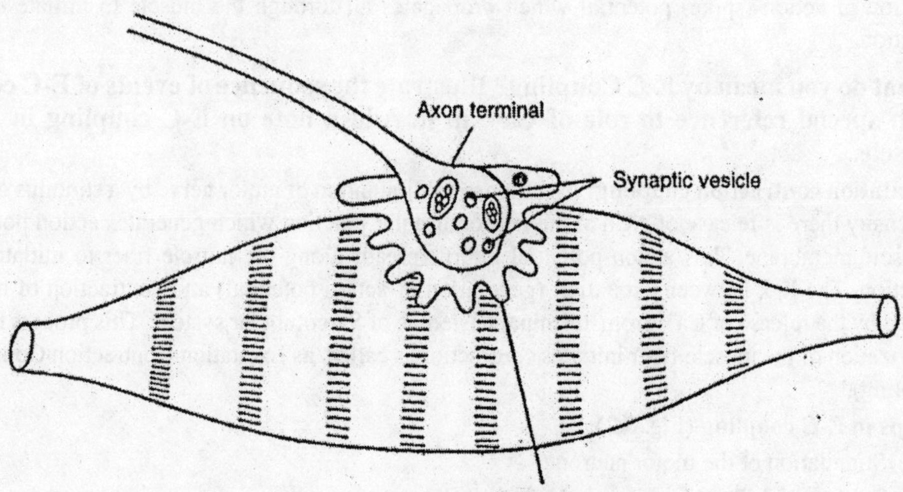

Fig. 3.1: Structure of Neuromuscular junction

- *Light microscopic*: While approaching to the muscle fiber each terminal branch of the motor nerve fiber looses it's myelin sheath close to the muscle and divides into a number of terminal buttons or end feet. Each of these terminal buttons invaginates inside the muscle fiber and makes a close and intensive contact with a specialised part of muscle sarcoplasm known as *Motor end plate*.
- *Electron microscopic*: The membrane of the nerve ending close to the muscle is called *pre synaptic membrane* whereas the muscle membrane is known as *post synaptic membrane*. The space between

these two membranes is called as ***Synaptic cleft***. At the terminal buttons there are many mitochondria and synaptic vesicles which contain the neurotransmitter substances Acetyl Choline (ACh). Mitochondria on the other hand contains ATP which provides the energy for the synthesis of ACh. Whereas the synaptic cleft contains basal lamina the matrix of which contains large quantity of enzyme acetyl cholinesterase which hydrolyses the ACh once it's action is over.

- Underneath the nerve endings, the muscle membrane of motor end plate is thrown into a number of folds called ***Palisades*** which increase the surface area on which ACh can act. Moreover on the post synaptic membrane there are some receptors which are stimulated by both ACh and Nicotine. These receptors are called as Nicotinic ACh receptors.

Mechanism of neuromuscular transmission:

The mechanism of neuromuscular transmission is represented sequentially by the following flow chart:

Propagation of action potential to presynaptic membrane of motor nerve ending → opening of voltage gated Ca^{++} channels of presynaptic membrane of motor nerve terminal → entry of Ca^{++} from ECF to terminal button → release of ACh from terminal button to the synaptic cleft by exocytosis → ACh diffuses quickly (within few hundred microseconds) to the post synaptic membrane → binding of ACh to the nicotinic ACh receptor present on the post synaptic membrane → opening of ligand gated Na^+ channels present on the post synaptic membrane → entry of Na^+ ions from ECF to muscle inside → depolarisation of post synaptic membrane to develop local potential called ***End Plate Potential*** (EPP) which is not propagatory in nature → when this EPP reaches to a threshold of – 40 to – 50 mv it causes generation of action (spike) potential which propagates all through the muscle to initiate muscular contraction.

2. What do you mean by E-C Coupling? Illustrate the sequence of events of E-C coupling with special reference to role of Ca^{2+} in it. Add a note on E-C coupling in cardiac muscle.

Excitation contraction coupling: In response to stimulation of motor nerve by a stimulus of threshold intensity there is release of ACh at the neuromuscular junction which generates action potential in the muscle membrane. This action potential inturn spreads along the muscle fiber to initiate muscle contraction. The link between excitation (generation of action potential) and contraction of muscle is provided by the release of Ca^{++} from Terminal Cisternae of Sarcotubular system. This process by which depolarization of the muscle fiber initiates contraction is called as Excitation Contraction Coupling (E-C coupling).

Steps in E-C coupling (Fig. 3.2):

1. Stimulation of the motor neurone.
2. Release of ACh at neuromuscular junction.
3. Binding of ACh to nicotinic ACh receptor.
4. Increased Na^+ conductance followed by K^+ conductance in muscle membrane.
5. Initiation of end plate potential.
6. Generation of action potential i.e. excitation of muscle membrane.
7. Inward spread of action potential along 'T' tubules.
8. Activation of ***dihydropyridine*** receptors present in 'T' tubule membrane which mainly serves as the voltage sensor.
9. Triggering of release of Ca^{++} in sarcoplasm from terminal cisternae via ***Ryanodine receptor*** which is related to IP_3 receptor i.e. Ligand gated Ca^{++} channels.
10. Diffusion of Ca^{++} to the myofilaments.

11. Binding of Ca^{++} to troponine 'C' to uncover the myosin binding site of actin.
12. Formation of cross bridge between myosin and actin and sliding of thin filaments on thick filaments.
13. Shortening of muscle i.e. muscle contraction.

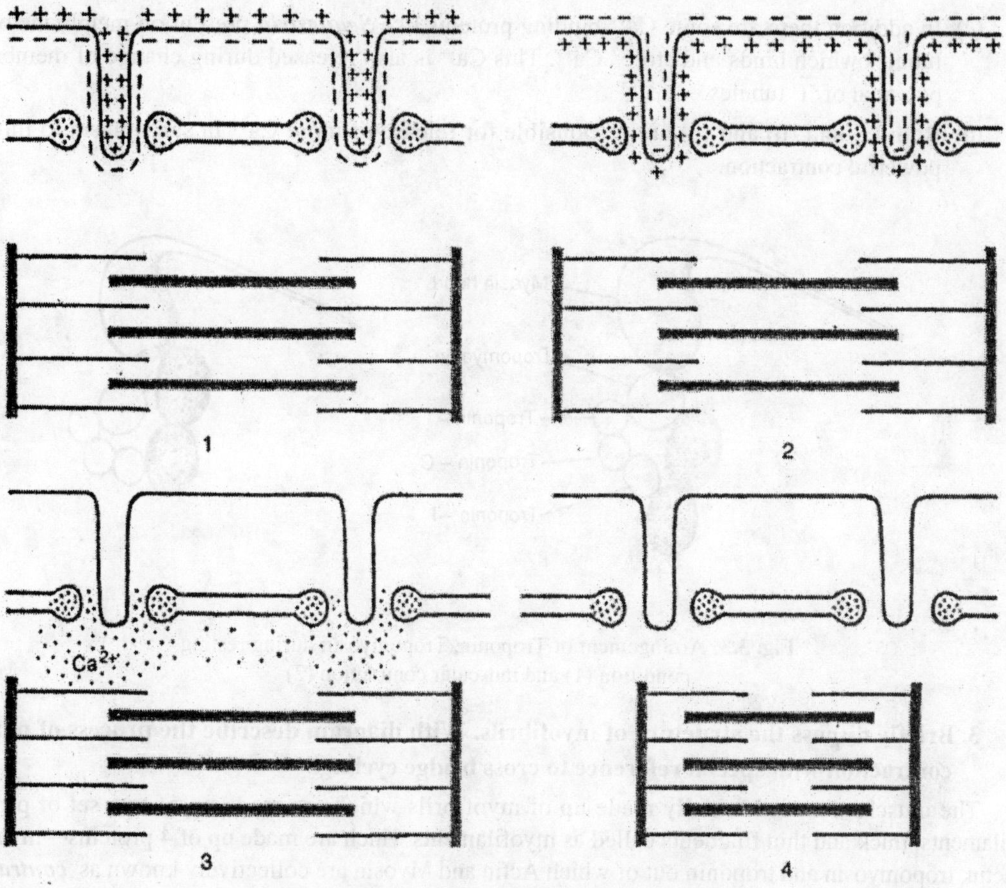

Fig. 3.2: Diagrammatic representation of EC Coupling

Role of Ca^{2+} in EC coupling: In response to stimulation (depolarization) of muscle membrane there is release of Ca^{++} in the sarcoplasm from the teminal cisternae. The Ca^{++} inturn binds with troponin-C molecule to result:

(a) Configurational and positional changes of troponin molecules which inturn pull tropomyosin molecule away from 'F' actin uncovering the binding sites for myosin heads on actin molecule (Fig. 3.3).

(b) Increased *ATPase* activity of myosin head to hydrolyze ATP for producing energy.

E-C coupling in cardiac muscle:

The basic mechanism of E-C coupling in cardiac muscle is similar to that in skeletal muscle. However there are some differences as follows:

In case of cardiac muscle terminal cisternae is not present or well developed as in skeletal muscle. Moreover the force of contraction of cardiac muscle is much more powerful. This is provided by following factors:

(a) ***Dihydropyridine*** receptors present in 'T' tubule membrane acts as a voltage gated Ca^{++} channels which cause release of Ca^{++} directly from, ECF to sarcoplasm.

(b) Influx of Ca^{++} via these channel triggers the release of Ca^{++} stored in the sarcoplasmic reticulum through the ligand gated Ca^{++} channel i.e. ***Ryanodine receptor***. This is known as **Ca^{++} induced Ca^{++} release (CICR)**.

(c) In addition there are some Ca^{++} binding proteins like ***Sequestrin*** present on membrane of 'T' tubules which binds and stores Ca^{++}. This Ca^{++} is also released during change of membrane potential of 'T' tubules.

(d) Both (a) and (b) and (c) are responsible for release of more Ca^{++} in sarcoplasm to initiate powerful contraction.

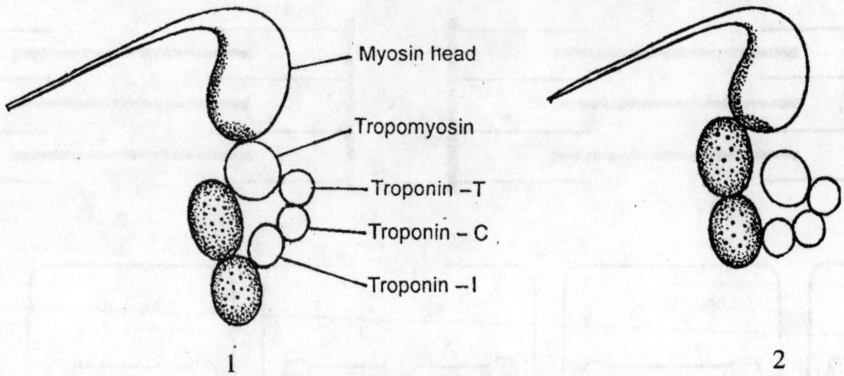

Fig. 3.3: Arrangement of Troponin, Tropomyosin during resting condition (1) and muscular contraction (2)

3. Briefly discuss the structure of myofibrils. With diagram describe the process of muscle contraction with special reference to cross bridge cycling.

The muscle fiber is basically made up of myofibrils which are made up of two set of protein filaments, thick and thin filaments called as myofilaments which are made up of 4 proteins—myosin , actin, tropomyosin and troponin out of which Actin and Myosin are collectively known as ***contractile elements*** or proteins of muscle whereas Troponin and Tropomyosin are referred as ***Regulatory proteins***.

A. ***Electron microscopic study of myofilaments*** **(Fig. 3.4):**

- E/M study of each sarcomere reveals that it is composed of many thread like protein filaments known as myofilaments. These myofilaments are of two types:

(a) *Thick filaments*:

- It is responsible for the A band and is made up of about 500 myosin molecules/thick filament.
- Each myosin molecule is formed by 6 polypeptide chains—2 heavy chains known as ***Heavy meromyosin*** (HMM) and 4 light chains of polypeptides known as ***Light meromyosin*** (LMM).
- The amino terminal end of two heavy chains are twisted against each other in the form a double helix. At the one end chain turns to one side and forms the globular head. Each myosin head has two sides—one is **for binding actin molecule** and another is for binding ATP to hydrolyse it known as **catalytic site**.
- To each part of the myosin head are attached 2 light chains which acts as a backbone for HMM.

- **Thus the amino terminal end of HMM and LMM constitute Head of myosin whereas two twisted (double helix like) carboxy terminal ends of HMM is known as Tail of myosin.**
- **The tail joins the globular head in the region which is known as *Myosin hinge*.**
- **The molecular weight of each heavy chain is 2,00,000 whereas the MW of each light chain is 20,000.**

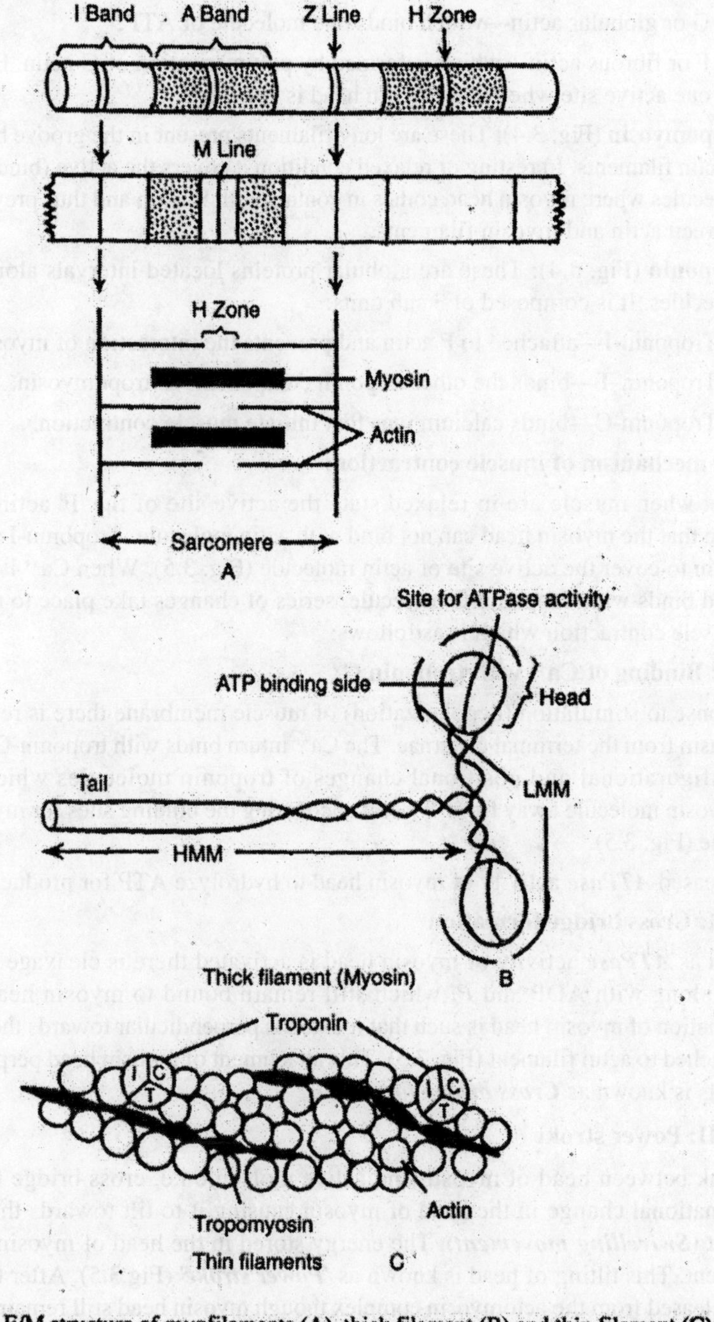

Fig. 3.4: E/M structure of myofilaments (A), thick filament (B) and thin filament (C)

(b) *Thin filaments*:

- It is made up of Actin, Tropomyosin and Troponin which arrange themselves to form 2 chain of globular proteins that form a long double helix. It forms the 'I' band.
- **Actin filaments** (Fig. 3.4): Each actin filament is made up of 300-400 actin molecules (MW of each molecule is 42,000) arranged in a double helix form. These actin molecules are of two types:
  - (i) G or globular actin—which binds one molecule of ATP.
  - (ii) F or fibrous actin—which is formed by polymerisation of G actin. Each F actin has got one active site where the myosin head is attached.
- **Tropomyosin** (Fig. 3.4): These are long filaments present in the groove between two strands of actin filaments. In resting or relaxed condition it covers the active (binding) sites of F-actin molecules where myosin head comes in contact with F-actin and thus prevents the interaction between actin and myosin filaments.
- **Troponin** (Fig. 3.4): These are globular proteins located intervals along the tropomyosin molecules. It is composed of 3 sub units:
  - i. Troponin-I—attached to F actin and prevents the interaction of myosin with actin.
  - ii. Troponin-T—binds the other troponin components to tropomyosin.
  - iii. Troponin-C—binds calcium ions that initiate muscle contraction.

Molecular mechanism of muscle contraction:

During rest when muscle are in relaxed state the active site of the 'F' actin is covered by the tropomyosin so that the myosin head can not bind with actin molecule. Troponin-I molecule also helps the tropomyosin to cover the active site of actin molecule (Fig. 3.5). When Ca^{++} is released inside the sarcoplasm and binds with Troponin C molecule, series of changes take place to result shortening of muscle i.e. muscle contraction which is as follows:

A. Stage I: Binding of Ca^{++} with troponin C

In response to stimulation (depolarization) of muscle membrane there is release of Ca^{++} in the sarcoplasm from the terminal cisternae. The Ca^{++} inturn binds with troponin-C molecule to result:
(a) Configurational and positional changes of troponin molecules which in turn pull and tropomyosin molecule away from 'F' actin uncovering the binding sites for myosin heads on actin molecule (Fig. 3.5).

(b) Increased ***ATPase*** activity of myosin head to hydrolyze ATP for producing energy.

B. Stage II: Cross bridge formation

As soon as ***ATPase*** activity of myosin head is activated there is cleavage of ATP to produce energy along with ADP and *Pi* which still remain bound to myosin head. In such a state, conformation of myosin head is such that it extends perpendicular towards the actin filament and gets attached to actin filament (Fig. 3.5). This attachment of myosin head perpendicularly to actin filaments is known as ***Cross bridge formation***

C. Stage III: Power stroke

The link between head of myosin and active molecule i.e. cross bridge formation causes a conformational change in the head of myosin causing it to tilt towards the center of myosin filament (***Swivelling movement***). The energy stored in the head of myosin is utilized for this movement. This tilting of head is known as ***'Power stroke'*** (Fig.3.5). After this event ADP and *pi* are released from the actomyosin complex though myosin head still remains attached to active site of actin filament.

D. Stage IV: Sliding of thin filaments over thick filaments

After the single cycle of tilting the head is over, new ATP molecule gets binds with myosin head. This decreases the affinity between myosin head and actin,so hea d of a cross bridge gets detached (Fig. 3.5). For next cycle to begin head of myosin again becomes perpendicular because of breakdown of ATP to ADP, *pi* and energy and gets attached to the new active site of actin molecule to repeat the cycle (Fig. 3.5).

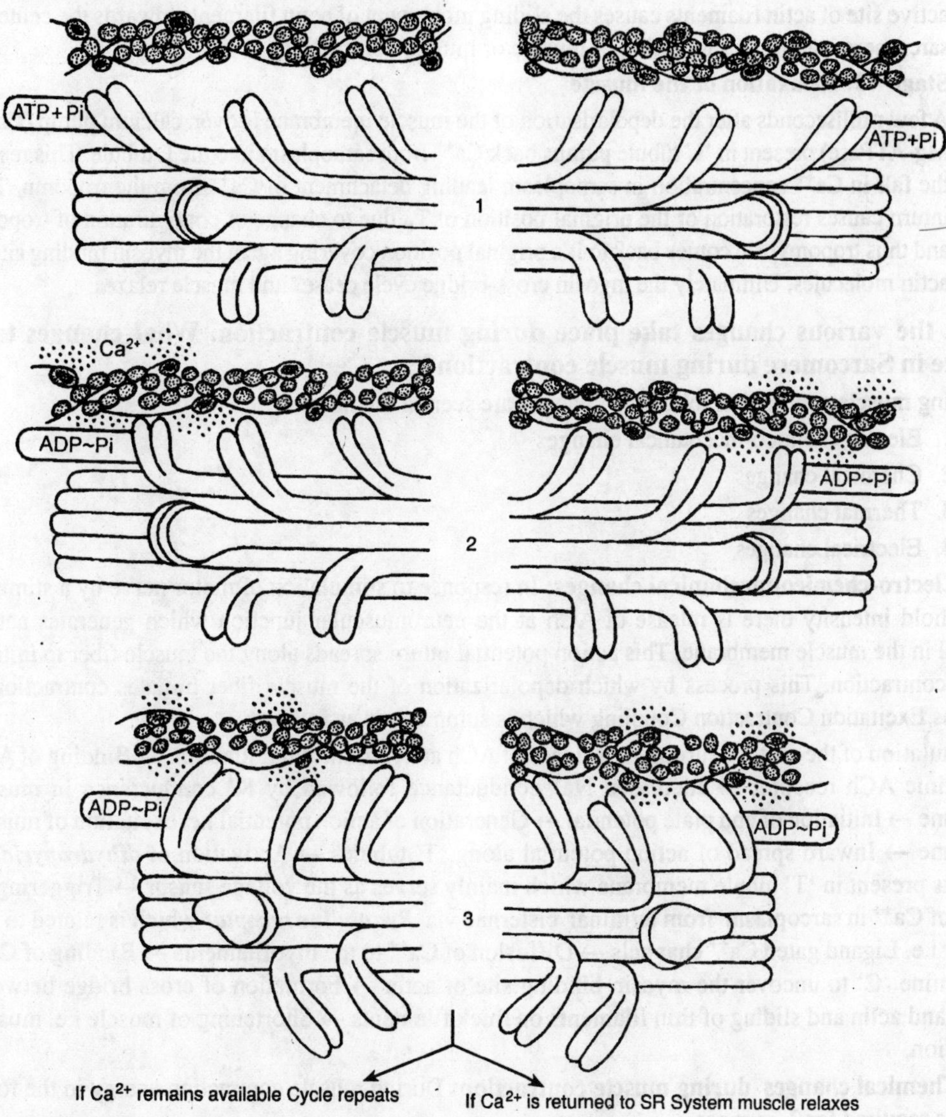

Fig. 3.5: Diagrammatic representation of steps in muscle contraction
(1 – *at rest, ATP binds to myosin head and is partially hydrolyzed to produce a high affinity binding site for actin on the myosin head. However, the head cannot bind the actin filament because of the blocking of the actin binding sites by tropomyosin.* 2 – *Ca^{2+} released from SR system in response to action potential binds to troponin-C, causing tropomyosin to move laterally and expose the myosin binding site on the actin molecule resulting Cross bridge formation.* 3 – *Power stroke which results sliding of actin filaments over myosin filaments*)

Thus with each cross bridge cycle actin filament is pulled towards the center of myosin. This process is known as **Sliding of thin filaments** i.e. actin filaments over thick filament. This event is first proposed by scientist. A.F. Huxley and H.E. Huxley in 1954 and therefore in known as ***Sliding filament theory of Huxley or Ratchet theory.***

E. Stage V: Shortening of the muscle

Repeated detachment of myosin head with old site of actin filament and reattachment with new active site of actin filaments causes the sliding movement of actin filaments towards the center of sarcomere leading to shortening of muscle or muscle contraction.

F. Stage VI: Relaxation of the muscle

A few milliseconds after the depolarisation of the muscle membrane is over, calcium pump (Ca^{++}–Mg-ATPase) present in 'L' tubule pumps back Ca^{++} from sarcoplasm into the L tubule. This results the fall in Ca^{++} concentration in sarcoplasm leading detachment of Ca^{++} from the troponin. This inturn causes restoration of the original position of T_I, due to change of configuration of troponin and thus tropomyosin comes back to it's original position covering again the myosin binding site of actin molecules. Ultimately the myosin cross-bridge cycle ceases and muscle relaxes.

4. List the various changes take place during muscle contraction. What changes take place in Sarcomere during muscle contraction?

During muscle contraction following changes are seen in the muscle:

1. Electro-chemico-mechanical changes
2. Chemical changes
3. Thermal changes
4. Electrical changes

1. Electro-chemico-mechanical changes: In response to stimulation of motor nerve by a stimulus of threshold intensity there is release of ACh at the neuromuscular junction which generates action potential in the muscle membrane. This action potential inturn spreads along the muscle fiber to initiate muscle contraction. This process by which depolarization of the muscle fiber initiates contraction is called as Excitation Contraction Coupling which is summarised as follows:

Stimulation of the motor neurone → Release of ACh at neuromuscular junction → Binding of ACh to nicotinic ACh receptor → Increased Na^+ conductance followed by K^+ conductance in muscle membrane → Initiation of end plate potential → Generation of action potential i.e. excitation of muscle membrane → Inward spread of action potential along 'T' tubules → Activation of ***dihydropyridine*** receptors present in 'T' tubule membrane which mainly serves as the voltage sensor → Triggering of release of Ca^{++} in sarcoplasm from terminal cisternae via ***Ryanodine receptor*** which is related to IP_3 receptor i.e. Ligand gated Ca^{++} channels → Diffusion of Ca^{++} to the myofilaments → Binding of Ca^{++} to troponine 'C' to uncover the myosin binding site of actin → Formation of cross bridge between myosin and actin and sliding of thin filaments on thick filaments → Shortening of muscle i.e. muscle contraction.

2. Chemical changes during muscle contraction: During muscle contraction energy in the form of ATP is required for 3 purposes:

(i) to energize the myosin head for cross bridge formation.

(ii) to dissociate cross bridge from actin to repeat the cross bridge cycle

(iii) to pump Ca^{++} inside the L tubules allowing the muscle fiber to relax.

This ATP is generally stored in the muscle and utilized after a few contractions. So for continuous muscle contraction (e.g. during exercise) ATP can be synthesized in the muscle from ADP (even during contractile activity) by different chemical mechanisms as follows:

(a) Phosphorylation of ADP by creatine phosphate (CP)

This is also known as ***Lohman's reaction*** in which Creatine kinase enzyme helps creatine phosphate (already stored in muscle) to react with ADP to from ATP:

$$ADP + CP \longrightarrow ADP + CP$$

The ATP formed by this mechanism is sufficient for contraction of the muscle for a few seconds only as amount of CP is limited.

(b) Synthesis of ATP from carbohydrate metabolism

In muscles an adequate amount of glycogen is stored and during the catabolism 2 molecules of ATP are produced along with 2 molecules of pyruvic acid from each molecule of glycogen in the process of ***Embden-Meyerhef (Glycolytic) Pathway***. From these pyruvic acids further ATP synthesis takes place in two following mechanisms depending on the availability of O_2.

(a) Oxidative phosphorylation in mitochondria: If O_2 is available the pyruvic acid enters into Krebs cycle to form 2 molecules of ATP and 16 atoms of Hydrogen. The hydrogen atoms are also responsible for synthesis of another 34 molecules of ATP in the mitochondria by the process known as ***oxidative phosphorylation***. Thus there are synthesis of 36 mol of ATP by the Kreb's cycle. For moderate level of exercise in which rate of ATP breakdown is moderate most of the energy is obtained by this mechanism. But in case of severe and rapid exercise the rate of ATP synthesis by this mechanism is not able to keep pace with rate of ATP breakdown.

(b) Anaerobic glycolysis: On the other hand if O_2 is unavailable (during rapid and intense exercise) pyruvic acid is converted to lactic acid. The lactic acid enters the blood and carried to liver to be converted into glucose after exercise. This glucose passes to muscle through blood and is converted to muscle glycogen. This is called ***Cori's cycle***. ATP is formed rapidly by anaerobic glycolysis of glucose obtained from muscle glycogen as well as through blood. ATP synthesis by this mechanism occurs at a very fast rate but amount of ATP synthesis is less but as the reaction occurs fast and anaerobical, the rate of ATP synthesis can keep pace with the rate of ATP breakdown though the muscle goes in ***O_2 debt***.

3. Thermal changes during muscle contraction: During muscle contraction energy is utilized and heat is produced which is liberated in different stages as follows:

A. ***Resting heat***: The heat produced by the muscle during rest due to basal metabolic process.

B. ***Initial heat***: Heat produced during contraction and relaxation is called Initial heat. This is made up of

(a) Activation heat (Maintenance heat): The heat that muscle produces whenever it is contracting is known as activation heat.

(b) Shortening heat: The heat produced during actual shortening of the muscle is known as shortening heat. It is due to structural changes within the muscle.

(c) Relaxation heat: The heat liberated during relaxation of the muscle.

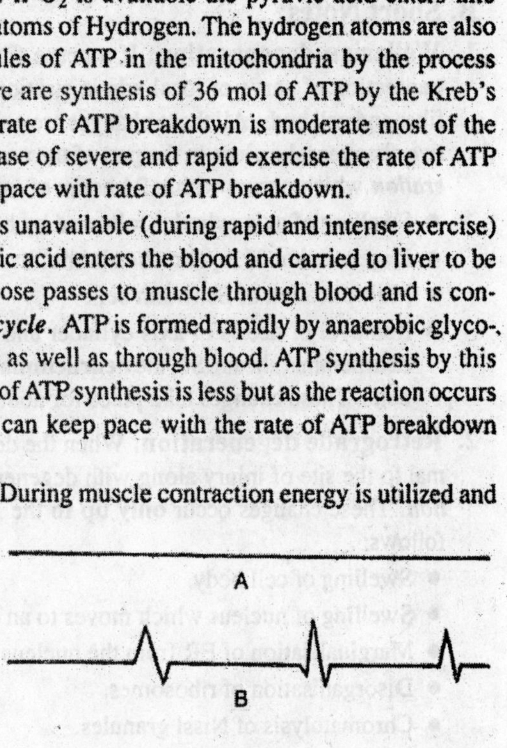

Fig. 3.6: Normal EMG during to muscular rest (A), during minimum muscular activity (B) and during maximum muscular activity (C)

C. ***Delayed heat or Recovery heat***: Heat produced after relaxation during recovery is called delayed heat or recovery heat. It is divided into 2 fractions.

i. Anaerobic heat: It is due to lactic acid formation from glycogen and resynthesis of phosphocreatine.

ii. Aerobic heat: It is due to oxidation of lactic acid to CO_2 and H_2O in presence of O_2.

4. Electrical changes: During resting condition no electrical activity is seen in the muscle. But as and when muscular contraction starts more number of motor unit potentials are recruited so that there is gradual increase in the number and amplitude of potentials (Fig. 3.6) which can be recorded as electromyogram or EMG.

Changes in Sarcomere during muscle contraction: These are;

- Reduction of length of sarcomere
- Reduction of length of I band
- Disappearence of H zone

B. Short Notes:

1. Wallerian degeneration: If a nerve fiber is injured either due to obstruction of blood flow or transection of nerve or local administration of toxic chemicals, various changes occur in the nerve fiber and cell body. All these changes are collectively called as **degenerative changes.** The degenerative changes take place in the part of the nerve fiber distal to the injury is named as ***Wallerian degeneration*** which occurs within 24 hours of injury. The changes are as follows:

- Swelling of axis cylinder followed by breaking up into smaller pieces.
- Degeneration of myelin sheath into fat droplets occur from 8th to 35th day.
- Multiplication of Schwann cell.
- Removal of debris of axis cylinder and fat droplets by invading macrophages without affecting neurilemmal sheath. So, the **neurilemmal tube** becomes empty and filled by cytoplasm of Schwann cells. These changes take place for about 2 months.

2. Retrograde degeneration: When the degenerative changes is seen in the part of the axon proximal to the site of injury along with degeneration of cell body, it is known as ***Retrograde degeneration***. These changes occur **only up to the 1st node of Ranvier near the injury.** The changes are as follows:

- Swelling of cell body.
- Swelling of nucleus which moves to an eccenteric position.
- Marginalisation of ER from the nucleus to periphery of cell body.
- Disorganisation of ribosomes.
- Chromatolysis of Nissl granules.

3. Regenerative Changes: The regeneration of injured nerve fiber takes place under some conditions and starts at 4th day after injury and is completed in about 80 days. The changes are as follows:

- Growth of schwann cell from the proximal and distal cut ends of the nerve in all direction to fill up the gap and leads to continuity of neurilemmal tube.
- Establishment of axis cylinder after 3 months of injury.
- Formation of myelin sheath within one year and increases it's diameter.
- Appearance of Nissl granules followed by golgi apparatus in cell body.
- Cell looses excess fluid and nucleus occupies the central position.

The factors affecting regenerative process are:

- Severity of the injury—The gap between proximal and distal parts if becomes more than 3 mm no regeneration takes place.

- Condition of the soma—If axonal damage is close to the cell body no regeneration occurs.
- Location of injury—In CNS regeneration is less.
- Neurotrophin release—The more the release of neurotrophins the more is the regeneration.

4. Synaptic delay: There is a delay of about 0.5 m sec during the transmission of impulse from one neurone to another via a single synapse. This is known as ***Synaptic delay*** which is due to :
- Time taken for release of NT.
- Time taken for movement of NT from presynaptic membrane to post synaptic membrane (PSM) via ECF of synaptic cleft.
- Time taken to open the ligand gated channels and entry of ions inside the cell membrane of PSM in response to binding of NT to receptor protein.

5. Occlusion and Subliminal fringe: When two afferent excitatory nerves (A and B) are stimulated simultaneously (Fig. 3.7 A) the sum total responses obtained is lesser than the responses obtained by

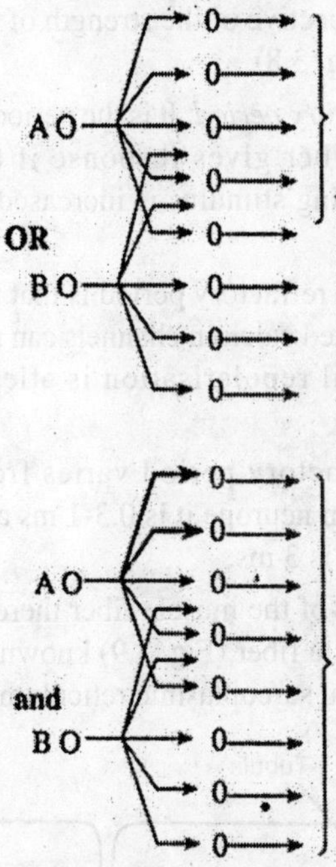

Fig. 3.7A: Demonstration of occlusion phenomenon

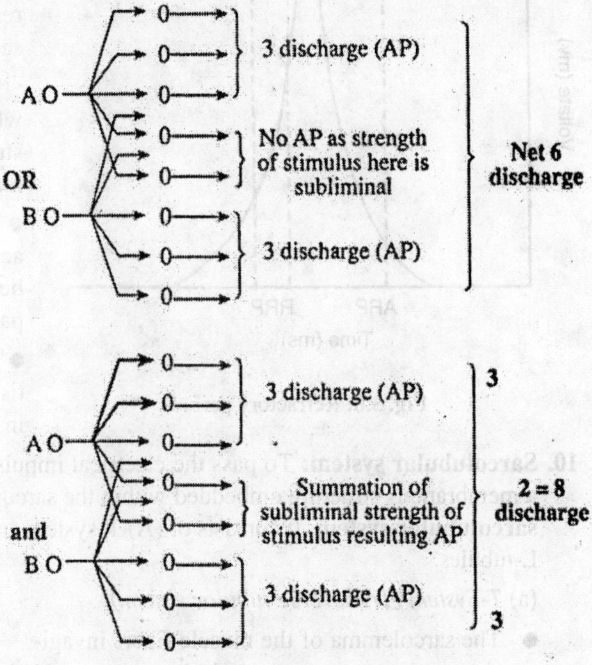

Fig. 3.7B: Demonstration of subliminal fringe effect

the individual nerve. This property is known as Occlusion. On the other hand when two afferent excitatory nerves are stimulated simultaneously (Fig. 3.7B) the sum total responses obtained is greater than the responses obtained by the individual nerve. This phenomenon is known as ***Subliminal Fringe.***

6. Heat production in nerve fiber: See thermal changes during muscle contraction of question no. 4.

7. Myasthenia gravis:
- **Definition:** It is a rare autoimmune disease characterised by rapid onset of fatigue with marked generalised weakness of muscles due to destruction of the nicotinic acelyl choline receptors on the post synaptic membrane of neuromuscular junction.

- *Cause*: Destruction of ACh receptors by the circulating antibodies to nicotinic ACh receptors.
- *Main site of occurrence*: Most affected muscles are: extraocular, facial, mastication and swallowing muscle.

8. Lambert Eaton syndrome:

- This is also characterised by generalised weakness of muscle due to the inability of Ca^{++} to influx into the terminal button of NM Junction and thereby there is no or decreased release of ACh.
- *Reason*: This is due to the damage of voltage gated Ca^{++} channels present on the presynaptic membrane of terminal button of NM Junction by the antibodies to Ca^{++} channel proteins.

9. Refractory Period:

- It is the brief period at which the nerve does not respond to the 2nd stimulus applied successively after 1st stimulus. It is of two types:

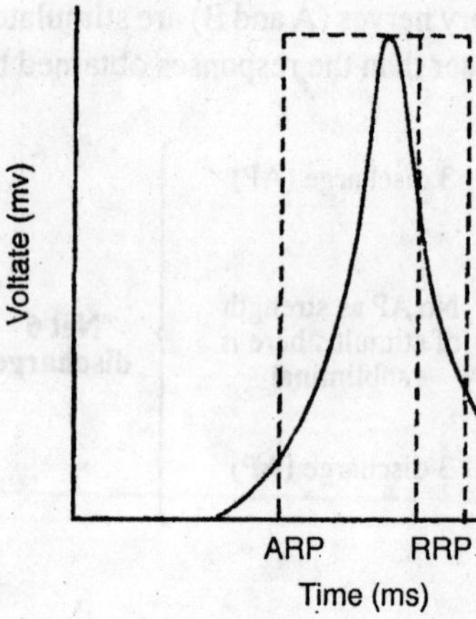

Fig. 3.8: Refractory period

■ *Absolute refractory period*: It is the period during which the nerve does not show any response at all irrespective of the strength of the second stimulus (Fig. 3.8).

■ *Relative refractory period*: It is the period at which the nerve fiber gives response if the strength of succeeding stimulus is increased to maximum.

- The ionic basis of refractory period is that the activated voltage gated calcium channels can not be reactivated until repolarisation is atleast partially completed.
- Duration of refractory period varies from tissue to tissue e.g. in neurone it is 0.3-1 ms and in skeletal muscle it is 3 ms.

10. Sarcotubular system: To pass the electrical impulse within the deep of the muscle fiber there is a membranous structure embedded within the sarcoplasm of the muscle fiber (Fig. 3.9) known as **sarcotubular system.** It consists of (A) T-system and (B) Longitudinal sarcoplasmic reticulum or L-tubules.

(a) *T-System (Transverse tubular system)*:

- The sarcolemma of the muscle fibers invaginate to form transverse tubular system and directed inwardly towards the muscle fiber at the A.I. Junction.
- These tubules penetrate the muscle cell through and through and open to the exterior of the muscle cell. Thus these tubules communicate with the ECE and therefore muscle fibrils are surrounded by the ECF.

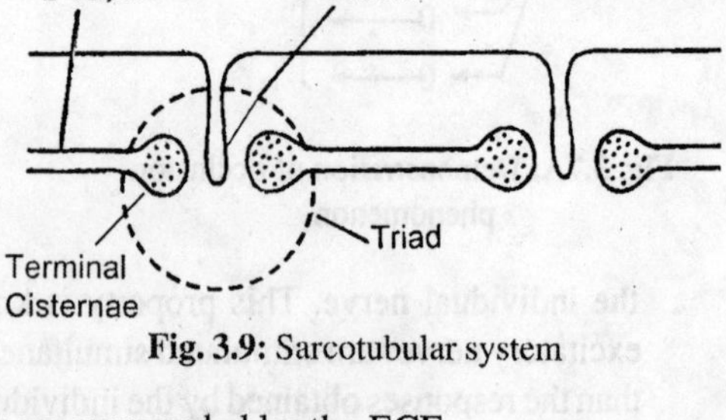

Fig. 3.9: Sarcotubular system

- This T-system facilitates the rapid transmission of electrical impulse to the myofibrils from the cell membrane.

(b) *Longitudinal Sarcoplasmic Reticulum ('L' tubules)*:

- These are like the endoplasmic reticulum of other cells with the exception of not having any ribosomes. Originating from sarcolemma there are also some closed tubular structures which run longitudinally and surround each myofibril.

- At regular intervals, the L-tubules dilate to form a pair of lateral sacs called ***terminal cisternae***. Each pair of terminal cisternae is lying close to T- tubule.
- These transverse tubule with two terminal external is called ***triad*** found at the A-I junction and thus there are **two triads per sarcomere in skeletal muscle.**
- The terminal cisternae contains Ca^{++} ion which are released into sarcoplasm when electrical impulse passes from T-tubule to the L-tubules. Ca^{++} are in turn initiates the muscle contraction.

11. Motor unit: A single ventral horn cell along with it's efferent fiber is known as the motor neuron and the single motor neuron, it's axon terminal and the muscle fibers innervated by it are collectively called as ***Motor Unit*** (Fig. 3.10).

Properties:

a. The number of muscle fibers in each motor unit varies and depends on the precision of movement performed by the muscles i.e.
   - The muscles controlling fine, graded and precise movements like laryngeal, pharyngeal and ocular muscles contains small number of muscle fibers in a single motor unit (3-6 muscle fibers / motor unit).
   - Whereas the muscles responsible for crude and coarse movements like muscles of leg and neck contain large number of muscle fibers in a single motor unit (120-165 muscle fiber / motor unit).

b. All the muscle fibers in a single motor unit are of same type i.e. each motor neuron supplies only one type of muscle fiber either type I **(Red muscles)** or type—II **(White muscle)** not both.

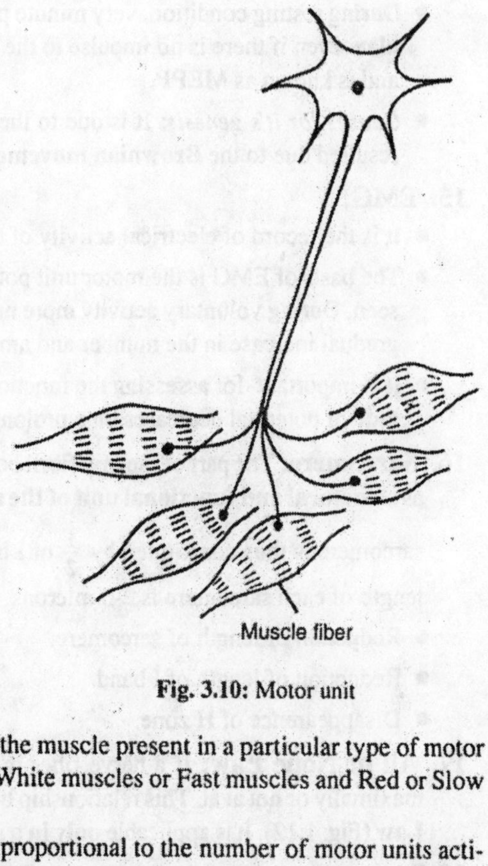

Fig. 3.10: Motor unit

c. Depending on the basis of contraction time of the muscle present in a particular type of motor unit, muscles of motor unit are of two types—White muscles or Fast muscles and Red or Slow muscle.

d. The graded response in the muscle is directly proportional to the number of motor units activated, i.e. if the strength of the stimulus is increased gradually there in gradual increase of motor response due to gradual increase of number of motor units involved in that response. This property is known as ***recruitment of motor units.***

12. Relaxing proteins:

- The troponin-tropomyosin complex is known as relaxing protein which prevents the muscle contraction during rest (Fig. 3.3).
- During resting condition Troponin-I is attached to myosin binding site on actin and partially covers the myosin binding site. Rest of myosin binding site is covered by tropomyosin filament. Thus tropomyosin molecule is held in this blocking position by troponin and thus prevents actin-myosin interaction to initiate muscle contraction.

13. End plate potential: In response to binding of ACh on the receptors present on post synaptic membrane there is entry of Na^+ which lead alteration of resting membrane potential of NM junction from – 90 mv to – 30 to – 40 mv. This change in the electrical potential (depolarisation) which is non prapagatory in nature is called ***End Plate Potential.***

Properties:

- It is nonpropagative in nature.
- It does not obey all or none law.
- It is monophasic.

14. Miniature end plate potential (MEPP):

- During resting condition, very minute potential changes (upto 0.5 mv) can occur in the motor end plate even if there is no impulse to the muscle. This is unable to produce EPP or action potential and is known as **MEPP.**
- *Causes for it's genesis*: It is due to the release of small quanta of ACh from the nerve terminal resulted due to the **Brownian movement** of flowing axoplasm.

15. EMG:

- It is the record of electrical activity of the muscle.
- The basis of EMG is the motor unit potential. So during resting condition no electrical activity is seen. During voluntary activity more number of motor unit potentials are recruited so that there is gradual increase in the number and amplitude of potentials (Fig. 3.6).
- It is important for assessing the function of the muscle. For example in myasthenia gravis amplitude of potential decreases on a prolonged voluntary effort.

16. Sarcomere: The part of the myofibril between two Z lines is called ***sarcomere*** which is considered as **structural and functional unit of the skeletal muscle** and is also called as **contractile unit.** This sarcomere is thus constituted by $\frac{1}{2}$ of I band + A band + $\frac{1}{2}$ of next I band (Fig. 3.4). The average length of each sarcomere is 2-3 microns. During muscle contraction following changes are seen:

- Reduction of length of sarcomere.
- Reduction of length of I band.
- Disappearence of H zone.

17. All or None Law: If a nerve fiber is stimulated by a stimulus it will be excited (depolarised) maximally or not at al. This relationship between the stimulus and response is known as **All or None** Law (Fig. 1.12). It is applicable **only in a single nerve/muscle fiber** not a nerve bundle/muscle mass.

18. Summation:

- The facilitatory response of the tissue to repeated stimulation by subminimal stimulus is called as summation.
- This property of the skeletal muscle can be demonstrated by-
  - Applying 2 or more subliminal stimulus of same strength at a rapid rate: When one subliminal stimulus is applied, it will not produce any response in the nerve fiber but if two or more these types of subliminal stimulus are applied within a short interval the response may be produced. This is due to the **summation of all subliminal stimuli.** This type of summation is called as ***Temporal Summation***. This is again two types:

    (i) **Incomplete summation** (superposition): When 2 successive stimuli is applied in such a way that the 2nd stimulus falls during the relaxation period of 1st curve then two curves are obtained but the 1st curve is superimposed by the 2nd curve (Fig. 3.11). This is called ***Incomplete summation*** or ***Superposition***. In this case also the height of 2nd curve is more than the 1st curve.

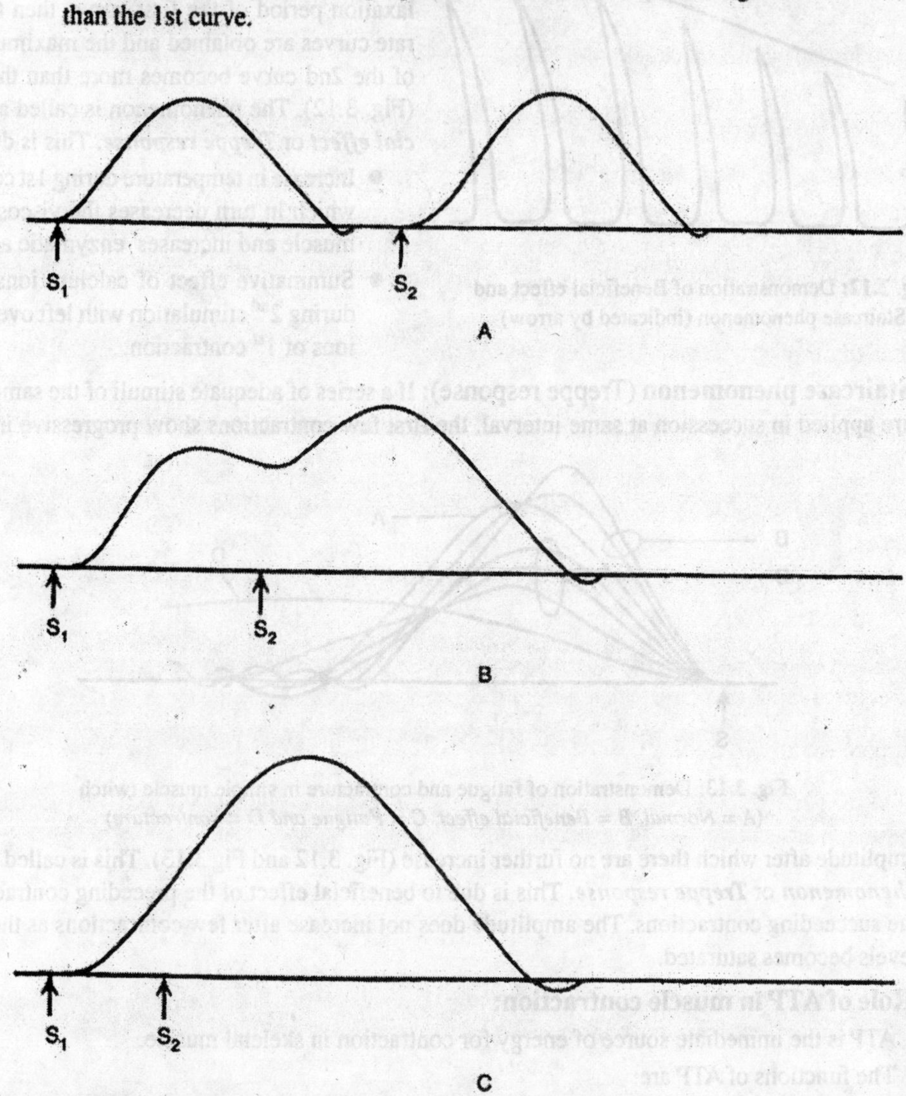

Fig. 3.11: Effect of two successive stimuli on muscle contraction. (*A = no separate response for 2nd stimulus* i.e. *S_2, B = incomplete summation (superposition) of 2nd response in which 2nd stimulus is applied during relaxation of 1st response and C = complete summation of 2nd response in which 2nd stimulus is applied during early contraction of 1st response*).

(ii) *Complete summation*: When 2 successive stimuli is applied in such a way that the 2nd stimulus falls during the contraction period of 1st curve then the two contractions are summated to give a single curve (Fig. 3.11) though the maximum height of this curve is greater than the height of normal curve. This is known as *Complete summation*.

- **Applying two or more subthreshold stimulus simultaneously at different but closely situated spots can also result the response which is known as *Spatial Summation*.**

19. **Beneficial effect:** When 2 successive stimuli are applied to a nerve muscle preparation in such a way that the 2nd stimulus is applied after the relaxation period of the first curve, then two separate curves are obtained and the maximum height of the 2nd curve becomes more than the 1st one (Fig. 3.12). The phenomenon is called as ***Beneficial effect*** or ***Treppe response***. This is due to:

- Increase in temperature during 1st contraction which in turn decreases the viscosity of the muscle and increases enzymatic activity.
- Summative effect of calcium ions released during 2nd stimulation with left over calcium ions of 1st contraction.

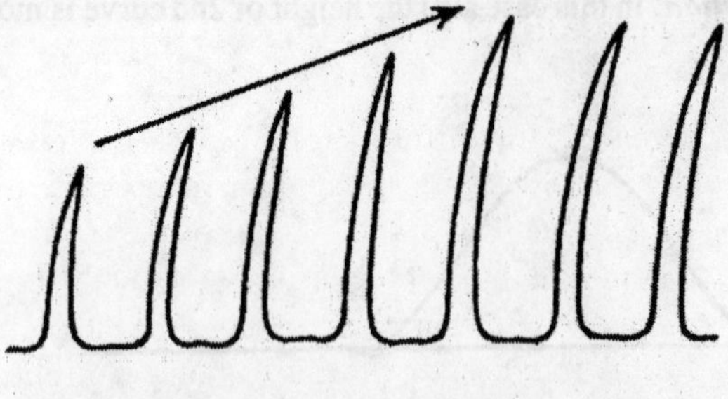

Fig. 3.12: Demonstration of Beneficial effect and Staircase phenomenon (indicated by arrow)

20. **Staircase phenomenon** (Treppe response)**:** If a series of adequate stimuli of the same strength are applied in succession at same interval, the first few contractions show progressive increase in amplitude after which there are no further increase (Fig. 3.12 and Fig 3.13). This is called ***Staircase phenomenon*** or ***Treppe response***. This is due to beneficial effect of the preceding contraction over the succeeding contractions. The amplitude does not increase after few contractions as the calcium levels becomes saturated.

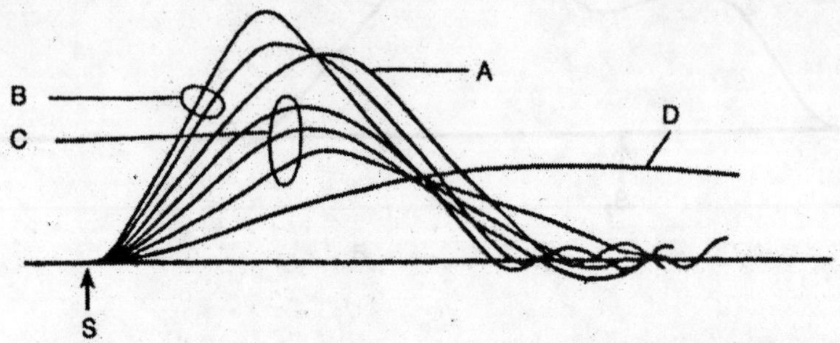

Fig. 3.13: Demonstration of fatigue and contracture in simple muscle twitch (*A = Normal, B = Beneficial effect, C = Fatigue and D = contracture*)

21. **Role of ATP in muscle contraction:**

- ATP is the immediate source of energy for contraction in skeletal muscle.
- The functions of ATP are:
  - It supplies the energy for crossbridge formation during muscle contraction.
  - ATP binding to myosin breaks the actin-myosin interaction and thus allows the cross bridge cycle to repeat.
  - Supplies energy to Ca^{++} – Mg^{++} ATPase to transport Ca^{++} back to the SR and thus helps in relaxation of muscle.
  - Supplies the energy to Na^+ – K^+ pump in the sarcolema to maintain membrane excitability (RMP).
- In resting muscle less ATP molecules are stored which are exhausted within fraction of a second after initiation of contraction. So to continue the further contraction ATP is synthesised by 3 mechanisms.

  (i) Phosphorylation of ADP by creatine phosphate.

(ii) Oxidative phosphorylation of ADP in mitochondria.

(iii) Phosphorylation of ADP by breakdown of glucose to CO_2 and H_2O.

22. Fatigue:

- ***Definition*:** If a muscle is stimulated with a series of stimuli for a prolonged period, after sometime, the muscle does not show any response. This decrease in muscular activity due to repeated stimuli for prolonged period is known as ***Fatigue*** (Fig. 3.13).
- In the genesis of fatigue curve there is increase in the amplitude of the curve initially (due to beneficial effect), then there is gradual fall of amplitude of the curve and also prolongation of latent period, contractile period etc. Just before the fatigueness, the muscle does not relax completely and remains in a partially contracted state which is known as ***Contracture.***
- **Cause of fatigue:** These are:
  - Exhaustion of ACh from N-M junction.
  - Accumulation of metabolites like lactic acid.
  - Lack of O_2 and nutrients like glycogen.
- Seat of fatigue:
  - In frog's Gastronemious muslce—nerve preparation:
    # N-M-Junction # Muscles
  - In human beings:
    # Pyramidal cells # Muscles # Anterior gray horn cells of spinal cord.
    # N-M-Junction
- Factors influencing fatigue are:
  - Rate of work — Directly related
  - Amount of work — Directly related
  - Type of muscle-fast muscles have more fatigueness
  - Blood supply — Inversely related
  - Sympathetic stimulation—delays fatigue by increasing motor end plate sensitivity.

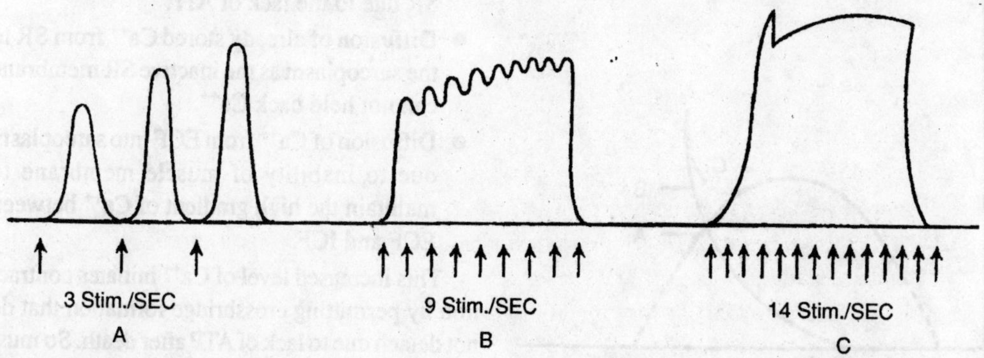

Fig. 3.14: Effect of multiple stimuli (*A = Treppe response, B = Incomplete tetanus and C = Complete tetanus)*

23. Tetanus: If a series of maximal stimuli are applied at a higher frequency i.e. the succeeding stimuli are applied during contraction period of previous twitch, the muscles remain in a state of sustained contraction due to fusion of contractions. This state of apparent sustained contraction of muscle evoked by repeated stimuli of higher frequency is known as ***Tetanus.*** It is of 2 types:

- Incomplete (Partial) Tetanus or clonus: When frequency of the stimulus is at low rates (15-30/sec in frog's gastroenemious sciatic preparation) the fusion of contractions is not complete resulting appearance of a wavy nature of the curve (Fig. 3.14). This is known as ***incomplete tetanus*** or ***clonus***.

- ❑ Complete tetanus: When frequency of the stimulus is at higher rates (over 30/sec in frog's Gastroenemious—sciatic nerve preparation) the fusion of contractions becomes complete resulting appearance of a sustained contraction (Fig. 3.14). This is known as ***complete tetanus***.

24. Muscle tone:

- **The living skeletal muscles are always in the state of partial sustained contraction. This is known as *muscle tone* and this property is known as *Tonicity*.**
- *Cause of tonicity*: It is due to continuous discharge of γ motor neurones to the muscle spindle.
- *Abnormalities of muscle tone*: The abnormalities of muscle tone are:

(1) Hypotonia:

- Decrease or loss of muscle tone is known as hypotonia.
- Cause: Lower motor neurone lesion.
- Result/Effect: It results flaccidity of the muscle which can not give response and undergoes wasting. This condition of the muscle is known as **flaccid paralysis** of the muscles.

(2) Hypertonia:

- It is state of muscle in which muscle tone becomes exaggerated.
- Cause: Upper motor neuron lesion which results increase in α motor discharge.
- Result: It results rigidity of the muscle and because of this muscle can not do it's function. This condition is known as **spastic paralysis** of the muscle.

25. Rigor mortis:

- ❑ ***Definition***: After death all the muscles of the body becomes rigid and remains in contractile state. This state of muscle is known as Rigor Mortis.
- ❑ ***Causes***: Following death the cytoplasmic Ca^{++} concentration remains elevated because of following reasons:

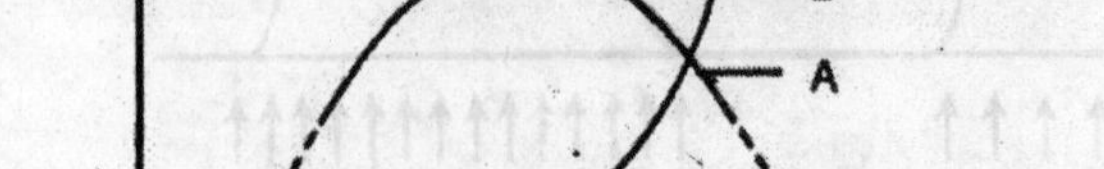

Fig. 3.15: Length tension relationship curve in skeletal muscle (*A = active tension, B = passive tension and C = total tension*)

- Absence of pumping back of Ca^{++} into the SR due to the lack of ATP.
- Diffusion of already stored Ca^{++} from SR to the sarcoplasm as the inactive SR membrane can not held back Ca^{++}.
- Diffusion of Ca^{++} from ECF into sarcoplasm due to inability of muscle membrane to maintain the high gradient of Ca^{++} between ECF and ICF.

This increased level of Ca^{++} initiates contraction by permitting crossbridge formation that do not detach due to lack of ATP after death. So muscle becomes stiff.

- ❑ It starts about 3-4 hour after death and gets completed in about 12 hour after death. The stiffness disappear 48-60 hours after death due to disintegration of muscle proteins.

26. Starling's law:

- ❑ The force of contraction of the muscle is directly related with initial length of the muscle fiber within a physiological limit. This is known as **Starling's law**. Thus the more is the initial length the greater is the force of contraction (Tension), up to a level beyond that tension falls. This relationship in between length and tension is as known as ***Length-Tension relationship*** or ***Length Tension curve*** (Fig. 3.15).

- In case of cardiac muscle it is known as Frank Starling's law of heart which states that within physiological limit the force of contraction of ventricular muscle is directly related with the end diastolic fiber length (EDFL) of the ventricular muscle.

27. O_2 dedt:

- During the reaction of anaerobic glycolysis muscle glycogen is converted into lactic acid. After the exercise, through Cori's cycle this lactate is again converted to glycogen to replenish the glycogen store in the muscle. Therefore, greater quantity of O_2 supply is necessary even after the exercise. This amount of extra O_2 consumed to remove muscle lactate, replenish ATP, CP and glycogen stores and also to replace small amount of O_2 that has been used from myoglobin is called ***O_2 debt.***
- For the requirement of this ***O_2 debt*** the respiratory rate remains in increased state for sometime even after the exercise according to the severity of the exercise.

28. After load and preload: In the experimental condition when load will act only when muscle contracts is known as after load. In after loaded condition the force of contraction and the physiological work done is less. Whereas when load will act not only when muscle contracts but also before it's contraction, it is known as free load. In free loaded condition the force of contraction and the physiological work done is more as in this condition the muscle fibers are stretched and the initial length of muscle fibers is increased, resulting increase of force of contraction as per Starling's law. This is why freeload is more beneficial than after load.

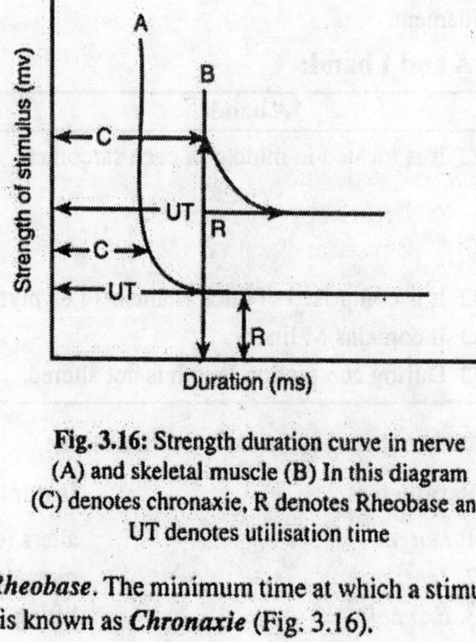

Fig. 3.16: Strength duration curve in nerve (A) and skeletal muscle (B) In this diagram (C) denotes chronaxie, R denotes Rheobase and UT denotes utilisation time

29. Chronaxie and Rheobase: To excite a muscle fiber a particular strength of the stimulus is required. The strength below this can not excite the cell whereas the strength above this level can not result more response beyond this. This minimum strength of the stimulus which is required to excite the tissue (skeletal muscle fiber) is known as ***Rheobase***. The minimum time at which a stimulus of twice of Rheobase voltage can excite a tissue is known as ***Chronaxie*** (Fig. 3.16).

C. Differentiate between:

Single unit smooth muscle	Multi unit smooth muscle
❑ Present in the walls of G-I tract and urogenital tract.	❑ Present in the walls of large arteries, intrinsic muscle of eyes, piloerector muscle and vas deferens.
❑ Have diffuse junctions.	❑ Have contact junctions.
❑ It obeys all or none law.	❑ It does not obey all or none law.
❑ It can be tonic or phasic.	❑ It is always phasic.
❑ It shows ephaptic conduction.	❑ It does not show ephaptic conduction.

Single unit smooth muscle	Multi unit smooth muscle
❑ It can get excited spontaneously.	❑ It can not get excited spontaneously.
❑ Can not be excited by generator potential.	❑ Can be excited by generator potential.
❑ It is excited by nerves and hormones, stretch and cold temperature.	❑ It is excited by nerves only.

Sensitisation	Habituation
❑ It is elicited by weak stimuli.	❑ It is elicited by strong and painful stimuli.
❑ It results gradual decrease in response.	❑ It results gradual increase in response.
❑ It is associated with decrease in neuro-transmitter release.	❑ It is associated with increase in neuro-transmitter release.
❑ It is due to inactivation of Ca^{2+} channels in presynaptic nerve endings.	❑ It is due to presynaptic facilitation by a 3rd neurone.
❑ It helps in avoiding fatigue.	❑ It helps in survival.

1. **G and F actin:** G actin is a globular protein that constitute F actin of thin filament of muscles. Whereas F actin is a double stranded alpha helical filament made up of G actin that form the backbone of thin filament.
2. **A and I band:**

A band	I band
❑ It is located in middle of each sarcomere	❑ It lies between ends of A bands of the adjacent sarcomere and includes the filaments that do not overlap the filaments.
❑ It is comprised of thick filaments i.e., myosin.	❑ It is comprised of thin filaments only.
❑ It contains M line	❑ It contains Z line.
❑ During contraction length is not altered.	❑ During contraction length is reduced.

3. **Isotonic and isometric contraction:**

Parameters	Isotonic contraction	Isometric contraction
1. *Length*	alters (decreases)	remains same
2. *Tension*	remains same	alters (increases)
3. *Example*	lifting a weight	trying to lift a weight
4. *External work*	present	absent
5. *Physiological work*	less	more
6. *Heat production*	less	more
7. Experimental Condition	after loaded	free loaded

4. **White and Red muscle:**

Parameters	White (fast) muscle	Red (slow) muscle
Diameter of muscle fiber	large	moderate
Length of muscle	long	short

Parameters	White (fast) muscle	Red (slow) muscle
Glycogen content	high	moderate
ATPase activity	high	low
Myoglobin content	less (so white)	more (so red)
Mitochondria content	less	more
Sarcoplasmic reticulum	more in number	less in number
Blood supply	less extensive	more extensive
Innervation	large and fast conducting motor neurones (So fast)	small and slow conducting motor neurone (so slow)
		[This property is known as ***'Size' principle.***]
Response	rapid	slow
Latent period	short	long
Contractile strength	powerful	less powerful
Fatiguability	easily	resistant
Function	for fine movements	for coarse and crude movements

5. **Heat rigor and rigor mortis:** Rigor mortis is the stiffness and rigidity of the muscle after death due to failure of muscles to relax because of lack of ATP. This has medicolegal importance to find out the time of death as it starts to appear after 4-5 hours and disappears in 24 hours. Whereas heat rigor is the state of rigidity of the muscles due to coagulation of muscle proteins resulted due to excessive temperature.
6. **Preload and afterload:** Vide answer of short notes question 28
7. **Duchne's and Becker's muscular dystrophy**

Duchne's muscular dystrophy	Becker's muscular dystrophy
❑ It is a type of muscular dystrophy resulted due to deletions of muscle protein dystrophin gene usually starts within first 5 years of age.	❑ It is a type of muscular dystrophy resulted due to deletions of muscle protein dystrophin gene usually seen in late childhood or early adulthood.
❑ Affected muscle are proximal and limb girdle.	❑ Affected muscle are proximal and limb girdle.
❑ It is the commonest form of muscular dystrophy.	❑ It is the rare form of muscular dystrophy.

8. **Skeletal, cardiac and smooth muscle:**

Parameters	Skeletal	Cardiac	Smooth
Location:	Attached to the bone or skeleton	Present in heart	Mostly in hollow viscera. e.g. GIT, Blood vessels, uterus etc.
Shape:	cylindrical	branched	fusiform / spindle shaped
Structure:			
(i) No. of Nucleus	Multi	Single	Single
(ii) Sarcolemma	Well defined and complete	Ill-defined and incomplete	Thin or deficient

(iii) 'T' tubule	Narrow and form 'Triad'	Large and form 'Diad'	Absent
(iv) S.R. System	Extensive	Less extensive	poorly developed
(v) Cell Junction	No gap junction and non syncitial	Intercalated disk and functional syncitial	Visceral smooth muscle - contains many gap junction Multiunit - Contains few gap junction
(vi) Striations	Present	Present	Absent
Control:	Voluntary	Involuntary	Involuntary
Electrophysiological aspects:			
RMP	–90 mv	–80 mv	–25 to –75 mv
type of AP	Spike	Plateau	Varies
Duration of AP	Small	Large	Varies
Mechanical aspect:			
Abs. refractory period	Short (1-3 m sec)	Long (180-200 m sec)	not defined
Duration of cont. period	Moderate	Long	Varies.

9. Contact junction and Diffuse junction: In multi unit smooth muscle synapse empassant come in close contact with individual cell known as contact junction, whereas in single unit smooth muscle there is a gap in between synapse empassant and sarcolema (so delay as that of NM junction of skeletal muscle). This is known as diffuse junction.

10. Fasciculation and Fibrillation potential: Fasciculation is an involuntary contraction of single motor unit resulting jerky visible twitch of a group of muscle fibers (seen in patient with chronic partial denervation). The motor unit potential that occur during fasciculation is known as fasciculation potential. On the otherhand fibrillation potential are action potential that arise spontaneously from single denervated muscle fibers.

11. Tonic and phasic smooth muscle: Smooth muscles of GI and urogenital sphincters remain mostly contracted and relax occasionally. Similarly smooth muscles in the walls of blood vessels and airways remain partially contracted. Such muscles are called as tonic smooth muscles. Whereas muscles of GI and urogenital tracts remain mostly relaxed and contract only in response to excitatory stimuli. These are phasic smooth muscles.

D. Brainstorming short answer type:

1. How blockade of NMJ can be achieved? Why it is required?

Blockade of NMJ can be done by

- inhibiting release of ACh by Botulinum toxin
- by antagonizing action of ACh on PSM by tubocurrarine (competitive inhibition) and succinyl choline (by persistent depolarizing).

Blockade of NMJ may be required to produce muscle relaxation thereby:

- helps in surgical operations providing a open field.
- reduces movements during electroconvulsive treatment of psychotic patients.

2. What is the safety factors for necessary neuromuscular transmission?

Though normally 60 quanta is released only 6 quanta is sufficient to produce neuromuscular transmission.

3. Classify the NM blockers.

- Drugs affecting ACh release: Botulinum toxin, hemicholinium etc.
- Drug inactivating ACh-E:
  - Reversible inhibitor: Neostigmine
  - Irreversible inhibitor: Organophosphate e.g. Malathione, Baygon, Nerve gas (Diisopropyl phosphofluridate)
- Drugs binding to ACh receptors:
  - Depolarizing NM blocker: Succinylcholine
  - Non depolarizing blocker: Tubocurarine, Bungarotoxin

4. What is Seddon's classification of nerve injury?

This is:

- Neuropraxia: minor nerve stretch/pressure → ischemic injury → conduction block without structural change.
- Axonotemesis: excessive stress injury to nerve → Wallerian degeneration.
- Neurotemesis: disruption of all sheaths.

5. What is synapse empassant?

The axon inervating the smooth muscle does not end at the site of innervation rather shows multiple swellings or varicosities along it's course that liberate neuotransmitters. These are called synapse empassant. These release ACh and norepinephrine.

6. Enumerate different mechanisms of EC coupling in smooth muscle.

(a) ***Electromechanical coupling***: Depolarising of sarcolemmal membrane → openning of volatage gated Ca^{++} channels → release of Ca^{++} from ECF to sarcoplasm → stimulate more release of Ca^{++} from SR (Ca^{++} induced Ca^{++} release) → binding of Ca^{++} to calmodulin → muscle contraction.

(b) ***Pharmaco mechanical coupling***: Chemical like neurotransmitters and hormones bind to sarcolemma → opening of ligand gated Ca^{++} channels → release of Ca^{++} from ECF to sarcoplasm → stimulate more release of Ca^{++} from SR (Ca^{++} induced Ca release) → binding of Ca^{++} to calmodulin → muscle contraction.

(c) ***Mechno mechanical coupling***: Stretching of muscle → opening of stretch sensitive Ca^{++} chanels → release of Ca^{++} from ECF to sarcoplasm → stimulate more release of Ca^{++} from SR (Ca^{++} induced Ca^{++} release) → binding of Ca^{++} to Calmodulin → muscle contraction.

7. Name the potential in NM transmission in smooth muscle junctional potential.

These are excitatory junctional potential (EJP) and inhibitory junctional potential (IJP).

8. Name the Automatic and Non –automatic fibers of the heart.

Automatic: Fibers of conducting systems

Non-automatic: Atrial and ventricular fibers.

9. What similarities of contraction exist in cardiac and smooth muscles?

Both shows automaticity, ephaptic conduction and also in both cases contractility is affected by hormones.

10. Enumerate the energy sources for muscle contraction.

These are:

- ATP for upto 3 secs
- Creatine phosphate for additional 5 secs
- ATP generated from glycolysis for additional upto 1 mins
- ATP (net 2 ATP) generated from glycolysis in absence of O_2 (through Cori's cycle) – additional 1min and 30 secs
- ATP (30 ATP) generated from glycolysis in presence of O_2 (through Kreb's cycle)–several hours.

11. What do you mean by recovery O_2?

After the muscle contraction it continues to take up extra O_2 which is equal to O_2 debt. This extra amount of O_2 is called as recovery O_2. This is used to—

- Replenish muscle store of ATP and phosphocreatine (fast component)
- Oxidize lactic acid (slow component).

12. What do you mean by motor unit potential (MUP)?

It is a compound potential that represents sum of individual action potential generated in those muscle fibers of the unit. The vertical line of EMG record is represented by MUP.

13. Mention the salient features of smooth muscle contraction.

These are:

- Has slower onset of smooth muscle contraction
- Lower energy requirements for contraction
- Can maintain a high tension without actively contracting (Latching)
- Has higher % age of shortening
- Can readjust it's resting length.

14. Briefly outline the cross bridge cycle in smooth muscle.

When sarcoplasmic Ca^{++} rises Ca^{++} binds to calmodulin → activation of enzyme myosin light chain kinase → phosphorylation of myosin regulatory chain proteins → acto-myosin complex formation → cross bridge cycle starts.

15. Mention the factors causing excitation and inhibition of smooth muscle.

- Multi unit smooth muscle regulated by nerves.
- Single unit smooth muscles are regulated by spontaneous excitation, ephaptic excitement, nerves, hormones, stretch and cold temperature.

E. MCQ:

1. Motor neurone have (i) long axons and long dendrites. (ii) long axons and short dendrites (iii) short axons and long dendrites (iv) short axons and short dendrites. (ii)
2. Sensory neurone have (i) long axons and short dendrites (ii) short axons and long dendrites (iii) short axons and short dendrites. (iii)
3. Nissl bodies are present except in following structure of the neurone (i) soma (ii) dendrites (iii) axon hillock (iv) none. (iii)
4. All are the examples of neuroglia except (i) microglia (ii) oligodendrocytes (iii) astrocytes (iv) Schwann cells. (iv)

5. The maximum rate of conduction of nerve impulse is in (i) Type A delta (ii) Type B (iii) Type C (iv) Type A alpha neurons. (iv)
6. The velocity of conduction of nerve impulse in Aα fiber is (i) 30-70 m/sec (ii) 70-120 m/sec (iii) 12-15 m/sec (iv) 15 m/sec. (iii)
7. The diameter of Aδ fiber is (i) 2-5 μ (ii) 6-12 μ (iii) 5-10 μ (iv) 12-20 μ. (i)
8. All or none law is not applicable in (i) single nerve fiber (ii) single muscle fiber (iii) cardiac muscle fiber (iv) none. (iii)
9. Maximum accommodation present in (i) sensory nerve fiber (ii) motor nerve fiber (iii) mixed nerve fiber (iv) all have same accommodation. (ii)
10. Retrograde degeneration occurs (i) only upto 1st node (ii) only upto the synapse (iii) only up to the 1st neurone (iv) only up to the cell body of affected neurone. (i)
11. All are the properties of synapse except (i) Bell –Megendie law (ii) Law of convergence (iii) Sub-liminal fringe (iv) Infatigability. (iv)
12. All are neuromuscular blockers except (i) Succinyl choline (ii) Botulinum toxin (iii) Neostigmine (iv) Curare. (iii)
13. All are nonpropagative except (i) EPP (ii) RMP (iii) Receptor potential (iv) Action potential. (iv)
14. All can be summated except (i) EPP (ii) RMP (iii) Receptor potential (iv) Action potential. (iv)
15. The T tubules are absent in (i) skeletal muscle (ii) smooth muscle (iii) cardiac muscle (iv) none. (iii)
16. SR system is poorly developed in (i) skeletal muscle (ii) smooth muscle (iii) cardiac muscle (iv) all. (i)
17. Relaxation of muscle is done due to activity of (i) Na^+ pump (ii) K^+ pump (iii) Ca^{++} pump (iv) Na^+–K^+ pump. (iii)
18. Seat of fatigue in intact man is (i) NM junction (ii) muscle (iii) CNS synapses (iv) all of the above. (iii)
19. In human body most muscle joint system are the type of (i) 1st class lever (ii) 2nd class liver (iii) 3rd class liver (iv) none of the above. (iii)
20. Resting O_2 utilisation /min of an young healthy person is nearly (i) 2 L (ii) 20 L (iii) 200 ml (iv) 20 ml. (iii)
21. During exercise (i) O_2 extraction from the capillaries of muscle rises (ii) recruitment of capillaries in the muscle develops (iii) both (iv) none of the above. (iii)
22. The most important cause of O_2 debt is (i) accumulation of lactic acid (ii) replenishment of ATP & CP (iii) restoration of glycogen store (iv) replacement of O_2 and myoglobin. (i)
23. Myelin sheath in peripheral nerve is formed by (i) Schwann cell (ii) Oligodendrocytes (iii) Astrocytes (iv) all of the above. (i)
24. The glial cell that constitute blood brain barrier is (i) Schwann cell (ii) Astrocytes (iii) Satelite cells (iv) Microglia. (ii)
25. The longest neurone present in our body is (i) reticulospinal tract. (ii) corticonuclear tract (iii) corticospinal tract (iv) fasciculus Gracilis. (iii)
26. The rate of regeneration of a nerve fiber is (i) 1-4 mm/day (ii) 8 mm/day (iii) 0.4 mm/day (iv) 1-4 mm/day. (ii)

Cardiovascular System

4

A. Long type:

1. Define cardiac cycle. Name the events of cardiac cycle. Enumerate the pressure changes during cardiac cycle.

The period from the end of one heart beat (contraction) to the end of the next heart contraction is called as *Cardiac cycle.*

Events of cardiac cycle: 4 major events (Fig. 4.1) take place during each cardiac cycle which are as follows:

A. Pressure changes	***B. Volume changes***
C. Production of heart sound	***D. Electrical changes (ECG)***

Pressure changes: The sequential contraction (systole) and relaxation (diastole) of the heart causes pressure changes in:

1. Atria	**2. Ventricles**
3. Aorta	**4. Pulmonary artery**

(a) Pressure changes in atria:

(i) During atrial diastole: During atrial diastole as atrial volume increases the pressure becomes very low. This results flow of blood from the great veins into the atria through superior and inferior vena cavae. Since the ventricles are also undergoing diastole at about the same time, the pressure in the ventricles is also low which results 70% of blood (flowing from great veins to atria) flow directly into ventricle.

(ii) During atrial systole: Due to the systole of atria the intra atrial pressure becomes high which results flow of remaining 30% of blood from the atria to the ventricles.

Atrial pressure changes can be recorded from external jugular vein which is directly connected to the atria. Such a record is known as ***Jugular venous pulse*** (JVP) in which following waves (Fig. 4.2) are seen:

(a) 'a' (atrial) wave: This is due to increase in intra atrial pressure during atrial systole.

(b) 'c' wave: This is again due to increase in intra atrial pressure due to bulging of tricuspid valves toward atria during ventricular systole.

(c) '*v*' wave: This is due to passive rise of pressure due to venous return.

(d) 'X' descents: This is due to fall of intra atrial pressure due to descent of the tricuspid valves.

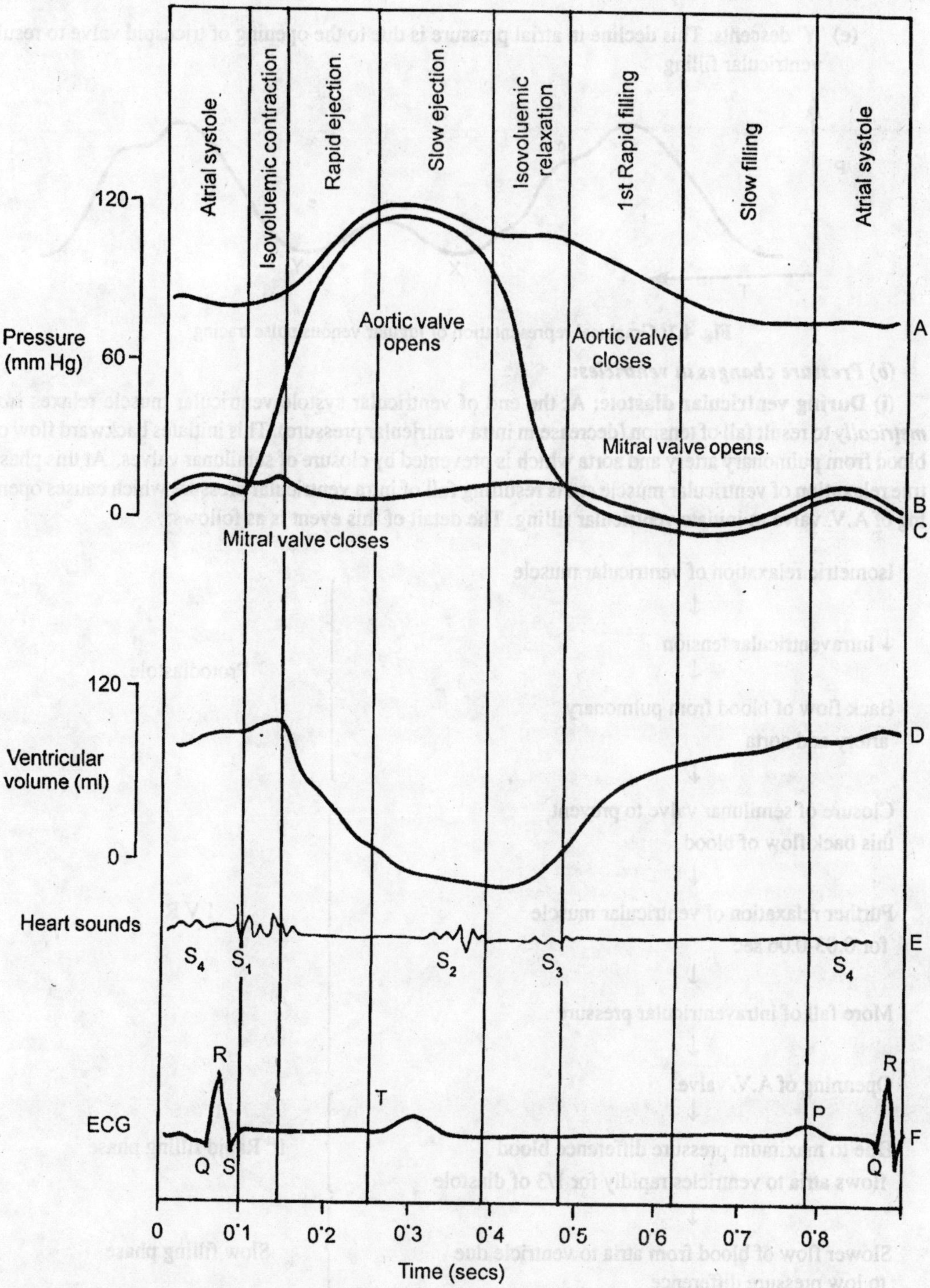

Fig. 4.1: Graphical representation of different events of cardiac cycle. (*A = Aortic pressure changes, B = Atrial pressure changes, C = Ventricular pressure changes, D = Intraventricular volume changes, E = Phono cardiogram, F = Normal ECG)*

(e) 'Y' descents: This decline in atrial pressure is due to the opening of tricuspid valve to result ventricular filling.

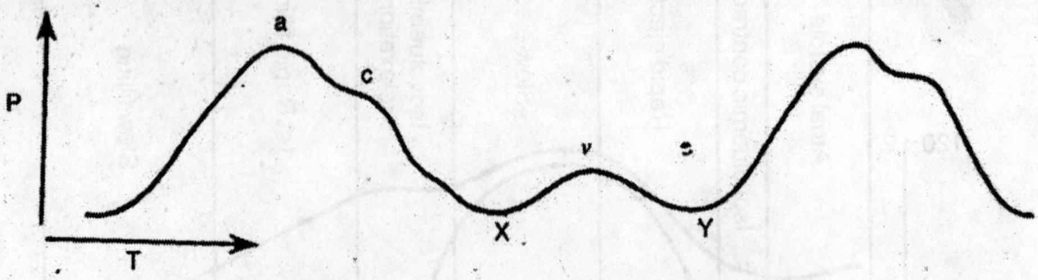

Fig. 4.2: Graphical representation of jugular venous pulse tracing

***(b) Pressure changes in ventricles*:**

(i) During ventricular diastole: At the end of ventricular systole ventricular muscle relaxes *isometrically* to result fall of tension (decrease in intra ventricular pressure). This initiates backward flow of blood from pulmonary artery and aorta which is prevented by closure of semilunar valves. At this phase true relaxation of ventricular muscle starts resulting fall of intra ventricular pressure which causes opening of A.V. valve to initiate ventricular filling. The detail of this event is as follows:

Event	Phase
Isometric relaxation of ventricular muscle ↓ ↓ Intraventricular tension ↓ Back flow of blood from pulmonary artery and aorta ↓	Protodiastole
Closure of semilunar valve to prevent this back flow of blood ↓ Further relaxation of ventricular muscle for 0.03-0.06 sec ↓ More fall of intraventricular pressure ↓ Openning of A.V. valve ↓	I V R
Due to maximum pressure difference blood flows atria to ventricles rapidly for 1/3 of diastole ↓	1st Rapid filling phase
Slower flow of blood from atria to ventricle due to low pressure difference ↓	Slow filling phase
Again rapid flow of blood from atria to ventricles due to increased pressure gradient during atrial systole	Last rapid filling phase

(ii) During ventricular systole: Immediately after ventricular diastole ventricular muscle undergoes *isometric* contraction. This result abrupt rise of ventricular pressure causing the closure of A-V valves. This initiates ventricular contraction with shortening of it's length to build up sufficient intra ventricular pressure to open the semilunar valves. Opening of these valves ultimately initiate ejection of blood into aorta and pulmonary artery. The detail of these sequence is described by the following flow chart:

Isometric contraction of ventricular muscle

↓

↑ Intraventricular tension

↓

Closure of A-V valve to prevent back flow of blood to atria from ventricles

↓

Further continuation of ventricular contraction (with muscle shortening) for 0.02 to 0.03 sec

— I V C Period

↓

More rise of intraventricular pressure

↓

Opening of semilunar valves

↓

Rapid ejection of blood for 1/3 rd of ejection phase due to more pressure gradient

— Rapid ejection

↓

Slow ejection during last 2/3rd of ejection phase due to fall of pressure difference

— Slow ejection

Maximum and Minimum pressure in chambers of heart		
Chamber	**Peak pressure in systole**	**Min. pressure in diastole**
Left ventricle	120 mm Hg	5-12 mm Hg
Right ventricle	25 mm Hg	2-6 mm Hg
Left atrium	15 mm Hg	5-8 mm Hg
Right atrium	6 mm Hg	1-5 mm Hg
Aorta	120 mm Hg	80 mm Hg
Pulmonary artery	25 mm Hg	5-12 mm Hg

(c) Pressure Changes in aorta*:** During ventricular systole the entry of blood into aorta causes stretching of wall of aorta and thus pressure in the aorta rises to a maximum of 120 mm Hg. At the end of systole as the intraventricular pressure drops there is a backward flow of blood from aorta towards ventricle which is prevented by closure of aortic valve. In the aortic pressure curve it is indicated by ***incisura. Even after closure of aorta the pressure in the aorta is maintained by the elastic stretch of wall of aorta which ultimately falls to minimum 80 mm Hg during the diastole of the ventricle because of the slow passing of stored blood from aorta to peripheral vessels i.e. arteries.

Aortic pressure changes can be studied from any of the peripheral arteries like, radial, carotid etc. which is known as ***arterial pulse.*** This arterial pulse (Fig. 4.3) consists of following waves:

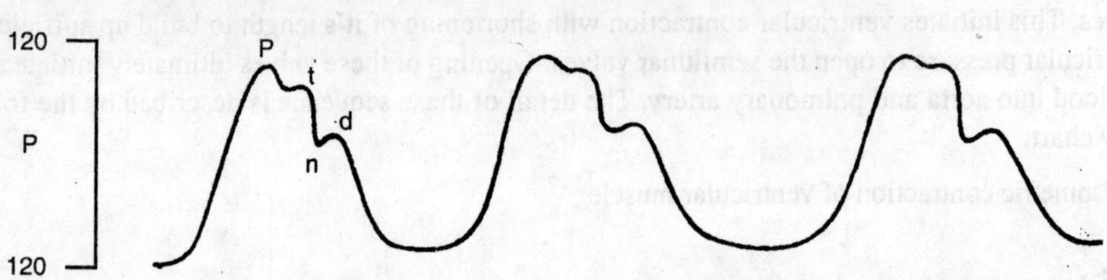

Fig. 4.3: Graphical records showing arterial pulse

- **Percussion (P) wave**: It is due to ejection of blood into aorta during ventricular systole.
- **Tidal (t) wave:** This wave is occassionaly seen which is due to elastic recoil of wall of aorta.
- **Dicortic (d) wave:** This is due to fall of pressure due to passage of blood to peripheral vessels during ventricular diastole after closure of aortic valve as indicated by a notch known as ***dicortic notch (n).***

(d) Pressure changes in pulmonary artery: The pressure changes in the pulmonary artery is similar to that in aorta though the pressure changes is approximately 1/6th of the pressure changes in aorta.

2. What is phonocardiogram? Describe the origin, cause and features of different heart sounds. What do you mean by auscultatory areas?

During each cardiac cycle the valves of the heart open and close. Opening of the valves is a slow process and does not produce any sound normally but the closure of the sound is a sudden process and causes vibration which results production of sounds. These sounds **recorded** graphically with the help of phonocardiograph are known as ***phonocardiogram***.

(a) Type of heart sound: There are 4 heart sounds – **1st** sound **(S_1)**, **2nd** sound **(S_2)**, **3rd** sound **(S_3)** and **4th** sound **(S_4)**. Out of which 1st two are easily heard by auscultation known as ***audible sound.*** Other two are not easily auscultated but can be recorded by means of phonocardiograph thus known as ***recorded sound.***

(b) Origin of different heart sounds:

- First heart sound: During closure of A–V (mitral and tricuspid) valves at the beginning of ventricular systole.
- 2nd heart sound: During closure of semilunar valves at the beginning of ventricular diastole.
- 3rd heart sound: During 1st rapid filling phase of ventricular diastole.
- 4th heart sound: During last rapid filling phase of ventricular diastole (atrial systole).

(c) Causes of different heart sounds:

S_1:

- Vibrations of A.V. valve due to it's closure at the beginning of ventricular-systole.
- Vibrations of blood surrounding the A-V valves.
- Vibrations of walls of heart.
- Vibrations of major blood vessels around the heart.

S_2:

- Vibrations of semilunar valve due to it's closure at the beginning of ventricular diastole.
- Vibrations of blood surrounding the semilunar valves.

- Vibrations of walls of heart.
- Vibrations of major blood vessels.

S_3: Vibrations of valves, blood, wall of heart and major blood vessels due to Ist rapid filling of blood into ventricles.

S_4: Vibrations of valves, blood, wall of heart and major blood vessels due to last rapid filling of blood into ventricles during atrial systole/last rapid filling phase of ventricular diastole.

(d) Characteristics of heart sound:

- S_1: It is:
  - Low pitched.
  - Long duration (0.14-0.17 sec) and soft in quality.
  - Represented by written word "LUBB".
  - Less frequency (25-45 Hz).
  - Best heard in mitral area and coincides with 'R' wave of ECG.
- S_2: It is:
  - High pitched and short duration (0.1-0.14 sec).
  - Loud and sharp in quality.
  - Represented by written word "DUB".
  - More frequency (50 Hz).
  - Best heart in aortic and pulmonary area.
  - Coincides with incisura of aortic pressure curve and end of 'T' wave in ECG.
- S_3: It is:
  - Not easily and normally audible.
  - "Recorded" sound.
  - So very soft in quality with short duration (0.1 sec).
  - Coincides with rapid filling phase of ventricular diastole.
  - Heard in children with thin chest wall and in patients with left ventricular failure, thyrotoxicosis etc.
- S_4: It is:
  - Normally not audible.
  - Recorded" sound.
  - Sometimes physiological in the elderly people.
  - Most common in hypertensive patient, aortic stenosis, hypertrophic cardiomopathy etc.

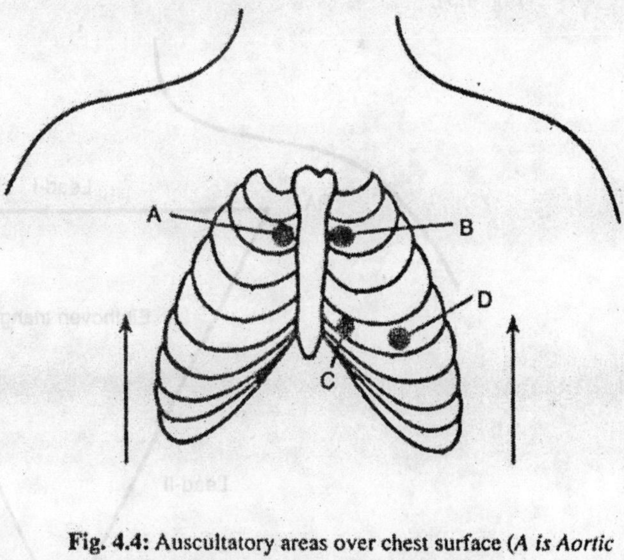

Fig. 4.4: Auscultatory areas over chest surface (*A is Aortic area, B is Pulmonary area, C is Bicuspid area and D is Tricuspid area*)

Auscultatory area:

- Though the heart sounds can be heard by placing directly over the chest wall in the neighbourhood of heart but the particular heart sounds are best heard over a particular area of the chest surface which are known as Auscultatory areas (Fig. 4.4).

- The auscultatory areas of different types of heart sounds are
  - In 2nd intercostal space at right sternal border the aortic component of 2nd heart sound is best heard.
  - In 2nd intercostal space at left sternal border the pulmonary component of 2nd heart sound is best heard.
  - In 5th intercostal space about 9 cm away from the midsternal line (Apex beat area) the mitral valve component (Mitral area) of 1st heart sound is best heard.
  - In the left of the lower end of sternum the tricuspid- valve component (Tricuspid area) of 1st heart sound is best heard.

3. Define electrocardiogram. Describe the normal ECG. Add a note on ECG leads.

Definition: It is the graphical record of electrical changes of heart during each cardiac cycle. The machine used to obtain the record i.e. electrocardiogram is known as electrocardiograph and the procedure is known as electrocardiography.

Electrical impulse generated by the heart can be recorded by placing suitable electrodes on the surface of the skin and connecting them to the electrocardiograph through the electrical wires. These electrodes along with the electrical wires connecting electrode to the machine is known as **electrocardiographic leads.**

***Lead*:** Generally two types of leads are used to record electrical potential changes of heart which are 1. Bipolar leads 2. Unipolar leads.

1. Bipolar leads: The ECG is recorded by placing two electrodes in two points of the body (Generally Limb)- one as a **'–' terminal** and another as a **'+' terminal,** then it is known as bipolar lead. It is also known as ***Standard Limb lead*** which are of 3 types as follows:

i. **Lead I:** Here one electrode is placed in right arm and another is at left arm. Negative terminal of the electrocardiograph is connected to the right and positive terminal is connected to the left arm (Fig. 4.5).

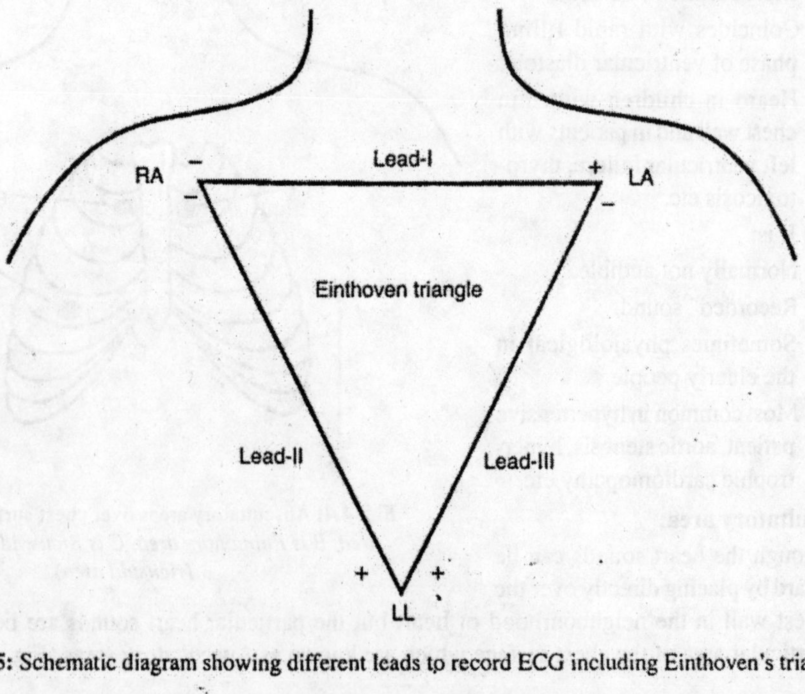

Fig. 4.5: Schematic diagram showing different leads to record ECG including Einthoven's triangle

ii. **Lead II:** Here negative terminal is connected to the electrode placed in right arm and positive terminal is connected to the electrode placed in left leg (Fig. 4.5).

iii. **Lead III:** Here negative terminal of the machine is connected to the left arm and positive terminal to the left leg (Fig. 4.5).

These leads are connected in such a way that for practical purposes they form an equilateral triangle center of which contains heart. This equilateral triangle is called ***Einthoven's triangle.***

2. Unipolar Leads:

- In this type of leads one electrode is kept at zero potential by connecting the electrodes (all three or any two) on right arm, left arm and left leg to a **central terminus** of the machine through a resistance. Thus this electrode does not pick electrical potential. That is why it is known as **indifferent electrode**. Other electrode (any one Limb lead or extra lead) is functional or active which is known as **exploring lead.**
- It is of 2 types: (i) Augmented Unipolar Limb Lead and (ii) Chest Leads.

(i) *Augmented unipolar limb lead*:

- Here any two of the limbs are connected through the resistance to the '–' terminal and 3rd one is connected to the '+' terminal of the electrocardiograph.
- It is of 3 types:
  - aVR: Right arm is '+' terminal and Left arm + Left Leg is at '–' terminal
  - aVL: Left arm is at '+' terminal and Right Arm and Left Leg is at '+' terminal
  - aVF: Left Leg is at '+' terminal and Left arm and Right arm is at '–' terminal.

(ii) *Chest (Precordial) Leads*:

- 3 limb leads are connected to central terminus through a resistance (5000 ohm).and attached to the '–' terminal and exploring electrode is placed on different surface of chest which is connected to the '+' terminal.
- As per the location of this exploring electrode it is of 6 types as follows:
  - V_1-In 4th intercostal space at right side of the sternum.
  - V_2-In 4th intercostal space at left side of the sternum.
  - V_3-In between V_2 and V_4.
  - V_4-In 5th left intercostal space and it's junction with mid clavicular line.
  - V_5-In 5th left intercostal space and it's junction with anterior axillary line.
  - V_6-In 5th left intercostal space and it's junction with mid axillary line.

Normal ECG curve: Normal ECG (Fig. 4.6) contains different waves like P wave, QRS complex, T wave and sometimes U wave. The features of different waves of normal ECG is as follows:

i. ***P wave:***

- It is '+' wave in Limb Lead-II.
- It is due to atrial depolarization.
- It represents spread of impulse from SA node to atrial muscles.
- It's normal duration is 0.1 Sec and voltage 0.5 mv.
- It occurs just before atrial systole.
- Prominent P wave indicates atrial hypertrophy and during atrial fibrillation 'P' wave is replaced by fine irregular oscillations known as **'F' wave.**

ii. ***QRS Complex:***

- It extends from beginning of Q to end of S wave.

- It is due to ventricular depolarization.
- It is a measure of intraventricular conduction time.
- It completes just before opening of semilunar valve.
- It's normal duration is 0.08-0.12 sec.

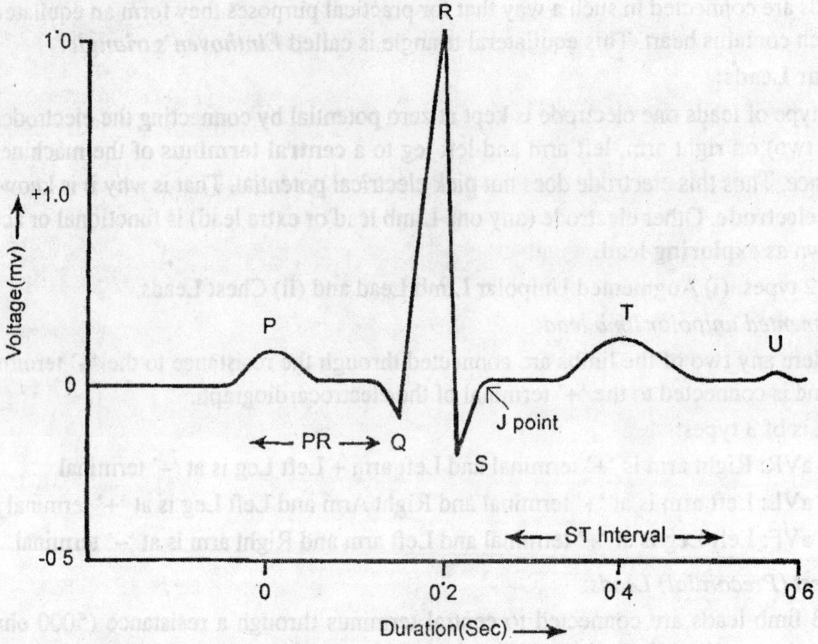

Fig. 4.6: Normal ECG

iii. ***T wave***:

- It represents ventricular repolarisation.
- End of T wave coincides with closure of semilunar valve.
- It's normal duration is 0.27 sec. and voltage is 0.5 mv.
- T wave is normally upright in Lead I and II. Inversion of T wave indicates myocardial ischaemia, bundle branch block and even ventricular hypertrophy.

iv. ***PR interval***:

- It is from the onset of P wave to the onset of Q/R wave.
- It represents atrial depolarisation and conduction of impulse to Bundle of His.
- It's normal duration varies from 0.12 to 0.2 sec.
- It's duration is increased during 1st and 2nd degree heart block.

v. ***QT interval***:

- It is measured from beginning of Q wave to the end of T wave.
- It represents ventricular depolarisation along with ventricular repolarisation.
- Normal duration is 0.35-0.42 sec.
- It indicates total systolic time of ventricles.

vi. ***ST interval***:

- It is from end of S wave to end of T wave.
- It represents ventricular repolarisation.
- Normal duration 0.32 sec.

vii. ***RR interval:***

- It is from the peak of one R wave to the peak of consecutive R wave.
- It varies with heart rate.
- It's normal value is 0.83 sec if the heart rate is 72 beats / min.

viii. ***ST segment:***

- It is the isoelectric line from end of S wave to beginning of T wave.
- It's normal duration is 0.04 to 0.08 sec.
- It's position is important to diagnose different cardiac abnormalities e.g. depression of ST segment > 2m below the isoelectric line indicates angina pectoris whereas elevation of ST segment >2 mm above the isoelectric line indicates the myocardial infarction (acute).

ix. ***J Point:*** The end point of QRS where the electrical potential is zero is known as 'J' point.

4. Define cardiac output. Give the normal value and variations of cardiac output. Explain the factors regulating cardiac output.

Definition: The amount of blood ejected by each ventricle in the circulation per minute is called ***minute volume*** or ***cardiac output.***

Normal Value: 5-6 lit/min

Variations:

Physiological variation:

a. **Physiological increase:** During following physiological conditions there is increase in C.O:

- *Emotional conditions* like anxiety, excitement, stress.
- *Muscular exercise*—rises upto 25-35 lit/min.
- *After meal*—After 1 hr. of meal there is 30% - 40% rise of cardiac output and declines after 3 hr.
- *Pregnancy*
- *High environmental temperature*
- *High PO_2 in the inspired air*
- *Low PCO_2 in the inspired air*

b. **Physiological decrease:** During following physiological conditions there is fall of C.O:

- *Sitting* or *standing from lying posture.*
- *Depression.*
- *It is less in elderly people due to decrease in heart rate and stroke volume.*
- *It is also less in female.*

Pathological variations:

a. Pathological increase: During hypertension

b. Pathological decrease: During hemorrhage, myocardial infarction, acidosis etc.

Factors influencing cardiac output: Cardiac output is primarily determined by two factors - Stroke volume and Heart rate (C.O = SV × HR). Different factors in turn either affect SV or / and HR to influence the cardiac output. These factors are:

(A) ***Stroke volume:*** Stroke volume is directly related with C.O (SV α HR) which is influenced by following factors:

(a) ***Contractility of the heart*** —This is directly related with SV and thus CO. Contractility of the heart is in turn dependent on:

(i) *End diastolic fiber length* (EDFL): It is the resting length of ventricular muscle at the end of diastole. Increase in EDFL increases the contractility i.e. the force of contraction of heart within physiological limit. This is known as **Frank starling's law of heart.** This is again directly related with venous return to the heart.

(ii) *Preload*: Preload is the degree to which the myocardium is stretched before it contracts. It is directly proportional to C.O. i.e. increase in preload increases the cardiac output.

(iii) *After load*: After load is the resistance against which blood is expelled and it decreases the cardiac output i.e. inversely related with C.O.

(iv) *ANS*: Both sympathetic and parasympathetic nervous system influence the contractility of the heart to affect stroke volume and thus C.O.

- Sympathetic stimulation → Increases C.O.
- Parasympathetic stimulation → Decreases C.O.

(b) ***Venous return (VR)***: Venous return to the heart is directly related with EDFL which in turn increases force of contraction of heart to increase C.O. Venous return in turn depends on:

(i) *Cardiac pump*—pumping activity of the heart regulates the venous return to the heart specially during exercise.

(ii) *Respiratory pump*—During inspiration–

- Intra thoracic pressure decreases → fall of pressure over and around large veins and arteries.
- Descent of diaphragm → increases of intra abdominal pressure → squeezing of blood out of abdomen.

Both these factors increases VR and similarly during expiration VR is decreased due to opposite event. This is known as **respiratory pump** which is one of the major factor to increase C.O. during exercise.

(iii) *Muscle pump*: During rhythmical contraction of skeletal muscle → squeezing of veins in the muscles → increase in venous return to the heart. Whereas during relaxation of skeletal muscle due to opposite fact venous return decreases. This factor also contributes during exercise.

(iv) *Blood volume*: Rise in blood volume increases venous return and thus cardiac output.

(c) ***Left ventricular size***: Increase in left ventricular size is directly related with force of contraction of heart and thus SV is increased to increase cardiac output.

(B) ***Heart rate***: Heart rate is also directly related with cardiac output (HR α C.O.). The factors which influence heart rate are: Sino-aortic reflex, Cardio-acceleratory reflex, Hypoxia, CO_2 excess, Adrenaline and thyroxin hormones.

5. What is cardiac index? Give an account of regulation of cardiac output.

Cardiac index: It is the amount of blood pumped out by each ventricle in each minute per sq. meter of body surface area. Normal value: 3.1 lit/sqm/min

Regulation / Control of cardiac output:

C.O is regulated by regulating heart rate which is known as **Extrinsic regulation** where as regulation of CO by controling stroke volume is known as **Intrinsic regulation.**

A. Extrinsic Regulation (Control through heart rate): Medullary vasomotor center by influencing ANS can control heart rate and thus cardiac output. This process involves mainly the baroreceptors and partly chemoreceptors as illustrated by flow chart FC 4A.

B. Intrinsic regulation: The normal heart that is not stimulated by ANS, can pump out maximum 13-15 lit blood per minute which is known as **permissive level of heart.** Upto this permissive level of heart cardiac output is controlled by two mechanism. In one mechanism end diastolic fiber length is

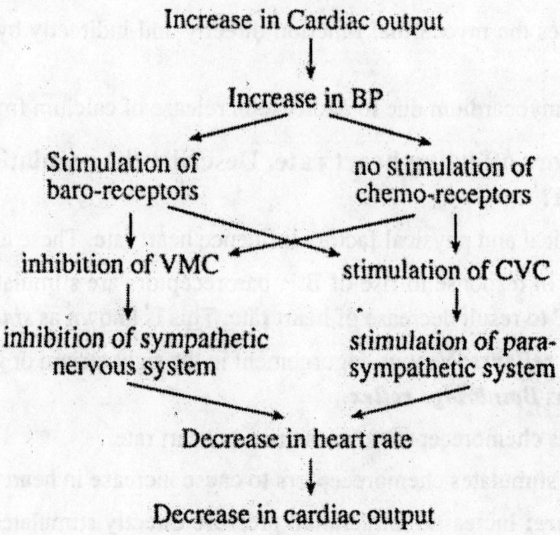

FC 4A: Extrinsic regulation of cardiac output

altered to alter stroke volume which is known as ***Heterometric regulation***. In another mechanism EDFL is not altered to alter the cardiac output which is known as ***Homometric regulation***.

(a) **Heterometric regulation:** This type of regulation of stroke volume and thereby cardiac output is under the influence of EDFL of ventricular muscle which is directly related with force of contraction within physiological limit (Frank Starling's Law). **Thus any factor which increases venous return (VR) → ↑ End diastolic volume → ↑ End diastolic fiber length → ↑ force of contraction → ↑ stroke volume → ↑ Cardiac output.**

(b) **Homometric regulation:** In this mechanism myocardial contractility changes without any change of EDFL. This is done by stimulating sympathetic or inhibiting parasympathetic nerves or by releasing catecholamines. The details of this mechanism is as follows:

- Stimulation of sympathetic nerves → ↑ myocardial contractility → ↑ stroke volume → ↑ cardiac output.
- Whereas stimulation of parasympathetic nerves → ↓ myocardial contractility → ↓ stroke volume → ↓ cardiac output.

Besides this CO can also be controlled by humoral mechanisms as follows which affect both the heart rate and stroke volume:

(a) ***Hormonal mechanisms***: It is mainly controlled by—

- ❑ catecholamines through increasing stroke volume and heart rate both.
- ❑ thyroid hormones by increasing myosin ATPase activity, number of beta receptors, protein synthesis in the myocardial cells etc.
- ❑ insulin by increasing force of contraction of heart.
- ❑ GH by influencing myocardial contractility.

(b) Chemical regulation: It is by—

- ❑ hypoxia decreases CO by directly suppressing myocardial contractility and by stimulating peripheral chemoreceptors.

- CO_2 excess depresses the myocardial function directly and indirectly by stimulating peripheral chemoreceptors.
- Acidosis depresses myocardium due to decrease in release of calcium from SR.

6. Enumerate the factors affecting heart rate. Describe the regulation of the heart rate. What is tachycardia?

Different neural, chemical and physical factors influence heart rate. These are:

A. ***Sino-aortic reflex*:** In response to rise of B.P. baroreceptors are stimulated which in turn sends impulse to VMC and CVC to result decrease of heart rate. This is known as ***sino-aortic reflex***.

B. ***Cardioacceleratory reflexes*:** Venous engorgement in the right atrium or great veins increases the heart rate. This is known as ***Bainbridge reflex***.

C. ***Hypoxia*:** Stimulates chemoreceptor to cause rise in heart rate.

D. ***CO_2 excess*:** It also stimulates chemoreceptors to cause increase in heart rate.

E. ***Intracranial pressure*:** Increased intracranial pressure directly stimulates the vagus nerve to reduce heart rate.

F. ***Adrenaline*:** Directly it increases the HR but reflexly it decreases heart rate due to the initiation of sino aortic reflex.

G. ***Thyroxin*:** Thyroxin increases heart rate by:

- stimulating sympathetic nerves.
- increasing BMR of the body.
- increasing metabolic rate of the SA Node.

Control of heart rate:

1. ***Neural control*:** Heart rate is regulated by medullary cardiovascular centers (VMC and CVC) through influencing ANS. Parasympathetic nerve inhibits and sympathetic nerve stimulates the heart rate though normally parasympathetic control of SA node dominates over the sympathetic control. Therefore the basal (normal) heart rate is less than the intrinsic heart rate i.e. heart rate in denervated heart. In response to any change of heart rate due to any factor the medullary centers are activated or inactivated by baroreceptors and chemoreceptors which in turn stimulate or inhibit sympathetic and parasympathetic nerves to control the heart rate. The detail mechanism is illustrated with the following flow chart (next page). Just opposite effect occurs when heart rate is reduced.

2. ***Hormonal control*:** Catecholamines and thyroid hormones increases the heart rate.

3. ***Chemical control*:** Hypoxia, CO_2 excess, acidosis decreases heart rate by stimulating peripheral chemoreceptors.

7. Define blood pressure. Enumerate the factors affecting BP. Describe the short term mechanism of regulation of B.P.

The blood pressure is defined as the lateral pressure exerted by the moving column of blood on the unit area of blood vessels.

Factors controlling BP: BP is the product of cardiac output and peripheral resistance i.e.

$$BP = CO \times PR$$

$$= SV \times HR \times PR$$

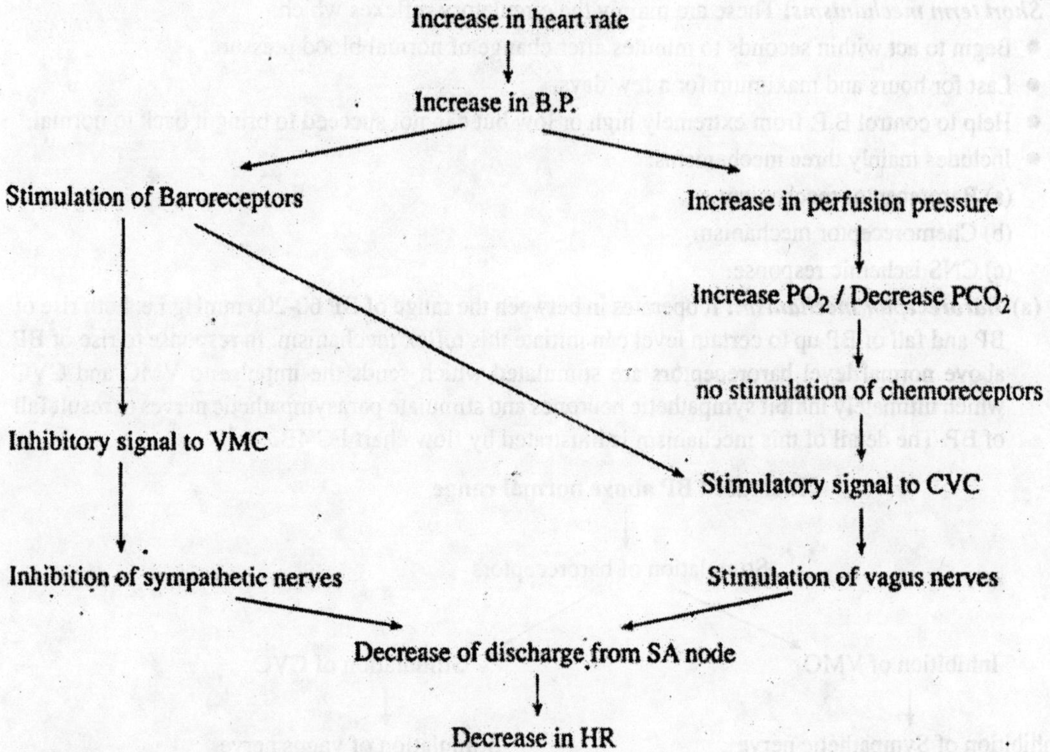

Thus BP is affected directly by stroke volume (SV), heart rate (HR) and peripheral resistance (PR).

***(A) Stroke volume*:**

- It is directly related with systolic blood pressure i.e. rise of SV means rise of SP. The factors which affect stroke volume and thus affect BP are:
  - contractility of heart which inturn dependent on EDFL (directly), preload (directly), after load (inversely) and ANS.
  - venous return directly
  - left ventricular size directly

***(B) Heart rate*:** It is directly related with generally DP though rise of HR up to certain extent also increases the SP.

***(C) Peripheral resistance*:** PR is directly related with DP i.e. increase in PR indicates rise of DP. Peripheral resistance in turn dependent on following factors:

- Velocity of blood → directly related with PR
- Viscosity of blood → directly related with PR
- Total amount of blood in arterial system → directly related with PR
- Elasticity of blood vessels → inversely related
- Length of the blood vessels → inversely related
- Diameter of the blood vessel-inversely related.

Short term regulation of BP: In response to any change in blood pressure beyond normal limit readjustment of the regulatory mechanism takes place to keep the blood pressure within normal range. This regulation is done by following mechanisms:

Short term mechanisms: These are mainly the circulatory reflexes which:

- Begin to act within seconds to minutes after change of normal blood pressure.
- Last for hours and maximum for a few days.
- Help to control B.P. from extremely high or low but can not succeed to bring it back to normal.
- Includes mainly three mechanisms:
  (a) Baroreceptor mechanism
  (b) Chemoreceptor mechanism
  (c) CNS ischemic response.

(a) ***Baroreceptor mechanism***: It operates in between the range of BP 60-200 mmHg i.e. both rise of BP and fall of BP up to certain level can initiate this reflex mechanism. In response to rise of BP above normal level baroreceptors are stimulated which sends the impulse to VMC and CVC which ultimately inhibit sympathetic neurones and stimulate parasympathetic nerves to result fall of BP. The detail of this mechanism is illustrated by flow chart FC 4B.

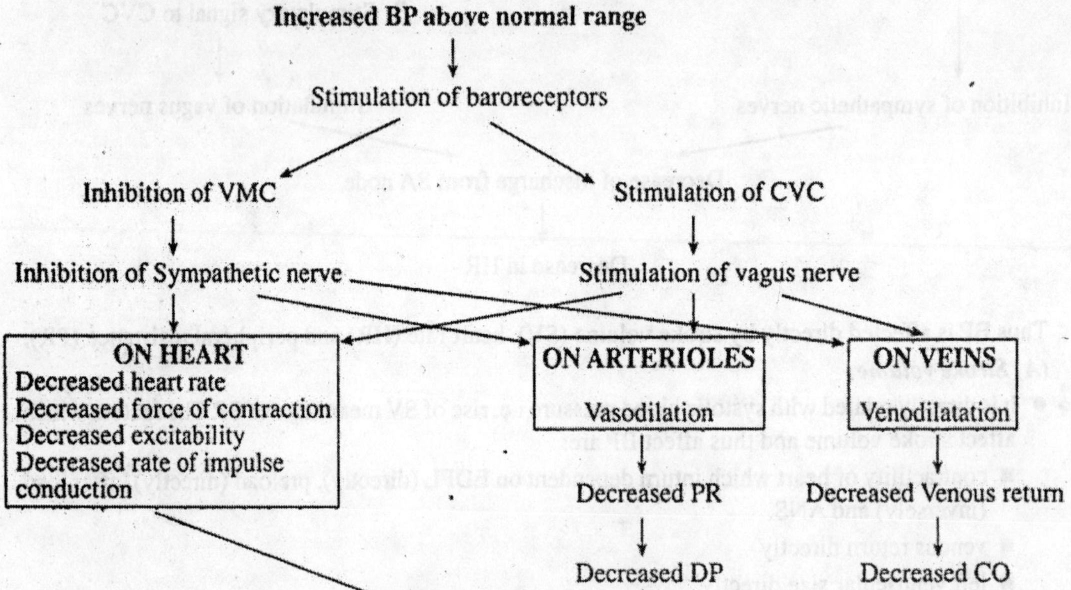

FC 4B: Flow chart showing Baroreceptor mechanism of Short term regulation of BP

In response to fall of blood pressure just opposite events take place to increase the blood pressure towards normal level.

(b) ***Chemoreceptor mechanism***: It is initiated when BP falls below 80 mm of Hg. So when BP falls chemoreceptors are stimulated which ultimately sends stimulatory signal to VMC and inhibitory signal to CVC to result stimulation of sympathetic nerves and inhibition of parasympathetic neurones (vagus nerve) and thus BP increases towards normal level. The detail of this mechanism is illustrated in Fig. FC 4C.

(c) ***CNS ischemic response***: This mechanism is the last ditch of effort to maintain the normal perfusion of brain tissue to prevent the death of the person in case of severe fall of BP. It acts in between 15-50 mmHg of mean blood pressure. The detail of the sequence of events is as follows:

Fall of BP below 50 mm of Hg → ischaemia of CNS → accumulation of CO_2 in VMC → stimulation of pressor area of VMC → strong stimulation of sympathetic neurons → ↑ HR, ↑ CO, ↑ PR → ↑ Blood pressure.

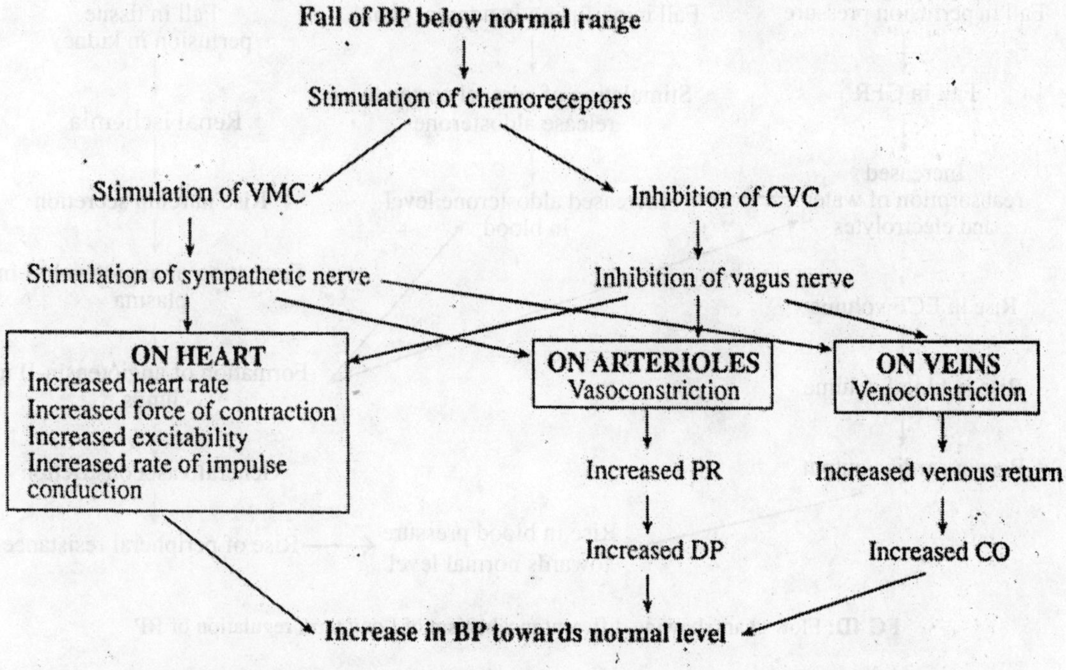

FC 4C: Flow chart showing chemoreceptor mechanism of short term regulation of BP

Tachycardia: Rise in heart rate beyond 90 beats per min is known as tachycardia.

8. Discuss the long term regulation of B. P. What is it's importance? Add a note on hypertension.

Long term mechanism: These are the most important mechanism which has got the ability to bring back the BP to normal level in response to any alteration of BP. These mechanisms:

- get initiate slowly i.e. it takes 3-10 days to activate these mechanisms fully.
- last over a period of days to years.
- are of 5 types:

(a) ***Renal fluid mechanism (Autoregulation of BP)***: In response to any alteration of BP kidney has got the ability to regulate GFR to control absorption of electrolytes and water. This in turn regulate the blood volume to control the blood pressure. This mechanism is also known as **Renal regulation of BP.**

(b) ***Renin-angiotensin mechanism***: As per this mechanism the blood pressure is regulated by regulating the secretion of an enzyme **renin** from JGA of kidney. This renin in turn activates plasma angiotensinogen to angiotensin I and then angiotensin-II which is a potent vasoconstrictor. Thus initiating vasoconstriction or vasodilatation BP is controlled.

(c) ***Renin-angiotensin aldosterone mechanism***: Angiotensin – II, not only by causing vasoconstriction but also by stimulating the release of aldosterone hormone from adrenal cortex controls the BP.

The detail of all these mechanisms are illustratef by flow chart FC 4D.

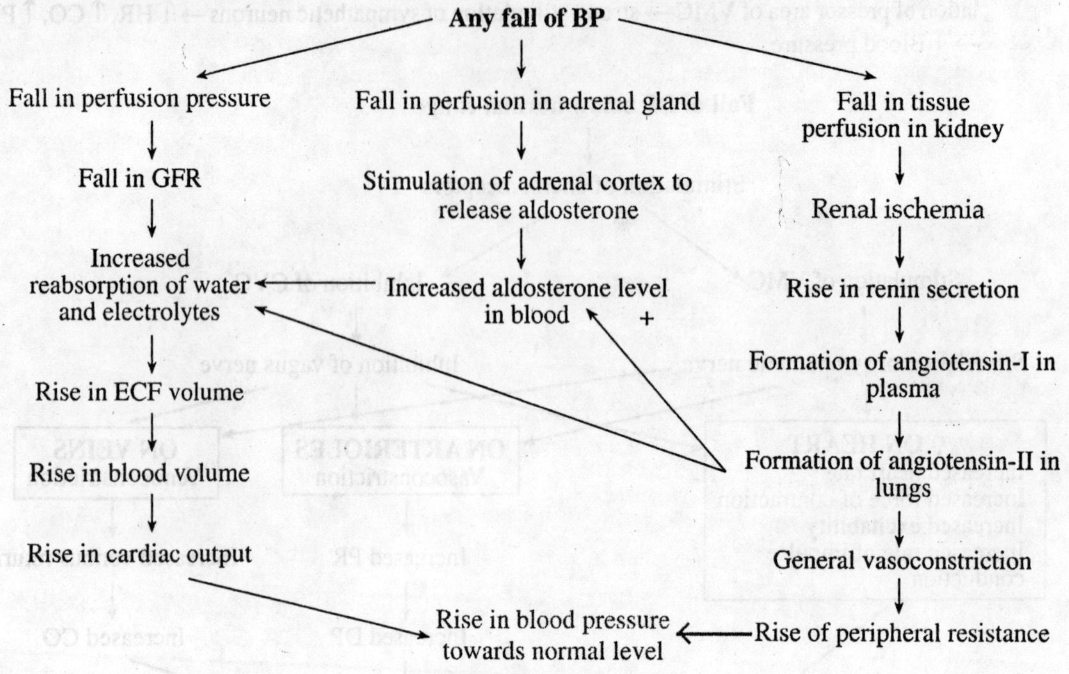

FC 4D: Flow chart showing different mechanism of Long term regulation of BP

(d) ***Osmoreceptor ADH mechanism***: Any fall of BP due to hypovolemia results rise in plasma osmolarity → stimulation of osmoreceptors present in hypothalamus → stimulate (1) thirst center of hypothalamus which inturn increases water intake (2) posterior pituitary to secrete the hormone ADH which increases water reabsorption by collecting duct → both of those factors correct the blood volume and thereby BP.

(e) ***Atrial natriuretic peptide mechanism***: Any rise of BP due to rise of plasma volume initiates this mechanism in which reabsorption of Na^+ and water (indirectly under osmotic effect) are controlled by the kidney and thus BP is controlled. The detail mechanism is as follows: Rise in plasma volume → increase in venous return → stimulation of stretch receptors present in atria due to overstretching → atrial natriuretic peptide secretion by the atrial cells → circulated through the blood and acts on renal tubules → decreases the absorption of Na^+ and water (indirectly) by the kidnbey → more passing out of electrolytes and water → decrease in plasma volume → decrease in BP.

Hypertension

- **Definition:** Sustained rise of blood pressure beyond the normal range is known as Hypertension i.e. the chronic rise of either SP above 140 mmHg or DP above 90 mmHg or both is termed as Hypertension. However, DP is a more significant parameter to be considered as marker of hypertension as it remains comparatively constant and does not vary with different conditions.
- ***Types***: It is of two types—

  A. *Primary or Essential hypertension*: The hypertension of unknown origin is known as Primary or Essential hypertension.

  B. *Secondary hypertension*: Hypertension of known origin is termed as Secondary hypertension e.g. Renal hypertension.

- ***Causes:***

Primary hypertension: Though the exact cause of this type of hypertension is not known, it is mainly due to hereditary factors and also very common to person with Type-A personalities and in some young men and is characterised by systolic hypertension, tachycardia and palpitations all indicators of sympathetic over stimulation. It may be transient phenomenon but all such patients ultimately develop increased peripheral resistance and therefore elevation of systolic and diastolic blood pressure.

Secondary hypertension:

- Renal diseases like nephritis, cystic renal disease etc.
- Thyrotoxicosis
- Pheochromocytoma i.e. adrenal medulla tumour
- Adrenal cortex tumour
- Severe polycythemia

9. Give the normal value of coronary blood flow. Mention the peculiarities of coronary circulation. Enumerate the factors affecting coronary blood flow.

Normal value of coronary blood flow:

During resting condition the coronary blood flow is **225 ml/min** i.e. **4-5%** of total cardiac output.

Peculiarities or features of coronary circulation:

A. Variation in dominance: There is a variation in dominance regarding the blood supply to myocardium. In man in majority of the cases (50%) the blood supply through right coronary artery predominates whereas in 20% individuals left artery predominates and in 30% cases there is a balanced supply through both the vessels.

B. Phasic changes in blood flow: Generally the blood supply to all the tissue is more during systole and less during diastole. This is reverse in case of heart muscle i.e. during systole the blood flow to the ventricular muscle falls to a very low level because of compression of small branches of coronary arteries by the contractile muscle. Whereas during diastole the cardiac muscle relaxes resulting dilatation of coronary arteries leading more blood flow (Fig. 4.7).

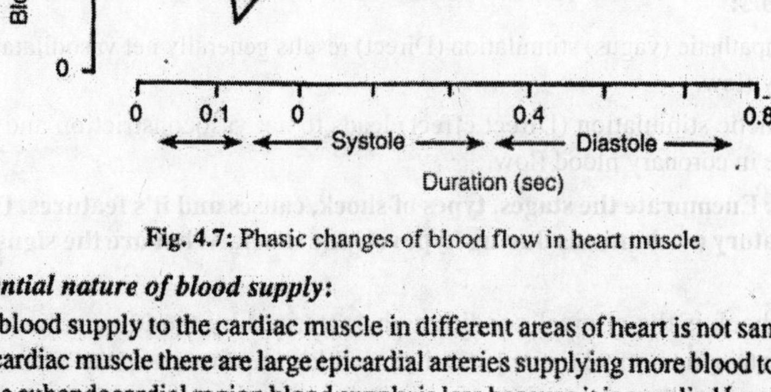

Fig. 4.7: Phasic changes of blood flow in heart muscle

C. Differential nature of blood supply:

- The blood supply to the cardiac muscle in different areas of heart is not same. On the surface of the cardiac muscle there are large epicardial arteries supplying more blood to those areas whereas in the subendocardial region blood supply is less because it is supplied by smaller intramuscular arteries and plexus of subendocardial artery the diameter of which are less. This blood supply to the subendocardial plexus is further reduced during systole. Therefore the **subendocardial region is more prone to mycardial infarction.**

- Again as the left ventrticular thickness is much more than that of right ventricle the occlusion is more severe in left ventricle. For this region **LV subendocardial region is more prone to MI.**

D. Presence of anastomotic channels: In the normal heart there are some collaterals among the smaller arteries which become active under abnormal conditions like myocardial ischemia. They open up within a few seconds after the sudden occlusion of larger artery and become double in number by the end of 2nd or 3rd day and reaches to normal by one month. When atherosclerosis causes constriction of coronary arteries slowly over a period of many years, collateral vessels develop restoring normal blood and thus the patient **never experiences acute episode of cardiac dysfunction.**

E. Autoregulation: Like some other organs the heart has the capacity to regulate it's own blood flow up to a certain limit in order to maintain an almost constant blood flow to the cardiac musculature in spite of any alteration of systemic blood flow. This property is known as ***autoregulation.***

Factors affecting coronary blood flow:

A. Phases of cardiac cycle: During systole coronary blood flow is reduced whereas in diastole the blood supply through the coronary vessels is increased.

B. Aortic blood pressure: Any increase in aortic pressure also increases the coronary blood flow.

C. The heart rate: The effect varies—

- If the diastolic time is not altered, the increase in heart rate leads to increase of coronary blood flow.
- If the diastolic time is reduced due to excessive increase in hearty rate the coronary blood flow is reduced due to reducition of stroke volume.

D. Exercise: It increases coronary blood flow.

E. Emotion: It also increases coronary blood flow.

F. Temperature: Warmth increases whereas cold reduces the coronary blood flow.

G. Hormones: Thyroid hormone increases whereas pituitrin decreases the coronary blood flow.

H. Neurohormonal factors:

- ADP, ATP, adenosin, histamin, bradykinin,PGs etc. cause vasodilatation and thereby increases coronary blood flow.
- Vasopressin, PGH_2 causes vasoconstriction → decreases coronary blood flow.

I. Neural factors:

- Parasympathetic (vagus) stimulation (Direct) results generally net vasodilatation → increases coronary flow.
- Sympathetic stimulation (Direct effect) leads to net vasoconstriction and thereby there is decrease in coronary blood flow.

10. Define shock. Enemurate the stages, types of shock, causes and it's features. Describe in brief the compensatory mechanisms during hypovolemic shock. What are the signs and symptoms of shock?

Definition: Shock is the clinical condition characterised by the low cardiac output which is inadequate to maintain the normal tissue perfusion resulting impairment of the normal body function.

Stages: Different manifestations of circulatory shock take place in 3 stages follows:

A. *Non progressive stage (Compensatory stage)*: In spite of the fall of cardiac output the blood supply to the vital organs like heart and brain remains normal due to operation of normal circulatory compensatory mechanisms to recover the condition without any help of outside therapy. This stage is known as **compensatory stage**.

B. *Progressive stage*: If the fall of cardiac output is so severe that compensatory mechanisms fails to recover the condition, then the severe symptoms start appearing and shock becomes steadily worse until death. This is known as **progressive stage** from which the recovery can be possible by outside therapy.

C. Irreversible stage: In this phase the shock progresses to such an extent that all forms of known outside therapy are insufficient to cause full recovery leading death due to cerebral or and cardiac failure.

Types: It is primarily of 4 types:

(A) Hypovolumic or cold shock

(B) Cardiogenic shock

(C) Vasogenic (warm) shock which inturn is of 3 types: (a) Neurogenic shock, (b) Anaphylactic shock, (c) Septic shock,

(D) Obstructive shock.

Causes of different types of shock:

The causes of different types of shock is tabulated as follows:

1. Hypovolemic shock: It is defined as the clinical condition in which amount of fluid in the vascular system is inadequate to fill it resulting decrease in circulatory blood volume that inturn leads to reduction in cardiac output. It is due to—

(i) External or internal hemorrhage due to any injury or fracture.

(ii) Blood or fluid loss due to diarrhoea, vomiting, burn, excessive swelling or surgery.

2. Cardiogenic shock: It is defined as the clinical condition in which cardiac output is markedly reduced due to inadequate pumping action of the heart. It is due to decreased pumping activity of the heart because of cardiac abnormalities like—

— MI – congestive heart failure –arrhythmias –valve dysfunction

3. Vasogenic shock: It is defined as the clinical condition in which size of the capacitance vessels is increased by vasodilatation that leads fall of cardiac output though the circulatory blood volume remains normal. It is due to—

(i) Neurogenic shock due to general or spinal anaesthesia, brain damage or emotional fainting.

(ii) Anaphylactic shock due to allergic reaction which release vasodilators and increase capillary permeability due to release of histamine etc.

(iii) Sepsis.

4. Obstructive shock: It is due to obstruction of blood flow in the lungs or heart due to pulmonary embolism, cardiac tumour, cardiac tamponade, tension pneumothorax etc.

Compensatory changes during hypovolemic shock: In hypovolemic shock there is reduction of blood volume and the circulatory system can recover if degree of reduction of blood loss is not severe due to various compensatory mechanisms set for maintaining cardiac output and blood pressure. These are : (1) Rapidly acting (2) Long term compensatory mechanism.

***A. Rapidly acting compensatory mechanisms*:** These are:

(a) *Baroreceptor reflex*

(b) *Chemoreceptor reflex*

(c) *CNS ischemic response*

Immediately during hypovolemia there is fall of BP which initiates all the above 3 mechanisms which promote the mass sympathetic stimulation which ultimately normalises the BP and also increases the perfusion pressure at tissue level. All these mechanisms take less than 30 secs to provide immediate recovery.

(d) *Reverse stress relaxation*: This causes blood vessels to constrict down so that available blood volume is adequately circulated.

(e) *Capillary fluid shift mech*anism: The fall in capillary pressure causes fluid from interstitial space to move into the capillaries and thus the circulatory blood volume is increased → ↑ venous return → ↑ C.O.

(f) *Stimulation of adrenal medulla*: Hemorrhage is the potent stimulator of secretion of adrenal medullary hormones i.e. epinephrine and norepinephrine. The increased blood levels of epinephrine and norepinephrine cause general vasoconstriction → ↑ BP.

All those mechanisms (d, e, f) require 10-60 mins to normalise the situation.

(g) *Renin angiotensin mechanism*: During hypovolemia due to ischemia there is a release of renin from kidney which increases level of angiotensin II in blood which inturn promotes:

- Generalized vasoconstriction
- Initiate thirst sensation
- Stimulate aldosterone secretion

All these mechanisms ultimately increase cardiac output and BP (For detail see in chapter 4.11). This angiotensin mediated response takes 1-48 hr for complete response.

(h) *Release of excess vasopressin* or ADH: Release of ADH causes retention of water by kidneys and thus helps in restoring ECF volume.

(B) Long term compensatory mechanisms:

(a) *Increased plasma protein synthesis*: After hemorrhage there is rapid entry of preformed albumin from extra vascular stores to the plasma, rest of the plasma protein losses are restored by hepatic synthesis over a period of 3-4 days.

(b) *Increased RBC count*: Hypovolemia increases the erythropoietin level in blood by stimulating the release of renal erythropoietic factors. This erythropoietein increases RBC count and thus normal RBC count is restored within 4 to 8 weeks.

Signs and symptoms:

Different signs and symptoms manifested during shock are as follows:

1. Reduction in arterial blood pressure
2. Reflex tachycardia and reduced stroke volume
3. Decrease pulse pressure and appearance of thready pulse
4. Reduction in velocity of blood flow producing stagnant hypoxia and cyanosis
5. Pale and cold skin due to reflex vasoconstriction
6. Decreased urinary output due to reduced renal blood flow and GFR
7. Fainting due to reduced blood flow to the brain tissue
8. Feeling of intense thirst if the patient is conscious
9. Rapid and shallow breathing
10. Metabolic acidosis due to excessive production of lactic acid by myocardium
11. Death due to cerebral or cardiac failure

11. Describe the cardiovascular and respiratory changes during exercise.

During exercise the metabolic need to the exercising muscle is increased. To meet this increased demand some cardiovascular and respiratory adjustments take place in the body which are as follows:

1. *Cardiovascular changes*: These include—

(a) Immediate changes: Following changes are seen—

(I) ***Increased heart rate*** mainly due to withdrawal of vagal stimulation and partly due to mass sympathetic discharge resulted from:

(i) Stimulation of vasomotor system by:

- increased PCO_2 in blood
- proprioceptive impulses to higher center

(ii) Rise in body temperature

(iii) Circulating catecholamines released during exercise.

(II) ***Increased cardiac output*** up to 35 lit/min due to increase in heart rate and stroke volume.

(III) ***Increased venous return***; due to increased—

(i) skeletal muscle pump

(ii) respiratory pump

(iii) Vis-a Tergo effect resulted from increased force of contraction of the left ventricle.

(iv) Vis-a Fronte effect due to increased negative pressure inside the right atrium which helps in suction of venous blood into the right atrium.

(IV) ***Increased strength of contraction of heart*** due to—

- Increased sympathetic activity on heart muscle.
- Increased end diastolic fiber length (EDFL) due to increase venous return resulted from cardiac pump activity, muscle pump activity, respiratory pump activity and splanchnic vasoconstriction.

This increased strength of contraction of heart leads to increase in stroke volume.

(V) ***Increased blood flow*** to the exercising muscles. This is due to the facts that (i) most of the peripheral vessels constrict during exercise except arterioles in the active muscle (by vasodilatation due to local effect and effect of adrenalin), increasing venous return to heart. Thus most of non-muscular areas except coronary and cerebral arteries of the body temporarily send their blood to muscles (ii) muscular wall of the veins and other capacitance vessels of the circulation are contracted powerfully. This promotes increased venous return and thereby increased cardiac output and thereby increased blood flow to the exercising muscles.

(b) Long term changes: These include—

(i) heart rate becomes less after training due to a high vagal tone.

(ii) resting stroke volume becomes more due to increased contraction of heart muscle due to its hypertrophy.

(iii) resting cardiac output becomes high.

(iv) resting BP becomes less.

(v) cardiac work efficiency is increased.

2. *Respiratory changes*: Following respiratory changes are seen especially during moderate muscular exercise:

(a) Increased pulmonary ventilation upto even 60 L/min due to—

(i) cortical stimulation activate respiratory center.
(ii) increased body temperature activate the respiratory center directly or by increasing the activity of reticular formation.
(iii) increased catecholamine release activate the respiratory center.

(b) Increased O_2 supply (upto 2.5 L/ min) to the tissue due to—
(i) rise in pulmonary ventilation
(ii) rise in O_2 uptake in lungs.
(iii) rise in blood flow to the tissues due to increased cardiac output.

(c) Increased respiratory quotient upto 0.88.
(d) Increased O_2 debt.

B. Short Notes:

1. Syncitium:

- A syncitium is defined as a tissue containing cells with no boundaries, thus it behaves like a single unit. In heart the myocardial fibers are separated from each other though they behave like a single unit due to presence of numerous gap junctions.
- Due to the presence of these **gap junction** there is the rapid transmission of impulse from one cell to another. Because of this rapidity in transmission of impulse even though there is no anatomical connection between two adjacent muscle fibers the cardiac muscle functions as a unit. This is why it is called as ***functional syncitium***.
- Heart is composed of 2 functional syncitiums - **atrial syncitium** and **ventricular syncitium**. The atrial syncitial nature permits both the atria to contract at a time whereas the ventricular syncitial nature permits both the ventricles to contract at a time. Of course atrial contraction takes place little ahead of ventricular contraction because of presence of **A-V delay** to permit complete filling of ventricles.

2. Valves: The heart valves allow the flow of blood through the heart in one direction. There are 4 valves-two in between the atria and ventricles known as atrio-ventricular valves and two are at the opening of the blood vessels arising from the ventricles.

(i) A-V valves:

- These are present in between the atria and ventricles.
- The valve present in between RA and RV is made up of 3 cusps and thus called ***Tricuspid valve.***
- The valve present in between LA and LV is made up of 2 cusps and thus called ***Bicuspid valves*** or ***Mitral valves.***
- These valves prevent the backflow of blood from ventricles to atria during ventricular systole.
- These valves open or close passively due to pressure gradient.

(ii) Semilunar Valves:

- Both the semilunar valves are made up of 3 cusps and thus known as ***tricuspid valves.***
- There are two semilunar valves namely ***Pulmonary valve*** and ***Aortic valve***.
- The pulmonary valve is present at pulmonary orifice which leads from RV to pulmonary artery.
- The aortic valve is present at aortic orifice which leads from LV to the aorta.
- These valves prevent the backflow of blood from pulmonary artery / aorta to heart during ventricular diastole.
- These valves open or close passively due to pressure gradient.

3. S-A node:

- It is located on the posterior aspect of heart at the junction of superior vena cava with right atria.
- It is innervated by both sympathetic and parasympathetic. Normal inhibition to the SA node function is due to it's autonomic innervation.
- It acts as a **pacemaker of heart** because the rate of impulse generation in normal heart is determined by this node because of it's highest rate of impulse generating capacity (75 ± 5 times/min) than other junctional tissues. This is why it is known as **cardiac pacemaker.**
- It acts as a pacemaker as it is composed of small round or oval cells called ***pacemaker cell*** or ***'P' cell*** which has got the ability to generate the impulse automatically and rhythmically.
- The impulse from SA node is transmitted to left atria through interatrial tract named Bachman's bundle and to AV node through three internodal tracts.
- The experimental proof to show that the SA node is the pacemaker is:

  (i) *By application of hot/cold saline*: Cooling of SA node slowers the heart rate and warming of SA node quickens it.

  (ii) *By applying Stannius ligature*:

  ■ First Stannius ligature applied over the sino-atrial groove (in between sinus venosus and atria) blocks the impulse and heart stops (Fig. 4.8). However after sometimes atria starts generating their own impulse which is then transmitted to ventricles. This results atria and ventricle start beating independent of sinus rhythm but at a slower rate.

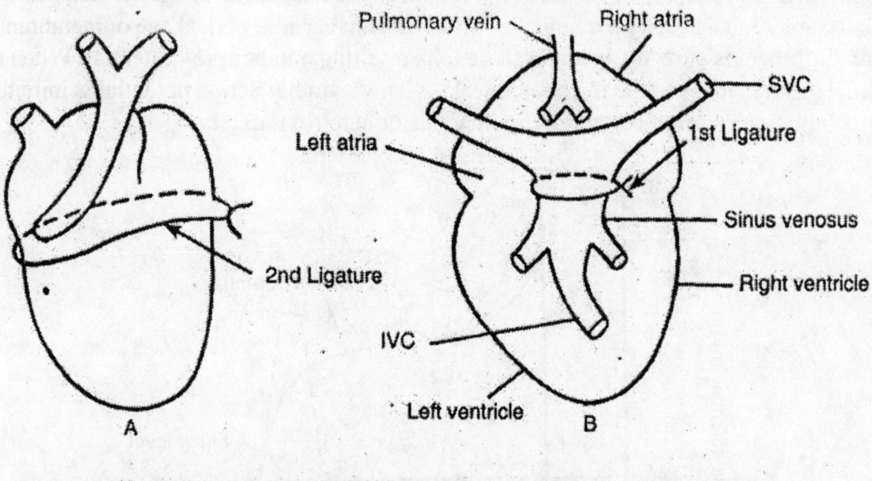

Fig. 4.8: Stannius ligature (*A = anterior view and B = posterior view*)

  ■ 2nd Stannius ligature applied over the A-V groove makes the atria to continue beating with it's own rhythm whereas the ventricle stops beating due to blockade of impulse from atria to ventricles. After sometimes ventricle generates it's own impulse and starts beating at much slower rate (Idioventricular Rhythm) (Fig. 4.9).

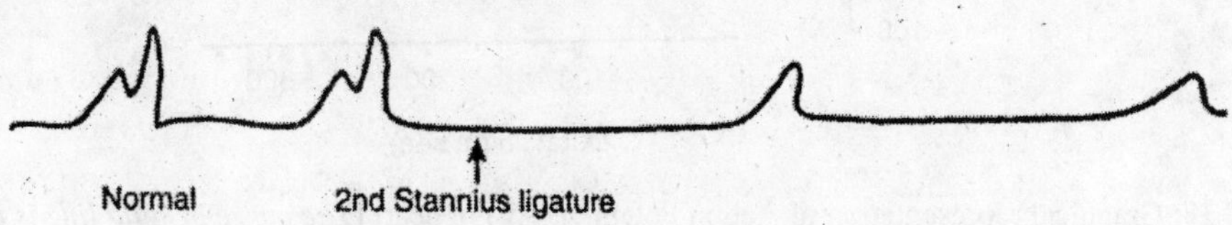

Fig. 4.9: Idioventricular rhythm

- When the pacemaker is other than SA Node (e.g. AV node etc.) it is called as ***ectopic pacemaker***.
- The causes of shift of pacemaker from SA nodes to other sites are:
  - More rate of impulse generation by other special junctional tissues.
  - Blockade of transmission of impulse from SA node to A-V node.
  - The ectopic pacemaker causes abnormal sequence of contraction of different parts of the heart.

4. Auto rhythmicity:

- The cardiac muscle fibers specially the special junctional tissues have got the capacity to generate their own impulse. This property is known as ***autorhythmicity.***
- In normal heart this rhythmicity is determined by SA node because of their highest rate of generation of impulse i.e. 75-80 times/min and thus SA node controls the rate of beating of heart. This is why it is called as ***cardiac pacemaker***.
- This ability of the SA node to generate the impulse rhythmically is due to the presence of ***'pacemaker cell'*** or ***'P'*** cell in it.
- The 'P' cell has **low resting membrane potential** (–50 to –55 mv) which is not steady but slow rising, This slow rising lower RMP is (Fig. 4.10) inside the Pacemaker cell is called as ***Pacemaker potential*** or ***pre-potential***. The early phase of this prepotential is mainly due to activation of unusual (**Funny**) channel called as **F channel** through which both Na ion and K ion can pass through. The Ca^{++} entry through **T type of voltage gated Ca^{++} channels** complete the pre-potential. When this pacemaker potential reaches at a threshold level (–40 mv) there is initiation of action potential because of sudden opening of **"L" type of voltage gated Ca^{++} channels** through which Ca^{++} enters inside to depolarise the membrane. Then at the end of depolarisation, voltage gated K^+ channels open and Ca^{++} channels close resulting K^+ efflux. This causes rapid repolarisation of the 'P' cell membrane to –55 mv. Again because of leakage of membrane to Na^+, K^+ and Ca^{++} there is slow diffusion of these ions resulting another pre- potential. When this pre-potential again reaches to the threshold level (–40 mv) another action potential is initiated. Thus there is initiation of impulses at regular intervals or auto rhythmicity.

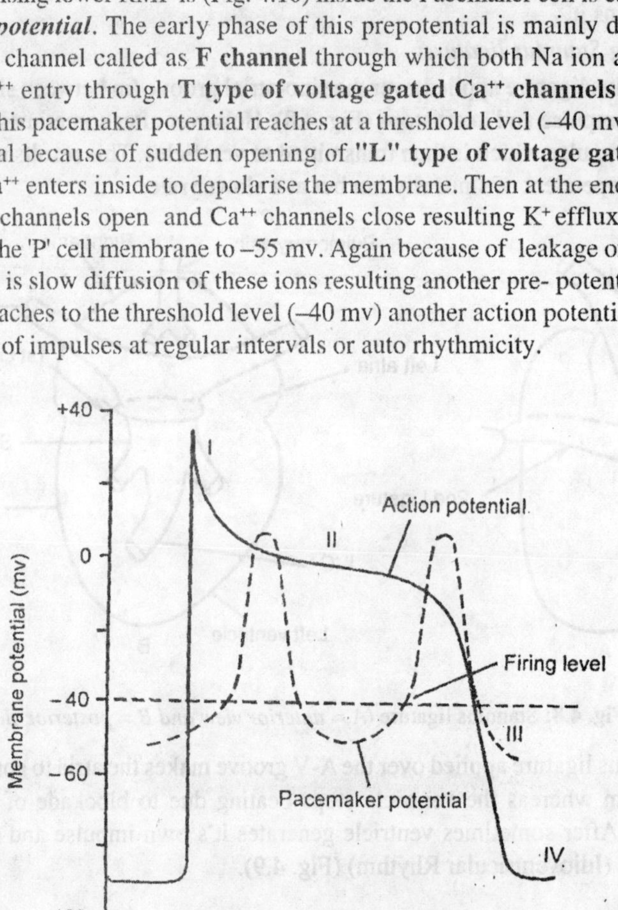

Fig. 4.10: Graphical representation of Action Potential (AP) in heart (*The curve in solid line is for AP in cardiac muscle and dotted line is for AP in SA Node i.e. pacemaker potential*)

5. **Pacemaker potential:** Vide last two points under autorhythmicity.
6. **Nodal rhythm:** Atrio-ventricular nodes take the charge of generating impulse rhythmically when SA node does not work. In this condition atria and ventricles beat almost simultaneously at the rate of 60 times per min. This rhythm of heart is known as ***Nodal rhythm.***
7. **A V delay:** In the A-V node there is a **delay of about 0.1 sec** to pass the information from A-V node. This time lag is known as ***A-V delay*** which has very important physiological significance i.e. it **permits the atria to contract little ahead of ventricular contraction** which allows filling of blood by the atria first before ventricular contraction.
8. **Windkessel vessels:**
   - Windkessel means an elastic reservoir.
   - The walls of the arteries are thick and contain a large portions of elastic tissue. By virtue of their elastic properties the expansion of large arteries during systole enables them to store blood which is then passed onward by recoiling during diastole maintaining blood flow during diastole. Thus the arteries act as **accessory pump** and this effect is called as the ***'Windkessel effect'*** (Fig. 4.11) **and *the arteries are called as windkessels vessels.***

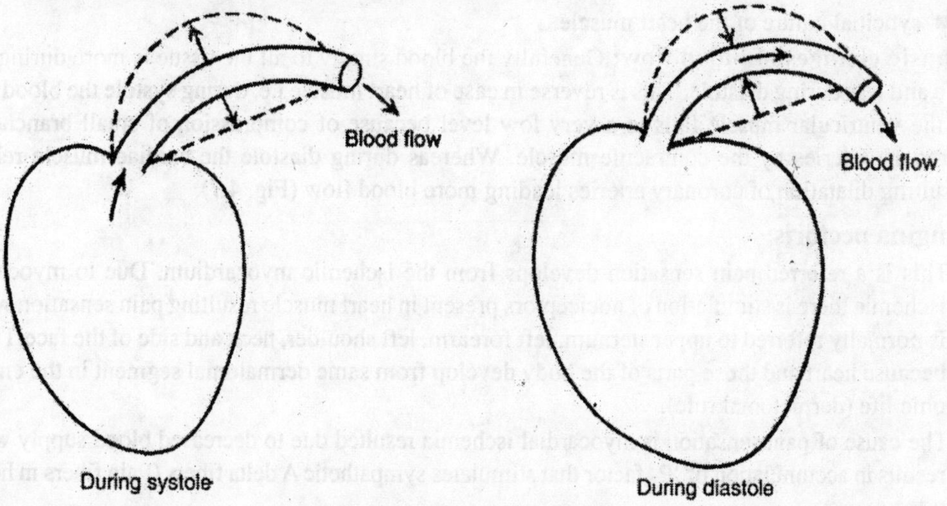

Fig. 4.11: Windkessel effect of arteries

   - Examples are aorta and it's main branches.
   - This Windkessel or recoiling effect pushes the blood in forward direction during diastole. Thus the blood flow is continuous during both systole and diastole. This continuous blood supply is essential for adequate tissue perfusion.
9. **Frank Starling's law of heart:**
   - German Physiologist Otto-Frank and English Physiologist Ernest Starling independently described the effect of preload on myocardial performance which is known as **Frank Starling's law of heart.**
   - It states that the greater the initial length of the ventricular muscle fiber or end diastolic length of muscle fiber, more is the force of contraction within physiological limit.
   - This influences force of contraction of heart which inturn influences stroke volume and thus cardiac output and thus BP.

- It is applicable only when all other condition remains same.
- Frank Starling's effect can be demonstrated even in denervated heart, therefore regulation by change in preload is a purely an intrinsic mechanism and such type of regulation of cardiac output by changing EDFL is known as heterometric autoregulation of the heart.
- The importance of Frank Starling's law are:
  - a life saving device in heart failure.
  - it helps to match the stroke volume of the ventricles so that there will not be any excess accumulation or complete emptying of blood in the pulmonary circulation as either of this is fatal.
  - it prevents venous engorgement by increasing stroke volume with increase in venous return.

10. All or none law in heart muscle:

- All or none law which states that if a stimulus is applied, whatever may be the strength of stimulus the cardiac muscle responds maximally or it does not give any response at all.
- It is applicable only in whole artrial muscle (i.e. atrial syncitium) or in whole ventricular muscle (i.e. ventricular syncitium) not **to a single cardiac muscle fiber.**
- It occurs due to—
  - all or none law of action potential
  - syncitial nature of the heart muscle.

11. Phasic changes of blood flow: Generally the blood supply to all the tissue is more during systole and less during diastole. This is reverse in case of heart muscle i.e. during systole the blood flow to the ventricular muscle falls to a very low level because of compression of small branches of coronary arteries by the contractile muscle. Whereas during diastole the cardiac muscle relaxes resulting dilatation of coronary arteries leading more blood flow (Fig. 4.7).

12. Angina pectoris:

- This is a referred pain sensation develops from the ischemic myocardium. Due to myocardial ischemia there is stimulation of nociceptors present in heart muscle resulting pain sensation which is normally referred to upper sternum, left forearm, left shoulder, neck and side of the face.This is because heart and those parts of the body develop from same dermatomal segment in the embryonic life (dermatomal rule).
- The cause of pain sensation is myocardial ischemia resulted due to decreased blood supply which results in accumulation of 'P' factor that stimulates sympathetic A delta fibers (Pain fibers in heart).
- It is of two types:
  - Stable angina that develops in exertion.
  - Unstable angina occurs even during rest.
- It is treated by drugs like nitrates, beta blockers and calcium channel blockers and surgery like coronary angioplasty and bypass surgery.

13. Myocardial infarction:

- Immediately after an acute coronary occlusion, the area of the muscle that has either no flow or little blood flow, can not sustain the normal cardiac muscle function. This results the irreversible damage of those area (necrosis). This clinical condition is known as *myocardial infarction (MI).*
- It may develop due to thromboembolism or due to prolonged vascular spasm arresting blood flow to the myocardium.
- It is characterised by—
  - elevation of ST segment in ECG studies

- severe chest pain radiating along the ulnar border of the hand
- excessive sweating
- increased level of creatine kinase and lactate dehydrogenase (LDH) enzymes and CK-MP isoenzyme and fraction –1 of LDH
- chronic diabetic mellitus pateint may have painless MI
- death in severe cases.

- Because of the MI death of the person can occur which is due to:
  - Cardiac shock
  - Damming of blood in venous system → increase in right and left atrial pressure → increase in capillary pressure → acute pulmonary oedema.
  - Rupture of infarcted area leading lost of blood → decrease in cardiac output and death.
  - Ventricular fibrillation which leads to incoordinated and ineffective contraction of heart → decrease in stroke volume → decrease in cardiac output → decrease in low cardiac output type of cardiac failure → death.

14. Stokes-Adams syndrome:

- It is a clinical condition characterised by periodic fainting and consciousness due to periodic stoppage of blood supply to the brain.
- This is resulted due to atrioventricular block (A-V Block) which may be resulted due to temporary stoppage of blood flow to the cardiac musculature.
- The mechanism by which periodic fainting and consciousness appears is as follows:

  Coronary occlusion → decrease in blood supply to heart muscle → decrease in blood supply to the intra atrial septum → A.V. Block → heart beat stops for 5-10 sec. → No blood supply to brain resulting fainting → discharge from BOH or purkinjee's fiber starts after 5-10 sec. → heart beat reappears. → improvement of blood supply to the heart → A-V block disappears. → normal heart beating restarts → normalisation of blood flow to the brain tissue → consciousness.

15. Idioventricular rhythm:

- In case of A-V nodal block or infranodal block (disease of conductive system below A-V node), a portion of ventricular muscle becomes pacemaker and generates the impulse resulting beating of ventricle at slower rate. In this case atrial beating and ventricular beating is different. This type of rhythm of heart beat is called as ***idioventricular rhythm*** (Fig. 4.9).
- In this case HR becomes 15-40 beats /min.
- This can be experimentally demonstrated by applying 2nd Stannius ligature on frog's heart.
- In this rhythm when the HR becomes as low as 15 beats /min it results Stokes-Adams syndrome.

16. Apex beat:

- It is the lowermost and outermost point of cardiac pulsation caused by the impact of the ventricles against the chest wall.
- It is normally located in the 5th intercostal space half inch medial to midclavicular line.
- It corresponds to mitral area from which the mitral component of 1st heart sound is best heard.
- It helps to diagnose the abnormal position of the heart (like pleural effusion, lung collapse, pericardial effusion, chest deformities etc.) and hypertrophy of the ventricles.
- In case of right ventricular hypertrophy it is shifted to the left, and left ventricular hypertrophy it is shifted downward and laterally, and in case of dextrocardia it is shifted on the right side of the thoracic cavity.

17. Heart sounds: See question no. 2.

18. End diastolic volume:

- During ventricular diastole the intra ventricular volume is increased which results filling of the ventricles. At the end of diastole the amount of blood filled by the ventricle is known as ***End diastole volume (EDV)***.
- It is normally about 120-130 ml.
- It determines the EDFL which inturn directly related with stroke volume and then cardiac output and thus systolic BP.
- It is directly affected by the preload which determines the contractility of the ventricular muscle.

19. Auscultatory areas: See question no. 2.

20. Marey's law:

- It was described by E. Marey in 1859.
- It states that heart rate is inversely proportional to blood pressure except in case of muscular exercise, emotions, exposure to hot environment in which situation HR is directly related with BP.
- Examples; hemorrhage, standing posture.
- It helps in short term regulation of BP and HR with the range of 60-160 mmHg of BP.

21. Murmur:

- These are the abnormal continuation of the sound over the heart and blood vessels due to the turbulence of blood flow.
- These differ from the heart sounds in that sense that these are of longer duration with higher frequency.
- These are of different types:
  - Systolic murmur- heard during systole in case of aortic stenosis, mitral valve incompetence and is of two types—1. *Pansystolic* that is heard when turbulent blood flow occurs across a valve throughout systole due to wide pressure difference between two chambers and 2. *Mid-systolic* that occurs when blood is ejected through a stenosed aortic or pulmonary valve.
  - Diastolic murmur-heard both during systole and diastole in case of patent ductus arterious.
  - Innocent murmur-physiological and seen in infants.
  - Thrills—felt over pericardium.
  - Bruits—heart over blood vessels.
  - Pericardial rub-heard in çase of pericarditis.
- These are useful in diagnosis of cardiac valvular disorders.

22. Protodiastole: At the beginning of ventricular diastole there is isometric relaxation of ventricular muscle → decrease in intra ventricular tension → back flow of blood from pulmonary artery and aorta → closure of semilunar valve to prevent this back flow of blood. This entire period is termed as protodiastole.

23. Stroke volume:

- During ventricular systole intra ventricular volume decreases which results increase in pressure thus ejection of blood out of ventricles. During each systole the amount of blood pumped out by each ventricle is known as ***Stroke volume (SV)***.
- Normal value : 70 ml/beat.
- It directly affects cardiac output and thus systolic BP.
- It is dependent on force of contraction of heart muscle, EDFL, preload, venous return, ANS and left ventricular size.
- It is inversely related with afterload.

24. Venous return:

- It is the amount of blood returned to the heart /min.
- Venous return to the heart is directly related with EDFL which inturn increases force of contraction of heart to increase C.O.
- Venous return inturn depends on:

(i) *Cardiac pump*: pumping activity of the heart regulates the venous return to the heart specially during exercise.

(ii) *Respiratory pump*: During inspiration

- Intra thoracic pressure decreases → fall of pressure over and around large veins and arteries.
- Descent of diaphragm → increases of intra abdominal pressure → squeezing of blood out of abdomen.

Both these factors increases venous return (VR) and similarly during expiration VR is decreased due to opposite event. This is known as **respiratory pump** which is one of the major factor to increase C.O. during exercise.

(iii) *Muscle pump*: During rhythmical contraction of skeletal muscle → squeezing of veins in the muscles → increase in venous return to the heart. Whereas during relaxation of skeletal muscle due to opposite fact venous return decreases. This factor also contributes during exercise.

(iv) *Blood volume*: Rise in blood volume increases venous return and thus cardiac output.

25. Peripheral resistance:

- It is the impediment to blood flow by the blood vessels.
- It can be calculated by modifying Ohm's law as follows: $R = \Delta P/Q$
- Unit of peripheral resistance is PRU and at rest total PR is 1 PRU which is increased upto 4 PRU during vasoconstriction and decreased upto 0.2 PRU during vasodilatation.
- PR is directly related with DP i.e. increase in PR indicates rise of DP. Peripheral resistance inturn dependent on following factors:
  - Velocity of blood → directly related with PR
  - Viscosity of blood → directly related with PR
  - Total amount of blood in arterial system → directly related with PR
  - Elasticity of blood vessels → inversely related
  - Length of the blood vessels → inversely related
  - Diameter of the blood vesselss which is inversely related with PR.

26. Heart block:

- Defect in conduction of impulse from atria to ventricles is called as A-V Block or heart block.
- It is classified as follows:

1. Partial (Incomplete) A-V block which are of 3 types—
   - 1st degree heart block characterised by prolongation of PR interval.
   - 2nd degree heart block which is characterised by gradual prolongation of PR interval followed by dropping of one beat (Wencheback phenomenon) or variable ratio of atrial and ventricular rate at 2 : 1 or 3 : 1 (2 : 1 or 3 : 1 block) or occasional failure of conduction of impulse resulting atrio-ventricular ratio 6 : 5 or 8 : 7 (Morbitz type–II block).
2. Complete or 3rd degree heart block characterised by complete dissociation of atrio-ventricular rhythm.

3. Bundle Branch Block: It is indicated by prolonged and deformed QRS complex which may be of 3 types—
   - Right Bundle Branch Block
   - Left Bundle Branch Block
   - Trifascicular block (Block in bundle of His)

27. Stannius ligature:

- This is the experimental basis in frog's heart to show that SA node is the normal pacemaker of heart.
- It is generally two types –1st and 2nd stannius ligature.
  - First stannius ligature applied over the sino-atrial groove (in between Sinus venosus and atria) blocks the impulse and heart stops (Fig. 4.8). However after sometimes atria starts generating their own impulse which is then transmitted to ventricles. This results atria and ventricle start beating independent of sinus rhythm but at a slower rate.
  - 2nd stannius ligature applied over the A-V groove (Fig. 4.8) makes the atria to continue beating with it's own rhythm whereas the ventricle stops beating due to blockade of impulse from atria to ventricles. After sometimes ventricle generates it's own impulse and starts beating at much slower rate (Idioventricular Rhythm) (Fig. 4.9).
- It can not be applied in mammalian heart as—
  - SA node is present inside the atrium, so 1st ligature is not possible.
  - Application of 2nd ligature obstruct the coronary blood supply resulting no beating of heart.

28. Extrasystole:

- When a strong stimulus is applied in the relative refractory period in an experimental recording of normal cardiogram an extra contractile response occurs before the normal response which is known as extrasystole (Fig. 4.12).

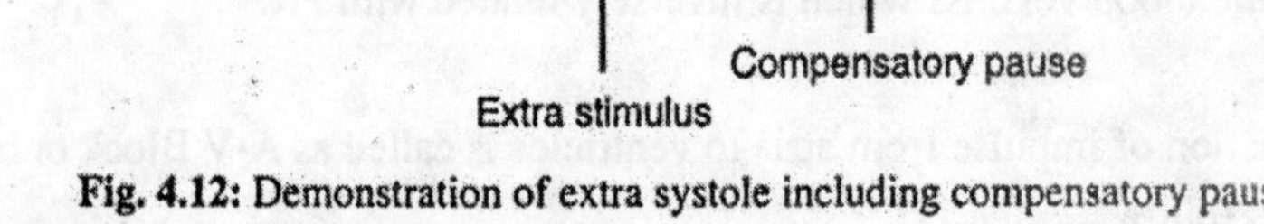

Fig. 4.12: Demonstration of extra systole including compensatory pause

- It is not always pathological as usually the extra stimulus arises from an ectopic focus in the ventricle.
- It is characterised by the less RR interval between normal beat and extra systole and more RR interval between extra systole and proceeding normal beat.

29. Arrhythmias:

- Abnormal rhythm of heart is known as arrhythmias.
- It may be developed due to—
  - disorders with the site and rate of impulse generation in heart.
  - conduction defects.

- Pathologically cardiac dysarrhythmias can be divided into—
  - disorders of SA node (Sick Sinus Syndrome)
  - atrial arrhythmias which includes extrasystole, paroxysmal supraventricular tachycardia, atrial flutter, atrial fibrillation.
  - ventricular arrhythmias
  - conduction disorders.
- It may also be physiological e.g. during respiratory cycle, sinus tachycardia and sinus bradycardia.

30. Einthoven's triangle:

- The standard limb lead-I, Lead –II and Lead-III are connected in such a way that for practical purposes they form an equilateral triangle center of which contains heart. This equilateral triangle is called *Einthoven's triangle* (Fig. 4.5).
- It is an equilateral triangle with each side representing the axis of one of the bipolar limb leads.
- It is an inverted triangle with apex pointing towards the groin and the base between two shoulders.
- It is used to calculate QRS axis of the heart.

31. Einthoven's Law:

- It states that if the electrical potentials of any two bipolar limb leads are known at a given instance the third one can be known mathematically by simply adding the 1st two considering '+' and '–' sign of the two values. *For example*: if Lead I records – 0.5 mv, and Lead II records + 1.5 mv, Then the voltage in Lead III = – (0.5) + (+1.5) = + 1mv.
- It was proposed by scientist Einthoven on the basis of a equilateral triangle known as ***Einthoven's triangle.***

32. Bipolar leads:

- Generally two types of leads are used to record electrical potential changes of heart which are 1. Bipolar leads 2. unipolar leads.
- Bipolar leads: When the ECG is recorded by placing two electrodes in two points of the body (Generally limb)- one as a **'–' terminal** and another as a **'+' terminal**, then it is known as bipolar lead. It is also known as ***Standard Limb lead*** which are of 3 types as follows:
  i. **Lead I:** Here one electrode is placed in right arm and another is at left arm. Negative terminal of the electrocardiograph is connected to the right and positive terminal is connected to the left arm (Fig. 4.5).
  ii. **Lead II:** Here negative terminal is connected to the electrode placed in right arm and positive terminal is connected to the electrode placed in left leg (Fig. 4.5).
  iii. **Lead III:** Here negative terminal of the machine is connected to the left arm and positive terminal to the left leg (Fig. 4.5).

33. Chest leads:

- These are the precordial leads present in the transverse plane on chest surface to record ECG.
- In this case 3 limb leads are connected to central terminus through a resistance (5000 ohm) and attached to the '–' terminal and exploring electrode is placed on different surface of chest which is connected to the '+' terminal.
- As per the location of this exploring electrode it is of 6 types as follows:
  - ☐ $V_1 \rightarrow$ In 4th intercostal space at right side of the sternum
  - ☐ $V_2 \rightarrow$ In 4th intercostal space at left side of the sternum
  - ☐ $V_3 \rightarrow$ In between V_2 and V_4

- ☐ V_4 → In 5th left intercostal space and it's junction with mid clavicular line
- ☐ V_5 → In 5th left intercostal space and it's junction with anterior axillary line
- ☐ V_6 → In 5th left intercostal space and it's junction with mid axillary line

- Lewis lead is a special bipolar chest lead used for recording ECG in atrial arrhythmias.

34. WPW syndrome:

- It is one type of conduction defects proposed by Wolff, Parkinson and White in which rate of conduction is accelerated.

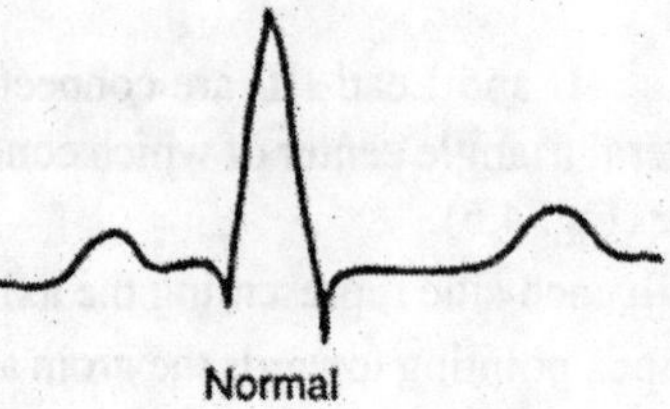

Normal

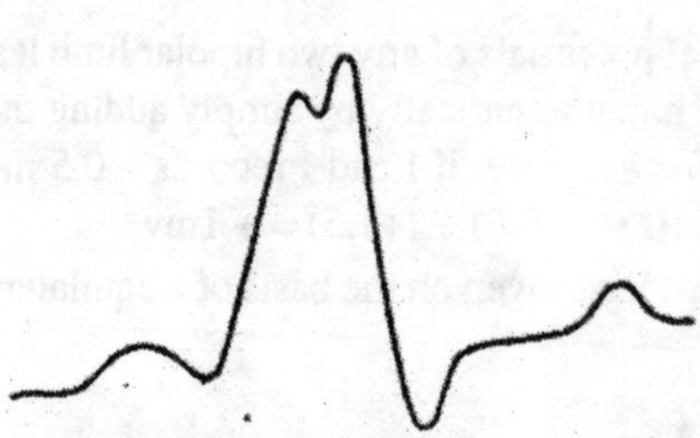

WPW syndrome

Fig. 4.13: ECG changes in WPW syndrome

- This is due to the presence of an aberrant internodal pathway named as Bundle of Kent in between atria and ventricle which transmits impulse in a faster rate than the usual transmission of impulse through the normal internodal pathways. This results early excitation of ventricles.
- It is characterised by more PR interval and widened QRS complex with slurred upstroke (Fig. 4.13). However PJ interval is normal.

35. Wencheback Phenomenon:

- In case of 2nd degree A-V block there is gradual prolongation of PR interval till there is missing of one ventricular beat (Fig. 4.14). This is known as Wencheback phenomenon.

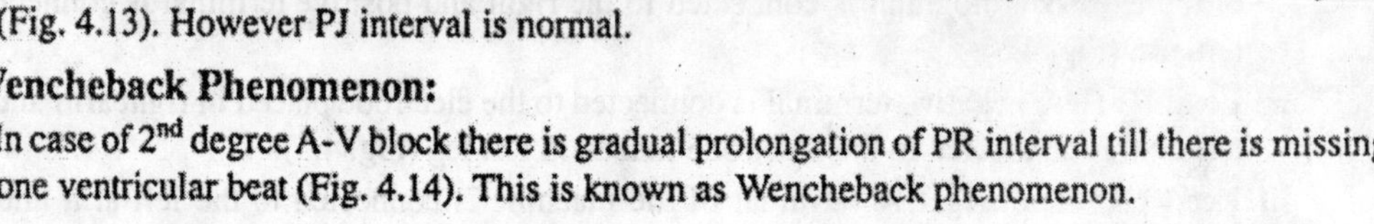

Fig. 4.14: ECG changes in Wencheback phenomenon

- This is usually seen in acute inferior myocardial infarction, acute carditis, digitalis toxicity and etc.

36. Right and Left axis deviation:

- The normal direction of the mean cardiac vector ranges between –30 to +110^0. If the axis falls to the left of –30° it is known as left axis deviation and if the axis falls to the right of +110° it is known as right axis deviation (Fig. 4.15).

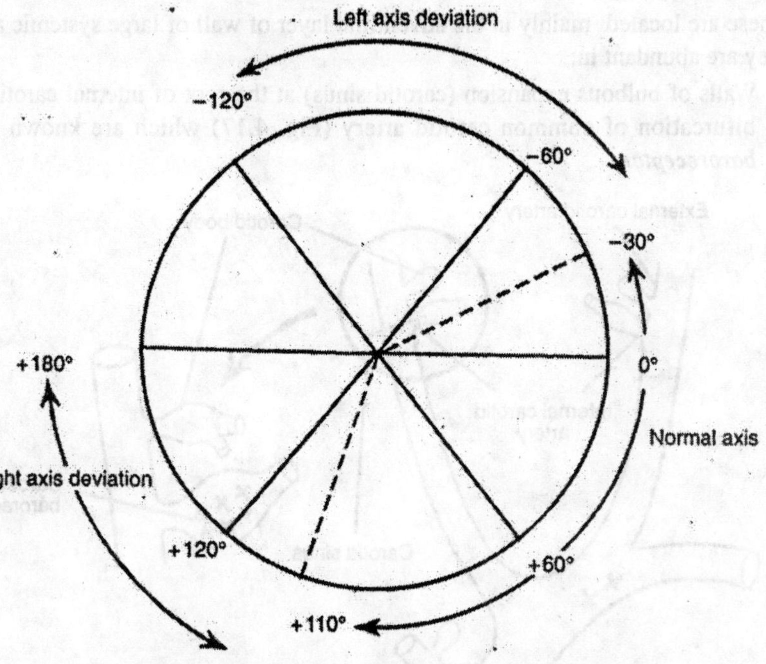

Fig. 4.15: Right and left axis deviation of cardiac vector

- It can be studied by roughly estimating QRS complex in lead –I and aVF. when the QRS complexes are predominantly upright in both the leads it is said to be normal. Whereas if the QRS complexes in lead –I is predominantly negative and in aVF it is predominantly positive it is said to be right axis deviation and the opposite is known as left axis deviation.
- Right axis deviation is seen in right ventricular hypertrophy, dextrocardia and left axis deviation is seen in left ventricular hypertrophy, inferior MI, obstructive airways disease etc.

37. Critical closing pressure:

- In blood vessels blood flow stops when pressure gradient is reduced beyond a point which is much more than zero. The pressure at which flow stops is called as critical closing pressure (Fig. 4.16).
- It does not follow the linear relationship between flow and pressure.
- It is explained by—
  - some pressure is required to push the RBCs to pass through capillaries.
  - intraluminar pressure should be more than the tissue pressure to resume the flow.

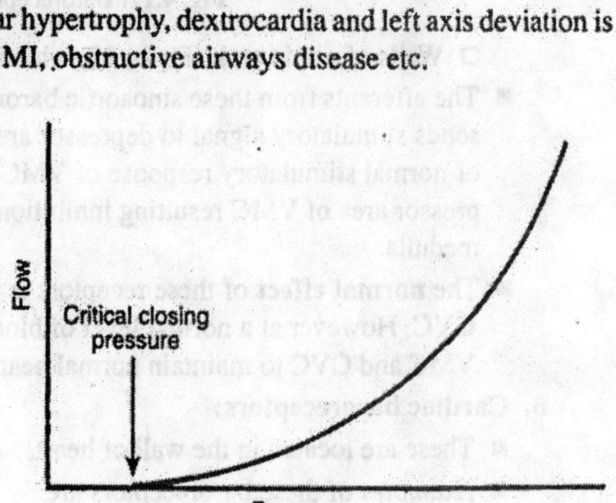

Fig. 4.16: Graphical representation of critical closing pressure

38. Baroreceptors:

- These are pressure / stretch / mechano receptors sensitive to stretch or deformation or distortion produced by pulsatile variations of blood pressure.

- These are two types: **Arterial baroreceptors** and **Cardiac baroreceptors** as per their location.

A. Arterial baroreceptors:

- These are located mainly in the adventitial layer of wall of large systemic arteries. However they are abundant in:
  - Walls of bulbous expansion (carotid sinus) at the root of internal carotid artery or at the bifurcation of common carotid artery (Fig. 4.17) which are known as ***carotid sinus baroreceptor.***

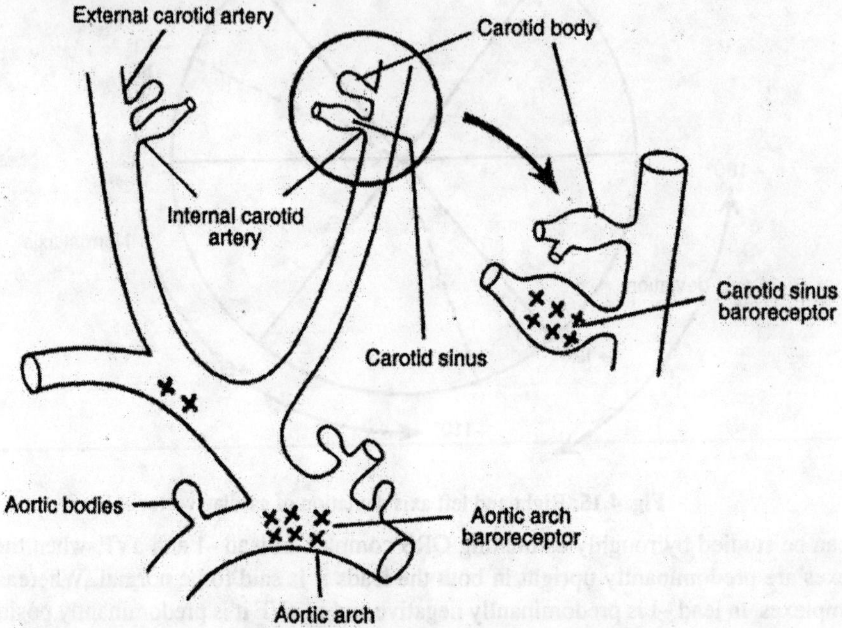

Fig. 4.17: Baroreceptors and chemoreceptors

  - Walls of aortic arch (Fig. 4.17) which are known as ***aortic arch baroreceptor.***
- The afferents from these sinoaortic baroreceptors synapse with NTS of medulla which in turn sends stimulatory signal to depressor area of **vasomotor center** (VMC) resulting withdrawal of normal stimulatory response of VMC (i.e. stimulation of baroreceptors result inhibition of pressor area of VMC resulting inhibition of sympathetic) and **cardiac vagal center** (CVS) of medulla.
- The **normal effect** of these receptors is **reflex inhibition of VMC** and **reflex stimulation of CVC**. However at a normal level of blood pressure these receptors discharge continuously to VMC and CVC to maintain normal heart rate and blood pressure.

B. Cardiac baroreceptors:

- These are located in the wall of heart.
- *Examples* of these baroreceptors are:
  - *Atrio-caval* and *pulmonary veno-atrial receptors*: These are responsible for initiation of ***'Bainbridge reflex'*** i.e. rapid perfusion of blood / saline in anaesthetised animals produces tachycardia if the initial heart rate is low.
  - *Atrial receptors*: Sensitive to rise of atrial pressure which results reflex vasodilatation especially in renal vascular circuit.

- *Ventricular receptors*: Sensitive to chemicals or partial occlusion of aorta or coronary artery which are responsible for profound bradycardia, hypotension and apnoea. This response is known as ***'Coronary chemo reflex'*** or ***Bezold Jarish reflex*** which is clinically associated with **Myocardial infarction or Vaso-vagal syncope.**

39. Chemoreceptors:

- These are stimulated in response to low PO_2 and high PCO_2 and H^+ concentration.
- These have normally no role in maintenance of B.P. but mainly responsible for regulating respiratory rate and depth. However in some abnormal condition like shock etc. it has a role in regulating B.P.
- These are of two types:
  - **Peripheral chemoreceptors:** These are again of 2 types
    - *Carotid body chemoreceptors*: Present in external carotid artery just above the bifurcation of common carotid artery (Fig. 4.17).
    - *Aortic body chemoreceptors*: Scattered around wall of arch of aorta (Fig. 4.17).
  - **Central chemoreceptors:** Present just beneath the ventral surface of medulla and are sensitive to changes of H^+ concentration of CSF and surrounding interstitial fluid. These are mainly responsible for regulating respiratory function.

40. Buffer nerves: The afferent nerves from carotid sinus baroreceptors and carotid body chemoreceptors is known as **carotid sinus** nerve or **Hering's nerve** which one is the branch of **glossopharyngeal nerve. Whereas** the afferent from aortic sinus baroreceptors and aortic body chemoreceptors is known as **aortic nerve** which ultimately **joins** to the **vagus nerve.** Both of those nerves are collectively known as ***sino-aortic nerve*** or ***buffer nerve*** as these nerves help to prevent any change of B.P.

41. Axon reflex:

- When the impulse is conducted from the site of injury antidromically to the blood vessels to cause arteriolar dilatation resulting spreading out of redness from the site of injury to the surrounding area it is called as axon reflex.
- It is responsible for flare of tripple response initiated due to firm stroke.

42. Bainbridge reflex:

- Bainbridge in 1915 demonstrated that rapid infusion of blood / saline in anaesthetised animals produces tachycardia if the initial heart rate is low.
- The receptors responsible for this reflex are in the atria at the veno-atrial junction known as tachycardia producing receptors (TPR).
- This reflex competes with baroreceptor reflex and tries to increase the heart rate.
- This reflex is abolished after vagotomy indicating that it is mediated by vagus nerve.
- It can also be initiated during inspiration due to: during inspiration decrease in intrathoracic pressure → increase in right atrial filling → stretching of right atria → stimulation of TPR → tachycardia.

43. Bezold Jarish reflex:

- Injection of veratridine or nicotine into the pulmonary circulation stimulates the pulmonary chemoreceptors which can cause bradycardia, hypotension and apnoea followed by tachypnoea (rapid, shallow breathing) called ***pulmonary chemoreflex***. Similar reflex originated due to stimulation of coronary chemoreceptors are known as ***coronary chemoreflex*** or ***Bezold Jarish reflex***.
- This has no physiological importance but occurs in pathological conditions like pulmonary congestion and after MI.

- It is abolished by vagotomy.

44. Cushing reflex:

- When intracranial pressure is high → there is decrease in blood flow to VMC due to compression of cerebral blood vessels → baroreceptor activation → stimulation of VMC → increase in sympathetic discharge → vasoconstriction → increase in BP → reflex bradycardia. This is known as cushing reflex.
- It is seen in case of brain tumor.

45. Fick principle:

- This principle states that the amount of a substance taken up by an organ or by whole body per unit time is equal to the arterial level of that substance minus the venous level (A-V difference) times the blood flow.

  i.e. **Blood flow / min = Amount of substance taken per min X 100 / (A-V difference of that substance)**
- On the basis of this principle cardiac output, coronary blood flow, renal blood flow, cerebral blood flow, body fluid volume etc. can be determined indirectly.

46. Indicator (Dye) dilution method:

- This is the indirect method followed as per **Stewart principle** which states that the volume of the fluid in a container can be calculated by adding a known amount of dye and measuring it's concentration after it has become evenly dispersed throughout the fluid medium.

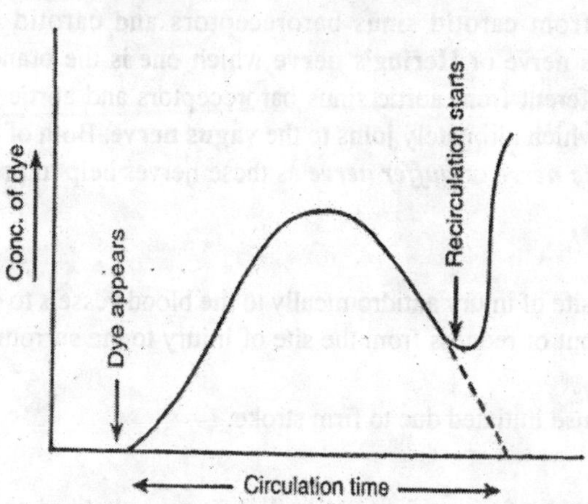

Fig. 4.18: Curve showing dye dilution method

- As per this principle a known amount of dye like cardiogreen, hypertonic saline etc. is injected into a vein. It will first pass through the heart and then pulmonary circulation and finally it will be evenly distributed in the blood stream. It's mean concentration during it's first passage (Fig. 4.18) through an artery can be determined from successive sample of blood taken from the artery. Now the blood flow in liters / sec (F) can by calculated from the formula:

  F = Q/Ct, (*Where Q = quantity of dye injected, c = mean concentration of dye, t = duration of 1st passage of the dye through the artery in sec).*
- Advantage of this method is that it is the accurate method for measuring cardiac output.
- Disadvantage: It should not be repeated in short time as the concentration of the dýe of the earlier use may give errors.

47. Respiratory pump: During inspiration—

- Intra thoracic pressure decreases → fall of pressure over and around large veins and arteries.
- Descent of diaphragm → Increases of intra abdominal pressure → squeezing of blood out of abdomen.

Both these factors increases VR and similarly during expiration VR is decreased due to opposite event. This is known as **respiratory pump** which is one of the major factor to increase C.O. during exercise.

48. Echo-cardiography:

- This is most advanced and non invasive method for study of heart in detail including measuring cardiac output, EDV, ESV etc.
- It is based on principle that if ultrasound waves are beamed at the heart, an echo is produced every time the wave passes an interface e.g. between muscle and blood. The returning echoes are picked up and is converted into electrical signal by suitable transducer. These electrical signals are displayed in CRO (Cathod Ray Oscilloscope) screen.
- It also gives a dyanamic view of cardiac function showing the movements of ventricular septum, valves, ventricular wall during cardiac cycle.
- It is a valuable investigation for valvular lesions and congenital heart diseases.
- 3 types of echocardiographic methods are used:
  (i) **'M' mode (imaging) echocardiography**—for anatomical imaging of the heart.
  (ii) **Doppler ultrasonography**—for assessment of abnormalities of blood flow.
  (iii) **Colour flow Doppler ultrasonography**—for dynamic representation of information of velocity of blood throughout the cardiac cycle.

49. Laminar and Turbulent blood flow:

- **Laminar or stream line flow:** It is fixed layer wise i.e. each layer of blood remains at the same distance from the wall blood vessels flowing through a long vessel and the velocity of blood is maximum in the core of the blood vessels and minimum in it's periphery or surface. This type of steady rate of blood flow is known as ***laminar blood flow*** (Fig. 4.19).

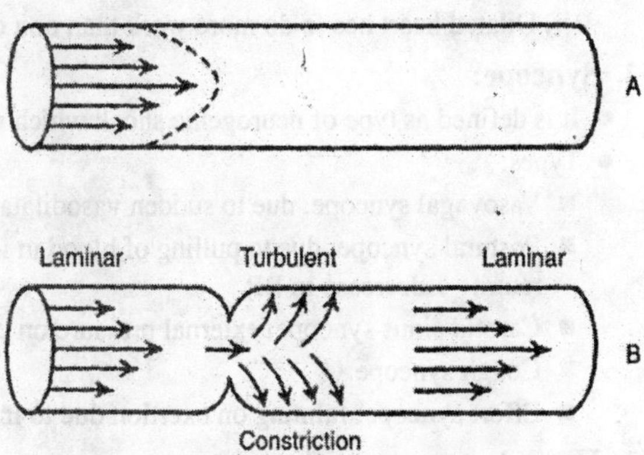

Fig. 4.19: Types of blood flow (*A = laminar and B = turbulent*)

- **Turbulent blood flow:**
  - When the blood flows crosswise in the vessels by forming whorls in the blood is called **eddy current.** This type of blood flow is known as ***turbulent blood flow*** (Fig. 4.19). It is produced by obstruction of vessels or when it takes sharp U turn. Turbulence of blood flow produces sound which can be heard by stethoscope.
  - *Factors influencing tendency of turbulent flow*: The tendency of the turbulence to occur is measured as **Reynold's number** which is calculated as follows:

    $Re = \rho DV/\eta$ *Where Re = Reynold's number, V = velocity of blood flow(cm/s), D = diameter of blood,* η *= viscosity of blood and* ρ *= density.*

    When Re is increased more than 2000-2500 turbulent blood flow will occur. In large artery even normally Re rises to 2000. Therefore there is always some turbulent flow.

50. Poiseuille's law (Poiseuille Hagen Formula): The relationship between the flow in a long narrow tube, the viscosity of the fluid and the radius of the tube is expressed mathematically in the Poiseuille Hagen formula: $Q = \pi \Delta P r 4/8 \eta l$.

Q = rate of blood flow, Δ*.P= pressure difference, r = radius,* η *= viscosity of blood, l = Length of the vessel.*

Thus, from this formula it can be stated that rate of blood flow is directly related with pressure difference and 4th power of the radius of blood vessels and inversely proportional to the viscosity of blood and length of the blood vessels. This interrelationship is known as Poiseuille's law. From this law it becomes clear that the diameter of the vessels plays a major role in determining the rate of blood flow. This is why the blood flow to a organ is so effectively regulated by small changes in the diameter of the arterioles and thus variations of arteriolar diameter have such great effect on systemic arterial blood pressure.

51. Law of Laplace:

- It is the relationship between distending pressure and tension on the wall in a hollow object.
- It states that the distending pressure (P) in a distensible hollow object is equal at equilibrium to the tension (T) in the wall of hollow object divided by two principal radii of curvature of the object (R_1 and R_2) i.e. $P = T (1/R_1 + 1/R_2)$
- In a sphere e.g. lung alveoli $R_1 = R_2$ so $P = 2T/R$ whereas in blood vessels as one radius is infinite, so $P = T/R$.
- ***Significance***:
  (i) As per this law the smaller the radius of the blood vessels lesser the tension in the wall necessary to balance the distending pressure. This is the reason because of which the minute, thin wall capillaries and delicate capillaries are less prone for rupture.
  (ii) Dilated heart has to do more work than non dilated heart.

52. Syncope:

- It is defined as type of neurogenic shock which results fainting and usually lasts for brief period.
- Types:
  - Vasovagal syncope: due to sudden vasodilatation due to parasympathetic (vagal) activation.
  - Postural syncope: due to pulling of blood in lower limbs upon standing → decrease in venous return → decrease in BP.
  - Carotid sinus syncope: external pressure on carotid sinus → vasodilatation → fainting.
  - Cough syncope.
  - Effort syncope: fainting on exertion due to inability to increase in cardiac output.

53. Heart lung preparation:

- It is the experimental protocol in usually dog to study the effect of preload and afterload on cardiac output.
- In this experiment heart and lungs in anaesthetised animals are canulated in such a way so that the blood from ventricles flow through a system of tubing and reservoirs to the right atria and thence through the heart and lungs back to the aorta.
- To study the effect of preload the reservoir of the fluid is raised to lower or volume of fluid inside it is changed. This results alteration of end diastolic volume → altered stroke volume → thereby altered cardiac output.
- To study the effect of afterload the calibre of the outflow tube decreases to increase peripheral resistance → accumulation of blood in the ventricle → increased stroke volume in next beat by Frank Starling's mechanism → thereby increased cardiac output.

54. Apex pulse deficit:

- Basically the value of **pulse rate and heart rate is same** but sometimes specially during premature beat or atrial fibrillation, ejection of blood from ventricle to aorta is less. This results poor contraction and relaxation of smooth muscles of wall of aorta which is too weak to palpate from peripheral artery. Thus a deficit in the number of pulses felt in the radial pulse in relation to number of heart beat is known as ***pulse deficit.***

- Pulse deficit usually seen in atrial fibrillation is more than 10 whereas in other arrhythmias and heart block it is less than 10.

55. Sino-aortic reflex:

- In response to rise of B.P. baroreceptors are stimulated which inturn sends impulse to VMC and CVC to result decrease of heart rate and BP. This is known as ***sino-aortic reflex.***
- The detail of this mechanism is as follows; In response to rise of BP above normal level baroreceptors are stimulated which sends the impulse to VMC and CVC which ultimately inhibit sympathetic neurones and stimulate parasympathetic nerves to result fall of BP. In response to fall of blood pressure just opposite events take place to increase the blood pressure towards normal level.
- This is named as buffer reflex as it neutralise the change in BP.
- It is also known as Marey's reflex.

56. Sinus arrhythmia:

- During inspiration HR is increased and during expiration HR is reduced. This phenomenon is called as ***Sinus Arrhythmia.***
- This is dominant in children and young adults.
- It is due to operation of 4 mechanisms:
  - alteration in autonomic activity i.e. during inspiration sympathetic stimulation and during expiration vagal stimulation affect the heart rate.
  - activation of Bainbridge reflex-during inspiration there is decrease in intrathoracic pressure → increase in venous return to right atria → stretching of right atria → stimulation of atrial tachycardia producing receptors → increase in heart rate.
  - irradiation from inspiration center to VMC directly.
  - activation of atrial stretch reflex → increase in venous return → stimulation of atrial stretch receptors → increase in heart rate.

57. Cardiac centers: These are responsible for ultimate control of cardiovascular response.

- Two types of centers are mainly involved as follows:

(I) ***Medullary center:*** Two types of cardiovascular centers are present in medulla—one is cardioacceleratory and another is cardioinhibitory. These are popularly known as:

1. Vasomotor Center:

- In the ventro lateral region of medulla contains some neurones which exert excitatory effects on spinal sympathetic neurones to produce presser effect on CVS like increase in heart rate, increase in stroke volume, vasoconstriction. These area is known as ***pressor area.***
- Near the caudal and medial part of IV ventricle in medulla there are another group of neurons which when stimulated produce inhibitory effect on spinal sympathetic neurones to produce depressor effect on CVS like fall of heart rate, stroke volume, vasodilatation. These are known as ***Depressor area.***
- Though two opposite effects are produced by VMC, normally the dominant action of VMC is **to stimulate sympathetic nervous system in response to it's stimulation.**

2. Cardiac vagal center (CVC):

- This is located in the nucleus ambiguus of medulla.
- Stimulation of these centers is responsible for stimulation of vagus nerve which is inhibitory to the heart and blood vessel.
- These centers are not tonically active like VMC.

3. **Others:** Some higher centers also control the cardiovascular response especially during emotion by controlling vasomotor center. These are-reticular substances of pons, mesencephalon, diencephalon, hypothalamus, cerebral cortex, limbic system etc.

58. Vagal tone:

- Normally the SA nodal activity is primarily under the control of vagus nerve which is known as vagal tone.
- The basal heart rate is determined by vagal tone which is lower than the intrinsic heart rate i.e. heart beat in denervated heart.
- In the normal resting heart vagal tone dominates over the sympathetic tone.

59. Autoregulation of blood flow: These mechanisms operate to maintain blood flow to an organ at relatively constant level in spite of change of blood pressure within physiological limit (Fig. 4.20).

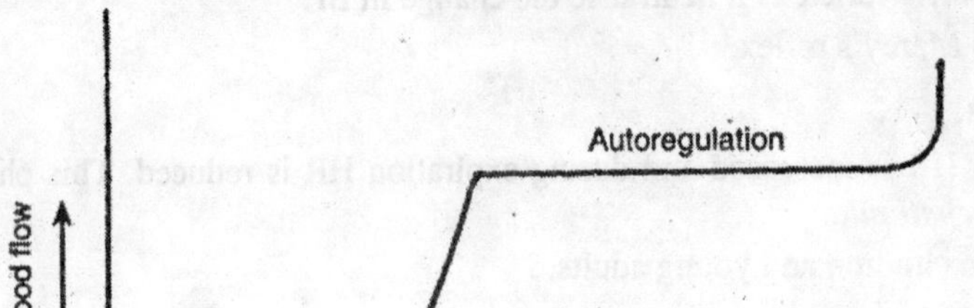

Fig. 4.20: Autoregulation of blood flow

By this mechanism local blood flow alters as per the alteration of rate of tissue metabolism. There are two theories for regulation of local blood flow—

a. Metabolic Theory: These depend on local metabolism of tissue, which is again of 2 types:

(i) **Vasodilator theory:** As per this theory some vasodilator substances are released in response to fall of blood supply to the tissue which in turn causes dilatation of vessels to increase blood flow to that particular tissue / organ. This is explained in detail by following flow chart:

Fall of blood flow to the organ with greater metabolic activity of that particular organ → lack of O_2 supply and other nutrients to the tissue → release of vasodilator substances like adenosine, lactic acid, bradykinin, prostaglandin, K^+, H^+ etc. → vasodilatation of the vessels supplying the blood to that organ → blood flow to that organ to normal level.

If there is rise of blood flow these vasodilator substances are washed out and thus there is no vasodilatation. So blood flow is reduced.

(ii) **O_2 demand theory:** O_2 is required to maintain vascular smooth muscle contraction. So in absence of adequate blood flow there is also inadequate O_2 supply to those vascular smooth muscle. This causes opening of precapillary sphincters and meta arterioles to result vasodilatation and thus blood flow is increased. The opposite effect occurs due to rise of blood flow.

b. Myogenic Theory: The blood vessels of some organs especially the vital organs has got intrinsic capacity to maintain the perfusion pressure at constant level even during alteration of blood flow to that organ. This is due to inherent myogenic activity of **pacemaker cells in the smooth muscle** of blood vessels which maintains a ***basal myogenic tone*** (BMT). By altering this tone there is alteration of diameter of the blood vessels and thus blood flow / perfusion pressure to that organ is maintained at almost normal level. This is known as **Myogenic theory**. The details of this process is as follows:

Increase in blood flow to the organ through the blood vessels → offers stretch to the pacemaker cell of the smooth muscle cell of blood vessels → stimulation of pacemaker cell → contraction of the smooth muscle cell of blood vessels to increase vascular resistance → reduction of blood flow to normal level. The opposite effect takes place when there is decrease of blood flow.

60. Arterial pulse:

- The arterial pulse is defined as the rhythmic expansion of the arterial wall due to transmission of pressure waves along the walls of the arteries during ventricular ejection of blood to aorta.
- Normally it is same as heart rate i.e. 60-90 times /min.
- Aortic pressure changes can be studied from any of the peripheral arteries like, radial, carotid etc. which is known as ***arterial pulse***. The arterial pulse if recorded is known as arterial pulse tracing which is represented by (Fig. 4.3). This arterial pulse consists of following waves:
  - **Percussion (P) wave:** It is due to ejection of blood into aorta during ventricular systole.
  - **Tidal (t) wave:** This wave is occasionally seen which is due to elastic recoil of wall of aorta.
  - **Dicortic (d) wave:** This is due to fall of pressure due to passage of blood to peripheral vessels during ventricular diastole after closure of aortic valve as indicated by a notch known as ***dicortic notch (n)***.
- **Clinical significance arterial pulse:** The rate, rhythm, character, volume and symmetry of arterial pulse and condition of the arterial wall gives idea about many cardio vascular disease. For example; the regularly irregular rhythm of heart beat indicates *Sinus arrhythmia* and irregularly irregular rhythm is seen in *atrial fibrillation.*

61. Jugular venous pulse:

- Atrial pressure changes can be recorded from external jugular vein which is directly connected to the atria. Such a record is known as ***Jugular venous pulse*** (JVP) as illustrated in (Fig. 4.2).
- In this JVP record following waves are seen:

  (a) **'a' (atrial) wave:** This is due to increase in intra atrial pressure during atrial systole.

  (b) **'c' wave:** This is again due to increase in intra atrial pressure due to bulging of tricuspid valves toward atria during ventricular systole.

  (c) **'v' wave:** This is due to passive rise of pressure due to venous return.

  (d) **'X' descents:** This is due to fall of intra atrial pressure due to descent of the tricuspid valves.

  (e) **'Y' descents:** This decline in atrial pressure is due to the opening of tricuspid valve to result ventricular filling.
- ***Clinical significance of JVP***: The normal upper limit where jugular venous pulse is seen is 4 cm vertically above the sternal angle and corresponds to pressure of 6 mm Hg. Elevation of the jugular venous pressure indicates elevation of the right atrial pressure indicating cardiac abnormalities like congestive heart failure, pulmonary embolism, tamponade, superior vena cava obstruction, right ventricular infarction etc.

62. Triple response:

- If the skin is stroked lightly with a sharp object the line of stroke shows a white streak which is known as white reaction whereas if a stronger stimulation is applied on the skin a three phased response is seen which is known as tripple response of Lewis.

- The phases are:
  - Red reaction: It is the redness to the injured site due to capillary dilatation which lasts for about 10 sec.
  - Whale: Local edema formation due to increased permeability of the capillaries and post capillary venules.
  - Flare: Spreading out of redness from the site of injury to the surroundings due to arteriolar dilatation resulted due to activation of axon reflex.

C. Differentiate between:

A-V valves	Semilunar valves
❑ Present in between atria and ventricles.	❑ Present at the openings of systemic aorta and pulmonary artery.
❑ Made up of 3 cusps or 2 cusps.	❑ Made up of always 3 cusps.
❑ It prevents back flow of blood from ventricles to atria.	❑ It prevents back flow of blood from pulmonary artery or aorta to heart.

1st heart sound	2nd heart sound
❑ Produced due to closure of AV valves.	❑ Produced due to closure of semilunar valves.
❑ Marks beginning of ventricular systole.	❑ Marks beginning of ventricular diastole.
❑ Low pitched sound (less than 50 Hz frequency).	❑ High pitched sharp sound (more than 50 Hz frequency).
❑ Continuous sound (LUBB).	❑ Splitted sound (DUB).
❑ Lasts for 0.14 sec to 0.17 sec.	❑ Lasts for 0.1 sec to 0.14 sec.
❑ Audible all over the chest surface though better heard in tricuspid and mitral areas.	❑ Audible all over the chest surface though better heard in aortic and pulmonary areas.
❑ Concides with R wave of ECG.	❑ Concides with end of T wave of ECG.

Lateral pressure	End pressure
❑ Pressure exerted by the blood laterally on the wall of the blood vessels is known as lateral pressure (Fig. 4.21).	❑ When the blood vessel is directly connected to a manometer the pressure exerted on the mercury column is known as End pressure (Fig. 4.21).
❑ It is comparatively less.	❑ It is more due to more kinetic energy.

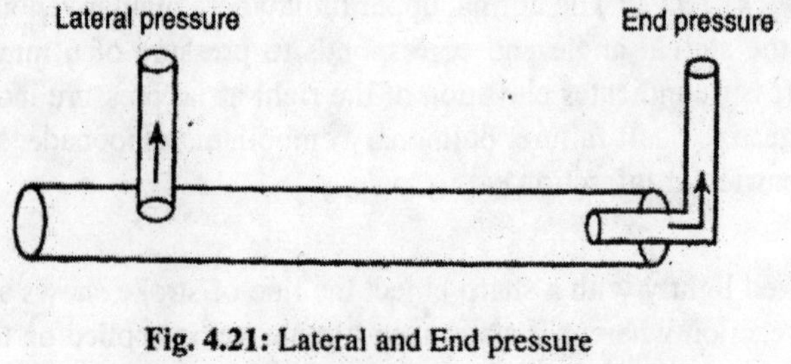

Fig. 4.21: Lateral and End pressure

1st degree heart block	2nd degree heart block
❑ It is characterised by simply prolongation of PR interval in ECG study.	❑ It is characterised by gradual prolongation of PR interval in ECG study.
❑ Successive PR intervals remain constant.	❑ PR intervals successively increases and thus do not remain constant.
❑ No missing of ventricular beat.	❑ Occasional missing of ventricular beat.

Incomplete heart block	Complete heart block
❑ Transmission of impulse from atria to ventricle is slowed down but not blocked completely.	❑ Impulse does not reach from SA node to ventricle due to blockade in between.
❑ Rhythm of heart beat is mostly regular and sometimes regularly irregular (2:1 or 3:1).	❑ No rhythm of heart beat i.e. idioventricular rhythm.
❑ Blood pressure remains normal.	❑ Blood pressure falls.
❑ Stokes—Adams syndrome does not occur.	❑ Stokes—Adams syndrome is common.

Sick sinus syndrome	Stokes—Adams syndrome
❑ It is characterised by dizziness and unconsciousness.	❑ It is characterised by periodic fainting and consciousness.
❑ It is due to sinus bradycardia.	❑ It is due to complete heart block.
❑ In this case the ECG remains normal.	❑ No rhythm in ECG.

Laminar blood flow	Turbulent blood flow
❑ It is the fixed layer wise flow.	❑ In this case blood flows cross wise in the vessels by forming whorls in the blood.
❑ It is seen in the normal vessels.	❑ It is seen when vessels are occluded or take sudden 'U' turn.
❑ No sound is produced in this type of flow.	❑ Sound is produced in this type of flow.
❑ It occurs only at velocities upto a critical level.	❑ It occurs when the velocities of blood flow increases above the critical level.

Arterial baroreceptor	Cardiac baroreceptor
❑ These are located in the adventitial layer of wall of large systemic arteries.	❑ These are located in the wall of heart.
❑ It is usually sensitive to high pressure.	❑ It is usually sensitive to low pressure or chemicals.

Vis-a-tergo	Vis-a-fronte
❑ Due to left ventricular contraction and ejection, the blood in the aorta and rest of the arterial system is pushed from behind to move forward which is known as Vis-a-tergo.	❑ Because of suction effect of respiratory pump and ventricular contraction, the venous blood is drawn towards the heart which is known as Vis-a-fronte.

Systemic circulation	Pulmonary circulation
❑ The blood flow from left ventricle to the various regions of the body through arteries and return of venous blood from various parts of the body through veins to right auricle is known as ***Systemic circulation.*** ❑ It is known as greater circulation. ❑ Blood is deoxygenated.	❑ The blood flow from right ventricle to lungs through the pulmonary artery and return of blood through pulmonary veins into left auricle is called ***pulmonary circulation.*** ❑ It is known as lesser circulation. ❑ Blood is oxygenated.

Extrinsic regulation of cardiac output	Intrinsic regulation of cardiac output
❑ In this case cardiac output is regulated through heart rate. ❑ It is dependent to cardiac innervation.	❑ In this case cardiac output is regulated through stroke volume. ❑ It is not fully dependent to cardiac innervation (by changing the EDFL mainly).

Heterometric Regulation	Homometric regulation
❑ Change of myocardial contractility is directly related with EDFL. ❑ It is independent to cardiac innervation.	❑ Change of myocardial contractility does nor vary with EDFL. ❑ It is dependent to cardiac innervation.

Primary hypertension	Secondary hypertension
❑ It is of unknown origin. ❑ It is mainly due to hereditary factors and psychological factors.	❑ It is of known origin. ❑ It is mainly due to organal defects.

Benign hypertension	Malignant hypertension
❑ In this situation the systolic blood pressure rises upto 200 mm Hg and diastolic pressure rises upto 100 mm Hg. ❑ It is less fatal.	❑ In this situation the systolic blood pressure rises above 250 mm Hg and diastolic pressure rises above 150 mm Hg. ❑ It is highly fatal.

Action of epinephrine in heart	Action of nor-epinephrine in heart
❑ It stimulates heart through beta receptor.	❑ It can not stimulate heart due to weak beta receptor activation.
❑ Peripheral resistance and DP remains normal or falls slightly due to stimulation of both alpha and beta receptor.	❑ Peripheral resistance and DP increase due to predominant stimulation of alpha receptor.
❑ Stroke volume and heart rate are increased due to direct stimulation on heart.	❑ Stroke volume and heart rate decrease due to reflex inhibition of sympathetic discharge produced due to high DP.

Peripheral chemoreceptors	Central chemoreceptors
❑ These are located near bifurcation at the carotid artery. ❑ These are stimulated by hypoxia. ❑ These are stimulated by PCO_2, pH and PO_2 of blood.	❑ These are located at ventral surface of medulla. ❑ These are inhibited by hypoxia. ❑ These are stimulated by PCO_2 and pH of blood and cerebral interstitial fluid.

D. Brainstorming short answer type:

1. Explain why anemia is associated with increased cardiac output?

Anemia → tissue hypoxia → vasodilatation → increase in venous return → increase in diastolic filling → increase in cardiac output as per as Starling's law of heart.

2. What is high and low cardiac output heart failure?

In the situation (e.g. thyrotoxicosis, wet beriberi) when, even the increased cardiac output is inadequate to provide tissue perfusion, it is known as high cardiac output failure. Whereas, when the heart failure is resulted due to low cardiac output because of decreased ventricular filling is known as low cardiac output failure.

3. What are salient clinical features of cardiac failure?

These are:

- Cardiomegaly resulted due to increased diastolic filling
- Prolonged circulation time due to ineffective cardiac pumping
- Pulmonary congestion
- Hepatomegally due to increased central venous pressure that leads to rise in pressure in hepatic portal vein
- Increase in JVP
- Edema and dysponea

4. What is plasma skimming?

Because of the cell free zone in the periphery of flowing blood vessels, that originate from the main blood vessels at a large angle, carries more plasma than cells. This phenomenon is called as plasma

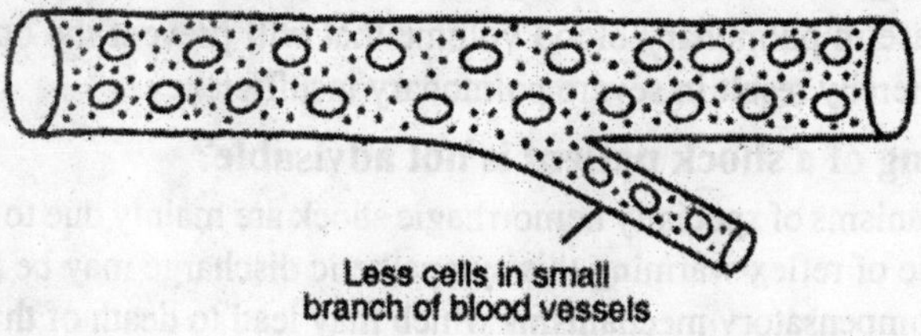

Fig. 4.22: Plasma skimming

skimming (Fig. 4.22). This is why the hematocrit of capillary blood is about 25% higher than the whole body hematocrit.

5. What are the arterio-venous shunts and where are they found?

These are the short channels that connect arterioles to venules bypassing the capillaries. These are present in the finger, pulms and ear lobes.

6. What are the cardiovascular changes associated with isometric exercise?

These are:

- Both heart rate and stroke volume increases but increase in stroke volume is much less as vagal inhibition is the major means of cardiac change.
- Systolic and diastolic BP increase sharply.
- Skeletal muscle blood flow is grossly reduced due to mechanical vasocompression.

7. Why shock patients are kept in cold room inspite of hypothermia?

Vide answer of question no.15

8. What are cardiovascular changes associated with a change of posture from lying to standing?

Immediately after standing there is fall in systolic BP by 20 mmHg due to venous pulling of blood in lower limbs due to gravitional effect though after few minutes it becomes to normal or mildly elevated due to baroreceptor mechanism.

9. Why the thin walled and delicate capillaries are less prone to rupture?

As per the law of Laplace the smaller the radius of the blood vessels lesser the tension in the wall necessary to balance the distending pressure. This is the reason because of which the minute, thin wall capillaries and delicate capillaries are less prone for rupture.

10. Give the functions of papillary muscles. What will happen if they get paralysed?

During ventricular contraction papillary muscles also contract and thus prevent the bulging of A-V valve into the atria. If these muscles are get paralysed the A-V valves tend to bulge backward resulting regurgitation of blood into the atria during ventricular systole.

11. Why heart sounds are not produced during opening of valves?

It is because of slow process which can not produce any noise.

12. How many extrasystoles / min are regarded as normal?

It is 2-4/ min

13. What will happen if nitric oxide deficiency occurs in the blood vessels?

It is associated with hypertension as it is helpful in relaxation of vascular smooth muscle.

14. What will happen if right ventricular output exceeds left ventricular output?

This will result in increase in pulmonary blood volume that will prevent the optimal exchange of gases across the lungs and thereby result in severe pulmonary insufficiency.

15. Why is reflex warming of a shock patient is not advisable?

The compensatory mechanisms of specially hemorrhagic shock are mainly due to the increased sympathetic discharge. So in case of reflex warming this sympathetic discharge may be abolished resulting failure of initiation of any compensatory mechanisms which may lead to death of that person.

16. How are lung alveoli kept dry?

Pulmonary capillary hydrostatic pressure is 8-10 mmHg whereas the plasma colloidal osmotic pressure is of 25 mmHg. This inwardly directed pressure gradient (15-17 mmHg) keeps the alveoli dry.

E. MCQ:

1. Pericardial fluid is present between (i) Endocardium and Myocardium (ii) Myocardium and Pericardium (iii) Pericardial and visceral layer of pericardium (iv) All of the above. (iii)
2. Pericardial fluid has following function (i) lubrication (ii) shock absorver (iii) all of the above (iv) none. (iii)
3. The cardiac pacemaker is (i) SA node (ii) AV node (iii) Bundle of His (iv) all of the above. (i)
4. Idioventricular rhythm is demonstrated in following experimental condition (i) by applying 1st Stannius ligature (ii) by applying 2nd Stannius ligature (iii) by applying both (iv) none of the above. (ii)
5. Windkessel effect is seen in (i) veins (ii) capillaries (iii) venules (iv) arteries. (iv)

6. The maximum gaseous exchange takes place through (i) arteries (ii) veins (iii) capillaries (iv) venules. (iii)
7. In cardiac muscle T tubule invaginates at (i) A band (ii) Z line (iii) M line (iv) A-I junction. (ii)
8. The RMP of pacemaker cell is (i) –50 mv (ii) –70 mv (iii) –90 mv (iv) 0 mv. (i)
9. The plateau phase of cardiac action potential is due to (i) influx of Na^+ (ii) efflux of K^+ (iii) efflux of Na^+ (iv) influx of Ca^{++}. (iv)
10. The total duration of action potential in cardiac muscle is approx (i) 250 m sec (ii) 120 m sec. (iii) 5 sec. (iv) 500 m sec. (i)
11. All or none law is applicable in all the cases except (i) a single skeletal muscle fiber (ii) a single cardiac muscle fiber (iii) a single nerve fiber (iv) none of the above. (ii)
12. At the AV node the AV delay is (i) 0.1 sec (ii) 0.1 ms (iii) 10 ms (iv) 10 s. (i)
13. The normal coronary blood flow is (i) 500 ml / min (ii) 5 L/min (iii) 225 ml/min (iv) 25 ml/min. (iii)
14. In case of angina pectoris the pain sensation is felt in the followings except (i) upper sternum (ii) epigastric region (iii) left shoulder (iv) left forearm. (ii)
15. Stokes-Adams syndrome is due to blockade of impulse in (i) SA node (ii) AV node (iii) internode (iv) Bundle of His. (ii)
16. The peak pressure in right ventricle during systole is (i) 120 mmHg (ii) 25 mmHg (iii) 50 mmHg (iv) 5 mmHg. (ii)
17. The minimum pressure in left ventricle during diastole (i) 80 mmHg (ii) 8 mmHg (iii) 40 mmHg (iv) 20 mmHg. (ii)
18. The peak pressure in right auricle during systole is (i) 6 mmHg (ii) 60 mmHg (iii) 16 mmHg (iv) 30 mmHg. (i)
19. The normal stroke volume is (i) 120 ml (ii) 50 ml (iii) 12 ml (iv) 70 ml (iv)
20. All are the waves seen in JVP except (i) P (ii) c (iii) v (iv) X. (i)
21. Normal duration of QRS complex is (i) 0.08s (ii) 0.8s (iii) 0.05s (iv) 0.15s. (i)
22. Normal duration of PR interval is (i) 0.012s (ii) 1.12s (iii) 0.12s (iv) 0.4s. (iii)
23. Normal duration of ST interval is (i) 0.4s (ii) 0.04s (iii) 0.035s (iv) 0.3s. (iv)
24. Following is not considered as buffer nerve for CVC regulation. (i) Hering's nerve (ii) sympathetic nerve (iii) aortic nerve (iv) vagus neve. (ii)
25. Following are the examples of baroreceptors except (i) Carotid sinus (ii) Aortic arch (iii) Atrio caval receptors (iv) Carotid body. (iv)
26. Following physiological factor do not affect cardiac output (i) pregnancy (ii) depression (iii) muscular exercise (iv) hypoxia. (iv)
27. Periperal resistance does not depend on (i) velocity (ii) viscosity of blood (iii) stroke volume (iv) volume of blood in arterial system. (iii)
28. All are the characteristics feature of hypokalaemia except (i) Tall and peaked T wave (ii) ST depression (iii) prominent U wave (iv) T wave inversion. (i)
29. WPW syndrome is due to faster conduction of impulse through following internodal pathway (i) Anterior Buchman's bundle (ii) Middle Buchman's bundle (ii) Posterior Buchman's bundle (iv) Bundle of Kent. (iv)
30. His Bundle electrogram does not constitute following wave (i) A deflection (ii) H deflection (iii) P deflection (iv) V deflection. (iii)
31. Diminution of 1st heart sound occurs in following cases except (i) shock (ii) anemia (iii) acute myocardial infarction (iv) pericardial effusion. (ii)

32. Normal ejection fraction is (i) 65% (ii) 80% (iii) 45% (iv) 75%. (i)

33. Normal cardiac reserve is (i) 15-25 L/min (ii) 30-40 L/min (iii) 15-25 ml/min (iv) 30-40 ml/min. (i)

34. Normal end systolic volume is (i) 70 ml (ii) 50 ml (iii) 100 ml (iv) 5 lit. (ii)

35. Normal cardiac index is (i) 4.5 L (ii) 8.2 L (iii) 3.2 L (iv) 5.4 L. (iii)

36. The dye used to determine cardiac output by dye dilution method is usually (i) radioactive inulin (ii) radioactive iodine (iii) Evan's blue (iv) tritium oxide. (iii)

37. Following hormone do not have any role in regulating cardiac output (i) insulin (ii) glucagon (iii) thyroxine (iv) oxytocin. (iv)

38. Venous return does not normally depend on following activity (i) atrial pump (ii) skeletal muscle pump (iii) thoracic pump (iv) abdominal pump. (i)

39. Vagal stimulation decreases cardiac output mainly by (i) decreasing cardiac contractility i.e. Stroke volume (ii) decreasing heart rate (iii) both (iv) none. (ii)

40. Afterload depends primarily on (i) vessel diameter (ii) viscosity of blood (iii) both (iv) none. (iii)

41. Pulse pressure is high in (i) arterioles (ii) capillaries (iii) veins (iv) aorta. (iv)

42. Normal central venous pressure is (i) 5 mmHg (ii) 10 mmHg (iii) –5 mmHg (iv) 50 mmHg. (i)

43. Preload is determined by (i) stroke volume (ii) end diastolic volume (iii) cardiac output (iv) all of them. (ii)

44. Following factors are positively inotropic except (i) sympathetic stimulation (ii) parasympathetic stimulation (iii) glucagon (iv) caffeine. (ii)

45. Vasomotor center receives inputs from (i) aortic and carotid baroreceptors (ii) carotid and aortic chemoreceptors (iii) both (iv) none. (iii)

46. Sino-aortic reflex basically is (i) baroreceptors reflex (ii) chemoreceptor reflex (iii) both (iv) none. (i)

47. The rate of O_2 consumption of heart is (i) 5.5 ml/100 gm of tissue (ii) 15.8 ml /100 gm of tissue (iii) 9.7 ml/100 gm of tissue (iv) 0.5 ml/100 gm of tissue. (iii)

48. Autoregulation of coronary blood flow occurs in the range of blood pressure which is about (i) 50-60 mmHg (ii) 120-140 mmHg (iii) 20-40 mmHg (iv) 70-110 mmHg. (iv)

49. All are the components of triple response except one (i) white reaction (ii) red reaction (iii) whale (iv) flare. (i)

50. Following is not the feature of hemorrhagic shock (i) hypotension (ii) bradycardia (iii) rapid and thready pulse (iv) thirst sensation. (ii)

51. High cardiac output failure is seen in following cases except (i) severe anemia (ii) Paget's disease (iii) hyperthyroidism (iv) myocardial infarction. (iv)

Respiration

5

A. Long type:1

1. Define mechanics of breathing. Explain the sequence of events take place during normal inspiration and expiration with special reference to pump handle and bucket handle movements of thoracic ribs and diaphragm.

The 1st step of respiration is **ventilation** in which exchange of gases takes place in between atmosphere and lungs by **bulk flow** from a region of high pressure to the region of low pressure. The **bulk flow** in case of lung can be determined by the following formula:

$$F = \frac{P_{atm} - P_{alv}}{R}$$

Where F = bulk flow, P_{atm} = atmospheric pressure, and P_{alv} = alveolar pressure

So when $\mathbf{P_{atm}}$ becomes more than $\mathbf{P_{alv}}$ then there is inward flow of air and when $\mathbf{P_{atm} < P_{alv}}$ then there is outward flow of air from lungs. This increase or decrease of intra alveolar air pressure is controlled by decreasing and increasing the volume of lungs which inturn is controlled by the movements of thoracic cage. This mechanical event is called as ***Mechanics of breathing***.

***Mechanism of quiet (Tidal) breathing (Normal respiration)*:** During tidal respiration expansion of the thoracic cavity during the phase of inspiration is mainly (90%) due to movement of diaphragm and partly due to movement of thoracic cage. This movement of diaphragm and thoracic cage during inspiration and expiration which results the gaseous exchange in between atmosphere and alveoli is a follows:

(a) Inspiration: Inspiration is initiated by:

(i) **Contraction of diaphragm,** *which draws* the central tendinous portion of diaphragm downward (Fig. 5.1) thereby increasing the vertical diameter of the thoracic cage.

(ii) **Contraction of external intercostal muscles of 2nd to 6th thoracic ribs** which causes

- Elevation of these ribs and also upward and forward movement of sternum (*Pump handle movement*) to increase antero-posterior diameter of the thoracic cage (Fig. 5.1).

- Upward and outward movements of the central part of these ribs which increases transverse diameter of the thoracic cage (*Bucket handle movement*).

(iii) **Contraction of external intercostal muscle of lower costal series (7th to 10th thoracic ribs),** which swings outward and upward to increase transverse diameter (***Bucket handle movement***) of the thoracic cage (Fig. 5.1).

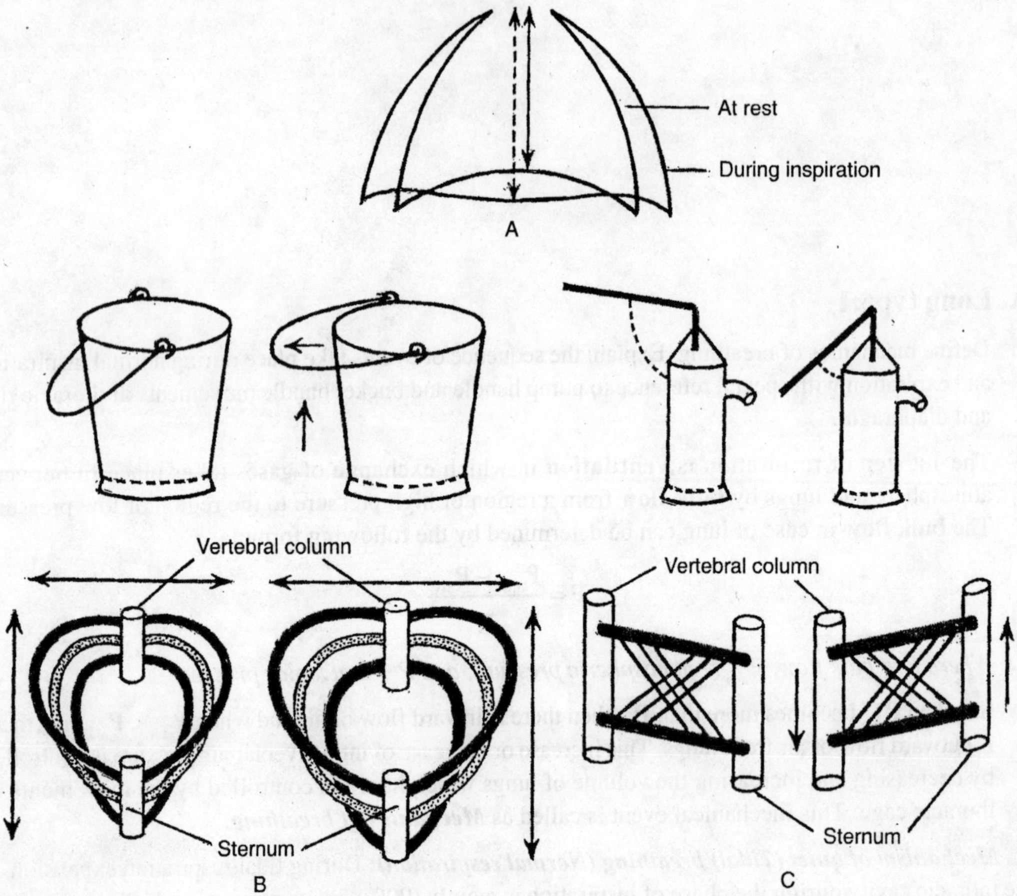

Fig. 5.1: Diagrammatic representation of diaphragm movement during inspiration (A), and ribs movements (B. *Bucket handle movement* and C. *Pump handle movement*)

Thus the increases of all three diameters of the thorax is responsible for increase of negative pressure in the thoracic cavity resulting expansion of the lungs and thus the pressure within the alveoli falls below the atmospheric pressure that causes the flow of air into the alveolus. The above mechanism is explained by the help of block diagram (Fig. FC 5A).

(b) Expiration: Expiration during tidal breathing is completely due to relaxation of the inspiratory muscles (i.e. passive process) because of which thoracic cage goes back to it's original position which inturn results compression of the lungs and thereby decrease in intra alveolar pressure. Rise of P_{alv} beyond P_{atm} causes the air to move out of lungs.

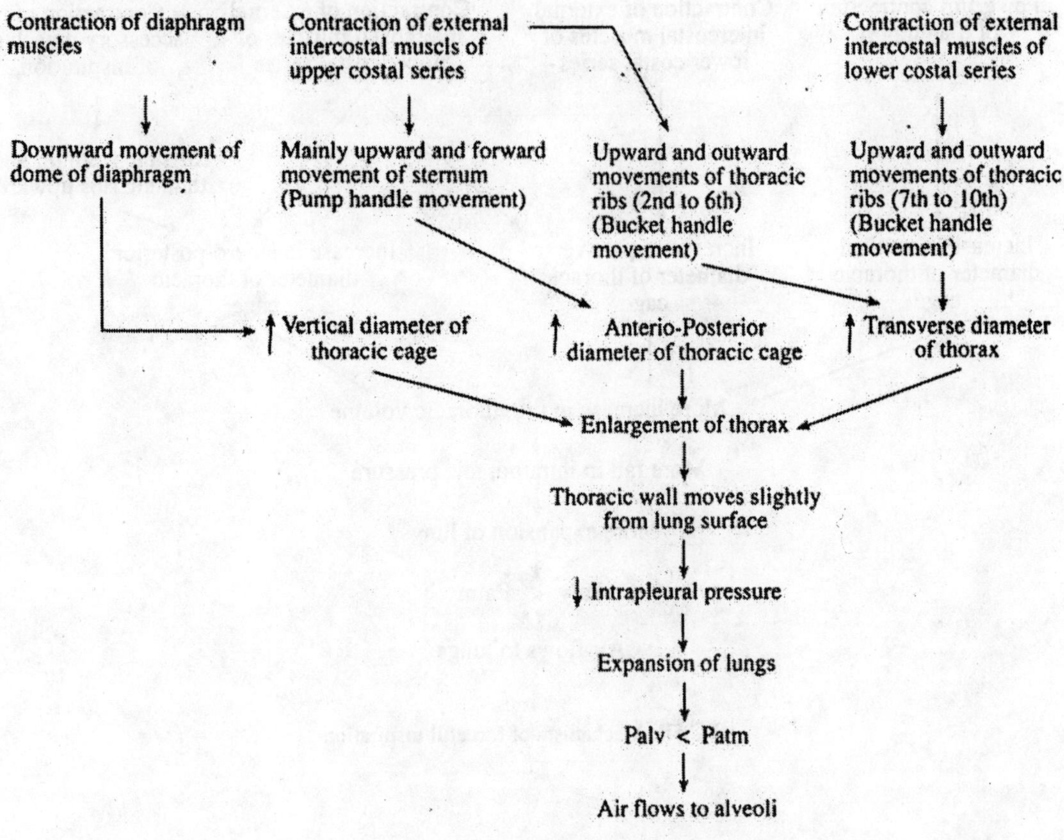

FC 5A: Mechanism of tidal respiration

2. Is the expiration active process? Briefly discuss the mechanism of forceful breathing during exercise.

Normal expiration is passive process as it does not require energy. It requires only relaxation of inspiratory muscles. But the forceful expiration is active process as during this involvement of additional expiratory muscles like internal intercostal muscles and abdominal muscles are required to bring the thoracic cage downward. The detail mechanism of forceful respiration is illustrated by flow chart as follows:

(a) Forceful inspiration: The detail mechanism is illustrated in flow chart (FC 5B).

(b) Forceful expiration: It is also the active process which is more powerful than quite expiration. The mechanism is described in flow chart (FC 5C).

3. In which form O_2 is transported from lungs to tissues? What is O_2 dissociation curve? Enumerate the factors affecting O_2 dissociation curve. What do you mean by Bohr's effect?

The forms in which O_2 is carried in the blood:

The O_2 in venous blood is transported from lungs to the tissues via heart in two forms:

(a) In dissolved form:

- Small amount of O_2 (0.3%) is carried in simple physical solution in plasma and water of RBC.

Powerfull contraction of diaphragm → Increase in vertical diameter of thoracic cage

Contraction of external intercostal muscles of lower costal series → Increase in transverse diameter of thoracic cage

Contraction of external intercostal muscles of upper costal series → Increase in transverse diameter of thoracic cage; Increase in antero-posterior diameter of thoracic cage

Contraction of accessory muscles of inspiration → Lifts the sternum and thoracic ribs upward → Increase in antero-posterior diameter of thoracic cage

↓

More increase in intrathoracic volume

↓

More fall in intrathoracic pressure

↓

More expansion of lungs

↓

Palv < Patm

↓

Air flows to lungs

FC 5B: Mechanism of forceful inspiration

Diaphragm relaxes → Dome moves upward into thoracic cavity

Abdominal muscles contract → Forced dome to move further upward

External intercostal muscles relax → Downward and inward movements of ribs

Internal intercostal muscles relax; Other accessory muscles of inspiration relax → Forced further downward and inward movements of ribs and sternum

↓

More decrease in thoracic volume

↓

More increase in intrapleural pressure

↓

More lung compression

↓

Palv > Patm

↓

Airflows out of alveoli

FC 5C: Mechanism of forceful expiration

- It's volume is 0.3 ml/100ml of blood/100 mmHg PO_2.
- The amount of O_2 dissolved in blood is directly proportional to the PO_2 of blood. It is known as **Henry's law.**
- Though the amount of O_2 transported through plasma is small in quantity it has utmost importance as partial pressure of O_2 in blood, which determines the amount of O_2 transported by hemoglobin, is determined by the dissolved O_2.

(b) **In combination with Hemoglobin (Hb):**

- O_2 combines with heme portions of hemoglobin in stepwise manner as follows to form oxyhemoglobin.

  (i) $Hb_4 + O_2 = Hb_4O_2$

  (ii) $Hb_4O_2 + O_2 = Hb_4O_4$

  (iii) $Hb_4O_4 + O_2 = Hb_4O_6$

  (iv) $Hb_4O_6 + O_2 = Hb_4O_8$

  This oxyhemoglobin is loose and reversible form and it's formation is dependent on partial pressure of O_2 i.e. in pulmonary capillaries as PO_2 is high O_2 binds with hemoglobin to form ***oxyhemoglobin*** whereas in tissue as PO_2 is low, the O_2 is released from oxyhemoglobin.

- One gram of Hb can combine with 1.34 ml of O_2 and at this stage Hb is considered as 100% saturated. Thus a person having Hb concentration of 15 mg% the 100 ml of his blood can carry $1.34 \times 15 = 20$ ml of O_2 at full saturation which is known as ***O_2 carrying capacity of blood.***

O_2 dissociation curve: Upto a limit the progressive increase of PO_2 causes the progressive increase of percentage of hemoglobin that binds with O_2 (Fig. 5.2). This is known as oxyhemoglobin dissociation curve.

Factors affecting the oxyhemoglobin dissociation curve: Different factors increase the affinity of hemoglobin for O_2 (Fig. 5.2) causing less release of O_2 in tissue and more uptake of O_2 in lungs which is known as ***Shift to the left.*** Similarly some other factors decrease the affinity of hemoglobin for O_2 (Fig. 5.2) causing more release of O_2 in tissue which is known a ***Shift to the right***.

(i) *The factors responsible for shifting of O_2 dissociation curve to the left*:

- ❑ **Decreased PCO_2 of blood:** Decrease in PCO_2 of blood causes the increase in affinity of Hb for O_2 resulting more uptake of O_2 in lungs and less release of O_2 in tissues.
- ❑ **Decreased H^+ concentration** in blood or increase pH of blood.
- ❑ **Decreased body temperature.**

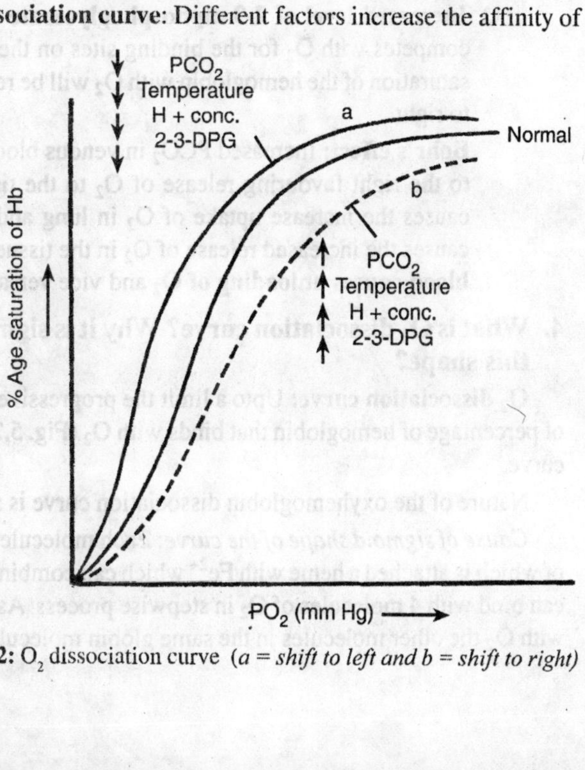

Fig. 5.2: O_2 dissociation curve *(a = shift to left and b = shift to right)*

- **Presence of carbon monoxide** shifts the curve to the left because of inhibition of 2-3 DPG formation. Though the uptake of O_2 by hemoglobin is not increased but decreased due to formation of more carboxy hemoglobin which has more affinity to bind with hemoglobin – i.e.

↑ PCO → inhibition of 2-3 DPG → More affinity of O_2 with Hb in tissue level

↓ (from inhibition of 2-3 DPG) More affinity of CO to bind with Hb

↓ More formation of carboxy-Hb

↓ unavailibility of Hb for O_2 carriage

↓ Less O_2 uptake

↓ (from More affinity of O_2 with Hb in tissue level) less O_2 release in tissue

- **Presence of fetal hemoglobin** (HbF) shifts the curve to the left because of less affinity of HbF for 2-3 DPG.

(ii) *Factors responsible for shifting of O_2-dissociation curve to the right*:

- **Increased PCO_2**—Increased PCO_2 in venous blood at tissue level shifts the O_2 - dissociation curve to the right favouring release of O_2 to the tissues. Thus reduced venous PCO_2 in the lungs causes the increase uptake of O_2 in lung and increased venous PCO_2 in the tissue capillary causes the increase release of O_2 in the tissue. This phenomenon in which **loading of CO_2 to blood causes unloading of O_2** and vice versa is known as ***Bohr's effect.***
- **Decreased pH of blood**
- **Increased temperature**
- **Increased level of 2-3 diphosphoglycerate** (2-3-DPG)—It is a product of glycolysis which competes with O_2 for the binding sites on the hemoglobin and thus at a given PO_2 the % age saturation of the hemoglobin with O_2 will be reduced in the presence of 2-3-DPG resulting shift to right.

  Bohr's effect: Increased PCO_2 in venous blood at tissue level shifts the O_2-dissociation curve to the right favouring release of O_2 to the tissues. Thus reduced venous PCO_2 in the lungs causes the increase uptake of O_2 in lung and increased venous PCO_2 in the tissue capillary causes the increased release of O_2 in the tissue. This phenomenon in which **loading of CO_2 to blood causes unloading of O_2** and vice versa is known as ***Bohr's effect.***

4. What is O_2 dissociation curve? Why it is sigmoid in shape? What are the advantages of this shape?

O_2 dissociation curve: Upto a limit the progressive increase of PO_2 causes the progressive increase of percentage of hemoglobin that binds with O_2 (Fig. 5.2). This is known as oxyhemoglobin dissociation curve.

Nature of the oxyhemoglobin dissociation curve is **sigmoid** i.e. 'S' shaped.

Cause of sigmoid shape of the curve: Each molecule of globin consists of 4 polypeptide chain to each of which is attached a heme with Fe^{2+} which can combine with one molecule of O_2. Thus one hemoglobin can bind with 4 molecules of O_2 in stepwise process. As soon as one of the molecules of heme combines with O_2 the other molecules in the same globin molecules acquires a great affinity for O_2 in steps. So O_2

rapidly combines with Fe^{2+} present in it. This is called as ***allosteric activation*** or ***allosteric modulation***. Thus the 'S' shape of this curve is due to shifting affinity of hemoglobin for O_2. The detail mechanism of allosteric medulation is as follows:

In deoxyhemoglobin, the iron atom is about 0.4 Å out of the porphyrin plane towards the proximal histidine. On oxygenation the iron atom moves into the plane of the porphyryin to form a strong bond with O_2 and the heme becomes more planner. Thus the iron atom pulls the proximal histidine with it when it moves into the plane of the porphyrin. This movement of histidine will ultimately cause the conformational change and there is the rupture of interchain salt bridges to switch the protein to the 'R' form. Thus a structural changes (oxygenation) within a subunit is translated into structural changes between other subunits. The binding of O_2 at one heme site is thereby communicated to parts of the molecule that are far away. This mechanism is called as ***allosteric modulation*** which can be further explained by the help of two models:

(i) Sequential model: In deoxyhemoglobin, Hb is in the T_4 state. The binding of O_2 to one of the subunits changes it's conformation from 'T' to 'R' but leaves then other subunits in the 'T' form. The O_2 binding affinity of unoccupied sites in RT_3 is higher than in T_4 because some salt bridges have been broken on binding the first O_2. So 2nd molecule of O_2 binds with 2nd subunit in a greater affinity to form R_2T_2 and thereby broke some salt bridges again. So R_2T_2 has greater affinity to O_2 than RT_3 and binds O_2 with greater affinity to form R_3T and ultimately R_4.

This model can be explained in terms of postage stamp analogy where two perforated edges must be torn to remove the 1st stamp and then one perforated edge must be torn to remove the 2nd and 3rd stamp and ultimately the 4th stamp will be free automatically.

(ii) Concerted or MWC model: According to this model all the subunits of a particular molecule must be in the 'T' form or 'R' form, hybrids e.g. TR are forbidden and ligands bind with low affinity to the T form and with high affinity to the R form. The binding of each ligand increases the probability that all subunits in that molecule are in the R form and thereby affinity of R form to O_2 is increased.

Advantage (physiological significance) of the sigmoid shape of O_2 dissociation curve:

(a) O_2 dissociation curve has the plateau above 60 mmHg. This flat upper part indicates that even if the PO_2 increases from 60 mmHg to 300 mmHg, the O_2 content of the blood will not vary significantly. Similarly the effect of O_2 lack on the body will not be manifested until the PO_2 goes down below 60 mmHg.

(b) The steep slope of the curve indicates that the slight decrease of PO_2 will cause greater release of O_2 from hemoglobin at the tissue level.

5. How does CO_2 is transported in blood? What is CO_2 dissociation curve?

CO_2 formed by the metabolic activity of the cell is taken up by the blood and transported to the lungs from where it is expelled out in the air. The CO_2 transport by the blood is described in following headings:

A. The uptake of CO_2 from the tissues:

In the arterial blood the PCO_2 is 40 mmHg and volume of CO_2 is 48% whereas in the venous blood the PCO_2 in 46 mmHg and volume is 52 ml%. Thus 4 ml (52-48) of CO_2 is transported from tissues to lungs by 100 ml of blood due to the pressure difference of CO_2.

B. Various forms in which CO_2 is transported: CO_2 is transported by the blood in mainly 3 forms:

(i) **Dissolved form (7%):**

- CO_2 diffuses into blood and dissolves in the plasma and water of RBC. In this form only 0.3 ml of CO_2 is transported per 100 ml of blood from tissues to lungs.

- Any rise of PCO_2 causes the rise of CO_2 in dissolved form in plasma which is known as **Henry's Law.**

(ii) In bicarbonate form (70%):

- Maximum amount of CO_2 (3 ml per 100 ml of blood) is transported from tissues to lungs in this form.
- The CO_2 enters in the blood of tissue capillary and reacts with water to form carbonic acid by the enzyme **Carbonic anhydrase which is rapidly ionised to form H^+ and HCO_3^- as follows:**

$$CO_2 + H_2O = H_2CO_3 = H^+ + HCO_3^-$$

H^+ formed in this reaction are buffered by plasma proteins and hemoglobin leading increased of HCO_3^- concentration inside the red cell as compared to that in plasma. Therefore HCO_3^- diffuses from RBC to plasma. As HCO_3^- is a negatively charged particles and the RBC membrane is relatively impermeable to cation the negatively charged Cl^- diffuses from plasma to RBC to maintain electrical neutrality. This phenomenon is called *Chloride Shift* or *Hamberger phenomenon* (Fig. 5.3). The reversal of this reaction occurs in blood of pulmonary capillaries i.e. When the blood reaches the alveoli → dissociation of $NaHCO_3$ in the plasma to form Na^+ and HCO_3^- → Bicarbonate moves in RBC to be reconverted back into CO_2 which is expelled out → Cl^- moves out of RBC to maintain electrical neutrality. This reversal of the reaction that takes place in lung capillaries is known as *reverse chloride shift.*

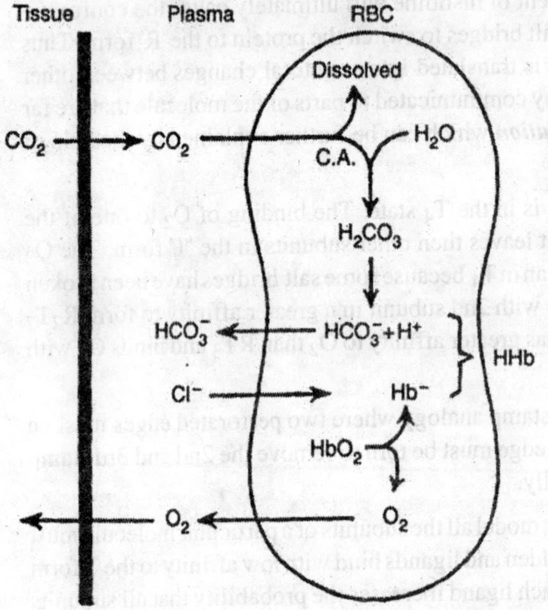

Fig. 5.3: Chloride shift

- Some of the H^+, liberated due to dissociation of H_2CO_3 are bound to reduced Hb in the red cell (i.e. $H^+ + HbO_2 = HHb + O_2$) as reduced Hb is better proton acceptor (less acid) than the oxy-hemoglobin. Thus the presence of reduced Hb in the peripheral blood helps in the loading of CO_2 and the oxygenation which occurs in pulmonary capillary helps in the unloading of CO_2 in the lungs. Thus an increase in CO_2 in the peripheral blood will cause O_2 to be released from oxy-hemoglobin in the tissues and similarly binding of O_2 with Hb in the lung capillaries tends to release CO_2 from the blood in the lung alveoli. This is called ***Haldane effect.***

(iii) As carbamino compounds (23%):

- 0.7 ml per 100 ml of blood of CO_2 is transported from tissues to lungs.
- CO_2 reacts with amino (NH_2) group of the proteins i.e. hemoglobin to form carbamino compounds in which form it is transported to the lungs.

C. The release of CO_2 from the blood in the lungs and it's expulsion:

In the lungs the PCO_2 of venous blood is 46 mmHg and PCO_2 in alveolor air is 40 mmHg. Due to this difference of partial pressure of CO_2, the CO_2 diffuses out from the blood into the alveolar air which is ultimately expelled out of alveolus again due to pressure difference existing in between alveolar air (CO_2) and atmospheric air (CO_2).

CO_2 dissociation curve:

The total quantity of CO_2 that combines with blood depends on PCO_2. If total CO_2 in blood in all forms are plotted against the PCO_2 of blood the curve obtained is called as **CO_2 dissociation curve** (Fig. 5.4).

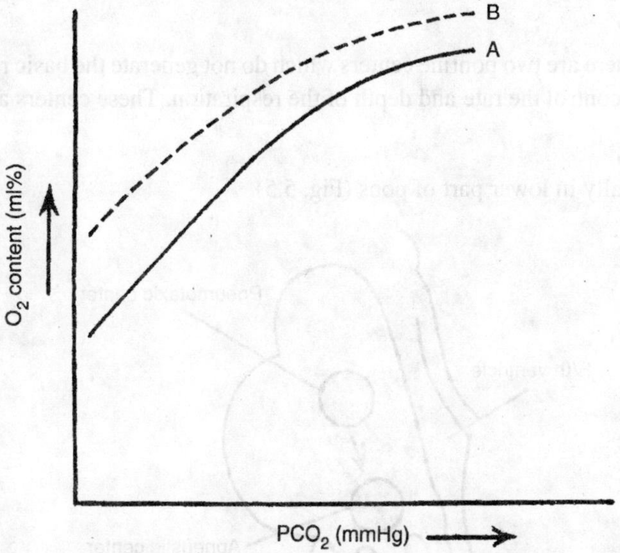

Fig. 5.4: CO_2 dissociation curve for whole blood (*A = oxygenated blood, B = deoxygenated blood*)

Factors affecting CO_2 dissociation curve: The rise of O_2 content in blood causes the shift of the CO_2 dissociation curve to the right resulting more release of CO_2 from Carboxy-hemoglobin.

6. Describe the components of respiratory regulatory mechanisms. Describe the nervous regulation of respiration.

There are 3 basic elements of the respiratory controlling mechanisms as follows:

*A. **Central controller***: The respiratory center is composed of several widely dispersed groups of neurones mainly located bilaterally in the medulla oblangata (**Medullary centers**) and pons (**Pontine centers**).

(a) **Medullary centers:** In the medulla 2 groups of neurones are there which are as follows:

(i) *Dorsal respiratory group (DRG) neurones*: Most of these neurones are located in the dorsal surface (within the nucleus of tractus solitarious and some are in adjacent to reticular substance) of medulla (Fig. 5.5). These neurones normally discharge the repetitive bursts of action potentials which is weak in the beginning and increases steadily for about 2 seconds followed by abrupt cessation of the impulse generation for next 3 secs. This type of signal is known as ***Ramp signal*** or ***Inspiratory ramp***. Because of this signal inspiration starts slowly and then reaches peak gradually followed by abrupt turning off of inspiration resulting quiet expiration. Until recently, it was thought the Dorsal respiratory group of neurons generate the basic rhythm of breathing. It is now believed that the breathing rhythm is generated by a network of neurons called the **Pre-Brotzinger complex** located near the upper end of the medullary respiratory centre.

(ii) *Ventral respiratory group (VRG) neurones*: The other group of neurones are present in ventrolateral surface (in nucleus ambiguus and nucleus retroambiguus of the medulla and known as VRG neurons, Fig. 5.5). These neurones remain inactive during quite breathing (thus quiet expiration is entirely due to inactivation of DRG neurones) and play a role only when there is increased pulmonary ventilation. This area contains the neurones responsible for both inspiration and expiration. Thus the DRG neurones and the part of VRG neurones which are responsible for inspirations are collectively known as **'I' neurones or inspiratory centers** whereas the remaining neurones of VRG groups which are responsible for expiration are known as **'E' neurones** or **expiratory center.**

(b) **Pontine center**: There are two pontine centers which do not generate the basic rhythm of impulse for inspiration but control the rate and depth of the respiration. These centers are:

(i) *Apneustic center*:

- It is located bilaterally in lower part of pons (Fig. 5.5).

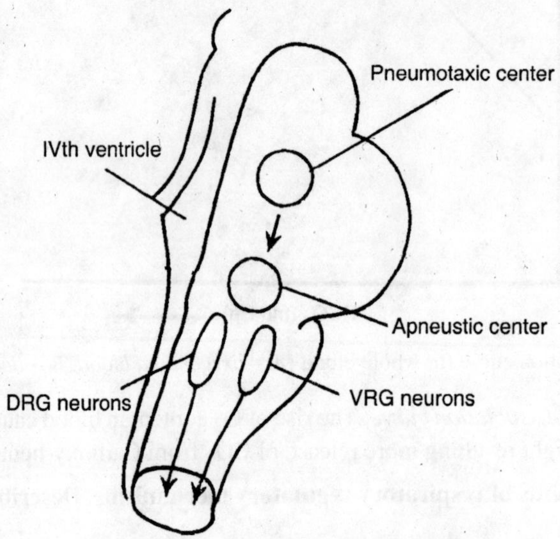

Fig. 5.5: Organisation of respiratory center

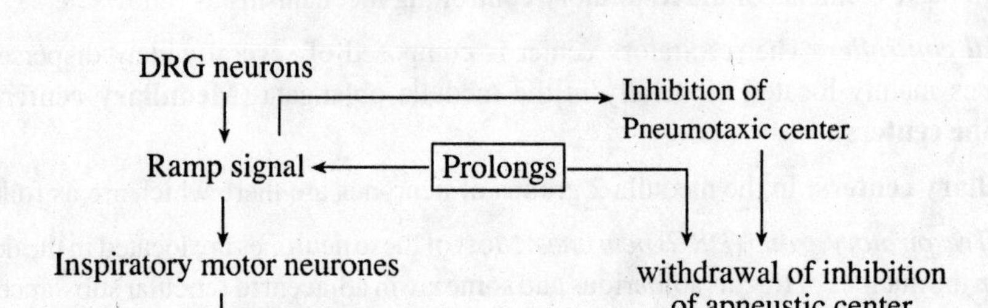

Fig. 5.6: Inspiration during Quiet breathing

- It sends signal to DRG neurones to prevent the **'switch off'** of the inspiratory ramp signal i.e. **it prolongs the inspiration.** This pattern of respiration is known as ***apneusis*** (prolonged inspiration with short expiratory gasp).

(ii) *Pneumotaxic center:*

- It is located bilaterally in nucleus parabrachialis of the upper pons (Fig. 5.5).
- Normally it inhibits the apneustic center and thus controls the 'switch off' point of inspiratory ramp, thus controlling the duration of inspiration.
- When pneumotaxic signal is strong the rate of respiration increases to 30-40 breaths / min because of rapid 'switching off' of ramp signals which reduces duration of inspiration and therefore also expiration.

(c) **Suprapontine centers:**

- Some neurones located in cerebral cortex, limbic lobe, amygdala, hypothalamus etc. also regulate the respiration.
- These higher centers can cause only temporary breath holding or temporary hyperventilation.

***B. Sensors*:** These are excited in response to any change of the environment and the sensation is carried to the respiratory centers which inturn signals the respiratory muscles to control the respiration. These sensors are of 2 types as follows:

(a) **Central chemoreceptors:**

- These are believed to be present about 200-400 μm below the ventral surface of medulla.
- These are surrounded by CSF which is separated from the blood by Blood-Brain Barrier which is impermeable to H^+ though molecular CO_2 diffuses across it easily.
- These are directly stimulated by increase of H^+ concentration in medullary interstitial fluid. When blood PCO_2 rises it diffuses to CSF and forms H^+ by following mechanism:

$$CO_2 + H_2O = H_2CO_3 = H^+ + HCO_3^-$$

- The main (70-80%) effect of CO_2 on respiration is due to it's effect on central chemoreceptor.

(b) **Peripheral chemoreceptors:**

- These are situated in carotid and aortic bodies.
- The nerve fiber which carries the sensation from peripheral chemoreceptors to respiratory center is **Carotid sinus nerve** or **Hering nerve** which joins the glossopharyngeal nerve.
- The stimuli which stimulates these receptors are
  - ↓ PO_2 (below 60 mmHg)
  - ↑ PCO_2 (by 10 mmHg)
  - ↓ pH (by 0.1 unit)

***C. Effectors*:** The respiratory muscles are the effectors which ultimately control the respiration.

Neural Regulation of respiration:

The **basic rhythm** of respiration (periodic inspiration and expiration) during quiet breathing is maintained by **periodic ramp signal** from the **DRG neurones.** When ramp signal is on, there is inspiration as illustrated in (Fig. 5.6) and when there is no ramp signal from the DRG neurones, there is expiration (Fig. 5.7) due to relaxation of inspiratory muscles. However this basic rhythm is modulated by pontine centers. During inspiration pneumotaxic centre remains inactivated leading withdrawl of it's inhibitory effect on apneustic center which results prolongation of inspiratory ramp generated by DRG neurones and thus inspiration tries to be prolonged whereas activation of pneumotaxic center during the peak impiratory ramp leads to inhibition of apneustic center and thus apneustic center switch off the inspiratory ramp resulting expiration. The detail of this mechanism is illustrated with the help of (Fig. 5.6) and (Fig. 5.7).

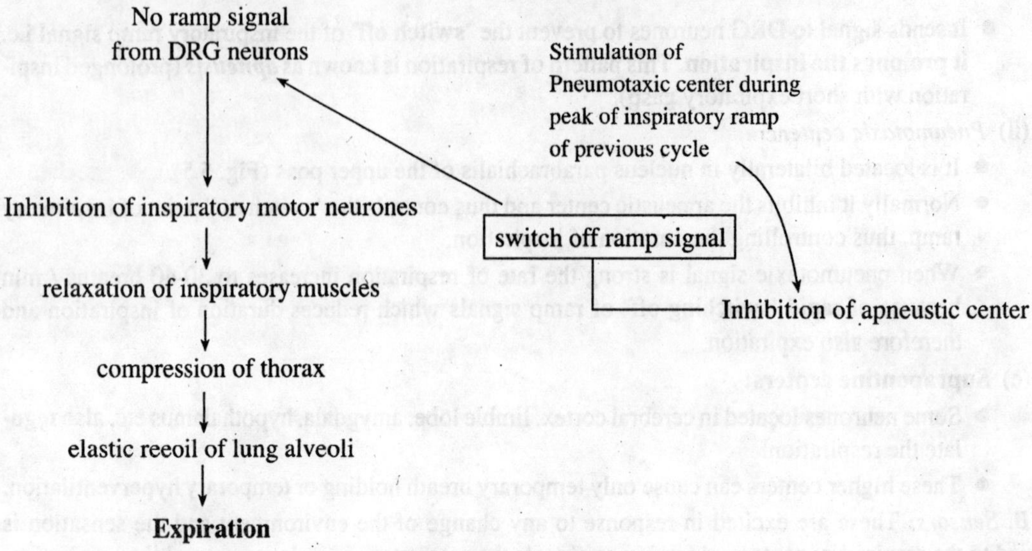

Fig. 5.7: Expiration during Quiet Breathing

7. Describe the chemical regulation of respiration.

Different chemical factors like PCO_2, PO_2 and H^+ alter the normal rate and depth of respiration by modulating different respiratory center either through central or peripheral or both chemoreceptors.

***a. PCO_2 on respiration*:**

- **Increase in PCO_2 increases the pulmonary ventilation irrespective of any change of PO_2 or pH or both in a following manner:**
  - **Increase in partial pressure of alveolar CO_2 beyond 35 mmHg increases the pulmonary ventilation (PV) even if alveolar PO_2 remains constant (Fig. 5.8).**
  - **Increase in partial pressure of arterial CO_2 beyond 40 mmHg increases the PV even if normal alveolar PO_2 is maintained i.e. 100 mmHg (Fig. 5.8).**

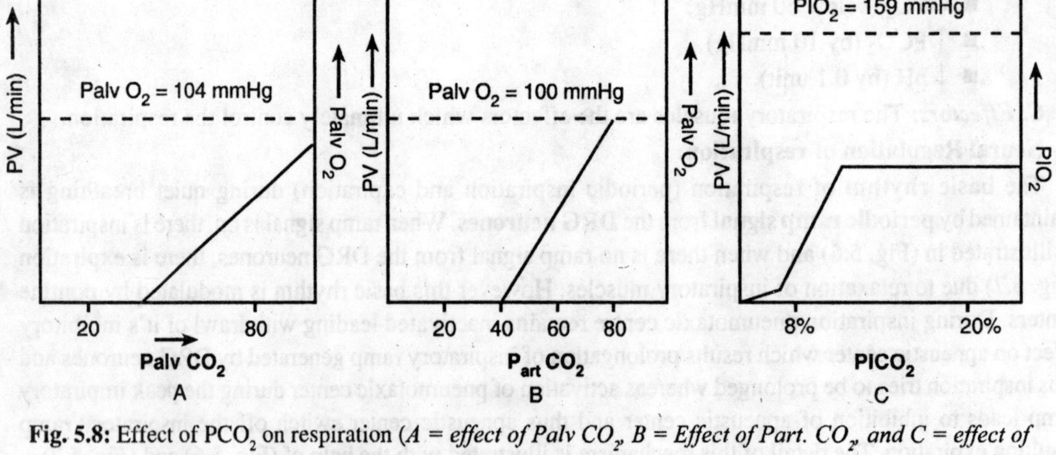

Fig. 5.8: Effect of PCO_2 on respiration (*A = effect of Palv CO_2, B = Effect of Part. CO_2, and C = effect of Pinspiratory air CO_2 on pulmonary ventilation*)

- Increase in partial pressure of inspiratory CO_2 (PI CO_2) beyond 0.3 to 4% increases slowly and up to 10% rise of PI CO_2 causes steep rise of ventilation (Fig. 5.8). Above 10% rise of PI CO_2 causes no further rise of PV and thereby results **CO_2 narcosis.**

- *Mode of regulation*: Increase in PCO_2 in blood increases both the rate of and depth of respiration directly by acting on peripheral chemoreceptors and indirectly by stimulating central chemoreceptor through H^+ as demonstrated by the flow chart of next page.

b. ***PO_2 on respiration*:**

- Decrease in PO_2 in arterial blood up to 60 mmHg do not affect ventilation but further fall of PO_2 (< 60 mmHg) increases pulmonary ventilation if the PCO_2 of arterial blood remains constant at 40 mmHg (Fig. 5.9).

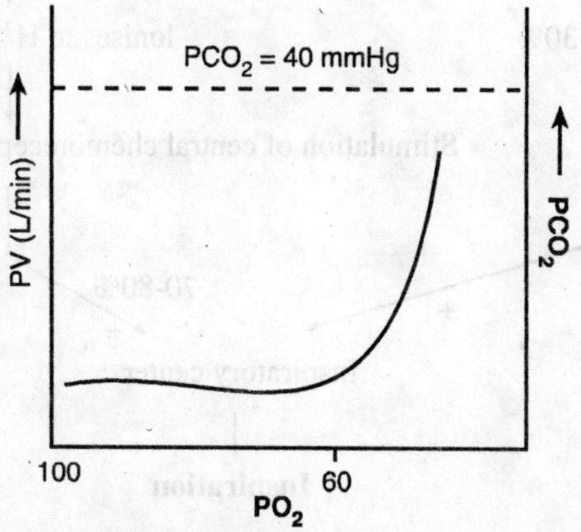

Fig. 5.9: Effect of PO_2 on pulmonary ventilation

- *Mode of regulation*: Any fall of PO_2 in blood beyond 60 mmHg results increase in rate and depth of respiration only by stimulating peripheral chemoreceptors. The detail mechanism is as follows: **Decrease in partial pressure of oxygen → Hypoxia to glomus cell → Stimulation of peripheral chemoreceptors → Impulse through vagus and glossopharyngeal → Stimulation of Inspiratory center → ↑ Inspiration.**

c. ***H^+ Concentration*:**

- Increase in H^+ concentration or decrease in pH due to any cause like respiratory, metabolic and renal acidosis results very slow rise of ventilation if the PCO_2 and PO_2 remains at normal level (Fig. 5.10).

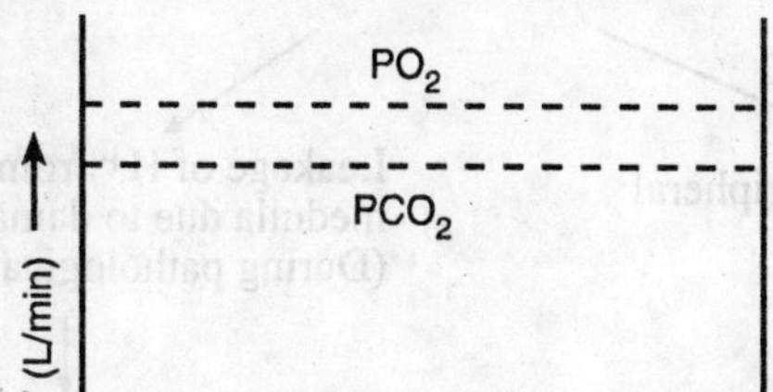

Fig. 5.10: Effect of pH on respiration

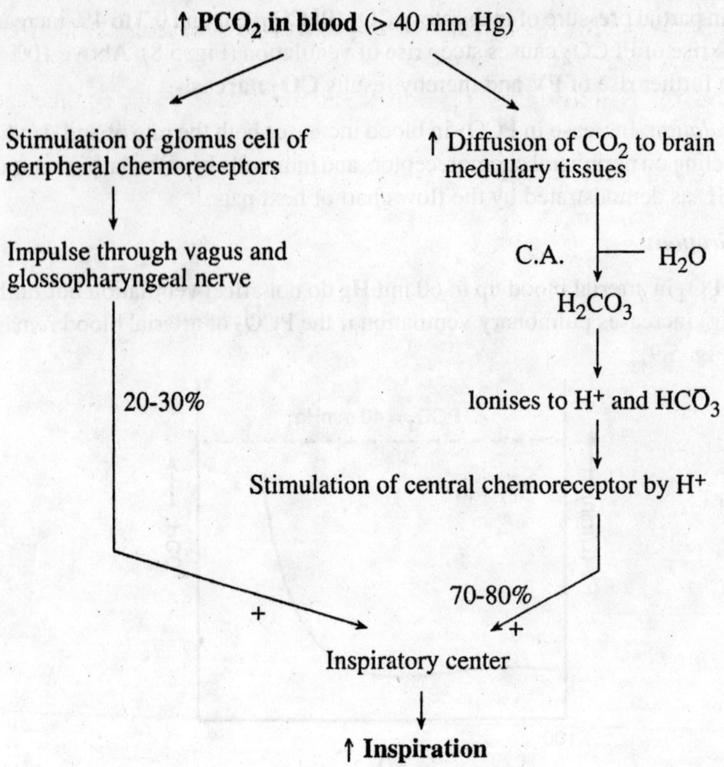

- *Mode of regulation*:Increase in H^+ in blood causes rise of inspiratory rate and depth through peripheral chemoreceptors. However, in case of excessive rise of H^+ in blood or damage of BBB there may be leakage of H^+ from blood to medullary interstitium and thus stimulate central chemoreceptor to affect inspiration directly. The detail mechanism is explained by flow chart above.

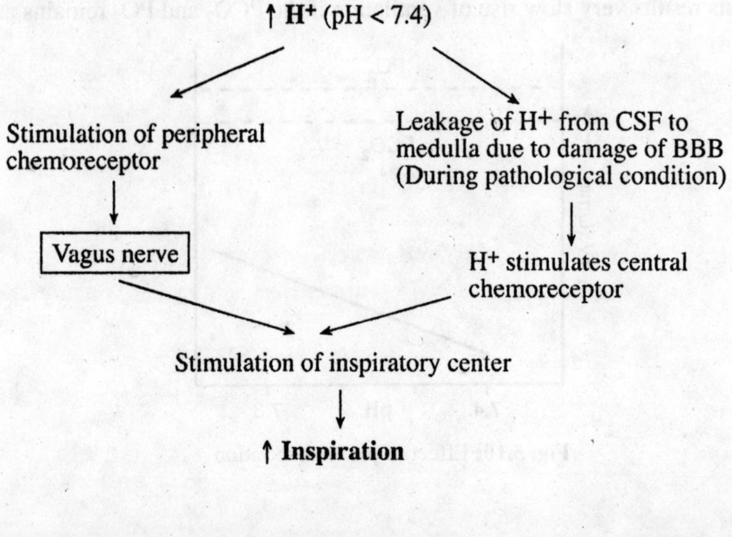

8. Define hypoxia. Describe the types, causes, signs and symptoms and effects of hypoxia. Add a note on O_2 therapy.

Definition*:** Lack of O_2 at tissue level is called as ***hypoxia whereas the complete absence of O_2 in tissue is termed as ***anoxia***.

***Types*:** It is four types as follows:

(a) Hypoxic or arterial

(b) Anaemic

(c) Hypokinetic or stagnant

(d) Histotoxic

(a) Hypoxic hypoxia:

- ***Definition*: The hypoxia in which the PO_2 of arterial blood is reduced but O_2 carrying capacity of blood and rate of blood flow is normal, is termed as hypoxic hypoxia.**
- ***Causes*: The causes / conditions are:**
  - **High altitude**
  - **Breathing of artificial gas mixture with low PO_2**
  - **Hypoventilation due to any cause e.g. damage of respiratory centers by drugs, Poliomyelitis etc.**
  - **Diffusion limitation due to loss of surface area of respiratory membrane**
  - **Imbalance of ventilation perfusion ratio ratio leading to physiological shunt formation.**
- ***Characteristic feature*: Vide table 5.a.**

(b) Anaemic hypoxia:

- ***Definition*: The hypoxia resulting due to decreased O_2 carrying capacity of the blood with normal PO_2 of arterial blood and normal rate of blood flow is known as anaemic hypoxia.**
- ***Causes*: Decreased hemoglobin content or altered hemoglobin which is incapable of O_2 carriage e.g. CO poisoning, methoemoglobin etc.**
- ***Characteristic features*: Vide table 5.a.**

(c) Stagnant hypoxia:

- ***Definition*: The hypoxia due to inadequate rate of blood flow to the tissue with normal PO_2 of arterial blood and O_2 carrying capacity of blood is known as stagnant hypoxia.**
- ***Causes*: Circulatory failure, congestive cardiac failure, atherosclerosis or thrombosis**
- ***Characteristic features* : Vide table 5.a.**

(d) Histotoxic hypoxia:

- ***Definition*: The decreased ability of tissues themselves to utilize O_2 is called as histotoxic hypoxia**
- ***Causes*: occurs due to cyanide poisoning**
- ***Characteristic features*—vide table 5.a.**

***Signs of hypoxia*: These are: Cyanosis (not always), Tachycardia, Tacypnoea and hyperapnoea.**

O_2 therapy: This is the important method to treat hypoxic patient. O_2 therapy can be done by two procedures e.g.

(i) Inhalation of 100% pure O_2 but this procedure has side effects like—

- **Nasal congestion, sore throat, sneezing, coughing, bronchoconstriction due to stimulation of irritant receptors in respiratory tract.**

- O_2 toxicity which is characterised by muscular twitching, dizziness, cog wheel (Jerking) respiration, convulsion, and unconsciousness. It is basically due to inhibition of tissue enzyme activity and cerebral vasoconstriction.

(ii) **Inhalation of 100% pure O_2 at high barometric pressure (hyperbaric O_2 therapy)** the main aim of which is to increase the amount of dissolved O_2 in plasma and thereby helps in all forms of hypoxic conditions except hypoxic hypoxia. However in early stages there may be ***O_2 toxicity***.

Table 5.a: Characteristic features of different hypoxia

Parameters	Hypoxic	Anemic	Histotoxic	Stagnant
1. Arterial PO_2	↓	N	N	N
2. Alveolar PO_2	↓	N	N	N
3. Arterial O_2 content	↓	↓	N	N
4. Hb content	N	↓	N	N
5. Rate of blood flow	N	N	↓	N
6. Cyanosis	present	absent	present	absent
7. Stim of peripheral chemoreceptors	Yes	No	Yes	Yes
8. A-V O_2 difference	↓	N	↓	0

↓ = decrease, ↑ = increase, N = Normal

B. Short Notes:

1. **Weibel's lung model:** Trachea divides into 2 Bronchi-left and right each of which ultimately divides into 6×10^4 terminal bronchioles (Fig. 5.11). As per Weibel's lung model, between the trachea and the alveolar sac, the air passage is divided into 23 times in which the trachea is numbered 'zero' generation, terminal bronchioles are **16th** generation and alveolar sac is **23rd** generation.

2. **Respiratory membrane:** The alveolar-capillary membrane through which diffusion of O_2 and CO_2 takes place is known as ***respiratory membrane***. It is basically formed by the epithelium of the respiratory unit and endothelium of pulmonary capillaries (Fig. 5.12). The different layers of respiratory membrane from inside to outside are as follows:
   (i) A layer of fluid lining the alveolus including surfactant.
   (ii) Alveolar epithelial cell layer.
   (iii) Basement membrane of alveolar epithelial cell layer.
   (iv) Interstitial space between alveolar epithelium and capillary basement membrane.
   (v) Capillary basement membrane
   (vi) Capillary endothelial cell layer.

The overall thickness of respiratory membrane is on an average 0.6 μ and total surface area is 70 M^2 in normal adult and total quantity of blood in the lung capillaries is 60-140 ml/cycle. So this small amount of blood spreads over the entire lung surface which increases the rapidity of diffusion.

3. **Non respiratory functions of lungs:** These are mainly mediated by respiratory tract.

A. Defense mechanism:

(a) **Filtering effect:** Different dust particles present in air are eliminated by different parts of the tract e.g.

- Large dust particles by hairs of nostrils

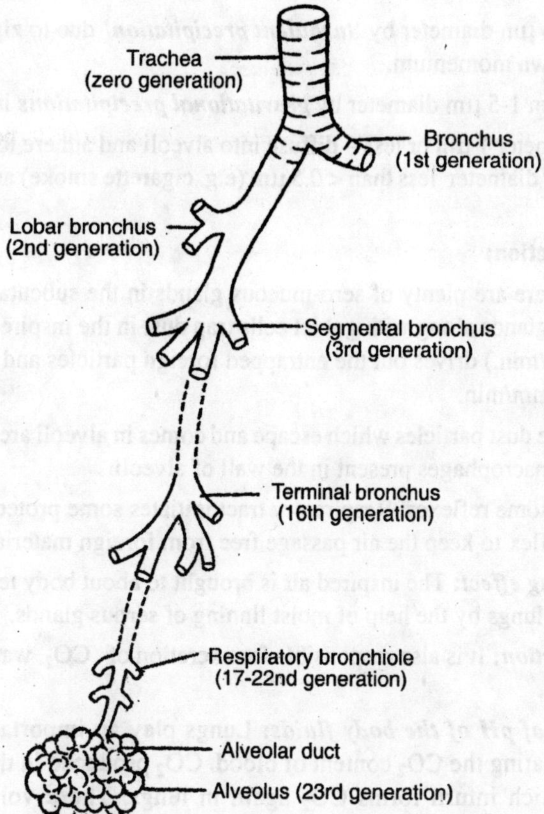

Fig. 5.11: Weibel's lung model

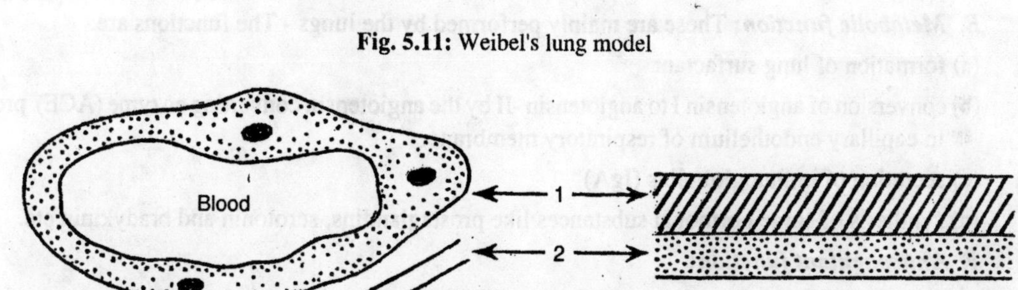

Fig. 5.12: Alveolar capillary membrane

(1 = Capillary endothelium layer, 2 = Basement membrane of capillary endothelium, 3 = Basement membrane of alveolar epithelium and *4 = Alveolar epithelium)*

- Particles up to 6 μm diameter by ***'turbulent precipitation'*** due to zigzag passage of nasal cavity and particles' own momentum.
- Particles between 1-5 μm diameter by ***gravitational precipitations*** in the smaller bronchioles.
- Particles of diameter 1 μm or less – diffuse into alveoli and adhere to the wall of alveoli however particles having diameter less than < 0.5 μm (e.g. cigarette smoke) are usually expired out (2/3 of total volume).

(b) **Protective function:**

(i) By trachea: There are plenty of sero-mucous glands in the subcutaneous coat of tracheal wall. These mucous glands along with goblet cells trap dust in the inspired air. Then the ciliary movement (20 times/min.) drives out the entrapped foreign particles and bacteria towards mouth at a velocity of 24 mm/min.

(ii) By alveoli: The dust particles which escape and comes in alveoli are destroyed by the phagocytic action of the macrophages present in the wall of alveoli.

(iii) By initiating some reflexes: Respiratory tract initiates some protective reflex like cough reflex and sneeze reflex to keep the air passage free from foreign materials.

***B. Air conditioning effect*:** The inspired air is brought to about body temperature and is humidified before it's entrance in lungs by the help of moist linning of serous glands.

***C. Excretory function*:** It is also responsible for excretion of CO_2, water vapor and certain volatile substance e.g. acetone.

***D. Maintenance of pH of the body fluids*:** Lungs play an important role in maintaining acid base balance by regulating the CO_2 content of blood. CO_2 produced in the tissues comes in blood to form bicarbonate which inturn forms CO_2 again in lungs. These volatile CO_2 is blown out by ventilation.

***E. Metabolic function*:** These are mainly performed by the lungs - The functions are:

(a) formation of lung surfactant

(b) conversion of angiotensin I to angiotensin -II by the angiotensin converting enzyme (ACE) present in capillary endothelium of respiratory membrane.

(c) secretion of immuoglobulins (IgA)

(d) synthesis of some hormonal substances like prostaglandins, serotonin and bradykinin etc.

***F. Anticoagulant function*:**

Lung contains the mast cells, which secrete heparin. Heparin, an anticoagulant, prevents the intravascular clotting.

G. Acts as left ventricular reservoir due to high compliance of pulmonary vessels.

4. Intrapleural or intra thoracic pressure:

- ***Definition*:** The lungs are covered by thin serous membrane called ***pleural membrane***. The pleural membrane is reflected from the root of each lung on the inner surface of the walls of the chest cavity and upper surface of the diaphragm. The membrane covering the lung is called **visceral pleura** and the thoracic wall and diaphragm is called the **parietal pleura**. These two layers thus form a closed membrane sac on each site of the chest called pleural cavity which contains a thin film of serous fluid that acts as a lubricant and helps the surface to glide over one another during respiratory movement. The pressure existing in the pleural cavity in known as **intrapleural pressure** (ip).

- **Normal values:**

Parameters	Intrapleural pressure(mmHg)	Intra-alveolar pressure
Normal Inspiration	– 5 to – 10	– 2 to – 4
Normal expiration	– 2 to – 5	6 to + 10
Forced Inspiration	– 40	– 40 to – 50
Forced expiration with closed glottis	50	10 to + 40

- **Why the intrapleural pressure is negative?** Intrapleural pressure is negative or subatmospheric due to 2 opposing forces:

  (i) The lung tries to collapse because of it's elasticity and surface tension in the alveoli.

  (ii) The chest wall always tries to expand.

  Thus the pleural layers becomes subjected to a force that tries to separate them resulting a suction pressure or negative pressure.

- **The circumstances in which ip becomes positive?**

  (i) When expiratory muscles are working against closed glottis (***Valsalva maneuvere***) e.g. during defaecation, coughing, lifting a heavy object.

  (ii) Injury of the chest causing exposure of pleural cavity to the exterior i.e. **pneumothrox**

  (iii) Collection of fluid in the pleural cavity (**Pleural effusion**) e.g. serous fluid (Hydro thorax) or pus formation (**pyothorax**) or collection of fluid stained with blood (**haemothorax**).

- **Significance of intrapleural pressure:** It has 2 important significance:

(i) As it is normally negative it prevents the collapse of lungs caused by elastic recoil of lung tissues.

(ii) It is responsible for the increased venous return during inspiration and exercise (respiratory pumps) as –During inspiration increase of negativity of intrapleural pressure → Increase in negativity of mediastinal pressure → expansion of larger veins and vena cava → Decrease of pressure in them → Sucking of blood into these veins from extrathoracic region → Increase in venous return → Increase in cardiac output.

5. **Airways resistance:** The resistance caused by friction of gas molecules between moving column of air and respiratory passages through which air pass to alveoli is known as *airways resistance*. It is due to **turbulent flow** of air.

Factors affecting airways resistance:

(i) **Cross sectional area of airways:** Airway resistance is inversely related with cross sectional area or diameter of the respiratory passages.

(ii) **Phases of respiration:** During inspiration the intrapleural and mediastinal negativity rises and as a result the bronchial diameter increases. Reverse occurs during expiration. Therefore resistance to airflow is normally low in inspiration and high in expiration. This is why in bronchial asthma inspiration may not be difficult but expiration becomes difficult. This explains why the "***Whezze***" in bronchial asthma is heard during expiration but not in inspiration.

(iii) **Tone of bronchial muscles:** Various factors can alter the tone of bronchial muscles and thereby airway resistance. For example:

- β_2 adrenergic stimulation → decrease in tone in bronchial muscle → increase in diameter of bronchioles → decrease in airways resistance.
- Histamin, PG, Ca^{2+} Channel blockers etc. → bronchospasm → decrease in diameter of airways → increase in airways resistance.

(iv) **Types of airflow:**

- High resistance during turbulent flow (during rapid breathing).
- Low resistance during laminar flow (during quiet breathing).

(v) **Rate of gas flow:** It is directly related with resistance i.e. the greater the rate, the greater is the resistance. Resistance offered by intermediate size bronchioles is highest because of it's velocity.

(vi) **Density of inspired air:** Directly related with airways resistance.

6. Pleural effusion:

- It is the collection of fluid in the pleural cavity due to Tuberculosis infection, Blockade of lymphatics, Heart diseases, Hypoproteinaemia etc.
- Significant pleural effusion limits lung expansion and thus decreases gas exchange.

7. Pneumonia:

- It is the condition in which there is collection of fluid and blood cells in the alveoli and consolidation of lungs because of porus alveolar cappillary membrane due to pneumococcal infection.
- It is a type of obstructive disease of lungs.

8. Emphysema:

- It is the degenerative disease in which there is permanent destruction of air spaces distal to terminal bronchioles due to destruction of alveolar septa.
- In this disease it is much easy to inflate lung i.e. the static lung compliance is higher but the elastic recoil of lungs is less due to which getting air out of lung is severely impaired. Therefore residual volume becomes abnormally high.
- This is characterised by:
  - More physiological dead space
  - Inadequate alveolar ventilation
  - Hypercapnoea in late stage
  - Barrel shaped chest
  - Pulmonary oedema
  - Difficulty in breathing
  - Enlargement of right side of heart (Cor-pulmonale)

9. Bronchial asthma:

- It is a paroxysmal episodic disorder at times with the attack commencing and ending abruptly and may become a chronic disorder.
- It is characterized by wheezing, feeling of tightess in the chest and difficulty to expire resulted due to brocho-constriction.
- It is due to:
  - inflammation of air passage releases various chemicals that cause bronchospasm.
  - hypersensitive reactions affecting the tracheo-bronchial tree.
  - pulmonary oedema in left ventricular failure which is known as cardiac asthma.
- In this case lung function is reduced drastically during the attack and otherwise remains normal.

10. Static lung volume and capacities: Lung volumes are defined as the fraction or subdivision of lung capacities.

A. There are 4 **static lung volumes:**

(a) **Tidal volume (TV):** It is the volume of air that can be breathed in or out during normal quiet breathing (Fig. 5.13). **Normal value:** 500-800 ml in normal adult.

(b) Inspiratory reserve volume (IRV): It is the maximum volume of air that can be breathed in over and above the tidal volume (Fig. 5.13) after normal inspiration. **Normal value:** 2000-3300 ml in normal adult male.

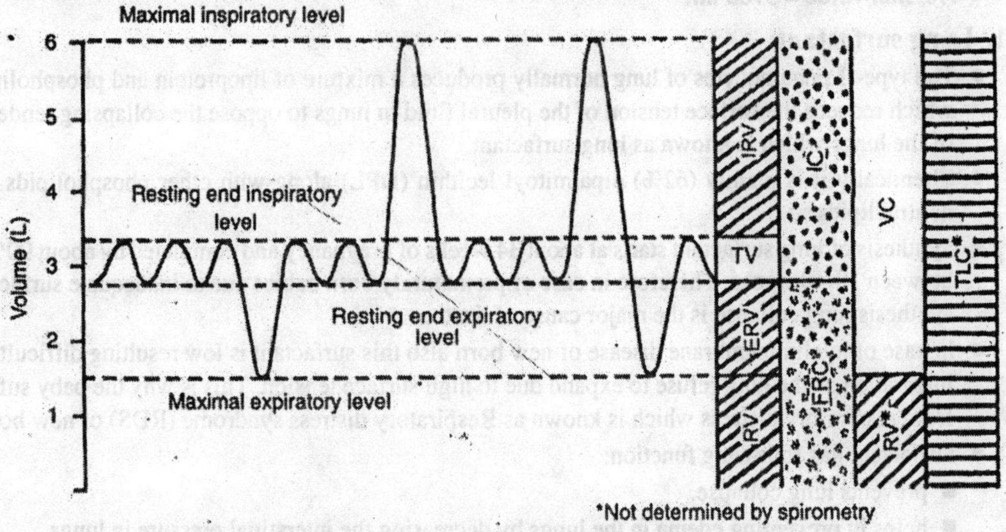

Fig. 5.13: Graphical representation of lung volume and capacities

(c) Expiratory reserve volume (ERV): It is the extra amount of air that can be breathed out by maximum expiratory effort after normal expiration (Fig. 5.13). **Normal value:** 1100 ml in normal adult male.

(d) Residual volume: It is the amount of air that remains in the lungs even after maximum expiratory effort. **Normal value:** 1200 ml in normal adult male.

B. Static lung capacity: Lung capacity is defined as the sum total of two or more lung volumes. There are 4 static lung capacities:

(a) Inspiratory capacity (IC): It is the maximum volume of air that can be breathed in from end expiratory position. It is calculated as IC = TV + IRV. **Normal value:** 3500 ml.

(b) Expiratory capacity (EC): It is the maximum volume of air that can be breathed out from end inspiratory position (Fig. 5.13).This is calculated as: EC = TV + ERV. **Normal value:** 1600 ml.

(c) Functional residual capacity (FRC):

- It is the volume of air remaining in the lungs after quiet expiration (Fig. 5.14). It is calculated as: FRC = RV + ERV
- **Normal value:** 2200 ml
- It cannot be measured directly by spirometry but by another 3 techniqnes: (i) **N_2 wash out techninqne.** (ii) **Body plethysmograph technique.** (iii) **Helium dilution technique.**
- The significance of FRC is that it helps the continuous exchange of gases even during expiration and thus concentration of O_2 and CO_2 in blood are maintained constant.
- It is increased in old age, emphysema, asthma and atelectasis.

(d) Vital Capacity (VC): It is the volume of air that can be breathed out by maximal expiratory effort after maximal inspiration.

- It is calculated as IC + ERV
- Normal value—4500 ml

(e) Total lung capacity:

- **It is the volume of air that lung can hold after a maximum possible inspiration.**
- It can be calculated as TLC = IC + FRC.
- **Normal value** = 5700 ml.

11. Lung surfactant:

- **The type-II pneumocytes of lung normally produces a mixture of lipoprotein and phospholipids which reduces the surface tension of the pleural fluid in lungs to oppose the collapsing tendency of the lungs which is known as lung surfactant.**
- Chemically it is mainly (62%) dipalmitoyl lecithin (DPL) along with other phospholipids and neutral lipids.
- Synthesis of lung surfactant starts at about 34 weeks of pregnancy and completed by about 90% in between 38-40 weeks. Therefore in case of prematurely born babies due to inadequate surfactant synthesis lung collapse is the major cause of death.
- In case of hyalin membrane disease of new born also this surfactant is low resulting difficulty in inspiration as the lung refuse to expand due to high surface tension. This is why the baby suffers from respiratory distress which is known as Respiratory distress syndrome (RDS) of new born.
- Surfactant has following function:
  - prevents lung collapse.
  - helps in preventing edema in the lungs by decreasing the interstitial pressure in lungs.
  - decreases the work of breathing so it becomes easier.
  - IgA and apoproteins of surfactants provide innate immunity.
  - promotes the alveolar stability by lowering surface tension proportionately more in smaller alveoli.
- Surfactant production is stimulated by vagal stimulation, thyroid hormones, glucocorticoids, insulin, growth hormone whereas it is inhibited by hypoxia, smoking and pure O_2 breathing.

12. Vital capacity:

- **It is the volume of air that can be breathed out by maximal expiratory effort after maximal inspiration.**
- It is calculated as IC + ERV.
- Normal value—4500 ml
- Significance: It gives the information about—
  - the strength of the respiratory muscles
  - the pulmonary functions through FEV1
- Factors affecting VC: The important factors that influence the vital capacity are:
  - **Physiological:**
    - ❑ **Sex:** Vital capacity is normally more in male due to:
      - increase in chest size
      - increase in muscle power
      - increase in body surface area
    - ❑ **Body build:** It is higher in tall and thin persons than in short and obese persons.
    - ❑ **Posture:** It is more in standing position than in lying position because in lying position abdominal contents push the diaphragm upward i.e. towards the thoracic cavity, causing lesser expansion of thorax.

- ❑ **Strength of the respiratory muscles:** It is directly related with VC.
- ❑ **Pregnancy:** During pregnancy VC is decreased as growing foetus push the diaphragm towards thoracic cavity causing less expansion of thorax.
- ❑ **Pathological:** During differernt lung diseases like poliomyelitis, fibrosis, emphysema, pulmonary oedema, pneumothorax, ascites etc. there is significant reduction of VC.

- Measurement: It is directly measured by Spirometry by asking the subjects to expire maximally through the mouthpiece of the *Spirometer* after taking maximum inspiration from air.

13. Lung compliance: It is the volume of expansion of lungs per unit change of pressure.

- **Normal values:**

(i) Compliance in relation to intra-alveolar pressure changes:

- Lungs along—220 ml/cm of H_2O
- Lungs and thorax—130 ml/cm of H_2O

(ii) Compliance in relation to intrapleural pressure changes:

- Lungs alone—200 ml/cm of H_2O
- Lungs and thorax—100 ml/cm of H_2O

- **Variations:**
  - ■ Reduction of lung compliance—In restrictive lung disease e.g. tuberculosis, lung abscess and respiratory distress syndrome.
  - ■ Increase of lungs compliance—In chronic obstructive lung disease e.g. emphysema.
- **Factors influencing compliance:**

1. ***Elasticity of lungs*:** It is inversely related with lung compliance i.e. decrease in elasticity of lungs causes increase in compliance e.g. emphysema.
2. ***Surface tension within alveoli*:** The alveoli contains a very thin film of fluid lining at their inner side. The individual molecules of this thin fluid attracts each other because of surface tension and the resultant effect is collapsing of lungs (Fig. 5.14). Thus surface tension is also inversely related with lung compliance.
3. ***Interdependence*:** When a few alveoli start to collapse the neighbouring alveoli also begin to be pulled because of their strong anatomical connection. This results the pulling of the walls of the collapsing alveoli due to Newton's 3rd law of motion and thus their collapse is opposed. This is called ***interdependence***.
4. ***Chest wall factors*:** Various diseases (e.g. kyphoscoliosis, ankylosing spondilitis) can cause immobility of chest wall and thereby result reduction in compliance.

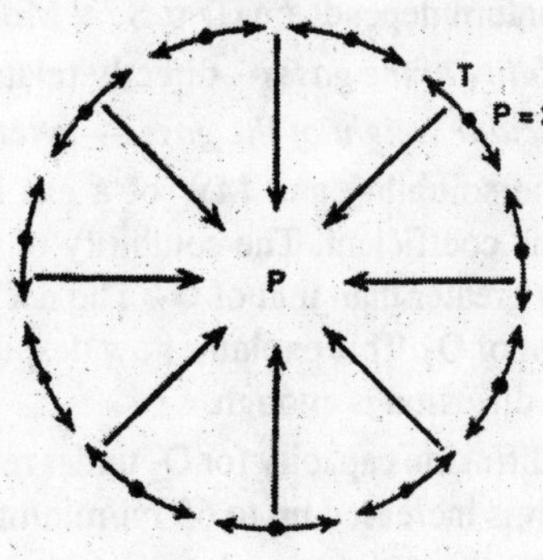

Fig. 5.14: Diagrammatic representation showing surface tension of alveoli (P = Pressure and T = Tension)

14. Ventilation perfusion ratio:

- The ventilation perfusion ratio is defined as the ratio of alveolar ventilation and the amount of blood that perfuses the alveoli / min.

- The gaseous exchange is maximum at the normal VA/Q ratio of 0.84. Any increase or decrease in ratio decreases the diffusion of gases through the membrane due to imbalance between alveolar ventilation and alveolar blood flow.
- Normal value: $\frac{\text{Alveolar ventilation}}{\text{Pulmonary blood flow}} = \frac{4200 \text{ ml / min}}{5000 \text{ ml / min}} = 0.84$
- It is high in the apex of lungs and low in the base of the lungs.
- Due to regional variations of ventilation perfusion tuberculosis occurs more commonly in the apex because of favourable environment for mycobacterium tuberculosis.
- Decrease in ventilation perfusion results fall of alveolar PO_2 and rise of alveolar PCO_2 and vice versa.

15. Diffusion capacity:

- It is the volume of gas that diffuses through the respiratory membrane per min. per mm Hg pressure difference.
- It is directly related with diffusion of gases i.e. the greater the diffusion capacity the more is the diffusion of gases.
- It depends on three factors as per following formula:

Diffusion Capacity = A/T × D

Where A = total surface area, T = thickness, D = Diffusion coefficient

(a) **Total surface area of respiratory membrane:** Rate of diffusion of gases is directly proportional to the surface area i.e. with decrease in surface area as occurs in bacterial infection like TB, the rate of diffusion of gases decreases.

(b) **Thickness of the respiratory membrane:** Rate of diffusion is inversely related with the thickness of the membrane. So any thickening of the respiratory membrane due to pulmonary edema or lung fibrosis results decrease in rate of diffusion of gases.

(c) **Diffusion coefficient:** The rate of diffusion is directly proportional to the diffusion coefficient which inturn depends on ($D \propto S / \sqrt{\text{Molecular weight of gases}}$):

- *Solubility of the gases*—directly related with diffusion coefficient.
- *Molecular weight of the gases*—inversely related with the root of it's MW

Thus the solubility and MW of a gas influences the diffusion capacity of a gas by affecting diffusion coefficient. The solubility of CO_2 is 25 times higher than that of O_2 but it's MW is slightly greater than that of O_2. The net result is—diffusibility of CO_2 is about 20 times greater than that of O_2. This explains how despite a smaller pressure difference compared to O_2, the rate of CO_2 diffusion is enough.

- The diffusion capacity for O_2 under resting condition in young male adult is 21ml/min/mm Hg which is increased up to 65 ml/min/mmHg during exercise due to:
  - opening of some previously dormant capillaries → ↑ surface area of respiratory membrane
  - better perfusion i.e. increase in ventilation—perfusion ratio (VA/Q).

16. Forced expiratory volume or forced expiratory vital capacity (FVC) or timed vital capacity:

- **Definition:** The volume of air that can be expired forcibly after a maximum inspiration in a given unit of time is called FEV or FVC.
- **Recording and measurement:** The person is first asked to take maximum inspiration and is then asked to expire in the Spirometer with maximum expiratory effort as rapidly and as completely as possible. The record is obtained (Fig. 5.15) on a fast moving drum.

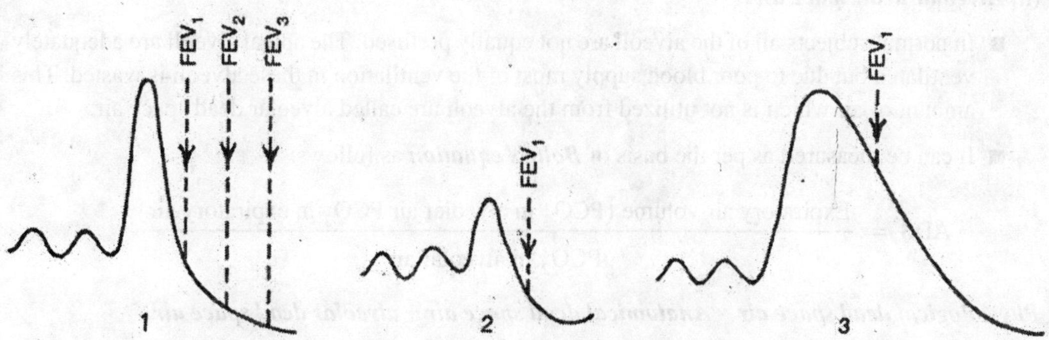

Fig. 5.15: Graphical representation of timed vital capacity

- **Fractions of FEV:**
  - Normally to expire the total amount of air that was inspired it takes 3 seconds out of which the amount of air that is expired in Ist second is known as FEV_1 and in 2nd sec is known as FEV_2 and in 3rd sec is known as FEV_3.
  - The normal values it FEV_1, FEV_2 and FEV_3 are:
    - ❑ FEV_1 = 75% to 85% of vital capacity
    - ❑ FEV_2 = upto 94% of VC
    - ❑ FEV_3 = upto 97% VC.
- **Significance:** The FEV_1 is useful to differenciate the restrictive type lung disease from the obstructive type of lungs disease as follows:
  - *In obstructive lungs disease*: FEV_1 = < 75% to 85% (normally about 40%) but VC = normal
  - *In restrictive lung disease*: FEV_1 = almost normal but VC is reduced.

17. Physiological shunt:

In some alveoli ventilation is more and alveolar blood flow is less. Available O_2 therefore is not transported due to lack of blood flow. So ventilation is wasted. This means that:

(a) all of the blood coming to the alveolus is net oxygenated. This unoxygenated portion of blood is called ***shunted blood***.

(b) also some additional blood flows through the bronchial vessels which is also unoxygenated. The total quantity (a + b) of blood per min is called ***physiological shunt***.

In chronic obstructive lung diseases (COLD) some areas have serious physiological shunt and some other are serious physiological dead space. So gas exchange in the lungs is severely effected leading to pulmonary disability. COLD is the most common cause of pulmonary disability.

18. Dead space air:

The amount of the air present in respiratory system which do not take part in gaseous exchange process and thus becomes a wastage is known as ***Total Dead space*** or ***Physiological dead space air***. It is constituted by two types of dead space air.

(i) Anatomical dead space air:

- The amount of air which is confined in the respiratory passages and thereby are not available for gaseous exchange process is known as anatomical dead space air.
- Normal value: 150 ml
- It can be measured by N_2 Washout technique

(ii) ***Alveolar dead space air:***

- In normal subjects all of the alveoli are not equally perfused. The apical alveoli are adequately ventilated but due to poor blood supply most of the ventilation in these alveoli is wasted. This amount of air which is not utilized from the alveoli are called alveolar dead space air.
- It can be measured as per the basis of ***Bohr's equation*** as follows:

$$ADS = \frac{\text{Expiratory air volume } (PCO_2 \text{ in alveolar air } PCO_2 \text{ in expiratory air})}{PCO_2 \text{ in alveolar air}}$$

Physiological dead space air = Anatomical dead space air + alveolar dead space air.

- Alveolar dead space in normal individual is negligible, so anatomical dead space is equal to physiological dead space.

19. O_2 carrying capacity:

One gram of Hb can combine with 1.34 ml of O_2 and at this stage Hb is considered as 100% saturated. Thus, a person having Hb concentration of 15mg % the 100 ml of his blood can carry 1.34 × 15 = 20ml of O_2 at full saturation which is known as ***O_2 carrying capacity of blood.***

20. Pulmonary ventilation Vs Alveolar ventilation:

As it is known that pulmonary ventilation is the total ventilation per minute i.e. RMV = TV × RR, the value of which is 6-7 lit. But in reality some amount of air (150 ml) is confined in the respiratory passages and thus not available for gas exchange process. So the actual ventilation is less than pulmonary ventilation. This amount of ventilation is known as alveolar ventilation. It can be calculated as:

Alveolar Ventilation = (TV-dead space volume) × RR
= (500–150) ml × 14/min
= 4.9 lit/min.

21. P_{50}:

- It is the level of PO_2 at which 50% of the hemoglobin is saturated with O_2.
- It assesses the binding affinity of hemoglobin for O_2.
- In adults at sea level the normal $\mathbf{P_{50}}$ is at PO_2 of 27 mmHg.
- If the P_{50} is high it signifies the decrease in affinity of hemoglobin for O_2 which is seen during shifting of O_2 dissociation curve to right and vice versa.

22. Pulmonary stretch receptors:

- These are slowly adapting myelinated nerves present in the wall of small airways.
- These are responsible for initiation of Hering-Breuer reflex.
- These receptors are activated only when the tidal volume exceeds 1000 ml and thus have no role in initiatin g Hering—Breuer reflex during quiet breathing, though these cause bronchodilatation and rise in respiration rate during exercise through initiating Hering-Breuer reflex.
- These are responsible for maintaining the basic respiratory rhythm and prevent overstretching of the lungs in the newborn and infants.

23. Non chemical stimuli stimulating respiratory center:

Though the chemoreceptors are mainly responsible for regulating respiration, there are some reflexes arising from upper airways and lungs initiated by non-chemical stimuli and other receptors from the other parts of the body which provide a feedback for fine tunning of breathing and also protect the lungs from environmental hazards. These are:

1. Pulmonary stretch receptors which are sensitive to change in lung volume. When stimulated they inhibit inspiration and prolong expiration which is known as Hering-Breuer reflex.

2. Non myelinated C fibers (J receptors described by Prof. A S Paintal)-present between the alveolar wall and the capillaries and are stimulated by accumulation of fluid between the capillary and alveolus in condition like exercise, pulmonary edema etc and cause hyperapnoea and dyspnoea.

3. Muscle spindle of inspiratory muscles (chest wall proprioceptors)-adjust respiration against high airway resistance and maintain tidal volume.

4. Pain receptors-sudden painful stimulus produces a reflex apnoea but sustained painful stimuli cause faster and deeper respiration.

5. Thermoreceptors also have role in controlling respiration. Sudden cold stimuli results reflex apnoea and warm stimuli results increase in breathing and ventilation.

6. Baroreceptors-sudden stimulation of baroreceptors inhibit respiration center to cause apnoea.

24. J-reflex: *J receptors*:

- ❑ It is believed to be present in the alveolar walls close to the capillaries (Juxta position to the capillaries, hence the name 'J' receptors) as described by Prof. A S Paintal.
- ❑ stimuli are engorgement of pulmonary capillary and increase in interstitial fluid volume of pulmonary tissue (pulmonary oedema)
- ❑ stimulation of these receptors causes hyper ventilation (during exercise) and dyspnoea (during left heart failure, pneumonia, etc.)

25. CO_2 narcosis:

- Increase in alveolar PCO_2 has almost a linear relationship with increase in ventilation but when CO_2 content of atmospheric air is too high (CO_2 content of inspiratory air is more than 7%) then PCO_2 of alveolar air and arterial blood increase abruptly. This results ineffective elimination of CO_2 from body and thus accumulation of CO_2 in the blood which is known as CO_2 narcosis.
- It results CNS depression.
- It is characterised by headache, mental confusion and ultimately coma.

26. Kussmaul breathing:

During some clinical conditions like diabetic ketoacidosis there is rapid and deep breathing eliminating CO_2 and bicarbonate. This type of rapid and shallow breathing is known as ***Kussmaul breathing***.

27. Breath holding time:

- Breathing can be inhibited for a period of 45-60 secs in normal healthy human beings voluntarily. This duration is known as **breath holding time (BHT)**. The point at which the breathing can no longer be stopped voluntarily is known as **breaking point**.
- BHT depends on—
  - phase of respiration during which breathing is arrested.
  - composition of air breathed-breathing with pure O_2 prolongs the BHT.
  - rate of respiration before breath holding.

28. Periodic breathing:

A. **Definition:** It is the repeated sequence of apnoea followed by normal respiration.

B. **Types:** It is of two types:

(a) *Cheyne—Stokes breathing*:

- It is defined as the repeated sequence of gradual onset of apnoea followed by gradual restoration of normal respiration (Fig. 5.16).

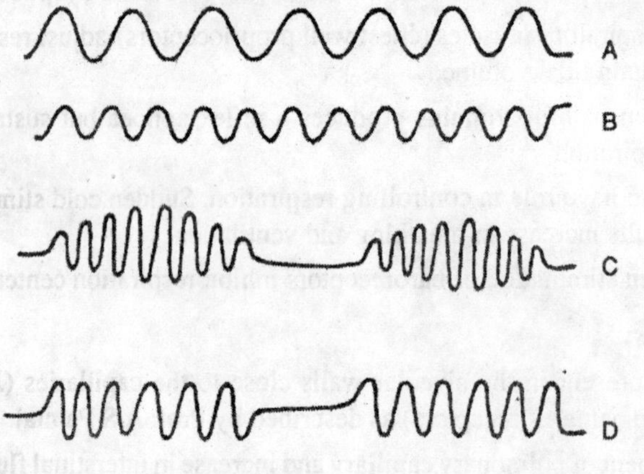

Fig. 5.16: Breathing pattern during different types of abnormal ventilation
(A = Normal breathing, B = Hyperventilation, C = Chyene Stoke's breathing and D = Biot's breathing)

- Causes:
  - **Physiological:**
    - Voluntary hyperventilation
    - High altitude
    - Sometimes during sleep in infants
  - **Pathological:**
    - Heart failure (Chronic)
    - Uremia
    - Brain damage

(b) *Biot's breathing*:

- It is the repeated sequence of 3-4 cycles of normal respiration followed by abrupt onset of apnoea further followed by abrupt onset of normal respiration (Fig. 5.16).
- It differs from Chyene-Stokes breathing in that—
  - it occurs at irregular intervals.
  - there is no waxing and waning of tidal volume during the period of respiratory activity.
  - it can never be physiological.
- Causes:
  - Meningitis
  - Medullary diseases (Brain)

29. Cough reflex:

Respiratory tract initiates some protective reflex to keep the air passage free from foreign materials. One of these reflexes is Cough reflex. Any physical or chemical irritation in the respiratory tract specially at the larynx and bifurcation of trachea causes the deep inspiration followed by forceful expiration resulting elimination of that particles at a great velocity. This is known as ***coughing***.

Mechanism: It is illustrated by following flow chart:

Foreign particles at larynx or bifurcation of trachea → physical or chemical irritation → stimulation of vagal afferents → sensation to medulla through vagus → deep inspiration is initiated → epiglottis, laryngeal opening get closed entrapping 2.5 lit of air into lungs → forcible contraction of abdominal and internal intercostal muscles. → increased intra alveolar pressure → sudden opening of glottis and vocal card → lung air comes out at a velocity of 160 km/hour → particles are thrown out of respiratory passages.

30. Mountain sickness: It is generally two types:

1. *Acute mountain sickness:*

- If a person who resides in sea level ascends to high altitude (>10,000 ft above sea level) he develops the sign and symptoms due to hypoxic hypoxia which are collectively called as ***high altitude sickness*** or ***Acute mountain sickness***.
- It is characterised by:
  - (a) starts 8-12 hrs after arrival in high altitude
  - (b) lasts for about 4-8 days
  - (c) *sign and symptoms*: headache, fatigue, nausea, vomiting, loss of appetite, dyspnoea, palpitation, sleep disturbances, insomnia etc. In some cases there may be even cerebral or pulmonary oedema.
- Treatment: (a) The person should immediately brought to low level (b) O_2 administration.

2. *Chronic mountain sickness (Monge's disease):* It is the disease occurring in case of failure of long-term acclimatization process to the residents of high altitude. The signs and symptoms are:

- extreme polycythemia
- ↑ viscosity of blood → fall of blood flow
- ↑ BP
- cyanosis, fatigue, exercise intolerance
- pulmonary oedema.

31. Acclimatization at high altitude (to low landers):

The acclimatization refers to the compensatory changes in the body to overcome the effect of hypoxic hypoxia in response to slow ascent in high altitude and/or long term exposure to hypoxia. These compensatory changes are:

a. Respiratory adjustments:

(i) Increase in pulmonary ventilation by 5-6 times primarily due to increase in tidal volume which may increase to 50% of vital capacity due to hypoxic stimulation of peripheral chemoreceptors i.e. high altitude (low barometric pressure) → hypoxia → stimulation of peripheral chemoreceptors → ↑ respiration → ↑ pulmonary ventilation.

(ii) Increase in diffusion capacity of lungs due to:

- expansion and dilatation of pulmonary capillaries
- increase in lung volume
- increase in blood volume
- increase in perfusion in apical part of alveoli
- increase in pulmonary arterial pressure

(iii) Shifting of O_2—dissociation curve to right due to increase 2-3 DPG concentration which favours unloading of O_2 in tissue.

(iv) Increase in maximum breathing capacity.

b. Cardio-vascular adjustments: These include:

(i) hypertrophy of right heart due to more work.

(ii) dilatation of blood capillaries to accommodate extra blood.

(iii) Increase in heart rate and force of contraction due to sympathetic stimulation → ↑ cardiac output.

(iv) Rise or fall of B.P.—vasoconstriction occurs due to stimulation of vasomotor center by hypoxia but is opposed by vasodilatation produced by local effects of hypoxia. The resultant of these two forces determines the outcome. The BP is also raised due to polycythemia in high altitude.

c. Hematological adjustments: These include:

(i) Increase in RBC count.

(ii) ↑ Blood volume up to 20-30%.

(iii) Increase in 2-3 DPG concentration in RBC.

d. Cellular changes:

(i) Increase in number of mitochondria

(ii) Increase in concentration of cellular oxidative enzymes.

32. Acclimatization to Natives (high lander):

The acclimatization that occurs in the residents who are residing in the high altitude permanently for generations after generations, are as follows:

(a) short body stature and large sized chest that results high ratio of ventilatory capacity to body mass

(b) hypertrophy of right heart

(c) polycythemia

(d) shifting of O_2 dissociation curve to right

(e) increase in size of carotid bodies.

33. Caissons disease:

- When the diver is working in the deep sea for a long time he is exposed to high alveolar gas pressure (high barometric pressure i.e. **hyperbarism**) to prevent the collapse of the lungs. The gas mixture administered to him contains O_2, CO_2 and N_2 with high pressure. Because of these a large amount of N_2 is dissolved in his body fluids and fats. Sudden exposure of that diver to low barometric pressure at sea level causes the formation of N_2 bubbles in body fluids and fatty tissues that may block capillaries, hearts and also affect nervous system badly. This results the development of some signs and symptoms which are collectively known as ***Decompression Sickness*** or ***Caisson disease*** or ***Dysbarism*** or ***Diver's palsy***. So this disease is basically due to effect of N_2 with high pressure known as ***N_2 narcosis***.
- *Signs and symptoms:*
  - Pain in joints, muscles of legs and arms.
  - Dizziness, paralysis, collapse, unconsciousness, temporary sensory and motor disturbances (if nervous system is affected).

- Bubble formation in lung vessels results into '**chokes**' characterised by shortness of breathing and pulmonary oedema.

- *Treatment*: Immediate recompression in a chamber and gradual decompression.
- *Prevention of decompression sickness*: It can be prevented by:

  (i) Gradual ascent from sea.

  (ii) Inhalation of O_2-helium mixture before the ascent. However at high atmospheric pressure it can produce ***high pressure nervous syndrome*** (NPNS) which is characterised by tremors, drowsiness and depression of a activity in EEG.

- Mild N_2 narcosis resembles alcohole intoxication and the person becomes very jovial, careless and fails to understand the seriousness of the situation. In severe cases the person develops lethergy, drowsiness, rapid onset of fatigue and loss of consciousness.

34. N_2 narcosis: See the answer of Caissons disease.

35. Artificial respiration:

A. ***Aim of artificial respiration***: These are—

a. avoiding asphyxia to brain

b. oxygenation of body tissue

c. ventilation of lung

d. stimulation of spontaneous breathing

B. ***The conditions when it is indicated?***

Artificial respiration is given to the subject in case of following conditions e.g.

(a) **Acute respiratory failure** due to

— overdose of anesthetic agent

— CO poisoning

— Drowning

— Electric shock

— Hanging

— Intake of narcotic drugs

— Resuscitation of new born

(b) **Chronic respiratory failure** due to

— Diphtheria

— Poliomyelitis

— Ascending paralysis

C. ***Methods of artificial respiration***: It is of 2 types Manual and Mechanical

(a) Manual:

— Mouth to mouth breathing

— Holger Neilson's Arm lift back pressure (ALBP) or BPAL method

— Other methods like Schafer's prone pressure method, Sylvester's method, Drinker's method.

(b) Mechanical: use of respiratory pump.

D. ***How long artificial respiration is to be continued?*** It should be continued untill

(i) The subject's own spontaneous respiration reappears.

(ii) The subject is hospitalised and appropriate treatment is started.

36. Resuscitation of new born:

- This is done to expand the lungs of newborn in case of premature birth of the child in which lungs is collapsed due to high surface tension which is not minimised because of lack of lung surfactant.
- Methods followed:
  - — Cutaneous stimulation e.g. slapping, warm or cold water application
  - — Mouth to mouth breathing
  - — ETI (endo-tracheal tube insertion) and insufflation of lungs with CO_2-O_2 mixture
- Artificial respiration should be continued until the subject develops normal rhythmic respiration.

37. VO_2 max:

- During resting condition the O_2 consumption by the whole body is about 250 ml/min which is increased up to 15-20 times during maximal exercise. The maximum amount of O_2 that can be consumed by an individual is called as maximal O_2 consumption or VO_2 max.
- The normal VO_2 in an adult is 3L/min and in athlet it is about 5L /min.
- It is an important indicator of the individuals capacity to carry out aerobic exercise.
- The factors affecting this are –cardiac output mainly, ability of tissue to extract O_2 and size of total muscle mass.
- It is maximum during adulthood and then declines with advancement of age.

38. O_2 therapy:

- It is indicated in acute and severe hypoxia especially when hypoxia is associated with dyspnoea.
- O_2 therapy can be done by two procedures e.g.

  (i) **Inhalation of 100% pure O_2** but this procedure has side effects like:

  - Nasal congestion, sore throat, sneezing, coughing, bronchoconstriction due to stimulation of irritant receptors in respiratory tract.
  - O_2 toxicity which is characterised by muscular twitching, dizziness, cog wheel (Jerking) respiration, convulsion, and unconsciousness. It is basically due to inhibition of tissue enzyme activity and cerebral vasoconstriction.

  (ii) **Inhalation of 100% pure O_2 at high barometric pressure (hyperbaric O_2 therapy):** The main aim of which is to increase the amount of dissolved O_2 in plasma and thereby helps in all forms of hypoxic conditions except hypoxic hypoxia. However in early stages there may be ***O_2 toxicity***.

  - O_2 therapy is very useful in hypoxic hypoxia and anemic hypoxia but not in stagnant hypoxia (as blood flow to the tissue is decreased in this condition) and histotoxic hypoxia (as tissue is unable to utilize O_2).

39. O_2 poisoning:

- During deep sea diving as O_2 is breathed at a higher pressure (100% O_2) the amount of O_2 dissolved in the tissue fluid becomes high. This may result fatal condition specially in CNS which is called as O_2 poisoning.

- It is characterised as nausea, dizziness, irritability, disturbed vision, disorientation and convulsions.
- It also begins to appear at 10 atm pressure of room air after more than 30 sec.
- To prevent the ill-effect of O_2 toxicity gas mixtures of O_2–helium is inhaled at high pressure in which O_2 concentration is reduced at about 20%.

40. Cyanosis:

- **Definition:** Bluish colouration of skin and or mucous membrane due to presence of at least 5 gm% of reduced Hb/100 ml of blood in capillaries is termed as ***cyanosis***.
- **Site:** Common site of occurrence are - Mucous membrane of undersurface of tongue, Lips, Nail bed and Tip of nose.
- **Causes:** The causes are:
  (a) Hypoxic hypoxia—Cyanosis results due to increased formation of reduced hemoglobin as arterial PO_2 is decreased.
  (b) Stagnant hypoxia—During this state there is decrease in rate of blood flow →↑ rate of extraction of O_2 by tissues →↑ formation of reduced Hb which leads to cyanosis.
  (c) In anaemic hypoxia there is reduction of formation of reduced Hb (as total Hb is low) and in histotoxic hypoxia O_2 is not used by the tissues. This is why during those hypoxic conditions cyanosis is absent.
  (d) Local factors:
  - Exposure to mild cold can result cyanosis due to vasoconstriction.
  - Exposure to severe cold → no cyanosis because of following reason:
    - decrease in O_2 consumption by tissues
    - Shift of O_2 dissociation curve to left → release of O_2 from Hb.
  - Meth-hemoglobinemia produced due to toxic dose of sulphanilamides or of acetanilamide.

41. Asphyxia:

- ***Definition***: Improper airation of the blood in which hypoxia is associated with hypercapnoea (↑CO_2 level) is called as ***asphyxia.***
- ***Causes***: similar to the causes of hypoxia
- ***Stages***: 3 stages:
  - stage of hyperapnoea
  - stage of convulsions
  - stage of collapse

42. Peak Expiratory flow rate (PERR):

- It is the maximum rate of air flow that is sustained for the period of 10 ms during forced expiration.
- **Normal value:**
  - In male = 400 – 600 L/min
  - In female = 300 – 400 L/min.
- **Significance:** It helps to asses the respiratory diseases. Generally it is reduced in all types of respiratory diseases however the reduction in obstructive diseases is more than in restrictive diseases.

- It can be recorded by using peak flow meter.
- It is an index of patency of airways.

43. Dyspnoea:

- ***Definition***: It is defined as **'a consciousness of necessity for increased respiratory effort'** or air **hunger** resulted due to difficulty in breathing.
- It is the clinical condition characterised by difficulty in breathing.
- Dyspnoea occurs when **Dyspnoeic index** falls below 60%. Therefore dyspnoea occurs when (i) MVV becomes less than normal (ii) ↓ VC, (iii) ↑ Pulmonary ventilation by 4.5 times.
- It occurs during respiratory disorders affecting ventilation, cardiac disorders affecting lung function and metabolic disorder like diabetic acidosis, uremia and etc.
- In the early stage, heart failure, dyspnoea occurs during exercise due to failure of LV output to meet the increased O_2 demand during exercise. This is known as dyspnoea on exertion whereas in the late stage of heart failure dyspnoea occurs even at rest due to increased venous pressure or due to gross inadequate ventricular pumping.
- During severe exercise also it is seen which is an example of physiological dyspnoea.

44. MBC and MVV:

- It is the maximum volume of air that can be taken in or given out in each minute.
- It is calculated as: MVV = VC × Respiratory rate.
- Normal value
  - ☐ In male = 150 – 170 liter/ min
  - ☐ In female = 80 – 100 liter/ min
- Significance: It is an overall index of ventilatory capacity. It's values may be altered by disease of the respiratory muscles of thoracic cage or by obstruction in airways like emphysema.
- The factors affecting MBC are respiratory muscle power, airway patency, compliance, elasticity and viscosity of lung.

45. Breathing reserve and dyspnoeic index:

Pulmonary reserve (PR) or Breathing reserve (BR)

- It is the maximum amount of air above the pulmonary ventilation that can be breathed in or out in one minute.
- It is calculated as: BR = MVV – RMV.

Dyspnoic index (DI)

- When BR is expressed as % of MVV it is known as DI.
- It is calculated as **DI = MVV – RMV × 100 / MVV**
  = BR × 100 / MV.
- **Normal value**—60% to 70%
- Significance: When this value reduces below 60% dyspnoea is present.

46. Vocal fremitus:

- It is one important palpatory device to asses the clinical condition of respiratory system.

- It is performed by placing the palm of the hand flatly on the chest surface and asking the subject to say ***one-two-three***. The vibrations transmitted to the chest wall felt by hand are called as vocal fremitus.
- Vocal fremitus is increased in consolidation of lung tissue and decreased in pleural effusion.

47. Respiratory minute volume (RMV) or Pulmonary ventilation (PV):

- It is defined as the volume of air that can be breathed in or breathed out per minute-during normal respiration.
- It is calculated as : RMV = TV × respiratory rate
- **Normal value** = 6-7 L/min.

48. Apnoea:

- ***Definition***: It is defined as the temporary stoppage of breathing.
- ***Causes***: The causes are
  - ❑ After hyperventilation
  - ❑ During sleep (sleep apnoea)
  - ❑ During deglutition (deglutition apnoea)
  - ❑ During Herring-Breuer deflation reflex
  - ❑ During Bezold Jarish reflex
  - ❑ Voluntary apnoea: A person can arrest his breathing for sometimes up to a certain period beyond which breathing starts automatically due to accumulation of O_2. This voluntary stoppage of breathing is known as voluntary apnoea and the period is called as breath holding time or BHT and the point beyond which it can no longer be held is known as breaking point.

49. Mouth to mouth breathing:

- It is one of the important manual method of artificial respiration preferably in adults.
- Procedure adopted is:
  - ❑ Subject is placed in the supine position.
  - ❑ Airways is cleaned and neck is extended (Fig. 5.17).
  - ❑ The nostrils of the patient is closed by pinching with the thumb and index finger of the performer.
  - ❑ Air is exhaled forcefully from the mouth of performer to the subjects mouth after taking a deep breath.
  - ❑ Chest expansion is noted.
  - ❑ Above steps are repeated at a rate of 10-15 /min.
- Advantages:
  - ❑ It can be applied immediately and simple technique.
  - ❑ Greater tidal volume (1000 ml) can be obtained.
  - ❑ CO_2 in expired air helps to stimulate the subject's respiratory center.
- Disadvantages:
  - ❑ There is a chance of infection in either direction.
  - ❑ Performer may go into exhaustion and thus can not be continued for long time.

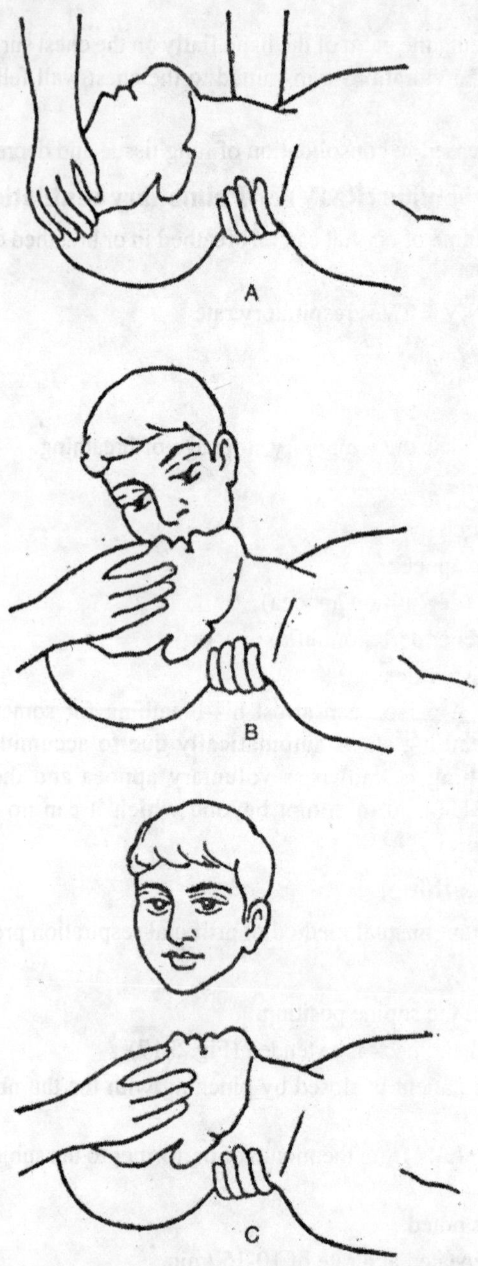

Fig. 5.17: Methods of artificial respiration. **Mouth to mouth breathing** (*A = the neck is extended by placing one hand under the neck and pressing the forehead with other hand, B = performer exhales the air into the patient's mouth by tightly placing his mouth over the patient's mouth keeping the nostrils of patient closed, C = allows the patient to exhale passively by unsealing nose and nostrils*)

50. Cardiopulmonary resuscitation:

- If the respiration fails along with stoppage of heart beat this procedure is followed till the person is not hospitalised for proper treatment.

- The basic life support is given by:
  - ❑ Cleaning of the airways
  - ❑ Mouth to mouth breathing at the rate of 16-18/m
  - ❑ External cardiac message by—
    - ■ pressing lower border of sternum by 4-5 cm at the rate of 30 times/min.
    - ■ after every 15 cardiac massage two mouth to mouth (15:2) breathing (if two subjects are present).
    - ■ after every 5 cardiac massage 1 mouth to mouth (5:1) breathing (if one subject is available).
- Advanced life support is given by defibrillation and airway management and O_2 therapy.

C. Differentiate between:

Terminal bronchi	**Respiratory bronchi**
❑ As per Weibel's lung model it is numbered as 16th generation. ❑ No gaseous exchange takes place in this zone. ❑ It is the conductive zone.	❑ As per Weibel's lung model it is numbered as 17th generation. ❑ Gaseous exchange takes place in this zone. ❑ It is the respiratory zone.
Conductive zone	**Respiratory zone**
❑ It is a pipe like structure of tracheobronchial tube through which air passes. ❑ It starts from Trachea (Zero generation as per Weibel's lung model) to 16th generation. ❑ Walls of this zone is thicker. ❑ Mean diameter is less. ❑ Velocity of air movement is high.	❑ It consists of balloon like structures in which gaseous exchange takes place. ❑ It starts from respiratory bronchiole to alveolar sac. ❑ Walls of this zone is thin. ❑ Mean diameter is more. ❑ Velocity of air movement is comparatively less.
External respiration	**Internal respiration**
❑ Respiration concerned with exchange of gases between environment and lungs is known as external respiration. ❑ No energy is liberated in this process.	❑ Respiration concerned with exchange of gases between the cells and the internal environment and it's use to provide energy is known as external respiration. ❑ Energy is liberated in this process.
Intrapleural pressure	**Intrapulmonary pressure**
❑ It is the pressure existing in the pleural cavity. ❑ Normally it is negative and positive only during forceful expiration. ❑ It helps to prevent collapsing of lungs.	❑ It is the pressure inside the alveolus. ❑ Normally it is positive and negative only during inspiration. ❑ It helps to drive air in and out of lungs and also controls the exchange of gases between alveolar air and blood.

Valsalva maneuver	Muller's maneuver
❑ It is the forced expiration against closed glottis. ❑ In this situation intraalveolar pressure increases beyond 100 mm Hg above the atmospheric pressure.	❑ It is the forced inspiration against closed glottis. ❑ In this situation intraalveolar pressure decreases below 80 mm Hg.

Static lung volume	Dynamic lung volume
❑ The lung volumes when not expressed in time is known as static lung volume. ❑ Clinically is not very much useful.	❑ The lung volumes when are expressed in time is known as Dynamic lung volume. ❑ Clinically is very much useful.

Alveolar ventilation	Pulmonary ventilation
❑ The amount of air that exchange through alveolus per min is called as alveolar ventilation. ❑ It excludes the dead space volume. ❑ It is thus less than pulmonary ventilation. ❑ Normal value—4.9 L / min.	❑ The amount of air that can be breathed in or out per min is called as pulmonary ventilation. ❑ It includes the dead space volume. ❑ It is thus more than alveolar ventilation. ❑ Normal value—6-7 L / min.

Fresh water drawning	Sea water drawning
❑ Water enters the lungs and thus quickly diffuses to blood due to hypotonicity of fresh water. ❑ It results hemodilution and thus hemolysis.	❑ Water in the lungs draws fluid from the vascular space of lung tissue resulting hypertonicity of body fluid. ❑ It results hemoconcentration and thus no hemolysis.

Hyperapnoea	Hyperventilation
❑ Increased pulmonary ventilation due to increase in force of respiration is known as hyperapnoea.	❑ Abnormal increase in pulmonary ventilation due to forced breathing which often leads to dizziness and sometimes chest pain is known as hyperventilation.

Vesicular breath sound	Bronchial breath sound
❑ It is produced by passage of air in and out of alveoli in the normal lung tissue. ❑ Normally it is heard over the healthy chest but most typically over the axillary and infrascapular region. ❑ Inspiratory sound is more loud.	❑ It is produced by passage of air in and out through the trachea and large bronchi. ❑ Normally it is heard over the trachea. ❑ Expiratory sound is more loud.

Vesicular breath sound	Bronchial breath sound
❑ No gap is present in between inspiration and expiration. ❑ Duration of inspiration sound is twice of expiratory sound.	❑ Silent gap is present in between inspiration and expiration. ❑ Duration is same.

Obstructive lung disease	Restrictive lung disease
❑ Any abnormal respiratory condition which makes it difficult to push the air outside the lungs (expiration) is called as obstructive lung disease. ❑ Examples: asthma, emphysema. ❑ Occurs due to abnormality in the respiratory tract. ❑ FEV1 is reduced in this condition but vital capacity is unaffected. ❑ Chest expansion is not restricted only expiration is obstructed.	❑ Any abnormal respiratory condition which makes it difficult to get the air into the lungs (inspiration) is called as restrictive lung disease. ❑ Examples: kyphosis, ankylosing spondilitis. ❑ Occurs due to abnormality in the lung, thoracic cavity and in the nervous system. ❑ FEV1 remains unaffected in this condition but vital capacity is reduced. ❑ Chest expansion is restricted.

High altitude native	Newcomer to high altitude
❑ Increase in pulmonary ventilation is more. ❑ Response to hypoxic stimulation is more. ❑ Urine is alkaline. ❑ Affinity of hemoglobin for O_2 is less. ❑ Vascularity is more. ❑ Mitochondria and myoglobin content is high. ❑ Diffusion capacity is more.	❑ Increase in pulmonary ventilation is less. ❑ Response to hypoxic stimulation is less. ❑ Urine is acidic. ❑ Affinity of hemoglobin for O_2 is more. ❑ Vascularity is less. ❑ Mitochondria and myoglobin content is less. ❑ Diffusion capacity is less.

D. Brainstorming short answer type:

1. **Why the combination of O_2 with hemoglobin is called as oxygenation and not oxidation?**
   It is because iron remains in ferrous form after combination with O_2.
2. **Why the O_2 carrying capacity of blood is 19 ml/ 100 ml of blood instead of 20.1 ml / 100 ml of blood?**
   It is because the hemoglobin is only 95% saturated with O_2.
3. **What is the O_2 carrying capacity of hemoglobin?**
   It is 1.34 ml i.e. 1 gm hemoglobin can carry 1.34 ml of O_2.
4. **Which protein is responsible for HCO_3^- and Cl^- exchange in RBC during Humburger phenomenon?**
   It is band 3 proteins which act like antiport in RBC.
5. **Why the amount of CO_2 transported through hemoglobin is more than that of plasma proteins?**
   It is because the quantity of plasma protein is only half of the quantity of hemoglobin.

6. How long the voluntary control of respiration (Voluntary apnoea) is possible?

It is for abouts 40 secs.

7. What is polypnoea?

Rapid shallow breathing resembling panting in dogs is known as polypnoea. Here only rate of respiration is increased but not force of respiration.

8. What is the efficacy of O_2 therapy in different types of hypoxia?

This is as follows:

- In hypoxic hypoxia: 100 % useful
- In anaemic hypoxia: 70 % useful
- In stagnant hypoxia: 50 % useful
- In histotoxic hypoxia: not at al

9. Why the airways resistance is high in conduction zone as compaired to the respiratory zone?

The resistance to the air flow is inversely related to the total cross sectional area of the respiratory passage i.e. the greater the cross sectional area, the lesser is the airways resistance. As the total cross sectional area is far more in respiratory zone the airways resistance is comparatively less than that of conductive zone.

10. Why the bronchial asthma is a disease of expiratory obstruction?

In bronchial asthma broncho-constriction develops resulting decrease in diameter of the airways that leads to increased airways resistance producing difficulty in breathing. Moreover during expiration these already constricted bronchioles further constrict resulting marked increase in airways resistance. This is why there is extreme difficulty in breathing during expiration.

11. Why the patients with defects in respiratory membrane suffer initially only hypoxic symptoms not of hypercapnia?

This is because the diffusion capacity of CO_2 is 20 times more than that of O_2 which result much CO_2 diffusion to the alveolus in comparison to O_2 diffusion to lungs capillaries inspite of decrease in diffusion capacity.

12. Which one is more dangerous situation rapid shallow respiration or slow deep respiration?

Rapid shallow breathing is more dangerous as during this type of breathing alveolar ventilation decreases though the pulmonary ventilation remains normal resulting less air available for gaseous exchange whereas in slow and deep respiration both the alveolar and pulmonary ventilation are normal.

13. Why PCV of venous blood is greater than that of arterial blood?

In the venous blood the HCO_3^- and Cl^- content in the RBC is far more because of fast operation of chloride shift → results hyper-osmolarity in RBC → more intake of water → more swelling of RBC → more rate of their settling in the tube → increase in PCV (hematocrit).

14. What will happen to respiration after bilateral vagotomy?

There will be regular normal respiration (Eupnoea) after bilateral vagotomy.

15. What will happen if peripheral chemoreceptors are removed?

There will be little change of respiration during rest but the ventilatory response in response to hypoxia, hypercapnoea and acidemia will be lost by approximately 30%.

16. What will happen to breath holding time after removal of carotid bodies?

It will be increased.

17. How mild to moderate hypoxia stimulation respiration but severe hypoxia depresses it?

Severe hypoxia depresses the respiration by directly inhibiting the respiratory center whereas the mild or moderate hypoxia stimulates respiration center by stimulating peripheral chemoreceptors.

18. Why respiratory chemoreceptors are not stimulated in anemia or CO poisoning?

Respiratory chemoreceptors are not stimulated in anemia and CO poisoning as the O_2 requirement of these receptors can be fulfilled largely by dissolved O_2 alone which used to be normal during those conditions.

19. Give physiological basis of pulmonary edema during rapid ascend?

During rapid ascend to high altitude → increase in sympathetic activity due to increase in physical work, cold and hypoxic stimulation of VMC → vasoconstriction → increase in pulmonary capillary hydrostatic pressure → diffusion of fluid to interstitial space of lungs from the pulmonary capillaries → pulmonary edema.

20. Give physiological basis of cerebral edema during slow ascent.

During slow ascend to high altitude → decrease in arterial PO_2 → when autoregulatory mechanism in cerebral blood flow is reached to it's highest limit there is increase in capillary pressure → transduation of fluid in brain tissue → cerebral edema.

21. Give physiological basis of alkaline urine in an acclimatized person.

In acclimatized person the alkalosis due to fall in arterial PCO_2 is compensated by actively excreting more HCO_3^- in urine to maintain normal pH. This results alkaline urine.

22. How one can not ascend high with 100% O_2 inhalation?

With 100% O_2 inhalation one can ascent upto 45000 ft only because above this height barometric pressure falls to 110 mmHg with only 33 mmHg PO_2. At this PO_2 there is impairement of mental function.

23. Explain: The dangers of high atmosphoric pressure are never due to high arterial PCO_2.

This is because body expires this excess CO_2 by hyperventilation.

24. Explain: O_2 therapy may cause death in an individual with severe respiratory failure.

This is because of the fact that whatever respiration is there, it will be due to hypoxic stimulation of peripheral chemoreceptors. So O_2 therapy in this condition will result withdrawal of hypoxic condition of peripheral chemoreceptors → leads direct depression of respiratory center by severe hypoxia and hypercapnoea → death.

25. Explain: Neonates should never be given 100% O_2 inhalation.

This is because it may result proliferation of retinal vessels with the formation of fibrous tissues leading permanent blindness.

26. Explain: Mild cold produces cyanosis but not seen in severe cold.

Mild cold → cutaneous vasoconstriction to preserve heat → decrease rate of blood flow in tissue → O_2 extraction by the tissue tends to remain normal due to slow passage of blood → increase in reduced hemoglobin → Cyanosis.

Whereas in severe cold there is decrease in O_2 consumption by the tissues and also shifting of O_2 dissociation curve to left leading less release of O_2 to the tissues → no significant rise of reduced hemoglobin → no cyanosis.

27. Explain: Cyanosis is not seen in anemic and histotoxic hypoxia.

In anemia total Hb content is low → no formation of enough reduced Hb → no cyanosis.

In histotoxic hypoxia O_2 is not taken up by the tissues → no significant formation of reduced Hb → no cyanosis.

E: MCQ:

1. The muscle takes part in normal inspiration is (i) diaphragm (ii) external intercostal muscle (iii) both (iv) none. (iii)
2. The muscle which do not take part in forceful expiration is (i) internal intercostal muscle (ii) external intercostal muscle (iii) abdominal muscle (iv) internal oblique muscle. (ii)
3. The Bucket Handle movement of the thoracic ribs are responsible for increase in (i) vertical diameter of thoracic cage (ii) antero-postero diameter (iii) transverse diameter (iv) all of the above. (iii)
4. The Pump Handle movement of the thoracic ribs are responsible for increase in (i) vertical diameter of thoracic cage (ii) antero-postero diameter (iii) transverse diameter (iv) all of the above. (ii)
5. The pump handle movement is contributed by intercostal muscles of thoracic ribs of (i) 2-6th (ii) 7-10th (iii) both (iv) none. (i)
6. The Bucket handle movement is contributed by intercostal muscles of thoracic ribs of (i) 2-6th (ii) 7-10th (iii) both (iv) none. (iii).
7. The vertical diameter of thoracic cage is altered by the movement of (i) external intercostal muscle of upper costal series (ii) external intercostal muscle of lower costal series (iii) diaphragm (iv) all of the above. (iii)
8. The normal intrapleural pressure during inspiration is (i) – 2 to – 5 mmHg (ii) – 40 to – 50 mmHg (iii) – 5 to – 10 mmHg (iv) 10 to 15 mmHg. (iii)
9. Cross sectional area of airways is (i) directly related (ii) inversely related (iii) not related anyway with airways resistance. (ii)
10. Normal residual volume is (i)1200 ml (ii) 2000 ml (iii) 500 ml (iv) 5000 ml. (i)
11. The normal value of FRC is (i) 1500 ml (ii) 2200 ml (iii) 3000 ml (iv) 5000 ml. (ii)
12. FEV_1 is reduced in (i) obstructive lung disease (ii) restrictive lung disease (iii) both (iv) none of the above. (i)
13. Normal RMV is (i) 4-5 lit (ii) 6-7 lit (iii) 8-10 lit (iv) 2500 ml. (ii)
14. The partial pressure of oxygen in alveolar air is (i) 100 mmHg (ii) 160 mmHg (iii) 104 mmHg (iv) 154 mmHg. (iii)
15. The CO_2 content in arterial blood is 52 ml% (ii) 0.04 ml% (iii) 48 ml% (iv) 19 ml%. (iii)
16. The normal ventilation perfusion is (i) 0.84 (ii) 1 (iii) 8.4 (iv) 0.1. (i)
17. The O_2 carrying capacity of blood is (i) 1.34 ml (ii) 20 ml (iii) 15 ml (iv) 1.72 ml. (ii)
18. Shift to the left of O_2 dissociation curve occurs in following conditions except (i) decrease in H^+ (ii) presence of CO (iii) decrease PO_2 of blood (iv) increased level of 2-3 DPG. (iv)
19. Shift to the right of O_2 dissociation curve does not occur in following conditions (i) increase in PCO_2 (ii) presence of HBF (iii) increase in temperature (iv) decrease in pH of blood. (ii)
20. The maximum amount of CO_2 is carried in (i) dissolved form (ii) bicarbonate form (iii) carbamino compound form (iv) only ii and iii. (ii)
21. Ramp signal is initiated by (i) Apneustic center (ii) Pneumotaxix center (iii) Suprapontine center (iv) DRG neurons. (iv)

22. The switching off of the inspiratory ramp signal is prevented by (i) Apneustic center (ii) Pneumotaxix center (iii) Suprapontine center (iv) DRG neurons. (i)
23. Central chemoreceptors are directly stimulated by (i) increase in H^+ in blood (ii) increase in H^+ con. in mudullary interstitial fluid (iii) decrease in H^+ in blood (iv) decrease in H^+ concentration in medullary interstitial fluid. (ii)
24. Arterial PO_2 is decreased in (i) hypoxic hypoxia (ii) anemic hypoxia (iii) stagnant hypoxia (iv) histotoxic hypoxia. (i)
25. Cynosis is present in (i) hypoxic hypoxia (ii) anemic hypoxia (iii) stagnant hypoxia (iv) histotoxic hypoxia. (i and iii)
26. Surfactant is produced in the alveoli by (i) Macrophage (ii) Type I cells (iii) Type II cells (iv) APUD. cells. (iii)
27. At high altitude the value of P_{50} is (i) less than sea level value (ii) more than sea level value (iii) same as that of sea level value. (ii)
28. The O_2 therapy is useful in (i) hypoxic hypoxia (ii) anemic hypoxia (iii) stagnant hypoxia (iv) histotoxic hypoxia. (i)
29. Cyanosis develops when there is (i) level of reduced Hb becomes 5 gm (ii) level of reduced Hb becomes 2 gm (iii) level of reduced Hb becomes 1 gm (iv) none. (i)
30. All the factors increase bronchial tone except (i) parasympathetic stimulation (ii) VIP (iii) exercise (iv) cold air. (ii)
31. At full term fetal lung surfactant maturation is facilitated by (i) glucocorticoid (ii) PTH (iii) ADH (iv) aldosterone. (i)
32. Closing volume is (i) less than RV (ii) more than RV (iii) equal of RV (iv) equal of FRC. (ii)
33. All except the followings can not be measured by spirometry (i) VC (ii) TV (iii) RV (iv) MVV. (iii)
34. Haldane effect facilitates (i) release of CO_2 in lung (ii) release of O_2 in tissue (iii) transport of O_2 by blood (iv) shift of O_2 dissociation curve to right. (i)
35. O_2 therapy is not useful in the following conditions except (i) hypoxia due to respiratory center depression (ii) hypoxia due to A-V shunts (ii) both (iv) hypoxia at high altitude. (iv)
36. Vagal stimulation causes (i) bronchial constriction (ii) increase in mucous secretion (iii) both (iv) bronchodilatation. (iii)
37. Pulmonary oedema is caused by (i) increased in capillary hydrostatic pressure (ii) decrease in oncotic pressure (iii) increase in capillary permeability (iv) decrease in capillary hydrostatic pressure. (iv)
38. Bohr's effect helps in (i) unloading of O_2 and loading of CO_2 (ii) loading of O_2 and unloading of CO_2 (iii) unloading of O_2 and CO_2 (iv) loading of O_2 and CO_2. (i)
39. Features of restrictive lung disease are as follows except (i) decrease in TLC (ii) decrease in VC (iii) decrease in RV (iv) decrease in FEV_1. (iv)
40. Following are the example of obstructive lung disease except (i) COPD (ii) Asthma (iii) Pulmonary fibrosis (iv) Cystic fibrosis. (iii)

6 Reproductive System

A. Long type:

1. How does sex is determined? How the sex is differentiated?

Sex determination and differentiation take place in 3 phases in which 1st phase takes place at the time of fertilisation of ovum by sperm whereas other two phases occur in embryonic life.

A. Determination of genetic (chromosomal) sex:

- Of the 23 pairs of chromosomes observed in human beings, 22 pairs are ***autosome*** which do not play any role in the determination of sex. The last pair is named as ***sex chromosome*** as they have a major role in sex determination.
- Sex chromosomes are labeled as X and Y chromosomes. The sex chromosomes in female are homologous i.e. **XX** whereas in male these are heterologous i.e. **XY.**
- During meiosis or reduction division of the primary spermatocyte or oocyte, half of the number of chromosomes pass to the daughter cell. As a result each daughter cell contains 22 autosomes and 1 sex chromosome. In male the sperm will thus contain 22 + Y chromosome or 22 + X and in female the ovum will contain 22 + X chromosome.
- In the process of fertilisation between sperm and ovum the resulting zygote would contain 22 pair autosomes and one pair sex chromosomes either XX or XY.
- Thus it has been observed that Y chromosome is necessary and sufficient for the production of testes, and masculine nature.

B. Determination of gonadal sex:

Once the genetic male is determined by the above mentioned process the gene present in the tip of the short arm of the human Y chromosome (which is known as **SRY chromosome**) plays an important role in determining gonadal sex. This SRY chromosome contains the **SRY gene** that encodes **Testis determining factor (TDF)**. A similar type of gene identical to SRY gene also encodes a histocompatibility antigen known as **H-Y antigen**. Both of those factors cause differentiation of indifferent or bipotential gonad to embryonic testis and thereby maleness in the following way—

- During the initial 5-6 weeks of fetal life a primitive gonad arises from the genital ridge, a condensation of tissue near the adrenal gland, on each side of the embryo. Until the 6th week after gestation this primitive gonad is identical in both sexes and thus is known as **Bipotential gonad** which consists of germ cells, coelomic epithelium and mesenchymal cells.

- During 7th to 8th week after gestation in genetic male under the influence of testis determining genes from SRY chromosome there is a development of fetal testis (Fig. 6.1).
- In case of genetic female because of the absence of SRY chromosome bipotential gonad is differentiated into fetal ovary (Fig. 6.1).

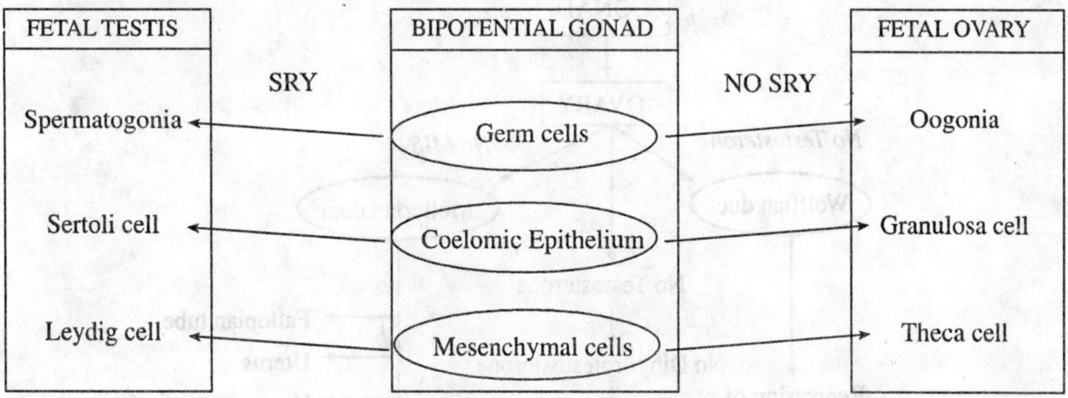

Fig. 6.1: Determination of gonadal sex

***C. Differentiation of phenotypic (Genital) Sex*:**

- During the sexually indifferent stage i.e. from 3-7 week after gestation, two genital ducts develop on each side—known as ***Wolffian*** duct and ***Mullerian*** duct. In 9-10 weeks when the development of fetal testis becomes complete, the sertoli cells of fetal testis secrete MIS (Mullerian Inhibitory Peptide or Factor) which causes the regression of mullerian duct where as the leydig cells secrete testosterone that causes differentiation of male genital tract and male external genitalia from the Wolffian duct (Fig. 6.2A).

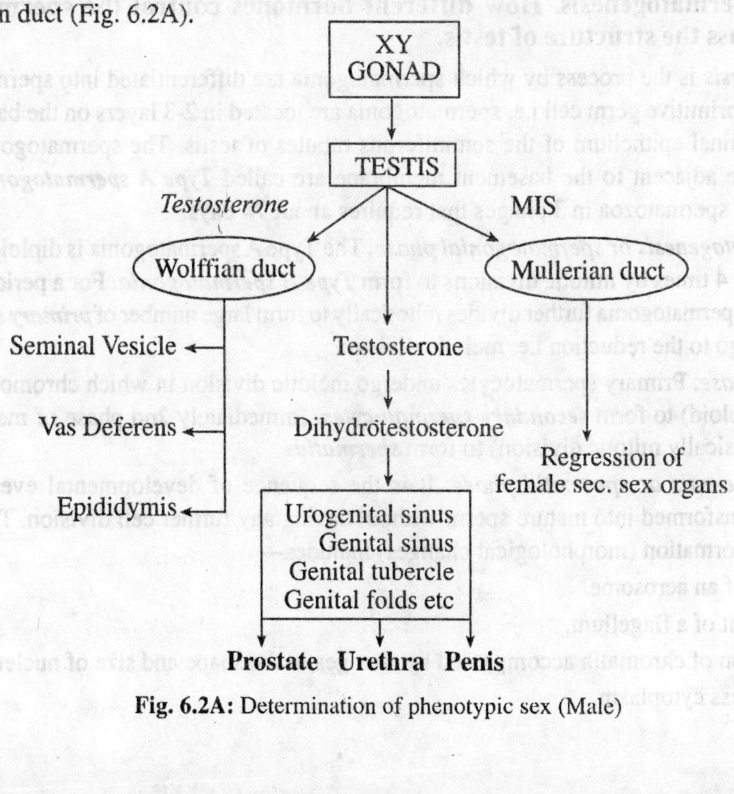

Fig. 6.2A: Determination of phenotypic sex (Male)

- If there is determination of genetic female there is no development of male gonad from bipotential gonad → differentiation of female gonad i.e. ovary → degeneration of Wolffian duct and development of Mullerian ducts to female external genitalia (Fig. 6.2B).

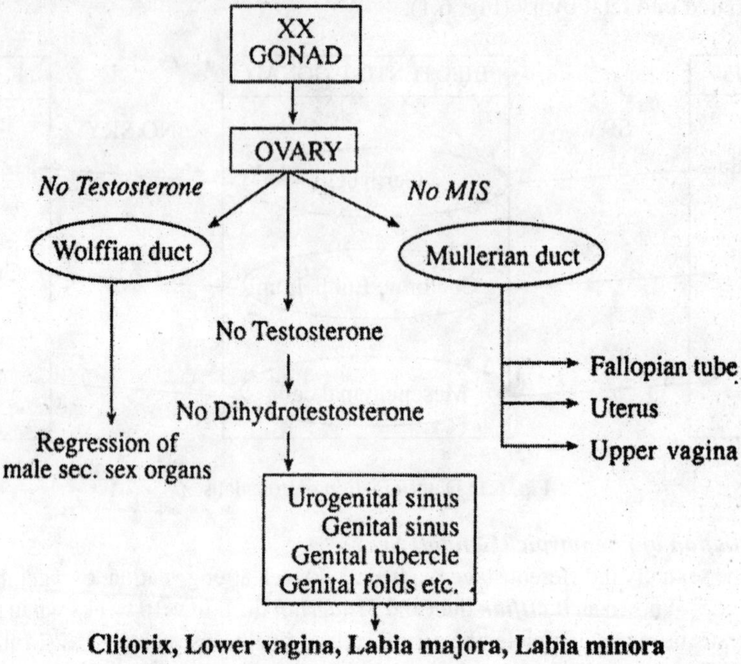

Fig. 6.2B: Determination of phenotypic sex (Female)

2. Describe spermatogenesis. How different hormones control the spermatogenesis? Briefly discuss the structure of testis.

Spermatogenesis is the process by which spermatogonia are differentiated into spermatozoa or viable sperms. The primitive germ cell i.e. spermatogonia are located in 2-3 layers on the basement membrane of the germinal epithelium of the seminiferous tubules of testis. The spermatogonia which are present immediate adjacent to the basement membrane are called ***Type A spermatogonia*** which are differentiated into spermatozoa in 3 phages that requires about 74 days.

(i) *Spermatocytogenesis or spermatogonial phase*: The Type A spermatogonia is diploid i.e. 44 + XY which proliferates 4 times by mitotic divisions to form ***Type B spermatogonia***. For a period of about 24 days each Type B spermatogonia further divides mitotically to form large number of ***primary spermatocytes*** which then undergo to the reduction i.e. meiotic division.

(ii) *Meiotic phase*: Primary spermatocytes undergo meiotic division in which chromosome number becomes half (haploid) to form ***secondary spermatocytes***. Immediately 2nd phase of meiotic division starts (which is basically mitotic division) to form ***spermatids***.

(iii) *Spermiogenesis or spermatid phase*: It is the sequence of developmental events by which spermatids are transformed into mature sperm without having any further cell division. The major features of this transformation (morphological changes) includes—

1. Formation of an acrosome.
2. Development of a flagellum.
3. Condensation of chromatin accompanied by changes in the shape and size of nucleus.
4. Loss of excess cytoplasm.

5. Synthesis of numerous proteins unique to the spermatozoa.

The sequence of changes converting the spherical spermatid into an elongated ***spermatozoa*** with complex intracellular reorganization is mediated by 4 sub phases (1) Golgi phase, (2) Cap phase, (3) Acrosomal phase and (4) Maturation phase. Full maturity and fertility power of sperm is acquired in female genital tract by the process known as Capacitation and Acrosomal reaction.

Hormonal regulation of spermatogenesis (Fig. 6.3): Spermatogenesis is regulated by hypothalamo-hypophyseal testicular axis through different hypothalamic, pituitary gonadotrophins and testicular hormones. Hypothalamus releases GnRH under the influence of which pituitary (anterior) secretes gonadotrophins i.e. FSH and LH. FSH acts on sertoli cells of testis to (i) stimulate formation of spermatogonia (ii) stimulate release of estrogen which stimulates **spermiogenesis** and maturation of sperm. (iii) stimulate release of inhibin (when spermatogenesis proceeds rapidly) which inhibits further secretion of mainly FSH and slightly GnRH and thus inhibit the spermatogenesis.

LH on the other hand stimulates leydig cell to form testosterone which inturn facilitates the formation of spermatozoa from spermatogonia. When testosterone level reaches to maximum it (1) inhibits the release of FSH, LH and GnRH to inhibit spermatogenesis, (2) stimulates release of inhibin (when spermatogenesis proceeds rapidly) which inturn inhibits further secretion of mainly FSH and slightly GnRH and thus inhibits the spermatogenesis.

Structure of testis:

- Each testis is enclosed by a white fibrous capsule called tunica albuginea, and located in a special sac outside the abdominal cavity called **Scrotum**.
- Tunica albuginea sends many septa into the interior, dividing it into a number of lobules each of which contains 3-4 coiled tubular structure known as ***Seminiferous tubules*** both end of which empty into rete testis and thence to ductuli efferents and finally into epididymis.
- **Seminiferous tubule** contains:
  - (i) Primitive germ cells called ***spermatogonia*** which give rise to the spermatozoa.
  - (ii) Germ cell line successor i.e. spermatocytes, spermatids and spermatozoa.
  - (iii) **Sertoli cells** which—
    - are rich in glycogen that nourishes the sperm.
    - secrete hormones estrogen, an androzen binding protein inhibin and activin and Mullerian inhibitory factor (in fetal testis).
    - acts as a **blood testis barrier** (because of presence of tight junctions in between adjacent sertoli cells) and thus prevents the entry of blood borne toxic substances that can damage germ cells and also prevent the release of spermatozoa to blood.
    - also destroys the damaged germ cells by phagocytosis.
  - Besides the seminiferous tubule, testis also contain endocrinal cells called **Interstitial cells of Leydig** or **Leydig cell** located in the connective tissue stroma of the testis between the seminiferous tubules. These cells secrete androgen i.e. testosterone hormone.

3. Name the male hormones. Describe the source, daily secretion, plasma level and functions of testosterone. Describe the regulation of testosterone.

Testis secretes mainly androgens and also estrogen in small amounts. The main androgen is testosterone though there are other form of androgens e.g. dihydroepiandro testosterone which is most active form of androgen and androstenedione.

Testosterone:

- *Source*: Interstitial cells of leydig of testis and also zona reticularis of adrenal gland.

- *Daily* secretion: In adult male—4-9 mg/day
  In female — 300-350 μgm/day
- *Plasma level*: In adult male — 500-600 ng% (Total)
- *Function*:

(i) **During fetal life:**

- Before 7th Week: In chromosomal male genital ridge secretes testosterone which is responsible for differentiation of fetal testis.
- During 8th Week: Fetal testis secretes testosterone which is responsible for differentiation of male genitalia and accessory sex organs.
- Last 2-3 months of pregnancy: It helps in descending down of testis in scrotum.

(ii) **During adult life:** After puberty it has following functions:

I. Growth and maturity of male accessory sex organs.

II. Differential distribution of body hairs: It causes growth of hair on face, chest, less often in back and also responsible for growth of male type pubic hair i.e. upward along the linea alba to the umbilicus or above. It is also responsible for anterolateral receding of hair line and also baldness.

III. Effect on larynx: It causes hypertrophy of laryngeal mucosa and enlargement of larynx resulting cracking voice initially which is gradually converted into typical adult masculine voice.

IV. Effect on skin:

- Increases thickness of skin.
- Increases secretion of sebaceous glands.

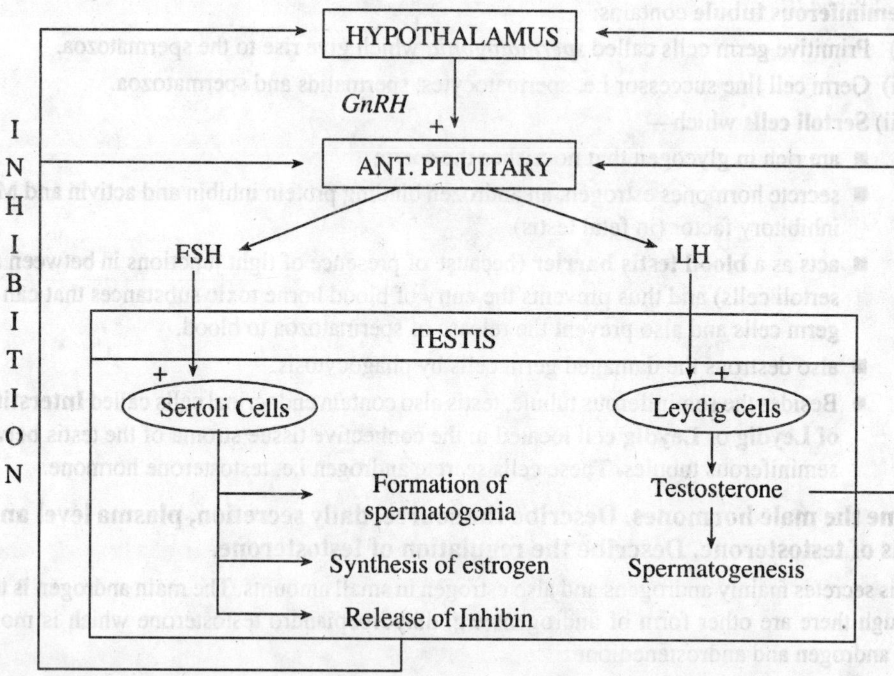

Fig. 6.3: Hormonal regulation of spermatogenesis through Hypothalamo-Hypophyseal Testicular Axis

V. Effect on muscle: Increases muscle mass due to increase in protein synthesis.

VI. Effect on bone:
- increases thickness of bone.
- increases deposition of Ca^{2+} salts.
- increases quantity of bone matrix.
- makes the pelvis funnel shaped.
- increases strength of entire pelvis and also causes the epiphyses to fuse to the long bone thus stops the linear growth.

VII. Effect on BMR: Increases BMR indirectly by increasing anabolic activity of protein.

VIII. Effect on RBCs:
- Increases RBC count by increasing the size of the kidney and partly by increasing the metabolic rate and partly by increasing erythropoiesis.

IX. Water and electrolytes balance: It increases retention of salt and water by the kidneys.

Regulation of testosterone secretion: The secretion of testosterone is regulated by mainly 2 ways:

(i) Hypothalamo hypophyseal testicular axis: Cells of arcuate nuclei of hypothalamus secretes GnRH which stimulate the release of FSH and LH from anterior pituitary gonadotrophic cells. LH in turn stimulates leydig cell to secrete testosterone (Fig. 6.3).

(ii) Negative feedback by testicular hormones:

I. **by testosterone:** When testosterone level in blood increases it inhibits both anterior pituitary and hypothalamus to release LH, FSH and GnRH (Fig. 6.3). Thus the further secretion of testosterone is controlled.

II. **by inhibin:** Under the influence of FSH sertoli cells secrete inhibin which inhibits mainly anterior pituitary to inhibit the release of FSH and LH and thus testosterone secretion gets inhibited (Fig. 6.3). Inhibin also inhibits the release of GnRH from hypothalamus but this role is not certain.

4. What are the female sex hormones? Discuss their source and functions. How the secretion of ovarian hormones are regulated?

There are 3 female sex hormones namely estrogen, progesterone and relaxin.

(a) Estrogen

(i) *Source*: Theca interna of graafian follicle (major), Granulosa cell of graafian follicle, placenta and adrenal cortex

(ii) *Functions*:

- **Effect on genital system:**
  - Increases size and functional capabilities of uterus, ovary, fallopian tube, vagina and also external genitalia like mons pubis, labia majora and minora.
  - Changes of cuboidal epithelial cells of vagina to stratified to increase resistant to trauma and infection.
  - Causes proliferation of endometrial stroma and endometrial glands of uterus.
  - Causes proliferation of glandular tissue of mucosal lining of fallopian tube, increase in number of cilliated epithelial cells—This inturn propels the fertilised ovum toward the uterus.
- **Effect on breast:**
  - Causes development of stromal tissues of breast
  - Causes growth of ductile-system

- Responsible for deposition of fat in the breast
- Initiates slight growth of lobules and alveoli of mammary gland

- **Effect on skeleton:**
  - It increases osteoblastic activity resulting rapid growth of female during her early reproductive year than her male counterpart.
  - It causes the union of the epiphyseal growth plate with the shafts of long bone. This is the reason that ultimate growth of female is less than her male counterpart.
  - After menopause fall of oestrogen results in decrease osteoblastic activity.
  - Decrease bone matrix due to increase osteoblastic activity and decrease deposition of bone calcium and phosphate.
- **On protein metabolism:** It has slight protein anabolic effect.
- **On BMR:** It increases BMR slightly.
- **On skin:**
  - It is responsible for soft texture of skin.
  - It is responsible for smoothness and increased vascularity of the skin.
- **On electrolyte balance:** It has slight aldosterone like activity.

***(b) Progesterone*:**

(i) *Source*: Corpus luteum, placenta, testis and adrenal cortex

(ii) *Functions*:

- **On uterus:**
  - On endometrium:
    - ☐ It produces secretory changes of oestrogen primed endometrium.
    - ☐ It causes elongation and secretion of endometrial glands.
  - On myometrium—decreases the frequency and amplitude of uterine contractions thus prevents abortion of fetus.
  - On cervix—secretion of thick and viscid mucous.
- **On breast:** It is responsible for—
  - Development of lobules and alveoli of mammary gland.
  - Secretory changes of alveoli though final changes occur under influence of prolactin.
  - Swelling of breast.
- **On Fallopian tube:** It is responsible for secretory changes necessary for nutrition of fertilised ovum.
- **On electrolyte balance:** It increases Na^+ and H_2O reabsorption from the distal tubules of the kidney.
- **Other function:** It increases basal body temperature and it inhibits ovulation by inhibiting release of GnRH.

(c) Relaxin:

- *Source*: Corpus luteum, uterus and placenta
- *Function*: It facilitates delivery of the fetus by—
  - relaxing the symphysis pubis and other pelvic joints.
  - softening of cervix.

Regulation of ovarian hormone secretion:

Regulation of ovarian hormones i.e. estrogen and progesterone is mediated by hypothalamo hypophyseal ovarian axis and also by negative feedback by plasma level of ovarian hormones similarly to testicular hormones.

A. ***Hypothalamo-Hypophyseal ovarian axis***: Under influence of hypothalamic GnRH anterior pituitary secretes FSH and LH. These inturn stimulate theca and granulosa cells to release estrogen and CL to secrete progesterone.

B. *Negative feedback effect*:

- *By estrogen and progesterone*: Increased plasma level of estrogen and progesterone inhibit hypothalamus and pituitary to secrete release of FSH and LH respectively.
- *By Inhibin*: Inhibin secreted by granulosa cells also exert inhibitory effect mainly on anterior pituitary to release FSH and LH and thus control estrogen and progesterone release.

5. What is menstrual cycle? Give an account of menstrual cycle. Add a note on hormonal regulation of menstrual cycle.

Definition: The normal reproductive years of the female are characterised by monthly rhythmical changes in the secretion of female hormone and corresponding changes in the ovaries (ovarian cycle) and uterus (uterine/menstrual cycle) and other sex organs. This rhythmical changes is called as the *female sexual cycle* or less accurately ***menstrual cycle.***

Normal duration: 28 ± 7 days, however it can even varies from 20 to 45 days in normal women.

Events of female sexual cycle: There are 3 events that take place during female sexual cycle as follows:

a. ***Ovarian cycle*** (ovarian changes)

b. ***Uterine cycle*** (uterine changes)

c. ***Changes in hormone production***

a. *Ovarian cycle*: Every month in each ovary more than one primordial follicle start undergoing maturation process but only one reaches maturity and rest undergo atresia. During fetal life some cells of the stroma become flattened and surround an primary oocyte. These cells are known as follicular cells and the ovum (Primary oocyte) surrounding follicular cells are known as **primordial follicle**. Numerous primordial follicles are present in the ovary at birth. At puberty further differentiation of primordial follicle takes place in two phases): (i) Follicular phase and (ii) Leuteal phase.

(i) *Follicular phase*:

Step 1: Under the influence of FSH mainly and LH the flattened follicular cells become columnar and at this stage follicles are known as **primary follicles** (Primary oocyte + surrounding columnar follicular cell).

Step 2: A homologues membrane i.e. zona pellucida appears in between follicular cells and oocyte. The follicle is now known as **multilaminar primary follicle.**

Step 3: Follicular cells now proliferate into several layers to form granulosa cells at this stage follicle (primary oocyte + granulosa cell) is now known as **secondary follicle**.

Step 4: There is now partial separation of glanulosa cell layer resulting appearance of follicular cavity filled with **liquor follicle** called ***antral fluid***.

Step 5: Enlargement of follicular cavity under the influence of ovarian hormone (estrogen) resulting thinning of granulosa cell layer at the wall of the follicle.

Step 6: Further expansion and formation of theca interna and theca externa surrounding the follicle occurs and at this stage the follicle is known as **Graafian follicles** (Mature follicle).

Step 7: Ultimately there is rupture of follicle and loosening of the cumulus oophorus resulting release of oocyte from the ovary (i.e. ***ovulation*)**.

(ii) *Luteal phase*:

The remaining part of the follicle undergoes changes that convert it into corpus luteum which secretes progesterone to proliferate the endometrial growth of uterus. The growth of the corpus luteum depends on fertilisation. If the ovum is not fertilized the corpus luteum (CL) persists for about 14 days which secretes progesterone to initiate endometrial growth required for implantation of zygote. These CL are small and known as **corpus luteum of menstruation**. After 14 days they degenerate to form corpus albican which no longer secretes progesterone.

If the ovum is fertilized and pregnancy results CL persists for 3-4 months and maintains the growth of endometrium. At this stage CL size is longer and known as **corpus luteum of pregnancy**. After 3-4 months it degenerates and it's function is taken over by the placenta.

b. Uterine changes (Endometrial / Uterine cycle):

Associated with the monthly cyclic production of estrogen and progesterone by the ovaries during ovarian cycle there is also development of endometrium in different phases.

(i) Menstruation (Bleeding) Phase:

- This phase starts from the day on which menstrual bleeding starts and continues as long as bleeding is present. It's normal duration is 3-5 days i.e. 1st to 5th day of menstrual cycle.
- In this phase the superficial part of the endometrium becomes ischemic resulting necrosis and shedding of superficial 2/3 of endometrium along with discharge of blood and mucous through vagina.
- Reason of menstrual bleeding: If the ovum is not fertilized the CL degenerates after 14 days → withdrawal of progesterone secretion → spasm of spiral arteries in the superficial layer of endometrium → fall of blood supply to superficial $2/3^{rd}$ of endometrium → necrosis of superficial $2/3^{rd}$ of endometrium → shedding and discharge of endometrial substance e.g. blood and mucus.

(ii) **Proliferative (Oestrogen) phase:** Immediately after bleeding the endometrium is < 2 mm thick and consists of only a thin layer of endometrium stroma and the epithelial cells present only in the deep of the glands and crypts of the endometrium. From 5th/6th to 13th/ till ovulation under the influence of estrogen proliferation of glands, blood vessels, stroma and superficial epithelium of endometrium occurs and the endometrium becomes 4 mm thick. Uterine glands also increase in length without secreting anything.

(iii) **Ovulatory phase:** At about 14th day ovum is released from the ovary without any significant changes of uterine endometrium. However there is increased secretion of watery fluid by cervical mucosa which is discharged through vagina and facilitate the easy entry of sperm inside the female genital tract.

(iv) **Secretory (progesteronal or luteal) phase:** After ovulation when CL is well formed and secretes progesterone then under the influence of progesterone following changes take place in uterus:

- Increase in length and diameter of endometrial glands which become more tortuous and filled with mucus.
- Proliferation and enlargement of stromal cells.
- Spiral artery becomes more coiled and dilated.
- Veins are filled with more blood.
- Cervical secretion becomes thick and constitute a barrier against sperm and infectious microorganism.

c. Hormonal changes including hormonal control of female sexual cycle:

At the end of menstrual cycle when CL degenerates there is fall of plasma level of estrogen and progesterone.

↓

This low estrogen + progesterone level by negative feedback way increases FSH and LH release from anterior pituitary directly and also indirectly via stimulating hypothalamic GnRH release.

↓

Under the influence of FSH multiple follicles begin to enlarge and secrete estrogen resulting rise of plasma estrogen level.

↓

Some how one follicle becomes dominant and secrets very large amount of oestrogen resulting further rise of estrogen level. It also starts secreting small amount of progesterone hormone.

↓

Very high blood level of estrogen + little progesterone together initiate a '+'ve feedback on anterior pituitary to increase the release of FSH and then LH. This peak rise of FSH and LH is known as ***FSH surge*** and ***LH surge*** respectively which occurs almost simultaneously.

↓

Increase LH level (LH Surge) causes ovulation and lead to formation and maintenance of CL which in turn secrete estrogen and mainly progesterone again resulting rise of plasma estrogen and progesterone.

↓

Both high level of estrogen + progesterone now by negative feedback way decreases secretion of both FSH and LH from anterior pituitary directly and also indirectly by inhibiting release of GnRH from hypothalamus.

↓

This fall of LH level causes degeneration of CL and thus withdrawl of progesterone and estrogen secretion resulting fall of plasma estrogen and progesterone.

↓

This fall of plasma estrogen and progesterone again increase FSH and LH release by negative feedback. Increased FSH again is responsible for growth of another ovum and thus initiates another cycle.

6. What is milk let down reflex? How milk is secreted? Add a note on the role of various hormones in the development of mammary gland and lactation.

The release and maintenance of milk out of breast (mammary gland) in response to suckling of the breast by the baby is known as ***lactation or milk let down reflex***.

Mechanism: The process of lactation can by divided into 4 phases e.g.

(a) Preparation of breast (***Mammogenesis***)

(b) Synthesis and secretion of milk by breast alveoli (***Lactogenesis***)

(c) Ejection of milk (***Galactokinesis***)

(d) Maintenance of lactation (***Galactopoiesis***).

Out of these 1st two phases (a and b) is termed as **initiation of lactation** and last 2 phases (c and d) can be termed as **milk ejection and maintenance.**

*(i) Initiation of Lactation-**Function of PRL***: Different hormones(e.g. estrogen, progesterone, GH, adrenal steroids, thyroids, PRL etc.) secreted from the stage of puberty to pregnancy initiate the growth of ductular system and lobulo-alveolar system of mammary gland. Out of which the main hormones responsible for formation of fully developed mammary gland is prolactin (PRL). However during pregnancy it's secretory action on the mammary gland is inhibited by high concentration of estrogen and progesterone from placenta. After the expulsion of baby and placenta there is a sharp decline in level of circulatory estrogen and progesterone which results prominent effects of PRL and the breast becomes ready to secrete milk in response to proper stimulation.

*(ii) Milk ejection: **Function of Oxytocin***-Milk is secreted continuously into the alveoli of the mammary gland under the influence of PRL but milk does not flow easily from the alveoli to the ductal system without appropriate stimulus. In response to suckling a combined neurogenic and hormonal reflex are initiated which cause release of posterior pituitary hormone oxytocin which leads to the contraction of myoepithelial cells (that surround the alveoli) to cause ejection of

milk. The process is called **let down of milk** or **milk ejection which is illustrated in detail by** following flow chart.

Suckling

↓

Stimulation of mechanoreceptors in areola and nipple

↓

Origin of spinally mediated reflex to stimulate hypothalamus

↙ ↘

↑ PRF release from hypothalamus	↑ Oxytocin secretion from post pituitory
↓	↓
↑ PRL release from anterior pituitory	↑ Plasma oxytocin
↓	↓
↑ Plasma PRL level	Contraction of myoepithelial cell
↓	↓
Stimulate glandular cell to synthesise milk	Milk ejection

B. Short Notes:

1. Puberty:

- ***Definition***: After birth the gonads of both sexes remain silent until they are activated by gonadotrophins i.e. FSH and LH which ultimately result the final maturation of reproductive system. This period of growth and maturation is known as puberty or adolescence. Thus puberty is defined **as the period when endocrine and gemetogenic functions of gonads have first developed to the point where reproduction is possible.**
- ***Onset of Puberty***:
  - **In male:** 9 years to 14 years.
  - **In female:** 8 years to 13 years.
- ***Pubertal changes***:
  - **In Boys:**
    - ❑ Enlargement of testis
    - ❑ Further growth of external and internal genitalia
    - ❑ Development of primary and secondary sex characters
    - ❑ Increase in height **(Height spurt)**
    - ❑ More musculature, more muscle power
    - ❑ Broad shoulder
    - ❑ Voice changes due to enlargement of larynx and thickening of vocal cords
    - ❑ Male type hair pattern i.e. **anterolateral receding of hairline on scalp**
    - ❑ Male pattern of pubic hair i.e. triangle with apex up
    - ❑ Increased adrenal hormone secretion **(Adrenerche)**
  - **In Girls:**
    - ❑ Appearance of breast (Thelarche)

- Development of axillary and pubic hair (puberche)
- Appearance of menstrual cycle (menarche)
- Maturity into adult type of genitalia
- Appearance of secondary sex characters like narrow shoulder, broad hips etc.

2. Capacitation:

- This is one of the process by which sperm becomes fully active and fertile in the female genital tract.
- When the sperm is released in female genital tract different factors in female genital fluid initiate different changes in the spermatozoa to activate the sperm for fertilization. These changes are collectively known as capacitation which includes:
  - Increase in sperm motility due to washing away of the inhibitory factors of semen by the uterine and fallopian tube fluids.
  - Loss of cholesterol vesicles from the head of sperm resulting weakening of membrane of head of sperm.
  - Release of acrosomal enzymes by increasing Ca_2^{++} permeability of the sperm head.

3. Acrosomal reaction: This is the process by which acrosomal enzymes are released by the sperm head which helps the sperm to penetrate zona pellucida of ovum to fertilize it. The detailed mechanism is described by following flow chart.

Once sperm becomes very close to ovum →↑ Ca_2^{++} permeability → release of acrosomal enzymes → dispersement and digestion of granulosa cells and corona radiata → attachment of sperm with sperm receptor on Zona protein (ZP_3) of Zona pellucida of ovum → rapid lysis of entire acrosomal membrane → more release of acrosomal enzyme → penetration of the zona pellucida by the sperm.

4. Structure of sperm: Mature spermatozoa is 55-65μ long consisting of head and tail (Fig. 6.4).

(a) ***Head***: It is composed of condensed nucleus within very thin cytoplasmic cell membrane around it. On the outer portion of 2/3rd of head there is a thick cap called acrosome formed mainly from golgi apparatus containing a number of enzymes like hyaluronidase, proteolytic enzymes etc.

(b) *Tail*: Tail of the sperm is flagellum which has 3 components—

(i) Axoneme: It is a central skeleton constructed of 11 microtubule.

(ii) Cell membrane covering axoneme.

(iii) Collection of mitochondria surrounding the axoneme in the proximal portion of the tail.

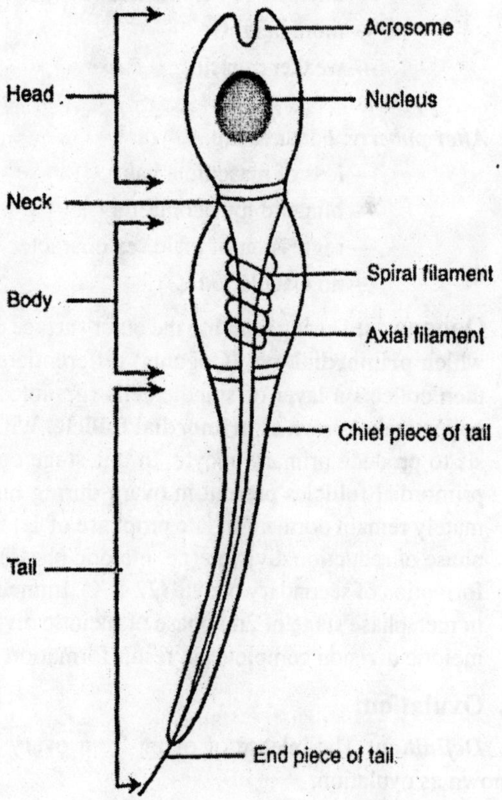

Fig. 6.4: Structure of sperm

5. Semen:

It is the fluid ejaculated from the penis at the time of orgasm. It is the product of sperm and secretions of seminal tracts and all related glands.

Composition:

- Colour: White opalescent
- Sp. gravity: 1.028
- pH: 7.35 to 7.50 (alkaline)
- Volume: 2.5 - 3.5 ml per ejaculate
- Sperm count: > 40 million / ml.
- Sperm motility: > 80%

Components of semen:

(i) Sperm: 10%

(ii) Seminal plasma: 90%

- Fructose (2-7 mg%):
- Others like PGs, ascorbic acid, citric acid, phospholipids, fibrinolysin, acid phosphatase, hyaluronidase, zinc, phosphate, bicarbonate, spermine etc.

6. Male hypogonadism:

Before puberty: Features are:

- — infantile sex characters (eunuchism)
- — child like voice
- — more height
- — thin and weak bone
- — weaker muscle
- — obesity (adiposo genital syndrome) due to abnormal feeding center.

After puberty: Features are:

- — loss of masculine hair
- — low masculinity
- — bilateral gynacomastia
- — atrophy of male sex organs
- — regression of male sex character
- — less sexual desire but not arrested
- — no ejaculation

7. Oogenesis: During fetal life the outer surface of the ovary is covered by a germinal epithelium from which **primordial ova** (Oogonia) differentiate and migrate into the ovarian cortex. Each oogonia then collects a layer of spindle cells (granulosa cells) from the ovarian stroma around it which is collectively known as **primordial follicle**. Within this primordial follicle it undergoes further mitosis to produce primary oocyte. In this stage oogenesis stops until puberty and there are number of primordial follicles present in ovary during birth. After birth reduction division starts which ultimately remain dormant in late prophase of 1st meiotic division. After puberty i.e. after ovulation 1st phase of reduction division (i.e. meiotic phase) completes resulting expulsion of 1st polar body and formation of secondary oocyte (22 + X). Immediately 2nd phase of meiotic division starts but it stops in metaphase stage of 2nd phase of meiotic division. When sperm penetrates the ovum then only the meiotic division completes to result formation of mature ovum.

8. Ovulation:

Definition: The release of ovum from ovary at approximately mid of the female sexual cycle is known as ovulation.

Day of ovulation:

- in case of 28 days cycle: It is on 14th day

- in case of less than/more than 28 days cycle: Depends e.g.
  - in case of 20 days cycle—ovulation will be at 20-14 = 6th day
  - in case of 40 days cycle—ovulation will be 40-14 = 26th day.

***Mechanism*:** Vide the follicular phase of ovarian cycle.

***Diagnosis*:**

1. **Basal Body Temperature test (BBT):** Body temperature is recorded in the morning as soon as awakening from 1st day of menstrual cycle (the day on which menstrual bleeding starts) till next cycles (1st day of next cycle) and the values are plotted in a graph paper. It is seen that there is gradual rise of body temperature from 96.5°F/97°F to 99°F with sudden rise of temperature of about 0.5°F which is maintained for some days (Fig. 6.5). The increase in temperature indicates that ovulation has taken place, which is due to more progesterone synthesis by CL.

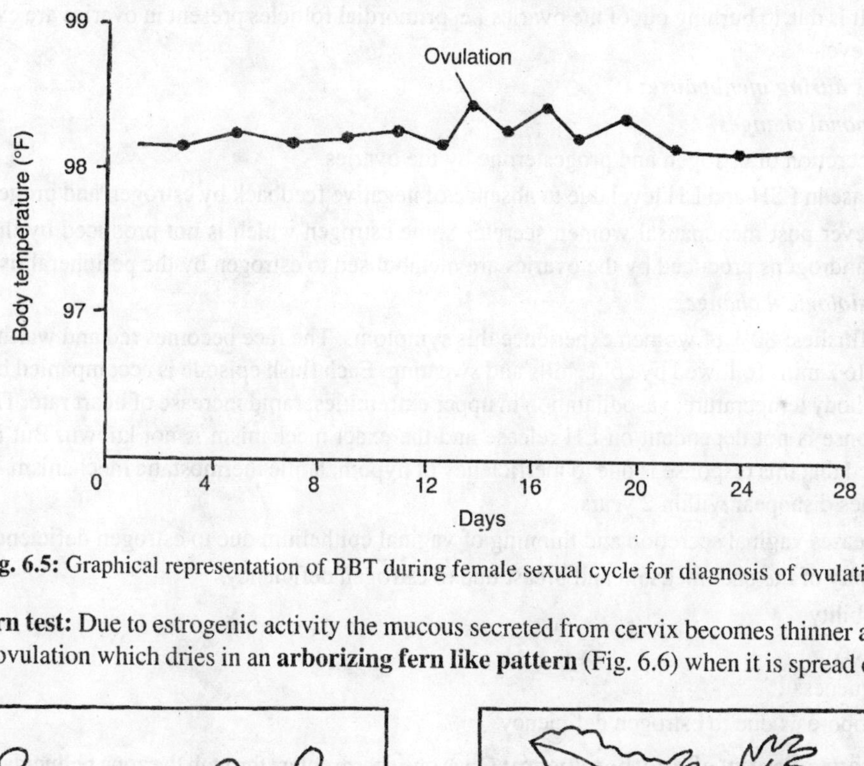

Fig. 6.5: Graphical representation of BBT during female sexual cycle for diagnosis of ovulation

2. **Fern test:** Due to estrogenic activity the mucous secreted from cervix becomes thinner at the time of ovulation which dries in an **arborizing fern like pattern** (Fig. 6.6) when it is spread on a slide.

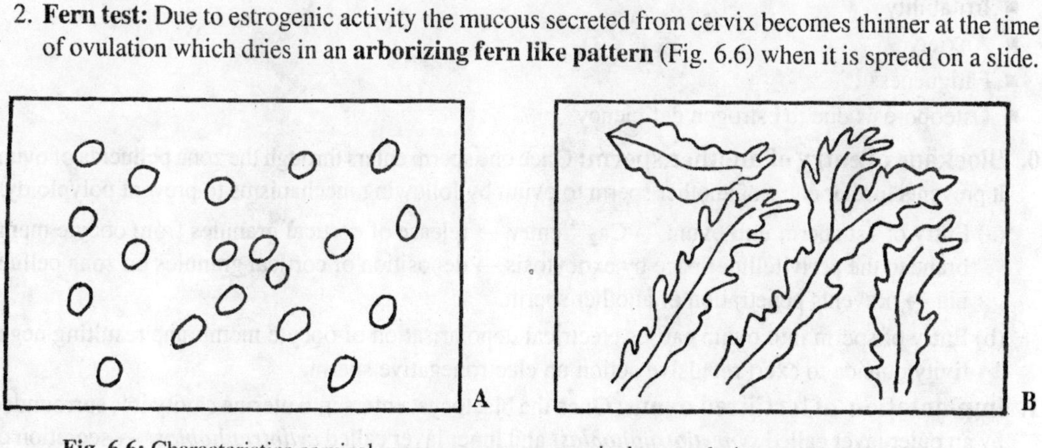

Fig. 6.6: Characteristics cervical mucous as seen on vaginal smear during menstruation cycle
(A = No fern pattern on secretory phase i.e. after ovulation and menstruation phase; B = Fern pattern on proliferate phase i.e. before ovulation)

Once corpus luteum is formed the mucous becomes thick due to progesterone activity and this thick mucous does not show fern like pattern in the slide. This is the basis of fern test. The absence fern like pattern (in between 6th-22nd days) indicates that the ovulation is going to happen.

3. **Measurement of urinary LH:** Ovulation is due to LH surge and during LH surge, LH is excreted through urine. So urinary measurement of LH hormone is also another method to detect whether ovulation has taken place or not.
4. Ultrasonography of follicular study and laproscopy are the most modern and useful method to detect the ovulation.

9. Menopause:

Definition*:** Within the period of 48-55 year (Avg. 51yr.) the female sexual cycles first becomes irregular and unovulatory which ultimately ceases and the secretions of female sex hormone diminishes rapidly to almost zero level. This period is known as ***menopause.

***Cause*:** It is due to burning out of the ovaries i.e. primordial follicles present in ovaries are exhausted to zero level.

***Changes during menopause*:**

(i) *Hormonal changes*:

- No secretion of estrogen and progesterone by the ovaries.
- Increase in FSH and LH level due to absence of negative feedback by estrogen and progesterone.
- However post menopausal women secretes some estrogen which is not produced by the ovary. The androgens produced by the ovaries are metabolised to estrogen by the peripheral tissue.

(ii) *Physiological changes*:

- **Hot flushes:** 80% of women experience this symptoms. The face becomes red and warm for few secs to 2 mins followed by cold chills and sweating. Each flush episode is accompanied by rise in core body temperature, vasodilatation in upper extremities, rapid increase of heart rate. This flush response is not dependant on LH release and the exact mechanism is not known. But it is presumed that this response is due to inefficiency of hypothalamic thermostatic mechanism. This hot flushes disappear within 2 years.
- Decreases vaginal secretion and thinning of vaginal epithelium due to estrogen deficiency.
- Atrophy of the endometrium and breast due to estrogen deficiency.
- Irritability
- Anxiety
- Fatigueness
- Osteoporosis due to estrogen deficiency.

10. **Blockade of entry of another sperm:** Once one sperm enters through the zona pellucida of ovum it prevents further entry of another sperm to ovum by following mechanisms to prevent polyploidy.

    (a) Entry of 1st sperm into ovum → Ca_2^{++} entry → release of cortical granules from oocyte membrane to the perivitelline space by exocytosis → deposition of cortical granules on zona pellucida → prevents penetration of another sperm.

    (b) Entry of sperm into ovum causes electrical depolarisation of oocyte membrane resulting negativity outside to exert repulsive action on electronegative sperm.

11. **Implantation of fertilized ovum:** Once the blastocyst enters into uterine cavity it is surrounded by an outer layer called ***syncytiotrophoblast*** and inner layer called ***cytiotrophoblast*** → secretion of proteolytic enzymes by the syncytiotrophoblast that digests the endometrium to help burrowing of blastocyst into deep of endometrium → separation of a cell layer of trophoblast from the initial

solid mass of blastocyst → microvilli of these cells interdigitate with those of endometrial cell to give the growing fetus a strong attachment with endometrium.

12. MRF/MIS:

- It is a peptide containing 536 amino acids secreted by sertoli cells of foetal testis.
- In males though the secretion of MIS starts at 8-10 weeks of gestation their plasma level reaches it's peak (50 ng/ml) at 1-2 years of age which then gradually declines and maintained at 2.5 ng/ml concentration throughout the rest of life.
- *Functions:*
  - During the sexually indifferent stage i.e. from 3-7 weeks after gestation, two genital ducts develop on each side—known as ***Wolffian*** duct and ***Mullerian*** duct. In 9-10 weeks when the development of fetal testis becomes complete, the sertoli cells of fetal testis secrete MIS which causes the regression of mullerian duct where as the leydig cells secrete testosterone that causes differentiation of male genital tract and male external genitalia from the Wolffian duct.
  - If there is determination of genetic female there is no development of male gonad from bipotential gonad → differentiation of female gonad i.e. ovary → degeneration of Wolffian duct and development of Mullerian ducts to female external genitalia. In late fetal life it helps in testicular descend.
  - It helps to maintain germ cells in both sexes.

13. Role of FSH in spermatogenesis:

- It has mainly indirect role on spermatogenesis by acting on sertoli cells.
- FSH acts on sertoli cells of testis to (i) stimulate formation of spermatogonia (ii) stimulate release of estrogen which stimulates **spermiogenesis** and maturation of sperm. (iii) stimulate release of inhibin (where spermatogenesis proceeds rapidly) which inhibits further secretion of mainly FSH and slightly GnRH and thus inhibit the spermatogenesis.
- It also stimulates production of Androgen binding protein (ABP) which maintains normal concentration of testosterone in the seminiferous tubule.
- It stimulates aromatase synthesis from sertoli cells which converts testosterone to estradiol which inturn influences spermatogenesis.

14. Relaxin:

- *Source*: Corpus luteum, placenta, uterus and breast tissue in females and prostate of males.
- *Function*:
  - It facilitates delivery of the fetus by relaxing the symphysis pubis and other pelvic joints and softening of cervix.
  - Inhibits uterine contraction in non pregnant women in the secretory phase and this quiscent uterus may facilitate implantation.
  - In male it facilitates sperm motility and penetration of ovum by sperm.

15. Inhibin:

- *Source*: Sertoli cells of testis and granulosa cells of ovaries.
- It is also produced by pituitary, brain, adrenal gland, corpus leteum and placenta.

- It inhibits FSH secretion from anterior pituitary gland.
- It inhibits androgen production.
- It's secretion is stimulated by FSH.

16. Fertile period and safe period:

- In 28 days regular menstrual cycle normal ovulation occurs between 12th and 16th (usually on 14th day) and sperm can survive for 2 days in female genital tract. So the period from 2 days before the ovulation and within 3 days after the ovulation there is maximum chance of fertilization. This period is known as ***fertile period*** and remaining period of the cycle is considered as ***Safe period***, during which no fertilization can take place.
- To avoid the pregnancy the unprotected intercourse is avoided during fertile period.
- Practically (specially in irregular cycle) there is no actual safe period as fertilization can take place in any time as it is difficult and tedious to know the date of ovulation.

17. Orgasm:

- It is the sexual act during sexual intercourse.
- Generally male sexual act or male orgasm is much more in sexual intercourse and female is the passive partner. However, the responses to intercourse in females are not passive.
- Male sexual act is a neural process but can be modified by hormones which is a 4 phased act as follows:
  - *Erection*: Erection of penis is initiated by dilatation of arterioles of the penis. As the erectile tissue of the penis fills with blood the veins are compressed blocking outflow of blood. This results increase in length and diameter of penis and it becomes rigid.
  - *Lubrication*: due to mucous secretion because of parasympathetic stimulation.
  - *Emission*: i.e. movement of semen into urethra.
  - *Ejaculation*: i.e. propelling the semen into urethra.
- Orgasm in female is associated with a pleasurable feeling accompanied by sudden increase in skeletal muscle activity, increase in heart rate, BP, rhythmic contraction of vaginal wall, engorgement of breast and erection of nipples, increased diameter and length of clitoris.
- For the best and happy conjugal life and to get maximum pleasure of sexual act orgasm of male and female should appear concurrently during sexual act.

18. Contraceptive pills:

- In this methods synthetic estrogen and/or progesterone is orally taken to—
  - prevent ovulation
  - prevent implantation of fertilized ovum
  - prevent entry of sperm into uterus
  - inhibit motility of sperm in female genital tract
- If correctly used it is most useful and successful non surgical method.

- These are of several types:
  - *Combined pill*: Large amount of progesterone and small amounts of oestrogen are given orally at bed time for 21 days starting from 5th day of menstrual bleeding and then stopped so that the next menstrual cycle starts due to withdrawal of progesterone (withdrawal bleeding).
  - *Sequential pill*: In this method large doses of oestrogen for 15 days from 5th day followed by combination of oestrogen and progesterone for 7 days is administered. This method is now withdrawn as it may result endometrial cancer.
  - *Mini pills*: In this case the low dose of progesterone pill are taken once daily for 21 days starting from 5th day.
  - *Post coital pills*: In this method high, and single dose of oestrogen and progesterone is given orally within 72 hours after coitus. This prevents the implantation of fertilized ovum in the uterus.

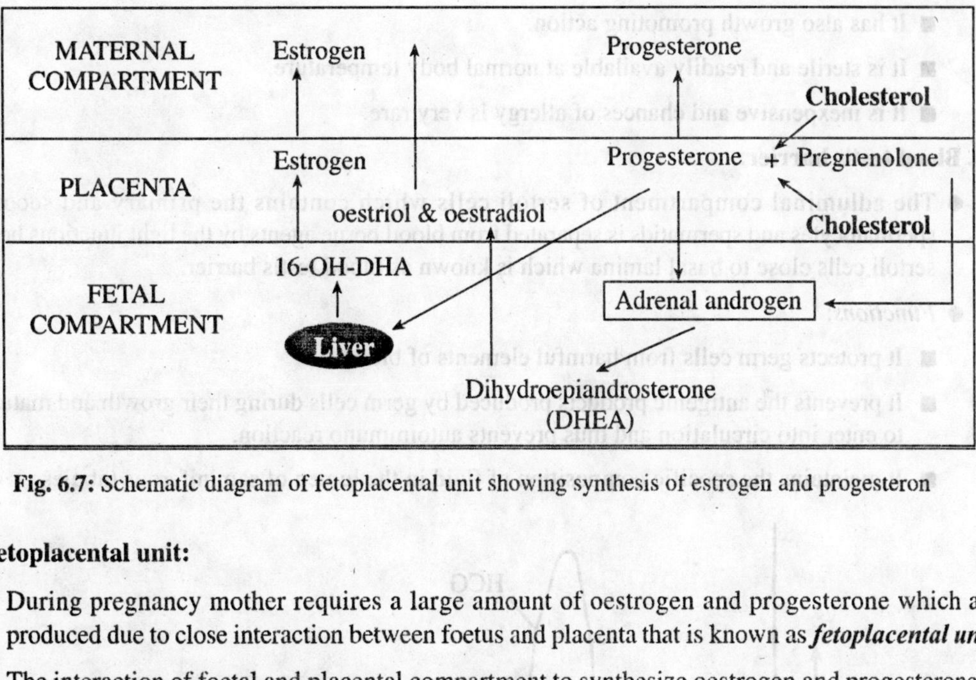

Fig. 6.7: Schematic diagram of fetoplacental unit showing synthesis of estrogen and progesteron

19. Fetoplacental unit:

- During pregnancy mother requires a large amount of oestrogen and progesterone which are produced due to close interaction between foetus and placenta that is known as ***fetoplacental unit.***
- The interaction of foetal and placental compartment to synthesize oestrogen and progesterone is schematically represented by following manner (Fig. 6.7).
- *Functions*:
  - Production of oestrogen and progesterone for maintenance of pregnancy.
  - Initiation of parturition in later phase of pregnancy.

20. Colostrum and breast milk:

- Immediately after delivery a watery fluid is secreted from breasts called ***colostrum*** which is rich in protein and immunoglobins.
- Colostrum secretion is replaced by milk in about 24-48 hours.

- Breast milk contains all nutrients in adequate quantity as follows:
  - Milk sugar, protein, fat, minerals, vitamins and water.
  - Antibodies for protecting newborn from infection.
  - Growth factors those help in physical development and maturation.
  - Large number of neuropeptides and endogenous opioids those facilitate brain development and behaviour of infant.
- Quantity of breast milk secreted is 1.5 to 2 lit/day.
- Duration of milk secretion is 1–5 years,
- Advantages of breast milk:
  - It is a natural and balanced diet.
  - Protects the newborns against infection as it contains leucocytes, lysozymes, immunoglobins.
  - Easily digested and assimilated.
  - It has also growth promoting action.
  - It is sterile and readily available at normal body temperature.
  - It is inexpensive and chances of allergy is very rare.

21. Blood testis barrier:

- The adluminal compartment of sertoli cells which contains the primary and secondary spermatocytes and spermatids is separated from blood borne agents by the tight junctions between sertoli cells close to basal lamina which is known as blood testis barrier.
- *Functions*:
  - It protects germ cells from harmful elements of blood.
  - It prevents the antigenic products produced by germ cells during their growth and maturation to enter into circulation and thus prevents autoimmuno reaction.
  - It maintains the specific composition of fluid in the lumen of seminiferous tubules.

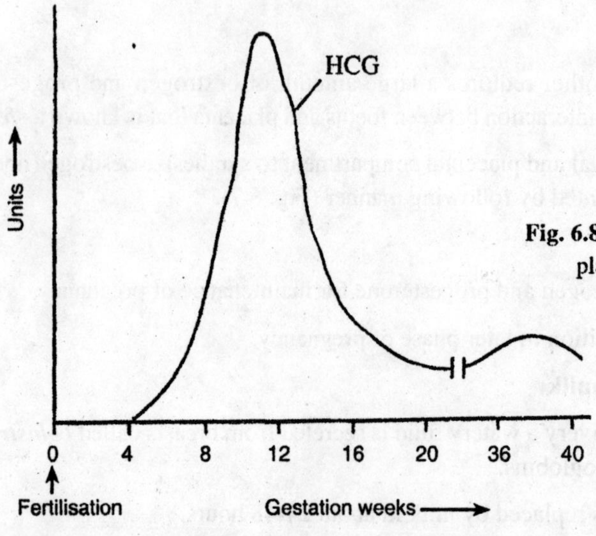

Fig. 6.8: Changes in blood level of placental hormone HCG

22. Dihydrotestosterone:

- Dihydrotestosterone is an active form of testosterone produced in the target tissues especially in prostate, scrotum, penis, skin and bones by 5 α-reductase.
  - It has 2-3 times more affinity than testosterone for binding with androgen receptors.
- DHT binds with androgen receptors in the nucleus and induces RNA transcription to produce various protein which inturn causes sexual maturation at puberty and external virilization.

23. Human chorionic gonadotropin (HCG):

- It is secreted by syncytio trophoblast cell immediately after implantation.
- Blood level of HCG gradually rises and reaches a peak in about 8 weeks after fertilization and then decline to a very low level by 12-16 weeks (Fig. 6.8). However, it is detected in the maternal blood **8-9 days after conception.**
- Urinary excretion of HCG starts **at 40-60 days after LMP**. It's detection in urine forms the basis for immunologic pregnancy test.
- Functions:
  - It acts like LH and has little FSH activity.
  - It maintains the corpus luteum to secrete estrogen and progesterone which has following effects:
    - maintains growth and proliferation of endometrium.
    - exerts negative feedback to pituitary and hypothalamus → no LH Surge → no ovulation and no menstruation.
  - It stimulates fetal testis to secrete testosterone prior to LH secretion from fetal pituitary.
  - It serves as a tropic hormone for fetal adrenal cortex.

24. Turner's syndrome (Gonadal dysgenesis):

- This is the abnormal sex differentiation due to non disjunction of sex chromosome; a phenomenon in which sex chromosomes fail to separate i.e. one gamete gets both sex chromosome other gets none.
- Characteristic features:
  - Genetically sexless.
  - Chromosomal configuration 44XO.
  - No gonadal sex i.e. neither testis nor ovary.
- Phenotypic features:
  - Female like appearance with delayed puberty.
  - Short stature and webbing of the neck.
  - No breast due to absence of estrogen.
  - No menstruation.
  - Sterile.

25. Klinefelter's Syndrome (Seminiferous tubule dysgenesis):

- This is the abnormal sex differentiation due to non disjunction of sex chromosome, a phenomenon in which sex chromosomes fail to separate i.e. one gamete gets both sex chromosome other gets none in which the gamet containing XX is fertilised by male gamet i.e. 22 + Y.

- Characteristic features:
  - ■ Genetic sex is female with chromosomal configuration 44 XXY.
  - ■ Atrophied testis (Gonadal sex).
- Phenotypic features:
  - ■ Male like appearance with feminine stigma
  - ■ Bilateral Gynaecomastia
  - ■ Small penis, testis, seminal vesicles etc.
  - ■ Sterile and impotent but secondary sex characters present
  - ■ Low or normal plasma testosterone level
  - ■ High serum LH but normal FSH level

26. Action of progesterone: See answer of question No.4.

27. LH surge and FSH surge:

- In the late follicular phase of ovarian cycle very high blood level of estrogen and little progesterone together initiate a '+'ve feedback on anterior pituitary to increase the release of FSH and then LH. This peak rise of FSH and LH is known as ***FSH surge*** and ***LH surge*** (Fig. 6.9) respectively which occurs almost simultaneously.
- Increase in LH level (LH Surge) causes ovulation and lead to formation and maintenance of CL which inturn secretes estrogen and mainly progesterone again resulting rise of plasma estrogen and progesterone.

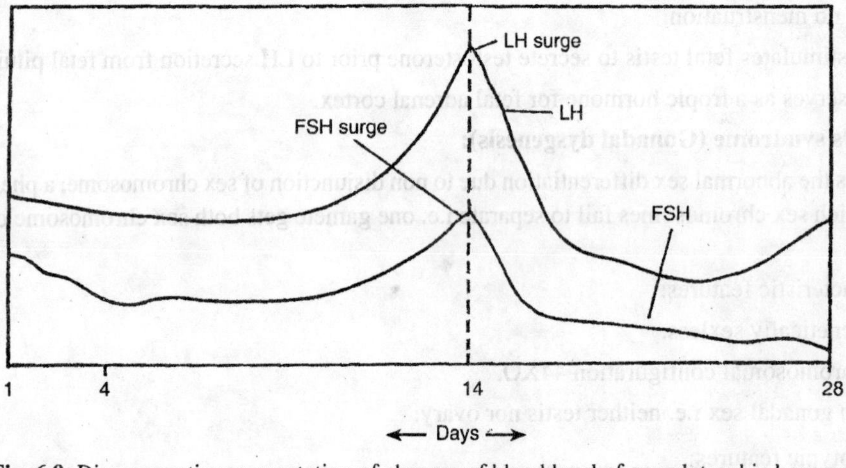

Fig. 6.9: Diagrammatic representation of changes of blood level of gonadotrophic hormones

28. Cryptorchidism:

- **Incomplete descent** of the **testis from abdominal cavity to scrotum in newborn** is known as ***cryptorchidism.*** In this case testis remain either in abdominal cavity or inguinal canal resulting degeneration of seminiferous tubule because of high temperature in those cavities compared to scrotum which is 2-3°C less than body temperature.
- **Features:**
  - ■ Spermatogenesis fails to occur and thus no sperm production resulting sterility.
  - ■ Normal male secondary sex characters because of normal testosterone secretion by leydig cells.
  - ■ Normal plasma level of testosterone.

29. Corpus hemorrhagicum:

- During the ovulation the ovum is released from graafian follicle and remaining part of graafian follicle becomes filled with blood which is called as corpus hemorrhagicum.
- The blood inside it clots slowly and thereafter is replaced by proliferation of granulosa cells to ultimately transform into corpus luteum.

30. Withdrawal bleeding:

- The endometrial shedding occurs due to sudden withdrawal of high plasma level of estrogen and progesterone is known as withdrawal bleeding.
- It is due to spasm in the spiral arteries supplying the superficial part of endometrial layer which results constriction of spiral arteries and consequently cutting- off the blood supply and thus necrosis of the superficial part of endometrium.
- Similar withdrawal bleeding is also seen 3-4 days after withdrawal of oral contraceptive pills.

31. Contraception

- ***Physiological basis***: contraception is physiologically based on the following facts:
  - prevention of release of sperm.
  - prevention of entry of sperm into female genital tract.
  - blockade of ovulation.
  - blockade of entry of ovum into fallopian tube.
  - prevention of implantation.
  - termination of pregnancy before term.
- ***Methods of contraception***: Methods of contraception may be divided into two groups: measures in males and female.

I. *In male*:

- Conventional methods (use of **condom**):
  - It's aim is to prevent release of live ejaculated sperm into the female genital tract.
  - It's advantages are:
    - easy to use
    - no side effects
    - provides protection against sexually transmitted diseases (STD) like AIDS.
- **Coitus interruptus:**
  - It means withdrawal of penis before ejaculation.
  - It is not safe as even a drop of semen can cause pregnancy.
- **Vasectomy:** It is the bilateral ligation of the vas deferens which prevents release of sperm from secondary storehouse into ejaculatory duct.
- **Drugs like:** Gossypol and synthetic testosterone can inhibit sperm formation and thus helpful for contraception.

II. *In female*:

- **Conventional method:** In this method either **Diaphragm** is inserted on the cervix or **Spermicidal jelly** or **Cream** is used during intercourse to prevent the entry of sperm into female genital tract or kill the sperm.

- **Calender method:** As per this method intercourse is limited to only during ***Safe period*** i.e. the period except from 3 days prior to 2 days after ovulation. This method has no practical value specially in case of irregular periods as time of ovulation is not fixed and also it is not easy to know the time of ovulation.
- **Tubectomy:** It is the surgical procedure in which bilateral ligation of the fallopian tube is done.
- **Intrauterine Device:**
  - It is the implantation of a foreign body (a piece of metal or plastic) into the uterine cavity to prevent implantation.
  - IUDs should be replaced periodically at intervals of 2–4 years otherwise their efficiency is lost or they can cause intrauterine infection.
- **Contraceptive pills**:
  - In this methods synthetic estrogen and/or progesterone is orally taken to—
    - prevent ovulation
    - prevent implantation of fertilized ovum
    - prevent entry of sperm into uterus
    - inhibit motility of sperm in female genital tract
  - If correctly used it is most useful and successful non surgical method.

32. Changes of mother during pregnancy: Pregnancy is divided into 3 trimesters (i) 1st trimesters (0-12 wk), (ii) 2nd trimesters (13-28 wk) and (iii) 3rd trimesters (29-40 wk). Total duration is 40 weeks from the 1st day of last menstrual period. During these phases following physiological changes takes place:

- ***On uterus*:**
  - Gross enlargement due to hypertrophy of endometrium and myometrium.
  - Formation of new fiber (hyperplasia).
  - Increase amount of connective and elastic tissues.
- ***On ovary*:** Suspension of ovarian cycle due to inhibition of FSH by negative feedback exerted by increased secretion of estrogen and progesterone from CL.
- ***On breast*:**
  - Enlargement and hyperplasia.
  - Growth of ductular and alveolar systems of mammary glands without secreting the milk.
  - Pigmentation of areola and nipple.
- ***On blood*:**
  - Increase in blood volume due to increased plasma volume. So there is decrease of RBC count and Hb% (**physiological anemia**)
  - Decrease plasma protein concentration
  - Increase in TLC specially neutrophil count
  - Increase in plasma fibrinogen level resulting increase of ESR
  - Fall in plasma iron level.
- ***On CVS*:**
  - Enlargement of heart.
  - Increase in cardiac output.

- Normal BP due to fall of peripheral resistance resulted from vasodilatation due to progesterone action on blood vessels.
- Increase in femoral venous pressure. This may result **edema in feet after prolonged standing.**

• ***On respiration***:

- Slight fall or no change of vital capacity.
- Increase in TV and pulmonary ventilation due to increase in sensitivity of respiratory centers to CO_2.
- Increase in O_2 consumption.

• ***On GIT***:

- Increase of stomach motility.
- Increase in acid secretion.
- Nausea and vomiting in 1st 2-3 months of pregnancy.

• ***On metabolism***:

- Weight gain (about 12 kg).
- Increase in total water content due to increase in Na^+ and H_2O retention.
- N_2 retention with positive nitrogen balance provided balanced diet is supplied.
- Tendency of glycosuria due to lowering of rental threshold of glucose.
- Increase in blood level of cholesterol, phospholipids, neutral fat.

33. Pregnancy diagnosis tests: Before any clinical signs or symptoms of pregnancy appear, it can be diagnosed by demonstrating the presence of HCG in urine or serum. However detection of HCG in urine is more popular but serum HCG can be detected by **ELISA** test very early i.e. about 8 days of missing period. The procedures used to diagnose pregnancy are:

A. Immunological test: These are based on the antigenic property of HCG. In this test urinary HCG is the basis of test which appears in urine after 14 days of missed period.

(a) ***Hem agglutination-inhibition test (Gravindex Test)***: Vide table 6.a.

(b) *Preg colour test*: In this method commercially available strip is dipped into the urine up to a certain level and kept it for 1 min. Appearance of single pink colour line means no pregnancy whereas appearance of double pink colour line denotes pregnancy.

Table 6a: Pregnancy (Gravindex) test

Procedure	Observation	Inference
STEP–I : One drop HCG antiserum is mixed with one drop of urine of a woman in a glass slide. **STEP–II :** HCG coated latex particles are added to the said content.	**IF –** presence of agglutination of latex particles due to antigen-antibody reaction between HCG in latex and non-neutralised HCG` antiserum by urine with no HCG.	**NO PREGNANCY**
	IF– absence of agglutination of latex particles due to no antigen-antibody reaction between HCG in latex and neutralised HCG antiserum by HCG of urine.	**PREGNANCY**

B. ***Biological test***: In the past HCG in urine used to be detected by bioassay technique which was first reported by Ascheim and Zondek in 1927. In India male frog test became very popular, however these tests are obsolete now.

(a) *Ascheim-zondek test*: 2-5 ml urine of women is injected to immature female mice twice or thrice a day for 2-3 days. On the 3rd day the abdomen is opened and ovaries are examined histologicaly. Presence of hemorrhagic corpora lutea indicates pregnancy.

(b) *Male frog test*: About 3-5 ml urine is injected into the dorsal lymph sac of the male frog. After $1^{1/2}$–2 hours urine is withdrawn from the cloacae and examined for the presence of sperms. Presence of shaded sperms indicates pregnancy.

34. Double Bohr's effect: This is represented by following flow chart:

Fetal blood entering placenta is having high PCO_2

↓

Diffusion of maternal compartment

↙ ↘

Maternal blood becomes more acidic | Fetal blood becomes alkaline

↓ ↓

Binding capacity of Hb to O_2 is decreased | Binding capacity of Hb to O_2 is increased

↓ ↓

More release of O_2 from maternal blood | More uptake of O_2 in fetal blood

↘ ↙

Sufficient picking up of O_2 in fetal blood from maternal blood

35. Respiratory system of a new born:

Foetal lungs are nonfunctioning as placenta provides the purification function of foetal blood. But after birth as the umbilical cord is cut off the lungs start functioning with the following changes in respiratory system:

- When placental blood flow is cut off there is sudden hypoxia and hypercapnoea which inturn stimulates the respiratory center of the newborn and thus respiration starts with gasping type of respiration followed by normal respiration.
- In foetal stage resistance of pulmonary vascular bed is very high causing little blood flow in foetal lungs. The first breath in the newborn causes expansion of lungs and thus reduction in the pulmonary vascular resistance and a sudden fall in pressure in pulmonary blood vessels. This results increased blood flow through pulmonary blood vessels.

36. Onset of puberty:

- During childhood the hypothalamus does not secrete significant quantities of GnRH because of inhibitory effect of sex steroids exerted on highly sensitive hypothalamus or other unknown factors. At puberty somehow the sensitivity of hypothalamus to this inhibitory effect of sex steroids decreases which results increase in GnRH release → increasde of gonadotrophins release from anterior pituitary → increased release of gonadal hormones → initiates change of external genitalia, accessory sex organs and other pubertal changes.
- It is predicted that before puberty the release of hypothalamic GnRH becomes inhibited by one hormone **'melatonin'** secreted from pineal gland. At puberty due to the calcification (?) of pineal gland it no longer secretes melatonin and thus inhibitory effects of melatonin is reversed or decreased to result more GnRH release.

C. Differentiate between:

Delayed puberty	Precocious puberty
❑ Onset of puberty is delayed beyond the age of 17 in girls and 20 in boys.	❑ Onset of puberty occurs before the age of 8.
❑ Occurs usually due to panhypopituitarism or gonadal dysgenesis.	❑ Occurs usually due to early secretion of gonadotropins from pituitary.

Leydig cell	Sertoli cells
❑ These are endocrinal cells present in the connective tissue stroma of the testis between the seminiferous tubule.	❑ It is the large and tall columner cells present within the seminiferous tubule of testis.
❑ It has no direct role in the production of sperm.	❑ It directly helps in the production of sperm.
❑ It secretes testosterone.	❑ It secretes inhibin, androgen binding protein, MIF and also responsible for conversion of testosterone to estrogen.

Spermatogenesis	Spermiogenesis
❑ It is the process by which spermatogonia are differentiated into spermatozoa.	❑ It is one of the phases of spermatogonia in which spermatids are transformed into mature sperm.
❑ Chromosomal configuration changes to 44 + XY to 22 + X or 22 + Y.	❑ No change of chromosomal configuration takes place in this phase.

FSH in spermatogenesis	LH in spermatogenesis
❑ Responsible for initiation of spermatogenesis.	❑ Responsible for secretion of testosterone from leydig cell and thus responsible for maintenance of spermatogenesis.

Testosterone	Dihydrotestosterone
❑ It is the prohormone.	❑ It is the active hormone formed from testosterone in the target tissue by 5-alpha reductase.
❑ It's affinity to bind androgen binding protein is less.	❑ It's affinity to bind androgen binding protein is 2-3 times more.
❑ It is secreted by leydig cells.	❑ It is synthesized in the target tissues.
❑ In fetal life it is responsible for differentiation of wolffian duct to male secondary sex organs like seminal vesicle, vas deferens, epididymis.	❑ In fetal life it is responsible for differentiation of urogenital sinus to prostate, urethra and penis.

Primary follicle	Secondary follicle
❑ It is the 1st stage of ovarian cycle in which follicular cells become columner.	❑ It is the the 3rd stage of ovarian cycle in which follicular cells become multi layered granulosa cells.
❑ It is primary oocyte plus columner follicular cells.	❑ It is primary oocyte plus granulosa cells.

Proliferative phase	Secretory phase
❑ It coincides with follicular phase of ovarian cycle.	❑ It coincides with luteal phase of ovarian cycle.
❑ Changes are due to mainly estrogenic activity.	❑ Changes are due to mainly progesterone activity.
❑ Characterised by endometrial proliferation and neovascularisation.	❑ Characterised by hyperemia, elongation and coiling of glands.
❑ Cervical mucous is thin and more alkaline.	❑ Cervical mucous is thick.
❑ Cervical mucous forms fern pattern.	❑ Cervical mucous does not form fern pattern.
❑ Mammary ducts proliferation is seen.	❑ Breast becomes swollen and tender due to interstitial edema, hyperemia and distention of ducts.

D. Short answer type:

1. Give physiological basis of the followings:

a. Number of males born are slightly greater than the females:

The human sperm containing Y chromosome is smaller than the sperm containing X chromosome → lighter sperm containing Y-chromosome swims fast in the female genital tract → more chance to fertilize the ovum. Thus male borns are slightly greater than the female.

b. Genetic sex is determined entirely by the sperm:

Y-chromosome of sperm if fertilizes X-chromosome of ovum there is genetic male and X- chromosome of sperm if fertilizes X-chromosome of ovum there is genetic female i.e. Y-chromosome is the factor which determines the determination of genetic female or male.

c. Sterility in male working in hot environment:

Long term exposure to high temperature there is degeneration of seminiferous tubules → no spermatogenesis → sterility.

d. Use of convenient contraceptive measure for about 2 months after vasectomy:

Vas deferens is the secondary store house of sperm and the ampula of vas deferens can store viable spermatozoa for 2 months. So first 2 months after vasectomy the spermatozoa can be released from ampula leading fertilization and thus pregnancy.

e. Androgen given orally are ineffective:

Androgen given orally is inactivated by liver to form less potent androsterone and DHEA.

f. Sperm count tends to be greater in winter:

Exposure to high temperature during summer causes degeneration of seminiferous tubules → less spermatogenesis → less sperm count.

g. Increase of BBT at the time of ovulation:

Increase in BBT at the time of ovulation is due to the peak rise of progesterone level which is thermogenic.

h. Menstrual blood does not normally contain clots:

Menstrual blood does not normally contain clots unless the bleeding is excessive because this blood promptly clot in the uterus but is liquidified by fibrinolysin in the vagina.

i. Tenderness and swelling of breast prior to menstruation:

This is because under the influence of cyclical changes of estrogen and progesterone level in the blood during menstruation there is considerable growth and branching of duct system of breast alveoli followed by regression.

j. Higher incidences of patent ductus arteroius in children with history of fetal distress:

Within few hours after birth there is usually closure of ductus arteroius (DA) due to contraction of smooth muscle in DA wall in response to increased availability of O_2 after birth. But in case of foetal distress O_2 availibility is not increased immediately even after birth → no contraction of smooth muscle in DA wall → no closure of DA → increases incidence of DA in such children.

k. Test tube babies:

In case of infertility due to fallopian tube obstruction ovum of that woman is isolated and fertilized in vitro by adding sperm and after few days the blastocyst is inserted into the progesterone primed uterus → birth of baby by this procedure is known as test tube baby.

l. Anemia and pregnancy:

During pregnancy the blood volume increases by 30% due to increase in plasma volume without any rise of blood cells → dilution of RBCs → relative decrease in RBC count, HB%, PCV → this is known as physiological anemia.

m. Prevention of fertilization of ovum by more than one sperm:

Once one sperm enters through the zona pellucida of ovum it prevents further entry of another sperm to ovum by following mechanisms to prevent polyploidy.

(a) Entry of 1st sperm into ovum → Ca^{2+} entry → release of cortical granules from oocyte membrane to the perivitelline space by exocytosis → deposition of cortical granules on zona pellucida → prevents penetration of another sperm.

(b) Entry of sperm into ovum causes electrical depolarisation of oocyte membrane resulting negativity outside to exert repulsive action on electronegative sperm.

n. Premature babies are kept in the incubator at neutral zone temperature (32.5-33.5 ^{0}C):

This is to minimize the higher O_2 consumption in case of newborn.

o. Low foetal weight in multilple pregnancies:

The weight of the infant is a direct function of weight of the placenta. So in case of multiple pregnancies placental function is distributed to all the foetus resulting low weight of foetus.

p. Hyperventilation in pregnant woman:

During pregnancy → increase in progesterone level → increase in sensitivity of respiration center to CO_2 → decrease in arterial PCO_2 → increase in TV and respiratory rate → increase in pulmonary ventilation. This is why pregnant woman hyperventilate to reduce alveolar PCO_2 to maintain normal PCO_2 in umbilical vein.

2. What will happen and why if?:

a. Fetal testis are removed at 8 weeks of intrauterine life:

It results development of female genitalia as in between 9th -10th week of gestation under the influence of testicular testosterone hormone, male external genitalia are differentiated from the wolffian duct along with regression of mullerian duct. So if the fetal testis are removed before 8 weeks of intra uterian life there will be no testosterone thereby no differentiation of male genitalia rather differentiation of female genitalia from the Mullerian duct.

b. Testis are removed in an individual before and after puberty:

Removal of testis before puberty results permanent sterility along with no pubertal changes (eunuchoidism). Whereas removal of testis after puberty results sterility and atrophy of seminal vesicle and prostate but voice changes, appearance of beard, mustache are normal and sexual desire and penile erection is little impaired but not arrested.

c. If ovaries are removed before and after puberty:

Removal of ovary before puberty results no pubertal changes, no menstruation and no secondary sex characters. Whereas removal of ovary after puberty results atrophy of genitalia, no menstruation, hot flushes though the sex desire is unaffected.

d. Corpus luteum fails to secrete it's hormone after fertilization:

If corpus luteum fails to secrete it's hormone progesterone after fertilization there is termination of pregnancy as growth of endometrium will be stopped to sustain the life of foetus.

e. Overectomy is done about 8 weeks of gestation:

This results no inturruption of pregnancy as the feto-placental unit takes charge to synthesise and secrete the oestrogen and progesterone.

3. How do the non motile sperms in seminiferous tubules reach the epididymis?

Ciliary movements and smooth muscle contraction of seminiferous tubules, rete testis, ductus efferentes propels the non motile sperm into epididymis.

4. How do the sperm penetrates through the cervical mucous plug?

The hyaluronidase enzyme present in the semen splits the mucopolysaccharides present in the cervical mucous of female genital tract that helps the sperm to penetrate through cervical mucous plug.

5. How long the sperm remains viable in female reproductive tract?

Sperms remain viable in female genital tract maximum 24-48 hours though the motility can persists upto 60 hours.

6. Why are so many sperms are released per ejaculation when only one sperm is required to fertilize the ovum?

So many sperms are ejaculated because penetration of zona pellucida layer surrounding the ovum depends on proteolytic activity of acrosomal enzymes present in sperm head (acrosomal reaction). As single sperm is not sufficient to release enough proteolytic enzyme the penetration of zona pellucida layer by single sperm may not be effective.

7. Can oestrogen be given to prevent the coronary artery disease?

No, because oestrogen in pharmacological doses promote thrombosis.

8. Justify—LH is an ovulatory hormone.

Ovulation occurs about 8-12 hours after LH surge. Therefore it can be said that the LH is an ovulatory hormone.

9. Why is parturition favoured by high oestrogen and low progesterone level?

Estrogen causes:

- Increased release of oxytocin from maternal pituitary.
- Increased synthesis of oxytocin receptors in myometrium and deciduas.

- Increased synthesis of prostaglandins in the deciduas which increase the formation of gap junctions in the myometrium, enabling coordinated muscle activity.
- Increased synthesis of myometrial contractile proteins.

Progesterone on the otherhand relaxes the uterine smooth muscles to facilitate the passage of foetus from the uterus.

E. MCQ:

1. The main source of testosterone in human is (i) seminiferous tubule (ii) epididymis (iii) Leydig cell of testis (iv) Sertoli cells of testis. (iii)
2. Klinefelter's syndrome has the following sex chromosomal configuration (i) XO (ii) YO (iii) XY (iv) XXY. (iv)
3. Following sex chromosomal combination is termed as Turner's syndrome (i) XO (ii) YO (iii) XY (iv) XXY. (i)
4. Barr body represents (i) active X chromosome (ii) inactive autosome (iii) inactive Y chromosome (iv) inactive X chromosome. (iv)
5. The bulk of semen is contributed by (i) seminiferous tubules (ii) bulbourethral gland (iii) prostate (iv) seminal vesicle. (iv)
6. FSH secretion in male is regulated by (i) inhibin (ii) testosterone (iii) oestrogen (iv) androgen binding protein. (i)
7. The normal duration of spermatogenesis is (i) 64 days (ii) 74 days (iii) 30 days (iv) 100 days. (ii)
8. Fertilization usually occurs in (i) vagina (ii) cervix (iii) uterus (iv) fallopian tube. (iv)
9. Presence of any of the following hormone in urine indicates pregnancy (i) FSH (ii) LH (iii) progesterone (iv) HCG. (iv)
10. All but one are secreted by sertoli cells of the testis (i) inhibin (ii) MIF (iii) estrogen (iv) testosterone. (iv)
11. Capacitation of sperm takes place in (i) male genital tract (ii) female genital tract (iii) both (iv) none of the above. (ii)
12. The length of mature sperm is (i) 55-65 μm (ii) 20-25 μm (iii) 50-60 mm (iv) 30-40 cm. (i)
13. Normal sperm count is (i) 80-120 ml/min (ii) 60-70 million per ml (iii) 20-40 million /ml (iv) 40 – 60 lakh /ml. (i)
14. Normal sperm motility is (i) > 50% (ii) > 80% (iii) less than 50% (iv) less than 80%. (ii)
15. All but one are the functions of testosteron (i) anterolateral receding of hair line (ii) increase in RBC count (iii) increase in muscle mass (iv) decreases salt and water retention. (iv)
16. In a 30 days menstrual cycle ovulation takes place in (i) 14 days (ii) 15 days (iii) 16 days. (iii)
17. Corpus luteum of pregnancy survives upto (i) 14 days after fertilization (ii) 3-4 months after fertilization. (iii) 6 months after fertilisation (iv) present till child birth. (ii)
18. LH surge is associated with following important function (i) fertilization (ii) sex differentiation (iii) ovulation (iv) mature follicle formation. (iii)
19. Menopause occurs in (i) 48-55 years of age (ii) > 60 yrs of age (iii) < 40 years of age (iv) 14 years of age. (i)
20. Urinary excretion of HCG starts at (i) 40-45 days after LMP (ii) 30 days after LMP (iii) 2-3 days after LMP (iv) at mid pregnancy. (i)
21. Which placental hormone is the marker of placental function (i) HCG (ii) HCS (iii) estrogen (iv) progesterone. (ii)

22. Which method of contraception is not reliable (i) use of condom (ii) tubectomy (iii) vasectomy (iv) coitus interruptus. (iv)
23. The average duration of pregnancy is (i) 284 days (ii) 270 days (iii) 384 days (iv) 262 days. (i)
24. Milk ejection is the function of (i) PRL (ii) estrogen (iii) progesterone (iv) oxytocin. (iv)
25. Following hormone is not secreted from placenta (i) HCG (ii) estrogen (iii) progesterone (iv) testosterone. (iv)

Gastro Intestinal System

7

A. Long type:

1. Classify the salivary glands. Describe the composition and functions of saliva. What is the mechanism and regulation of salivary secretion? What do you mean by Xerostomia?

There are 3 pairs of major salivary glands:

(i) **Parotid gland**—Situated at the side of the face just below and in front of the ear.

(ii) **Sub maxillary gland**—Situated in sub maxillary triangle medial to mandible.

(iii) **Sublingual gland**—Situated in mucosa at the floor of the mouth.

Composition of saliva: In the oral cavity saliva is secreted by the salivary glands. It's composition is:

- Volume—1000-1500 ml/ day
  —1 ml/min
- Reaction—Slightly acidic (pH-6.35-6.85)
- Specific gravity—1.002-1.012
- Constituents:

(a) Water-99.5%

(b) Solid- 0.5%

(i) *Organic compounds* (0.3%):

- Enzymes like salivary amylase (ptyalin), phosphatase, lysozyme, ribonuclease, kallikrein etc.
- Mucin
- Small traces of urea, amino acids, cholesterol
- Other proteins like nerve growth factors, epidermal growth factor, blood group antigens.

(i) *Inorganic substances* (0.2.%): NaCl, KCl, sodium phosphate, calcium carbonate, calcium phosphate, potassium thiocyanate.

(ii) *Cellular constituents*—Yeast cells, bacteria, protozoa, polymorphonuclear leucocytes, desquamated epithelial cells etc.

(iii) *Gases* like O_2, CO_2, N_2

Functions of saliva:

(a) *Protective function:*

- It decreases the risk of buccal infection and dental carries and thus maintain oral hygiene by:
  - Continuous secretion of saliva that washes away food debris and pathogenic bacteria.
  - The enzymes lysozyme and thiocyanate which kill some bacteria like Staphylococcus, Streptococcus and Brucella.
  - The protein antibodies which destroy bacteria including the bacteria causing dental carries.
- It dilutes hot and irritant food thus preventing injury to oral mucosa of mouth.

(b) *Digestive function:*

- The salivary amylase of saliva digests boiled starch, glycogen and dextrin. The starch is digested to maltose.
- Some traces of maltase present in saliva convert some amount of maltose to glucose.

(c) *Mechanical function:*

- It aids in mastication process.
- It also helps in swallowing by lubricating the mouth.
- It also helps in speech by keeping the soft mouth part and lips moistened and lubricated.

(d) *Excretory function:*

- Many substances like mercury, leads, thiocyanate, KI are excreted through saliva.
- It also excretes out some viruses like rabies and mumps virus.
- In some pathological conditions it excretes some substances e.g. urea (in nephritis), sugar (in DM) and Ca^{2+} (in hyper parathyroidism).

(e) *Regulation of water balance:* It also influences water intake by decreasing salivary secretion in response to dehydration which results dryness of the mouth. The dryness of the month inturn initiates thirst and thereby water intake is increased.

(f) It helps to apprehend taste sensation by dissolving the food stuffs.

Salivary secretion:

(a) *Mechanism of salivary secretion:*

(i) Mechanism of water and electrolyte secretion: The mechanism of salivary water and electrolyte secretion occurs in two stages:

1. The secretary end piece (acinar part) along with intercalated ducts secrete a primary secretion (Fig. 7.1) containing ions in concentration almost the same as in ECF.

2. While passing through the excretory and striated ducts, these secretions are modified to secondary secretion by absorbing Na^+ from saliva and by adding K^+ and HCO_3^- to the saliva.

Therefore as saliva flows down the ducts it comes progressively hypotonic. In presence of excess aldosterone there is increased reabsorption of Na^+ and Cl^- from salivary ducts resulting fall of Na^+ and Cl^- level and rise of K^+ concentration in saliva.

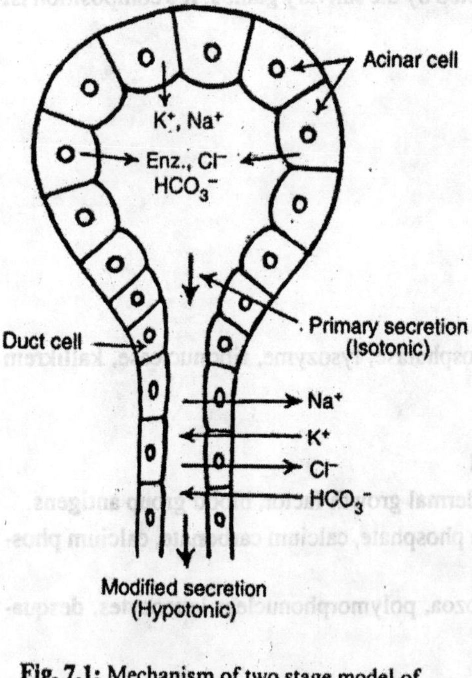

Fig. 7.1: Mechanism of two stage model of salivary secretion

(ii) Secretion of salivary amylase: In their apical cytoplasm, serous acinar cells have zymogen granules that contain salivary amylase and mucins. When the gland is stimulated, the zymogen granules fuse with the plasma membrane and the contents are released into the lumen as primary secretions by exocytosis.

(b) *Regulation of salivary secretion*:

- The primary physiological control of salivary secretion is mediated through ANS whereas the role of hormone is insignificant.
- Stimulation of sympathetic and parasympathetic nerves to these glands stimulate salivary secretion through the effects of parasympathetic are stronger and long lasting.
- Sympathetic stimulation causes contraction of myoepithelial cells, vasoconstriction, direct stimulation of glandular epithelial secretion and results in scanty, viscid secretion.
- Parasympathetic stimulation results vasodilatation, stimulation of glandular tissue and leads profuse watery secretion.
- The types of reflex are involved in salivation: *Conditioned* or *Acquired* and *Unconditioned* or in born reflex.
- Salivation controlled by unconditioned reflex: The detail unconditioned reflex mechanism of salivation is illustrated by flow chart FC 7A.
- Salivation due to conditioned reflex: The existence of this reflex is proved by the fact that even the sight or smell of food can stimulate salivation. Pavlov first experimented this type of salivation by using a sound stimulus to dog before the food is given. The experimental protocol is :

(i)	Only sound	→	No salivation
(ii)	Sound followed by food	→	Salivation
(iii)	Only sound without giving food after repeating protocol (ii) for some days	→	Salivation

In this case the sound acts as a conditioned stimulus, which can initiate salivation.

Xerostomia: Temporary or permanent reduction of salivary secretion due to the congenital absence or hyperplasia of salivary glands is known as Aptyalism or Xerostomia.

2. Enumerate the composition and functions of gastric juice. Add a note on gastric secretion along with it's phase and the factors affecting it.

Composition of gastric juices:

- Total quantity — 1200-1500 ml/day
- Reaction — slightly acidic
- Constituents:

Water — 99.45%

Total solid — 0.55%

Inorganic (0.15%) — NaCl, KCl, $CaCl_2$, bicarbonate, phosphate, sulphate etc.

Organic (0.40%):

(a) Mucin

(b) Intrinsic factor

(c) Enzymes:

- Proteolytic-pepsin, cathepsin etc.
- Lipolytic-Gastric Lipase
- Gastric renin
- Lysosyme, urease, carbonic anhydrase

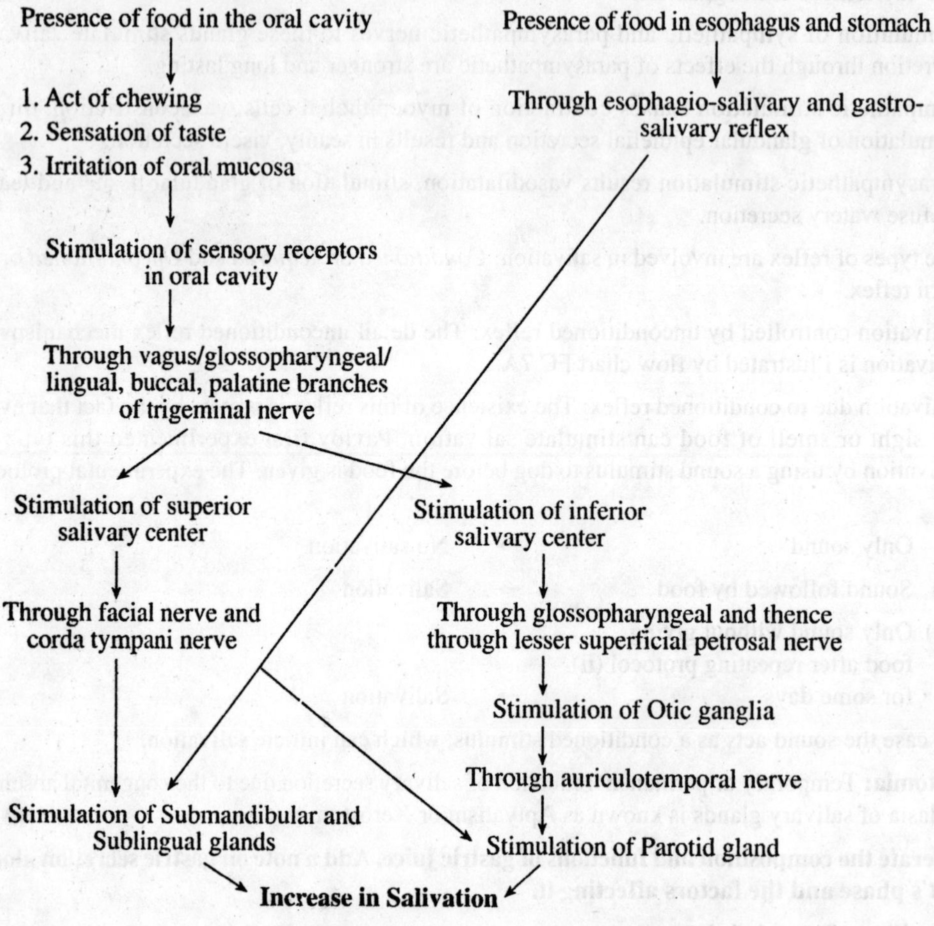

FC 7A: Mechanism of salivation initiated by unconditioned reflex

Functions of gastric juice:

1. The enzyme pepsin digests proteins up to the stage of peptide.
2. Gastric lipase digests fat to some degree.
3. HCl acts as an antiseptic and causes some hydrolysis of all the foodstuffs. It also provides optimum pH i.e. 2-3 for pepsin activity.
4. Renin coagulates casinogen of milk.
5. Helps in absorption of Vit-B_{12} in small intestine by secreting intrinsic factor from it's oxyntic cells.
6. It also helps to excrete out toxins, heavy metals, certain alkaloids.

Secretion of gastric Juice:

***A. Mechanism of secretion of HCl*:**

- HCl is secreted in the intracellular canaliculi of parietal cells separately as H+ and Cl– which ultimately opens into the lumen of the gastric gland (Fig. 7.2). In the lumen H+ and Cl– combines to form HCl. Thereby no HCl is formed in the cytoplasm of the cell to prevent cell injury.

- CO_2 formed due to cell metabolism or entering the cell from the blood combines with H_2O to form H_2CO_3 by the enzyme carbonic anhydrase. H_2CO_3 is then rapidly ionized to form H^+ and HCO_3^-

- H^+ are actively secreted into the canaliculi in exchange of K^+ by $H^+ - K^+$ ATPase present in the luminal surface.

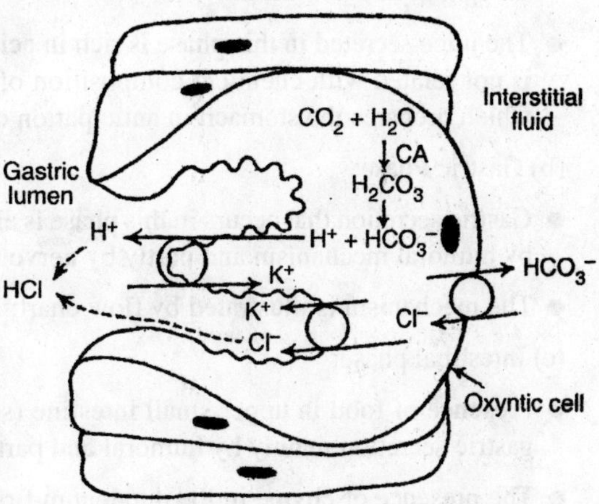

Fig. 7.2: Mechanism of HC1 secretion

- HCO_3– on the other hand is reabsorbed from the cell to the blood in exchanger of secretion of Cl^- to the parietal cell via HCO_3^- – Cl^- exchanger mechanism operated in the basal surface. Due to this absorption of HCO_3^- to the blood, the alkalinity of then blood is increased specially after meal. This results excretion of excess HCO_3– through urine, the condition known as ***post prandial alkaline tide.***

- The HCO_3^- on the other is reabsorbed from the cell to the blood in exchange of secretion of Cl^- on the parietal cell via HCO_3^- – Cl^- exchanger mechanism operated in the basal surface. Due to this absorption of HCO_3^- to the blood, the alkalinity of the blood is increased specially after meal. This results excretion of excess HCO_3^- through urine, the condition known as ***post prandial alkaline tide.***

- The Cl^- secreted into the cell from the blood now actively transported to the canaliculi resulting an electrical gradient. This leads passive flow of K^+ and small amount of Na^+ from cytoplasm to the canaliculi.

- In the canaliculi secreted H^+ and Cl^- reacts with each other to form HCl.

***B. Mechanism of secretion of pepsin*:** Pepsin is synthesized in chief cell and contained in membrane bound zymogen granules. In response to any stimulation it is released as pepsinogen by exocytosis. In gastric acidic pH pepsinogen is activated to form pepsin.

***C. Phases and control of HCl secretion*:** After a meal the rate of acid secretion by the stomach increases promptly in 3 phases—Cephalic phase, Gastric phase and Intestinal phase.

(a) Cephalic phase:

- In this phase gastric secretion occurs even before the food enters into the stomach. The secretion is elicited by sight, smell or taste of food primarily through nervous mechanism.

- The mechanism of gastric secretion in this phase is : Sight/smell/taste of food → sensation to either cerebral cortex or appetite center of hypothalamus or amygdala → stimulation of vagal efferents → release of ACh, gastrin, histamin etc. at gastric glands → release of HCl and pepsin.

- Two types of reflex is involved in this mechanism:
  1. *Unconditioned reflex* in which the reflex stimulation of gastric glands takes place in response to chewing and swallowing of food.
  2. *Conditioned reflex* in which the reflex arises due to vision or smell or taste of food.
- The secretion in this phase starts with a latency of < 5 minutes and continues for 30-120 mins at the rate of 250-750 ml/hr.
- The juice secreted in this phase is rich in acid and pepsin and has got high digestive capacity. It is not related with chemical composition of food and is called ***Psychic juice*** or ***appetite juice*** which prepares the stomach in anticipation of a meal.

(b) Gastric Phase:

- Gastric secretion that occurs in this phase is elicited by the presence of food in the stomach mainly by humoral mechanism and partly by nervous mechanism.
- The mechanism is illustrated by flow chart: FC 7B.

(c) Intestinal phase:

- Presence of food in upper small intestine (specially duodenum and upper jejunum) stimulates gastric secretion mainly by humoral and partly by neural mechanism.
- The presence of chyme in the duodenum first stimulates and then inhibits acid secretion. Early in gastric emptying when pH of gastric chyme is above 3, the stimulatory influences predominate, whereas in later stage when pH of chyme is decreased the inhibitory influence predominates.

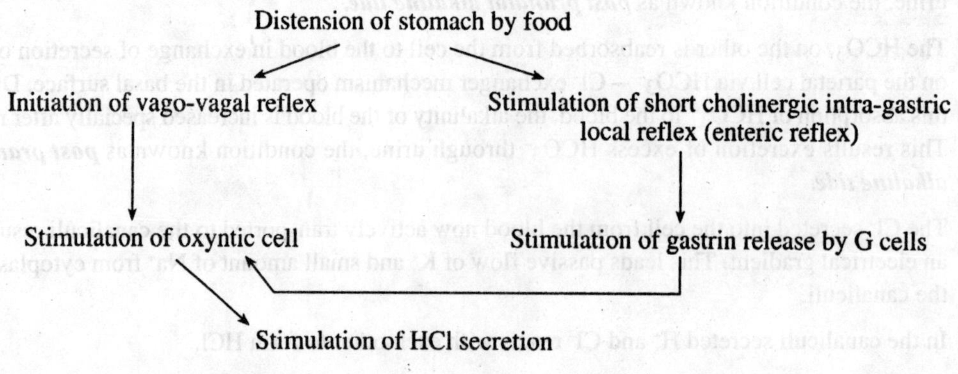

FC 7B: Mechanism of HCl secretion in gastric phase

***D. Factors affecting gastric secretion*:**

(a) In cephalic phase: Different factors increase gastric secretion in this phase are:

— Vagal stimulation — Noradrenalin — GABA
— Gastrin — Neurotensin — Calcitonin
— Chronic exposure to TRH — Nicotine

(b) In gastric phase: The factors influencing the gastric secretion in this phase are:

- Presence of amino acids in the stomach → leads gastrin release → increases HCl secretion.
- Presence of caffeine and tea → cAMP production → ↑ HCl secretion.

- Increased acidity → increase in HCl secretion.
- Presence of fatty acid in stomach → inhibit HCl secretion.
- Distension of small interstine → decreases gastric secretion.
- Presence of acid or protein breakdown product or fat etc. in small intestine → release of secretion, CCK, gastric inhibitory peptide, VIP etc. → inhibit gastric secretion.

(c) In intestinal phase: Differet factors influencing gastric secretion in intestinal phase are:

- Distension of duodenum → secretes gastrin → ↑ HCl secretion.
- Peptide and amino acid in duodenum → secretes gastrin →↑ HCl secretion.
- Fatty acids in small intestine → secretes GIP →↑ gastric secretion.

3. Describe the composition, function and regulation of secretion of pancreatic juice with special reference to its mechanism of secretion.

Composition and character of pancreatic juice:

- Total quantity — 1500 ml/day
- Reaction — alkaline
- pH – 8.0–8.3
- Constituents:
  - Water – 98%
  - Solids (2%)
    - Organic (0.8%)—
      (a) Amylolytic enzymes—Pancreatic amylase.
      (b) Proteolytic enzymes—Trypsin, chymotrypsin, carboxypeptidase, elastase, collagenase etc.
      (c) Lipolytic enzymes—Pancreatic lipsase, cholesterol esterase, phospholipase A_2, lecithinaser, colipase (cofactor for lipase).
      (d) Other enzymes—lysosomal enzymes, alkaline phosphatase, nuclease.
      (e) Other components—Small amount of immunoglobulins, kallikrein, mucins.
    - Inorganic (12%) — Na^+, K^+, Ca^{2+}, Mg^{++}, Zn^{++}, HCO_3, Cl^-

Function of pancreatic juice:

(i) ***Digestive function***: Different enzymes present in pancreatic juice take part in digestion of proteins, lipids and also carbohydrates. For example:

- Trypsin converts protein to proteases and polypeptide.
- Chymotrypsin converts proteins into polypeptides.
- Carboxypeptidase converts polypeptides into amino acids.
- Nuclease converts nucleic acids into mononucleotides.
- Pancreatic lipase converts triglycerides into monoglycerides and fatty acids.
- Phospholipase converts lecithin into lysolecithin and thence to phosphatidyl choline.
- Pancreatic amylase converts starch into maltose.

(ii) **Neutralisation** of acid mixed gastric chyme by the bicarbonate present in it.

Secretion of pancreatic Juice:

A. Mechanism of secretion:

(a) *Cellular mechanism of bicarbonate rich secretion*: The proposed mechanism of bicarbonate rich secretion is as follows:

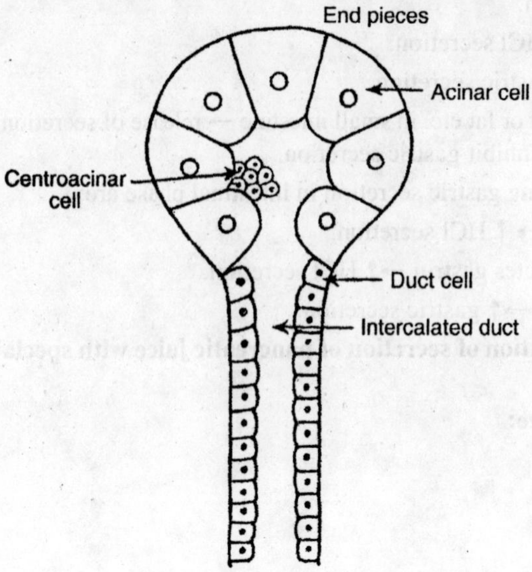

Fig. 7.3: Pancreatic acinus

- CO_2 diffuses from blood to the acinar cell which combines with water to form H_2CO_3 in presence of enzyme carbonic anhydrase (Fig. 7.3).
- H_2CO_3 rapidly dissociates into H^+ and HCO_3^-.
- HCO_3^- is —
  - mainly actively transported to the lumen in exchange of Cl^- to the cell by Cl^{-1}/HCO_3^- exchanger mechanism.
  - also transported to the lumen through the anionic channels.
- H^+ on the other hand is transported to the capillaries in exchange of Na^+ to the cell. The Na^+ then enters to the lumen due to concentration gradient.
- Thus the secretion of HCO_3^-, Na^+ to the lumen exerts osmotic effect which results entry of water to the lumen from the cell by osmosis.

(b) *Cellular mechanism of NaCl rich secretion*:

- At the basolateral surface of the acinar or ductular cell there is $Na^+ - K^+ - Cl^-$ pump which actively pumps in 2 mol of Cl^- along with 1 mol K^+ and 1 mol of Na^+ from ECF to the cell interior (Fig. 7.4).
- Na^+ then diffuses to the ductular lumen due to concentration gradient. Some Na^+ goes back to the ECF in exchange of K^+ from ECF.
- Cl^- enters the lumen through the anionic channel due to concentration gradient.

(c) *Secretion of enzymatic component*: Pancreatic acinar cells (Fig. 7.3) contain numerous membrane bound zymogen granules in their apical cytoplasm. These granules contain most of the pancreatic enzymes. In response to appropriate stimulation the zymogen granules fuse with the plasma membrane to dump their content into the duct by exocytosis.

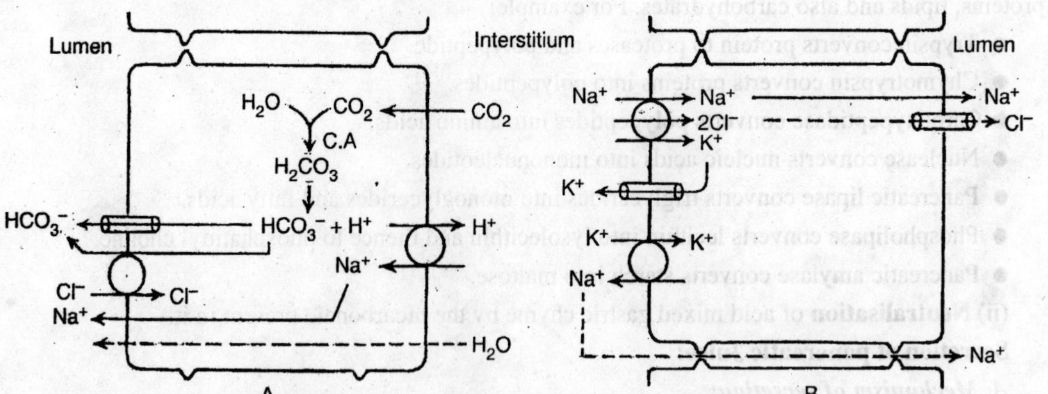

Fig. 7.4: Postulated mechanism of pancreatic secretion
(*A = Bicarbonate rich secretion* and *B = NaCl rich secretion*)

B. Phase of pancreatic secretion along with it's control : The secretion of pancreatic juice occurs in 3 phases-cephalic, gastric and intrestinal phase.

(a) Cephalic phase:

- Ingestion of the food inside the mouth initiates the unconditioned reflex which inturn stimulates vagus nerve to result increase in pancreatic secretion.
- Sight, smell and thought of the food also initiate the conditioned reflex which inturn stimulates vagus nerve that causes increase in pancreatic secretion.
- Vagal stimulation increases the pancreatic secretion not only by releasing ACh which stimulates acinar cell to release enzymes but also increases gastrin and other hormone (CCK/VIP) release which also increases pancreatic secretion.

(b) Gastric phase:

- It results from the stimuli acting in the stomach when food comes into the stomach.
- Distension of stomach initiates a nervous signal through vaginal fibers which releases ACh on pancreatic acinar cells.
- Gastric distension also causes the release of gastrin which also increases pancreatic secretion.

(c) Intestinal phase:

- After chyme enters the small intestine a variety of intraluminal stimulants can act on the intestinal mucosa to stimulate pancreatic secretion through both neural (Vago-vagal reflex) and hormonal (CCK and Secretin) mechanism.
- Presence of fatty acids, amino acids, H^+ and Ca^{++} in intestine activates vagovagal reflex which increases both pancreatic enzyme and electrolyte secretion.
- Presence of highly acid mixed chyme in duodenum release **secretin** which via blood comes to pancreas to increase the secretion of large quantities of fluid containing high concentration of HCO_3^- but low Cl^- with little enzymes. Alkaline pancreatic juice neutralises the acid chyme and provides proper medium for digestion (***hydrelatic effect***).
- Whereas presence of fatty acids, peptides and amino acids in the intestine causes release of CCK from Duodenal 'I' cells which mainly causes secretion of pancreatic juice with high enzyme contents and NaCl rich fluid (***ecbolic effect***).

4. Enumerate the functions of liver. What is the composition of bile? What is the difference between liver bile and gall bladder bile? What do you mean by enterohepatic circulation?

Function of liver:

A. ***Hematological function***: Liver has varied hematological functions e.g.

(a) It is the site of RBC formation in fetal life.

(b) It is the site of RBC destruction in adult life.

(c) It serves as a store house of blood and also takes part in regulation of blood volume.

(d) It is also responsible for blood cleansing action by Kupffer cells.

B. ***Synthetic function***: It is responsible for synthesis of different substances e.g.

(a) Plasma proteins like albumin.

(b) Clotting factors like fibrinogen, prothrombin, factor V, VII, IX and X.

(c) Enzymes like SGOT and SGPT.

(d) Urea.

(e) Cholesterol.

C. Metabolic function:

(a) **In carbohydrate metabolism:** Liver helps in synthesis, storage and release of glucose by glycogenesis, glycogenolysis and gluconeogenesis.

(b) **In protein metabolism:** Liver helps in synthesising plasma proteins, blood clotting factors, enzymes etc. from amino acids.

(c) **In fat metabolism:**

- It is a site at β oxidation and thereby forms active acetate by oxidising the fatty acids.
- It takes part in synthesis of cholesterol and saturated fatty acids from active acetate.
- It also helps in synthesis of lipoproteins like, HDL, LDL, chylomicrons etc.

(d) **In alcohol metabolism:** Liver converts the alcohol into fatty acids.

(e) **In hormone metabolism:**

- It decreases the circulatory adrenal cortical and sex steroids.
- It also helps in inactivation of insulin, glucagon, ADH and anterior pituitary hormones.

(f) **In vitamin metabolism:**

- It helps in formation of Vit -A.
- It is the storehouse of Vit A, B_{12} and D.
- It converts folate to it's active form i.e. tetrahydrofolate.

D. Excretory function: Liver also excretes some toxic products like, heavy metals, bacterial toxins, drugs, cholesterol and bile pigments.

E. Detoxifying or protective function: By the process of oxidation, hydrolysis, reduction and conjugation it detoxifies different substances either produced in the body or taken along with the food.

F. Thermal function: It takes part in heat regulation by producing large amount of heat.

Composition of bile:

- Total quantity–800-1200 ml/day.
- Reaction–alkaline
- pH–8-8.6
- Constituents: Vide table 7a.

Table 7a: Difference of composition of Liver and Gall bladder bile

Constituents	Liver bile (%)	Gall bladder bile (%)
(i) Water	98%	89%
(ii) Solids	2%	11%
— Inorganic salts	0.75%	0.8%
• Na^+	145 (meq/lit)	135 (meq/lit)
• K^+	5%	12%
• Ca^{++}	5%	23%
• Cl^-	100%	25%
• HCO_3^-	28%	10%
— Bile salts	0.9%	6%
— Bile pigments	0.4%	3%
— Cholesterol	0.06%	0.38%
— Fats and FA	0.07%	0.82%

Enterohepatic circulation:

- The substances undergoing enterohepatic circulation are bile acids, bile pigments, Vit. D, B_{12} etc. which are secreted by the liver and enter into the intestine via gall bladder. From the intestine most of these are absorbed back into the blood and presented to the liver to be excreted again. Thus by this enterohepatic circulation (Fig. 7.5) same substances are utilised again and again.
- The bile pigments present in the bile are transported directly to the interstine or via gall bladder. In the intestine these are reduced to form mesobilirubin and then mesobilirubinogen and finally urobilinogen (stercobilinogen) by colonic bacteria. Some of these urobilinogen is excreted through urine, some are excreted through faces as stercobilinogen and most (80%-90%) of them are reabsorbed from the terminal ileum to go back to the liver to be concverted again into bilirubin.

5. What are the functions of bile? How the bile is formed, stored and emptied from the gall bladder? Discuss the control of secretion of bile from the gall bladder.

Functions of bile:

A. Digestion: The bile salts of the bile are responsible for digestion of mainly fat in the intestine by—

- Reducing the surface tensions of the lipid to make it water soluble so that lipolytic enzymes can act on it. This action of bile salts is known as ***emulsification of fat.***
- Increasing the surface area for the activity of lipase enzymes.
- Activating different lipases.
- Acting as a good solvent for fat.

B. Absorption: Bile salts help in fat absorptionm and also in absorption of fat soluble vitamins.

C. Excretion: Some metals like copper, zinc and mercury and toxins of bacteria and bile pigments are excreted through bile.

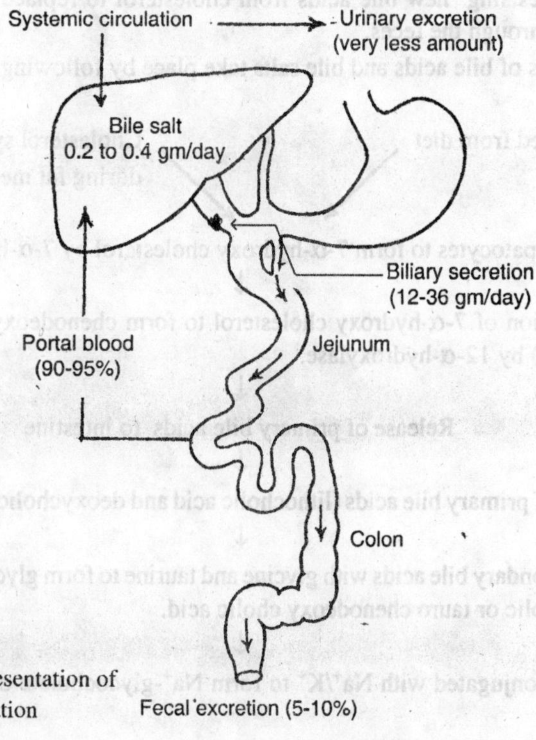

Fig. 7.5: Diagrammatic representation of enterohepatic circulation

D. ***Laxative action***: Bile salts stimulate peristaltic activity of colon which facilitates smooth and easy evacuation of bowels.

E. ***Chologogue action***: Bile salts act as it's own stimulant and thereby release of bile from gall bladder is enhanced. This cholagogue action of bile is mediated through the release of the hormones like CCK-PZ which inturn contracts gall bladder to initiate bile secretion.

F. ***Maintenance of pH***: It maintains the suitable pH in duodenum for proper activity of digestive enzymes.

G. ***Lubricating action***: The mucin of bile acts as a lubricant for the chyme to pass through intestine.

H. ***Cholerectic action***: Bile salts also stimulate the secretion of bile from the liver.

I. ***Protection of gastric mucosa***: Regurgitation of bile into stomach helps to neutralise gastric acidity, which prevents injurious effects of acids on gastric mucosa.

Bile formation:

- Bile contains 4 major ingredients—
  - (a) Bile acids and bile salts,
  - (b) Bile pigments,
  - (c) Phospholipids, cholesterol,
  - (d) Inorganic salts,
- Out of these 4 elements (i), (ii) and (iii) are secreted by hepatocytes and (iv) are secreted by the epithelial cell lining of the bile ducts.

A. ***Formation of bile acids and bile salts***:

- Bile acids are secreted by the liver hepatocytes from 2 sources—
  - (i) by absorbing bile acids from intestine through enterohepatic circulation (60-85%) (200-500ng/day).
  - (ii) by synthesising new bile acids from cholesterol to replace the daily loss of these substances through the feces.
- The synthesis of bile acids and bile salts take place by following mechanism:

Cholesterol absorbed from diet ↘ ↙ Cholesterol synthesized in hepatocytes during fat metabolism.

Hydroxylated in hepatocytes to form 7-α-hydroxy cholesterol by 7-α-hydroxylase.

↓

Further hydroxylation of 7-α-hydroxy cholesterol to form chenodeoxycholic acid and cholic acid (Primary bile acids) by 12-α-hydroxylase.

↓

Release of primary bile acids to intestine

↓

Dehydroxylation of primary bile acids (lithocholic acid and deoxycholic acids) by intestinal bacteria.

↓

Conjugation of secondary bile acids with glycine and taurine to form glycocholic or glycochenodeoxy cholic and taurocholic or tauro chenodeoxy cholic acid.

↓

These are further conjugated with Na^+/K^+ to form Na^+-glycocholate or Na^+ taurocholates and etc. (bile salts).

***B. Formation of bile pigments*:**

- **Biliverdin and bilirubin are the principal bile pigments which are excretory products of heme metabolism.**
- **During the destruction of old or damaged RBC in the reticuloendothelial cells the hemoglobin liberated from the RBC is hydrolysed to form globin and iron containing porphyrin *'heme'*.**
- **The iron moiety of the heme is now removed to form biliverdin some of which are converted to bilirubin by reduction in the R-E system. Thus one gram of Hb yields about 35 gm of bilirubin.**
- **This bilirubin is now released into plasma to bind with plasma albumin.**
- **This bilirubin-albumin complex is transported to the hepatocytes to result following events:**

Uptake of bilirubin in to hepatocytes through a protein *'ligandin'* present in the hepatocyte membrane

↓

Esterification of bilirubin with glucoronic acid by transferase enzyme to form bilirubin diglucoronide (known as conjugated bilirubin)

↓

Secretion of bilirubin diglucoronide in the bile

- **3rd ingredients of bile is phospholipids and cholesterol which are secreted by hepatocytes after collecting these from the blood.**
- **4th ingredients are inorganic salt of bicarbonate and chloride those are also secreted by the bile duct epithelial cells from the plasma.**

Storage and concentration of bile ingall bladder:

- **Gall bladder concentrates, acidifies, stores and discharges bile whenever needed.**
- **The gall bladder concentrates the bile by absorbing Na^+,Cl^-, HCO_3^- and water from liver bile so that the bile acids, salts, pigments and phospholipids can be concentrated by 5-20 times.**
- **The mechanism of reabsorption of different substances are illustrated by (Fig. 7.6). This diagram depicts that:**

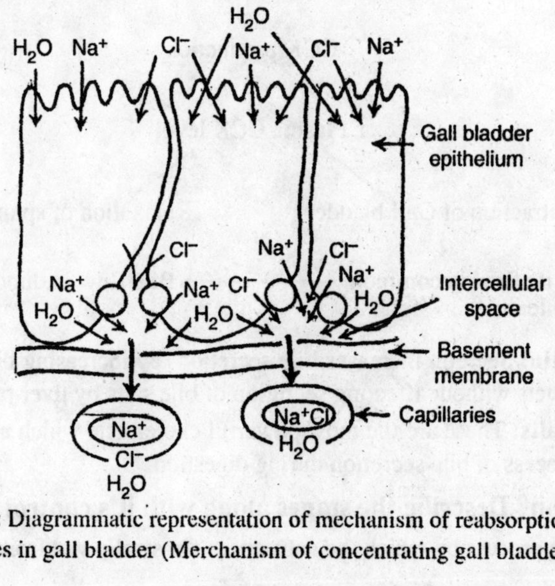

Fig. 7.6: Diagrammatic representation of mechanism of reabsorption of electrolytes in gall bladder (Merchanism of concentrating gall bladder bile)

- Most of the Na^+ is reabsorbed by the epithelial layer of gall bladder actively secreted into bile in exchange of H^+.
- This movement of Na^+ into cells results passive movement (absorption of Cl^- and HCO_3^-) by the epithelial cell to maintain electrical neutrality.
- Movement of ions inside the cell now generate osmotic gradient which leads passive flow of water from lumen into inter cellular space and thence to cell inside.
- The movement of water into the inter cellular spaces now increases the hydrostatic pressure which inturn causes further absorption of Na^+, Cl^-, Ca^{2+} through the porous basement membrane into the capillaries.

Mechanism of secretion of bile-emptying by gall bladder:

- Emptying of the gall bladder contents into the duodenum begins several minutes after the start of a meal.
- During gastric and cephalic phases of digestion vagal discharges initiate gall bladder contraction and relaxation of sphincter of oddi to result bile discharge into duodenum.
- Contraction of gall bladder during both of these phase also initiate peristaltic waves which is transmitted to the sphincter of oddi down the common bile duct to result relaxation of sphincter.
- Relaxation of sphincter of oddi also takes place due to the transmission phase of the intestinal peristaltic wave over the wall of duodenum.
- Thus all these actions help to discharge $2/3^{rd}$ of it's content during Ist hour of digestion. During digestion the gall bladder remains in a contractile state so that hepatic bile is not stored but employed directly to the intestine.

Control of secretion:

- Bile secretion is practically independent of neural influence and depends on chemicals especially hormonal influence.
- The control of bile secretion is mainly mediated by CCK and also by secretin in some extent. Other agents are bile salts which also influence the bile secretion.
  - **Role of CCK:** CCK helps in bile secretion by following mechanism:

Fatty acids in duodenum
↓
↑ CCK production
↓
↑ Plasma CCK level
↙ ↘
Contraction of Gall bladder → ↓ → ↑ Bile flow in common bile duct → ↑ Bile flow in duodenum
Relaxation of sphincter → ↓ → ↑ Bile flow in duodenum

  - **Role of secretin:** Secretin increases bile secretion by increasing bicarbonate from epithelia cells of bile ducts without affecting secretion of bile salts by liver parenchymal cells.
  - **Role of bile salts:** These are the most powerful cholerectic which act as the main stimulus ir the normal process of bile secretion during digestion.

6. What is deglutition? Describe the stages along with it's control of deglutition.

Definition: It is the process by which the substances are swallowed from the oral cavity.

Stages of Diglutitions : Diglutition occurs in 3 stages:

(i) *Oral stage* takes place in mouth mainly and is voluntary in nature.

(ii) *Pharyngeal stage*— takes place in pharynx and involuntary in nature.

(iii) *Oesophageal stage*—occurs in esophagus and involuntary.

***Mechanism of deglutition*:**

(i) ***Oral stage*:** It is a voluntary stage which initiates the swallowing process in a following manner:

(a) Rolling of food on upper surface of tongue to form a bolus by tongue movement.

(b) Sealing of nasopharynx and thus prevention of nasal regurgitation by the movement of soft plate and nasopharynx to be close together. During bulbar poliomyelitis and diphtheria there is paralysis of the muscle of soft palate resulting no sealing off the nasopharynx → regurgitation of fluid through nasal cavity.

(c) Reflex stoppage of respiration (***deglutition apnea***) to prevent entry of food to the respiratory tract.

(d) Elevation and retraction of the tongue due to action of myelohyoid, styloglossus and hypoglossus muscles, which forces the bolus towards the pharynx.

(ii) ***Pharyngeal stage*:** When bolus moves from mouth to pharynx receptors present in the pharynx are stimulated and the sensation goes to deglutition center which initiates series of muscular contractions that lead following events:

(a) Pushing of the bolus to epiglottis by the tongue movement.

(b) Palato pharyngeal folds on either side of the pharynx approximate to make a slit like opening for food, allowing only properly masticated food to pass through.

(c) Closure of laryngeal opening that prevents entry of food to trachea.

(d) Relaxation of upper esophageal sphincter to allow the food to enter into the esophagus

(e) Contraction of entire muscular wall of pharynx generating a fast peristaltic wave which pushes the food into esophagus.

(iii) ***Esophageal stage***: In this phase food enters from esophagus to stomach by:

(a) Propelling the food to the lower end of esophagus by the peristaltic movement of esophagus.

(b) Relaxation of lower esophageal sphincter to allow the food enter into stomach.

***Control of deglutition*:**

(a) ***Oral stage*:** It is mainly voluntarily controlled.

(b) ***Pharyngeal stage: Structure*** in the back of the mouth like anterior pillars of pharynx, base of the tongue, soft palate are highly sensitive to touch. As soon as the bolus touches these structures, swallowing reflex starts. The detail control is illustrated as follows:

In response to touch sensation in the above mentioned areas by the bolus, the tactile receptors are stimulated → The afferent impulse is conducted to the medullary swallowing center by superior laryngeal (branch of vagus), glossopharyngeal and also trigeminal nerve → The efferent impulses from the deglutition center is passed to the structure from pharynx to LES of esophagus by hypoglossal, glossopharyngeal, vagus and facial nerves → Appropriate function to divert the food from pharynx to esophagus.

(c) ***Esophageal stage*:**

- It is reflexly controlled, by the deglutition center generated when the bolus comes into esophagus. The efferent pathway is mediated mainly through the vagus.
- Reflex stimulation of deglutition center initiate primary peristalsis whereas the local reflex (initiated due to distention of upper esophagus by food) initiates secondary peristalsis → forces the bolus down.
- Reflex relaxation of LES helps in the entry of bolus to stomach.

7. Enumerate the small intestinal movements. What is Starling's law of intestine?

Small intestinal motility: In addition to the movements caused by MMC the small intestine shows various movement like:

(a) **Segmentation:**

- Pendular movement
- Peristalsis

(b) **Segmentation:**

- These are ring like contractions that appear at fairly regular intervals along the gut involving a localised segment of 1-2 cm.
- It involves two types of contraction- Eccentric and Concentric contraction.
- By this movements, food is divided and mixed together with digestive enzymes thoroughly.
- These types of movements are seen even in absence of intrinsic nerves, due to ***Basic Electric Rhythm*** (BER) in the smooth muscle and hence are also called as ***myogenic contraction***.
- These contractions are initiated and controlled by ***Pacemaker cell*** present in 2nd part of duodenum near the entry in common bile duct. A basic electrical rhythm (BER) generated by these cells are conducted caudally by the longitudinal muscle layer under the influence of myenteric plexus.
- The frequency of their contraction is directly related with the frequency of the BER and strength is directly related with the frequency of the spike generated by BER.
- The slow wave (BER) amplitude is increased by G-I hormones like gastrin, CCK-PZ, motilin and decreased by secretin and glucagon.

(c) **Pendular movement:**

- In this movement a long segment (20 cm) of intestine sweeps it's content to and fro with the regularity of a pendulum and hence called ***pendular movement***.
- It also helps in mixing the intestinal contents with digestive juice.

(d) **Peristalsis:**

- It is a propulsive movement which is responsible for pushing the chyme normally towards the aboral end of intestine.
- It is first described by Starling and Bayliss which involves a ring like contraction in one segment and receptive relaxation of immediately distal segment that results propulsion of food.
- The sequence of events that take place in this type of movement is illustrated in flow chart FC 7C from next page.
- In this type of movement food can move in either direction from a stimulated point but it normally dies out rapidly in oral direction but continue towards the anus. This is called ***Polarity of the intestine*** or ***Law of the gut***.
- Peristalsis is initiated and conducted with the help of the intrinsic nerves however the extrinsic nerves have profound influences on peristalsis so also the different hormones like gastrin, CCK –PZ, serototin, secretin.
- Peristalsis can be of 3 types:

  (i) Types—I -This moves slowly (2 cm/sec).

  (ii) Types—II (**Peristaltic rush**):

  - It does not occur in normal individual.

Entry of mass of chyme into small intestine

↓

Distension of wall of small intestine

↓

Initiation of local reflex by intrinsic plexus which causes

Left branch:
- **Contraction of circular muscle layer behind the chyme**
- ↓
- **Constriction of lumen behind the mass of chyme**

Right branch:
- **Contraction of longitudinal muscle layer in front of chyme**
- ↓
- **Shortening of tract in front of chyme**

↓

Forward movement of chyme to a new position

↓

Distension of wall in new position

↓

Initiation of another reflex

↓

Continuation of same events

↓

Ultimately chyme enters large intestine

FC 7C: Sequence of events occur during peristalsis

- In response to localised mechanical obstruction of small intestine very intense peristaltic wave is initiated called as ***Peristaltic rush***.
- This type of powerful contraction begins in duodenum and passes through entire length of small intestine finally reaches the ileocecal valve within a few minutes.
- During this type of movement segment proximal to obstruction dilates and becomes filled with gas and fluid → leads increase in pressure in the segment → results compression of blood vessel in it's wall → leads local ischemia → stimulation of visceral afferent nerve fiber to cause pain, sweating, hypotension and severe vomiting.

(iii) Type III peristalsis (***Antiperistalsis***):

- It normally occurs in duodenum in abnormal conditions as in vomiting.
- It is similar to peristalsis but in oral direction.

B. Short Notes:

1. Crypts of Liberkuhn:

- In between the villi of small intestine the intestinal glands open into lumen of the intestine. These intestinal glands are simple tubular in structure which secrete mainly electrolytes. These glands are known as **Crypts of Lieberkuhn** which are lined by columnar cell.
- These are seen mainly in jejunum and ileum.

2. Bruner's gland:

- In addition to intestinal glands, the first part of duodenum contains some mucous glands called Bruner's gland, which secrete mucous and traces of some enzymes.
- These are present in the submucous layer.

3. Villi:

- The mucous membrane of small intestine is covered by minute projections called villi which are lined by—
  - (i) Columnar cells called enterocytes which secrete different enzymes.
  - (ii) Goblet cells that produce mucus.
  - (iii) Paneth cells—are phagocytic.
  - (iv) Argentaffin cells—produce serotonin.
- Each enterocyte gives rise many projections called microvilli. These villi and microvilli increases the surface area of mucous membrane facilitating absorption of different substances.
- The intestinal epithelial cell at the base of the villus are actively mitotic and are continually replaced by new cells. About 17 billions of cells are replaced every day and the entire intestinal epithelial is replaced in every 5 days.
- Each villus contains a arteriole, a venule and a communicating capillary plexus which acts as a countercurrent system to help water reabsorption.
- Within each villi there is central channel called **lacteal** that opens into lymphatic and blood vessels and are concerned with absorption of fat.

4. Enteric nervous system:

- It is the intrinsic nervous system of the G-I tract which forms the anatomical basis of local G-I reflexes for which it is also known as 3rd division of ANS.
- ENS consists of approximately 100 millions of neurones including sensory, motor and interneuron. Therefore it is loosely called as the mini brain of the gut.
- It includes—

(i) Myenteric plexus or Auerbach's plexus:
  - (a) It lies between longitudinal and circular smooth muscle layer.
  - (b) It is mainly motor in function.
  - (c) It is concerned with the peristaltic activity of the gut by increasing tone of gut wall, intensity of rhythmic contractions, rate of rhythmic contraction, velocity of conduction of excitatory waves along the gut wall.

(ii) Submucous plexus (Meissner's plexus):
  - (a) It lies between the submucous layer and inner circular smooth muscle layer.
  - (b) It is mainly sensory and is concerned with control of exocrine and endocrine function of GIT.

- These two plexuses are interconnected and are under the control of extrinsic (autonomic nervous system).
- Afferent fibers of these intrinsic nervous system bring sensation from the mucous layer due to either distension or chemicals.

5. Deglutition apnoea:

- In the pharyngeal phase of deglutition respiration is reflexly inhibited due to inhibition of respiration centers which is known as deglutition apnoea.
- It helps to prevent entry of food into the respiratory tract.

6. Achalasia cardia:

- Normally when food enters oesophagus, esophagial peristaltic movement pushes the food into the stomach through the opened lower esophageal sphincter (LES). But in case of any abnormality of opening of LES due to **excessive tone** of LES causes difficulty in exit of food from stomach → leads distension of esophagus which is clinically known as ***Achalasia*** or ***megaesophagus.***
- It is due to —

  (i) degeneration of myenteric plexus in lower part of esophagus.

  (ii) increased sensitivity of LES to gastrin.

  (iii) inadequate release of inhibitory neurotransmitter — VIP and nitric oxide by intrinsic neurons.
- In severe cases the esophagus gets dilated due to accumulation of food which is known as megaesophagus.

7. Experiments to study gastric secretion:

Gastric secretion in different phases are studied experimentally in animals are:

Sham feeding:

- In this study the food is chewed and swallowed but not reached to the stomach as it is diverted to outside of the body by one oesophageal fistula proposed in the dog.
- A canula is fitted in the stomach to drain out the gastric juice.
- When dog swallows the food it, is diverted outside rather reaching to the stomach. Even though the gastric secretion is increased.
- This experiment proves the cephalic phase of gastric secretion.

Pavlov's pouch:

- The scientist **Pavlov** prepared a pocket in the stomach of dog (Fig. 7.7) with the nerve supply and blood supply keeping intact.

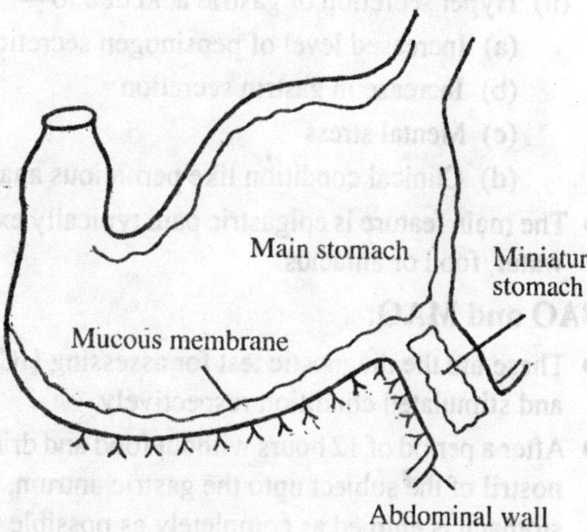

Fig.7.7: Experiments showing study of HCl secretion in *Pavlov's pouch*

- A canula is also fitted in the Pavlov's pouch to collect the gastric juice.
- From the pouch, juice is collected with different stimuli and can be analysed.
- It helps to study different factors influencing the secretion including the different types of food.

Heidenhan's pouch:

- It is same as Pavlov's pouch but here the pouch in denervated keeping the blood supply intact.
- Secretion from the pouch occurs only by the influence of blood borne chemical, so it helps to study the hormonal control on gastric secretion.

8. Peptic ulcer:

- ***Definition***: Peptic ulcer is a disorder resulting form autodigestion of the gastric or duodenal mucosa by gastric juice.
- ***Pathophysiology of peptic ulcer***: Normally this autodigestion of gastric or duodenal mucosa do not occur due to protective device present in the mucosal layer of stomach and duodenum. This protective device is known as ***Gastric-mucosal-bicarbonate barrier*** which constitutes—

(i) Soluble mucous layer secreted from mucous neck cell.
(ii) Visible mucous secreted from surface epithelial cell.
(iii) Prostaglandins present in the stomach.
(iv) Continual renewal of the mucosal cells lining the stomach.
(v) Higher bicarbonate level secreted from surface epithelial cell.

- Breakdown of these layer results the damage and ulceration of gastric/duodenal mucosa.
- ***Pathogenesis***: Peptic ulcer may be resulted due to—
  (i) Damage of gastric mucosal barrier by—
    (a) infection with H. pylori bacteria
    (b) ethanol
    (c) bile salts
    (d) non steroidal anti inflammatory drug like aspirin
    (e) smoking
  (ii) Hyper secretion of gastric acid due to—
    (a) Increased level of pepsinogen secretion
    (b) Increase in gastrin secretion
    (c) Mental stress
    (d) Clinical condition like pernicious anaemia and Z-E syndrome.
- The main feature is epigastric pain typically experienced in empty stomach and releived by taking water, food or antacids.

9. BAO and MAO:

- These are the diagnostic test for assessing HCl secretion by the stomach during resting condition and stimulated condition respectively.
- After a period of 12 hours without food and drink a nasogastric tube (Ryle's tube) is passed through nostril of the subject upto the gastric antrum. Patient is placed in a semi recumbent position and stomach is empied as completely as possible with a hand syringe.
- This specimen collected is labeled as fasting contents.
- Then 15 min samples are collected to give the basal secretion of acid known as ***Basal acid output*** **(BAO)** which is defined as micromoles of HCl secreted per hour under basal condition.
- Then stimulation of gastric glands are done by:
  (i) Subcutaneous injection of histamine (Histamine test)
  (ii) Intra muscular injection of pentagastrin (Pentagastrin test)
  (iii) Intravenous injection of soluble inulin (Inulin test)
  (iv) and the juice is collected by continuous suction through a Ryle's tube. This secretion of HCl/hour under maximally stimulated condition is known as ***Maximal acid output*** **(MAO)**.

Normal rate of BAO is 0.5 –2 meq/hr and MAO is 40 –60 meq/hr.

10. Bile salts:

- Bile salts are Na^+ /K^+ salts of bile acids conjugated with taurine and glycine e.g: Na^+/ K^+ glyco-cholate, Na^+/ K^+ taurocholate.
- Functions of bile salts are:
  (i) Responsible for emulsification of lipids to facilitate lipid digestion.
  (ii) Increases secretion of lipolytic enzymes from pancreas through CCK-PZ, thus helping in digestion of lipids.

(iii) Helps in micelle formation to facilitate fat absorption.

(iv) Increases the motility of G-I tract to facilitate quick passage of foodstuffs through the intestine (luxative action).

(v) Inhibits the growth of certain bacteria and facilitate their expulsion through faeces.

(vi) Stimulates the secretions of bile from the liver (cholerectic action).

(vii) Prevents the gall stone formation by keeping the cholesterol and lecithin in solution.

(viii) Stimulates gall bladder emptying (cholagogue action).

11. Gastric emptying:

- When the food enters into the pylorus of the stomach it initiates a more powerful contraction of pyloric region known as ***systolic contraction*** without opening the pyloric sphincter. This results most of the antral contents to **rebound back** towards body of stomach. This phenomenon is known as ***retropulsion***.
- In later stages of systolic contraction the pyloric sphincter relaxes resulting opening of sphincter that leads chyme to enter into duodenum. This is known as ***gastric emptying***.
- The factors affecting gastric emptying are as follows:

(i) Acidity of duodenal content inhibits gastric emptying via neural (vagus) and hormonal (secretin) mechanism.

(ii) Product of lipid digestion inhibits gastric emptying by hormone enterogastrone.

(iii) Stretching of duodenum inhibits gastric emptying by enterogastric reflex mechanism by chyme.

(iv) Osmolarity in the duodenum inhibits gastric emptying.

(v) Hormones like CCK, secretin, GIP, motilin inhibit gastric emptying.

(vi) Parasympathetic stimulation increases rate of gastric emptying.

(viii) Emotion like excitement increases rate of gastric emptying.

(viii) Emotion like depression, fear decreases rate of gastric emptying.

12. Mastication:

- ***Definition***: The grinding of food into smaller particles with the help of teeth and jaw muscles is known as mastication.
- ***Importance of mastication***: There are several importance e.g.
  - This process breaks the food into smaller particles and thereby increases the surface area and hence the rate of digestion.
  - It causes mixing of food particles with saliva and thereby (a) facilitates the digestion of unboiled starch by salivary amylase (b) lubricating the bolus to facilitate inward transmission of food towards stomach.
  - It also breaks the indigestible cellulose membrane present around the fruits and raw vegetables.
  - Grinding of food to very fine particles prevent the damage of G-I mucosa by the rough food particles.
  - Chewing brings the food in contact with taste and olfactory receptors to generate taste sensation and also olfaction which inturn increases pleasure of eating and stimulates gastric secretion.
- ***Muscles of mastication***: masseter, temporalis, pterygoit, digastric.
- ***Mechanism of mastication (chewing reflex)***: Mastication is voluntary process though it is initiated and co-ordinated by a reflex mechanism known as ***chewing reflex***.

Presence of food in oral cavity → reflex inhibition of mastication muscles → downward motion of lower jaw → stretching of the muscles of mastication → contraction of mastication muscle (masseter, temporalis, pterygoid) due to initiation of stretch reflex → raising the jaw to original position, thereby closing the mouth → compression of bolus against the lining of mouth which inhibits jaw muscle once again → repetition of the previous event to cause mastication.

- ***Role of teeth in mastication***: Different teeth helps in mastication for example:
  - Incisors provide strong cutting action.
  - Canines help in tearing action.
  - Premolars and molars have grinding action.

13. APUD cells:

- The cells of the G-I tract which secrete the gastrointestinal hormones are similar in structure and all of them take up a precursor substance of an amine which is then decarboxylated to form an amine. From this amine the hormones are synthesised. These cells are therefore called as ***Amino Precursor Uptake Decarboxylation (APUD) cells***. Apart from G-I tract these types of cells are also found in brain and in some other endocrine glands.
- These originate in the neural crest and migrate to the pancreas and GIT and get located in the mucosal layer.
- The hormone containing granules are concentrated at the base of the cells close to the capillaries.
- The major hormones secreted by these cells classified into 3 groups—
  - Gastrin family—that includes Gastrin and CCK-PZ.
  - Secretin family—that includes secretin, GIP, VIP, gut glucagon.
  - Others—that includes Somatostatin, Bombesin, Motilin and Substance-P.
- The important functions of these hormones are to regulate the secretion of the various digestive juices and the movement of the G-I tract.

14. Peristalsis:

- It is a propulsive movement which is responsible for pushing the chyme normally towards the aboral end of intestine.
- It is first described by Starling and Bayliss which involves a ring like contraction in one segment and receptive relaxation of immediately distal segment that results propulsion of food.
- The sequence of events that take place in this type of movement is illustrated in flow chart FC 7C.
- In this type of movement food can move in either direction from a stimulated point but it normally dies out rapidly in oral direction but continue towards the anus. This is called ***Polarity of the intestine*** or ***Law of the gut***.
- Peristalsis is initiated and conducted with the help of the intrinsic nerves however the extrinsic nerves have profound influences on peristalsis so also the different hormones like gastrin, CCK – PZ, serototin, secretin.
- Peristalsis can be of 3 types:
  - (i) Types—This moves slowly (2 cm/sec).
  - (ii) Types—II (Peristaltic rush):
    - It does not occur in normal individual.
    - In response to localised mechanical obstruction of small intestine very intense peristaltic wave is initiated called as ***Peristaltic rash***.
    - This type of powerful contraction begins in duodenum and passes through entire length of small intestine finally reaches the ileocecal valve within a few minutes.

- During this type of movement segment proximal to obstruction dilates and becomes filled with gas and fluid → leads increase in pressure in the segment → results compression of blood vessel in it's wall → leads local ischemia → stimulation of visceral afferent nerve fiber to cause pain, sweating, hypotension and severe vomiting.

(iii) Type III peristalsis (***Antiperistalsis***):

- It normally occurs in duodenum in abnormal conditions as in vomiting.
- It is similar to peristalsis but in oral direction.

15. Basal electrical rhythm (BER):

- It is initiated by stellate muscle like pacemaker cell in the circular muscle layer near the myenteric plexus.
- It is seen in whole G-I tract even if the intrinsic and extrinsic nerves supply is sectioned.
- It's rate of discharge is 12 times /min in duodenum and 8 times/min in ileum.
- It rarely causes muscle contraction but spike potential due to entry of Ca^{2+} ions.
- It is responsible for segmentation contraction in small intestine.

16. Migrating motor complex (MMC):

- It is a type of peristalsis which occurs in stomach and small intestine during fasting.
- During fasting condition the periods of digestion is characterised by modified electrical and motor activity of GIT which migrates from stomach to distal ileum in circular manner. This cycle is known as *MMC.*
- It starts with a—

  (i) Quiescent period (Phase-I)

  (ii) Continuous with a period of irregular electrical and mechanical activity (Phase II)

  (iii) Ends with a burst of regular activity (Phase-III)
- Rate of transmission is 5 cm/min.
- Occurs at intervals of approx. 90 min.
- Functions are not clear but it is presumed that it has got role in gastric secretion, bile flow and pancreatic secretion. It also sweeps the excessive digestive secretions into the colon and prevents the accumulation of the secretions in stomach and intestine.

17. Postprandial alkaline tide:

- During HCl secretion H^+ are actively secreted into the canaliculi in exchange of K^+ by $H^+ - K^+$ ATPase present in the luminal surface whereas HCO_3^- is reabsorbed from the cell to the blood in exchange of secretion of Cl^- to the parietal cell via $HCO_3^- - Cl^-$ exchanger mechanism operated in the basal surface. Due to this absorption of HCO_3^- to the blood, the alkalinity of the blood is increased specially after meal. This results excretion of excess HCO_3^- through urine, the condition known as ***post prandial alkaline tide.***

18. Steatorrhoea:

- It is a condition characterised by passage of fatty, bulky, clay coloured stool due to excretion of excess fat.
- It occurs due to—
  - deficiency of pancreatic lipase.
  - impaired reabsorption of bile salts in the distal ileum which increases lipid absorption.
  - increased gastric acid secretion which results decreased duodenal pH and thus inhibition of pancreatic lipase.

19. Enterohepatic circulation:

- The substances undergoing enterohepatic circulation are bile acids, bile pigments, Vit. D, B_{12}, etc. which are secreted by the liver and enter into the intestine via gall bladder. From the intestine most of these are absorbed back into the blood and presented to the liver to be excreted again. Thus by this enterohepatic circulation (Fig. 7.6) same substances are utilised again and again.
- The bile pigments present in the bile are transported directly to the intestine or via gall bladder. In the intestine these are reduced to form mesobilirubin, mesobilirubinogen and then urobilinogen (stercobilinogen) by colonic bacteria. Some of these urobilinogen is excreted through urine, some are excreted through faeces as stercobilinogen and most (80%-90%) of them are reabsorbed from the terminal ileum to go back to the liver to be converted again into bilirubin.

20. Jaundice:

- ***Definition***: It is the clinical condition characterised by yellowish pigmentation of the skin, mucous membrane and deeper tissues due to presence of more than 2 mg% serum bilirubin.
- ***Classification*** (based on physiology of bilirubin): It is of 3 types:

(i) Hemolytic jaundice:

- **Cause:** due to excessive destruction of RBC which results excessive formation of bilirubin.
- **Sign and symptoms:**
  - High serum level of unconjugated bilirubin
  - Yellowish colouration of skin
  - More urobilinogen in urine resulting dark urine on standing
  - No fat in faeces
  - Yellow or dark colour stool
  - No bleeding disorder
  - No bile salts in urine
  - Normal level of alkaline phosphatase.
- **Pathophysiology:** The pathophysiology of signs and symptoms of jaundice is illustrated with flow chart FC 7D from next page.

(ii) Obstructive jaundice:

- **Cause:** It is due to obstruction of bile duct so that the secretion of bile pigments is disturbed.
- **Sign and symptoms:**
  - High serum level of conjugated bilirubin.
  - Presence of conjugated bilirubin and bile salts in urine resulting dark yellowish urine.
  - White coloured stool with steatorrhoea.
  - Bleeding disorder present.
  - Increased alkaline phosphatase activity.
- **Pathophysiology:** The pathophysiology of different signs and symptoms of obstructive jaundice is illustrated in flow chart FC 7E from next page.

(iii) Hepatic or hepatio cellular jaundice:

- **Cause:** Infective (viral or bacterial) or toxic damage of liver and inability to excrete conjugated bilirubin, and also congenital defect or absent of UDR glucoronosyl tranferase (Gilbert's syndrome, Crigler Najjar syndrome and Dubin Johnson's syndrome).

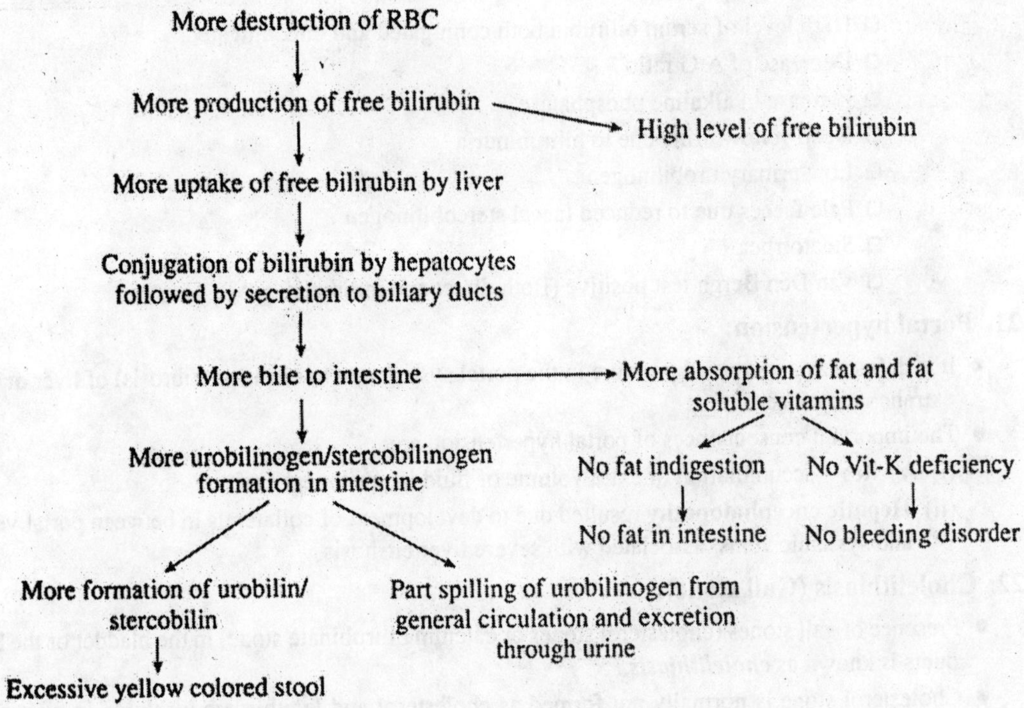

FC 7D: Pathophysiology of signs and symptoms during hemolytic jaundice

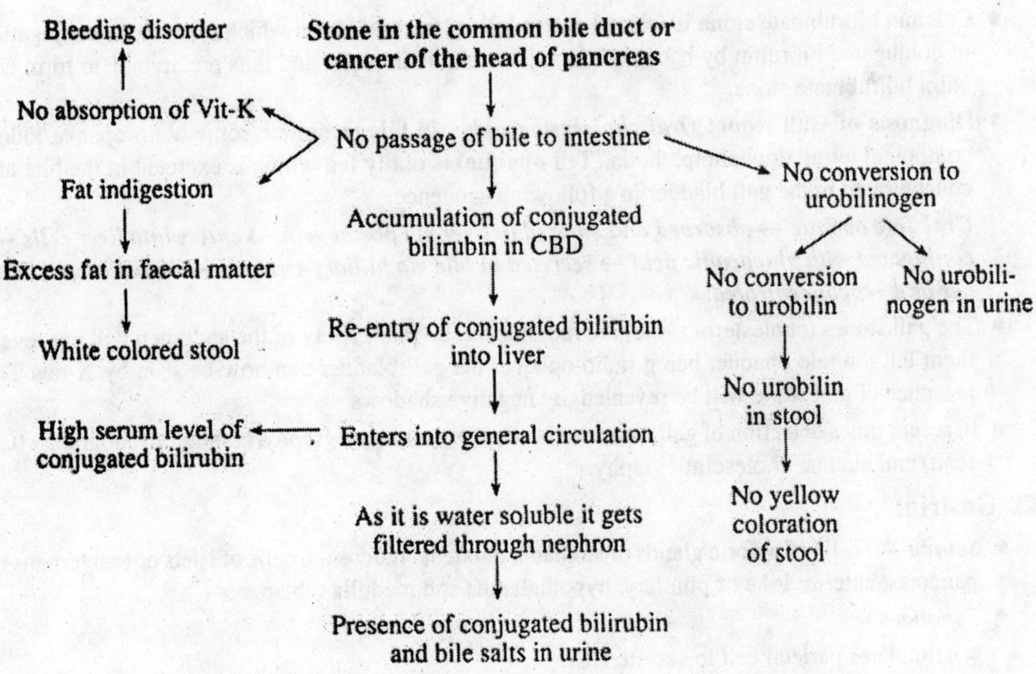

FC 7E: Pathophysiology of signs and symptoms during obstructive jaundice

- **Sign and symptoms:**
  - High level of serum bilirubin both conjugated and unconjugated.
  - Decrease of A:G ratio
  - Increase in alkaline phosphatase
  - Deep yellow urine due to bilirubinuria
  - Low urinary urobilinogen
  - Pale faeces due to reduced faecal stercobilinogen
  - Steatorrhea
  - Van Den Bergh test positive (Both direct and indirect).

21. Portal hypertension:

- It is defined as a increased pressure in the portal system due to cirrhoris (fibrosis) of liver or any extrahepatic cause.
- The important consequences of portal hypertension are:
  (i) **Ascites**—accumulation of extra volume of fluid in peritoneal cavity.
  (ii) **Hepatic encephalopathy** resulted due to development of collaterals in between portal veins and systemic veins associated with severe liver cirrhosis.

22. Cholelithiasis (Gall stone):

- Presence of gall stones (cholesterol stones or calcium bilirubinate stone) in the bladder or the bile ducts is known as ***cholelithiasis.***
- Cholesterol stone is normally not formed as cholesterol and lecithin are insoluble in water but they are kept in solution because of formation of micelles of bile salts. When proportion of lecithin, cholesterol and bile salts are altered, cholesterol crystalises leading to stone formation. These stones are radiolucence.
- Calcium bilirubinate stone is formed due to biliary tract infection which leads to de-conjugation of conjugated bilirubin by bacteria which is insoluble in water and thus precipitate to form calcium bilirubinate stone.
- **Diagnosis of Gall stone: *Oral cholecystography***: In this technique some radio-opaque iodine compound tetraiodophenolphthelin (**Teli opaque**) is orally fed which is excreted in the bile and concentrated in the gall bladder in a following sequence:
  Oral Tale opaque → absorbed and entered in liver via portal vein → enters into liver cells → conjugated with glucoronic acid → secreted in bile via billiary channel → stored in gall bladder and get concentrated.
- The gall stones (cholesterol stone) are radiolucent. So plain X ray of the abdomen will not reveal them but the tale opaque, being radio-opaque, the gall bladder can now be seen by X-ray. The presence of gall stone will be revealed by negative shadows.
- In recent times detection of gall stone can be done by ultrasonography, computed tonography (CT scan) and nuclear cholescintiography.

23. Gastrin:

- *Source*—G cells of pyloric glands of stomach, duodenal mucosa, δ cells of islets of Langerhans of pancreas, anterior lobe of pituitary, hypothalamus and medulla oblangata
- *Functions*
  - stimulates parietal cell to secrete HCl.
  - stimulates peptic cell to secrete pepsinogen.

- stimulates the growth of mucosa of the stomach and intestine.
- stimulates gastric motility.
- causes contraction of LES.
- stimulates insulin and glucagon secretion.
- stimulates pancreas to secrete bicarbonate rich fluid and enzymes.
- enhances rate of gastric emptying.

- *Factors affecting gastrin secretion*:
  (i) **Luminal factors:**
  - **Presence of peptides and amino acid** *in G-I tract* increases gastrin secretion.
  - **Distension of pyloric antrum** increases gastrin secretion.
  - **Acidity** increases gastrin release.

  (ii) **Neural factors: Vagal stimulation** increases gastrin release.

  (iii) **Blood borne factors:**
  - Calcium and epinephrine increase gastrin release.
  - Secretin / GIP /VIP etc. decreases gastrin secretion.

24. Cholecystokinin – Pancreozymin (CCK-PZ):

These are having similar function on both gall bladder and pancreas and thus collectively called as CCK-PZ.

- *Source*: 'I' cells of duodenum and jejunum, brain and enteric nervous system.
- *Function*:
  - Increases release of pancreatic enzymes.
  - Increases secretion of enterokinase enzyme from duodenum.
  - Increases contraction of gall bladder to release bile.
  - Causes contraction of pyloric sphincter and delays gastric emptying thus prevents reflux of duodenal contents into stomach.
  - Augments the function of secretin.
- *Factor affecting secretion of CCK-PZ*:
  - Acidity in duodenal content increases CCK-PZ release.
  - Products of carbohydrates, protein and fat digestion also increases CCK-PZ secretion.
  - Vagal stimulation increases CCK-PZ secretion.

25. Lactose intolerance:

- It is the clinical condition characterised by diarrhoea in response to intake of lactose.
- It occurs due to deficiency of lactase in the brush border of enterocytes resulting no digestion and absorption of lactose from the intestinal lumen.
- The lactose enters the colon where it produces gas and different metabolites by the action of colonic bacteria.
- The gas production results in borboygami and abdominal distension whereas the metabolites increase colonic motility and diarrhoea.

26. Diarrhoea:

- It is the clinical condition characterised by the increase frequency of passing the stool.
- Physiologically it occurs either due to increased GI motility or due to increased secretions from GI tract as occurs in cholera.

- It may result dehydration and hypovolemia for which oral rehydration therapy is often required to prevent it.

27. Hirschprung's disease:

- Due to congenital absence of intrinsic auerbach's plexus in the pelvi-rectal junction normal defecation cannot occur → resulting collection of huge amount of stool in the sigmoid colon → leads to enlargement of sigmoid colon which is called as mega colon.
- It is characterised by abdominal distension, anorexia and lassitude. In severe cases symptoms appear in new borns as early as 3rd day after birth.
- It is usually treated by surgical dilatation.

28. Intestinal flora:

- In the intestine specially in the colon and rectum there is higher amount of bacterial flora which includes *E. coli*, Enterobacteria, aerogens etc.
- These are normally not harmful and supply some vitamin K, and B complex to the body.
- They also can degrade certain materials in the stool and thus decrease the stool mass.
- They can produce the gasses like CO_2, N_2, H_2S, methane etc. which contribute to the flatulus. They also produce the fowl smelling of stool.
- If the bacterial population increases it does harm to the body by consuming many important nutrients like Vit-C, B_2, destroying bile salts etc.

29. Blind loop syndrome:

- Though normal bacterial flora is essential for health, overgrowth of bacteria is harmful. Such overgrowth occurs when there is stasis of intestinal contents commonly observed in patients with surgically created blind loops in small intestine which is known as blind loop syndrome.
- It is characterised by macrocytic anemia due to malabsorption of Vit-B_{12} and steatorrhoea due to excessive breakdown of bile salts by the intestinal bacteria.

30. BMR:

- It is defined as the energy expenditure of body at basal condition.
- Normal value 40Kg/hr/m^2 + 400mg.
- The factors affecting BMR are-Age, Sex, Pregnancy, Exercise, type of food, hormones like T_4, catecholamines, environmental temperature, fever, sleep, anxiety, emotions etc.

31. Vomiting:

- **Definition:** It is the process by which the contents of the upper gut is expelled to the exterior of the mouth.
- **Center for vomiting:** Center is situated bilaterally in medulla oblongata near the tractus solitarius. This center is situated near the salivary center for which reason the vomiting is usually associated with salivation.
- **Mechanism of vomiting:** Vomiting occurs when different stimuli like distension or irritation of stomach, tricking in throat etc. are transmitted to the vomiting center through vagus and sympathetic afferent fibers. Whereas the vomiting induced by drugs like morphine, apomorphine etc. or induced by motion sickness, the afferent impulses reaches to the vomiting center through a specialized zone present in the floor of IV ventricle called ***chemoreceptor trigger zone*** (CTZ).

  The motor impulses causing act of vomiting are transmitted from vomiting center to the upper part of GIT through V, VII, IX, X and XII cranial nerves and to diaphragm and abdominal muscles through spinal nerves. The detail mechanism of act of vomiting is illustrated by the flow chart FC 7F.

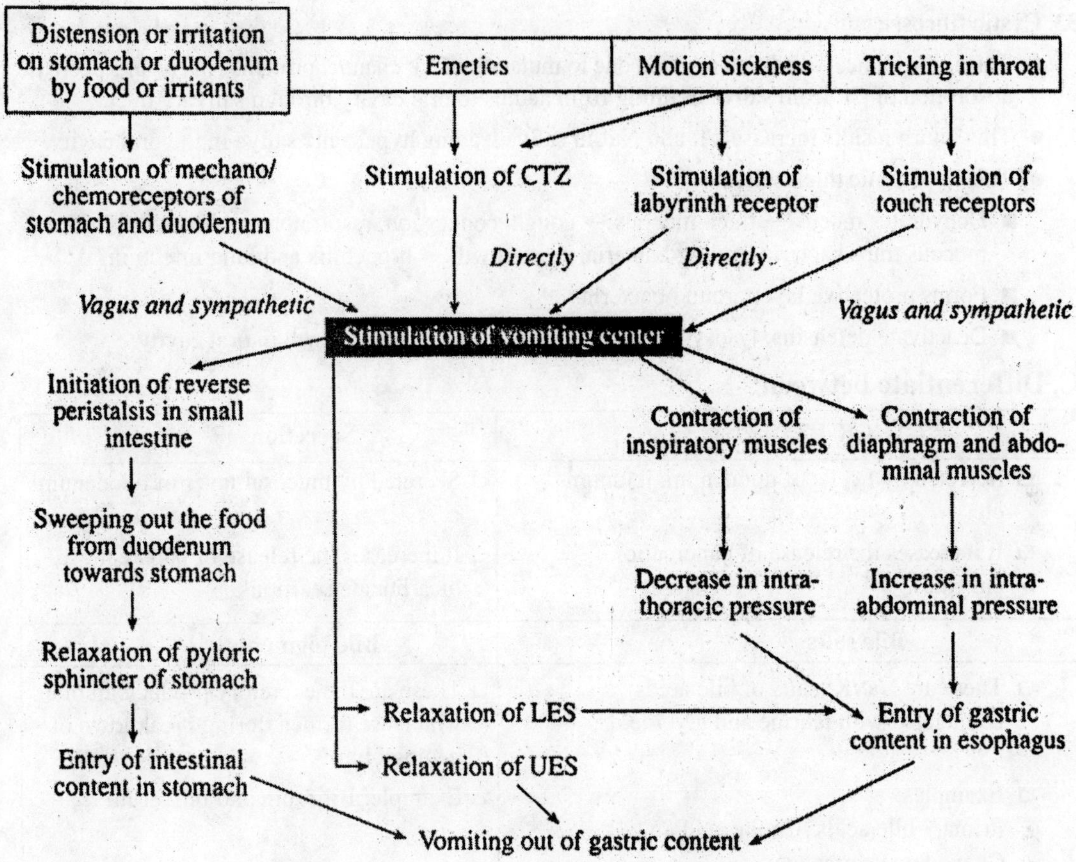

FC 7F: Flow chart showing mechanism of vomiting

32. Gastric glands:

- The entire stomach mucosa has got two types of tubular glands:

(i) ***Oxyntic*** or ***gastric glands*:**

- mainly located in the fundus and body of the stomach.
- It contains 3 types of cells:
  - **Mucous neck cell:** that secretes mainly mucous and little pepsinogen.
  - **Peptic or chief cell** that secretes large amount of pepsinogen.
  - **Parietal or oxyntic cell** that secretes HCl and intrinsic factor.
  - Other cells like APUD cells, Argentaffin cell etc.

(ii) ***Pyloric glands*:**

- mainly located in the pyloric and antral region of stomach.
- It contains 4 types of cells:
  - Mucous neck cell in large amount
  - Peptic cell in small amount

- ❑ Oxyntic cell in small amount
- ❑ G cell that secretes hormone gastrin
- ❑ D cells that secretes somatostatin

33. Cystic fibrosis:

- This is the clinical condition resulted due to mutation of Cl^- channel protein. This results decrease absorption of Cl^- from saliva draining from acinus to oral cavity through salivary duct.
- This inturn results increase Cl^- and Na^+ in saliva leading hypertonic saliva in the oral cavity.
- This hypertonic thick saliva :
  - ■ Dehydrates mucus → thick mucous → cough, congestion, respiratory problem and thick mucous traps bacteria leading bacterial overgrowth → bronchitis and lung infection.
  - ■ Forms protective layer around bacteria.
  - ■ Deactivate defensins, lysosymes etc. that lead bacterial overgrowth in oral cavity.

C. Differentiate between:

CCK-PZ	Secretion
❑ Secreted by I cells of duodenum, jejunum etc. ❑ It increases the release of pancreatic enzymes.	❑ Secreted by mucosal layer of duodenum. ❑ It increases the release of pancreatic bicarbonate secrtions.
Bile salts	**Bile pigments**
❑ These are Na^+/K^+ salts of bile acids conjugated with taurine and glycine. ❑ Examples: Primary bile acids: Cholic acid and Chenodeoxycholic acid. Secondary bile acids: Deoxycholic acid and lithocholic acid.	❑ These are the excretory products in bile which are formed during breakdown of hemoglobin. ❑ Example: Bilirubin and biliverdin.
Primary bile acids	**Secondary bile acids**
❑ These are formed from cholesterol of liver. ❑ These are not directly related with bile salts formation. ❑ Example: Cholic acid and Chenodeoxycholic acid.	❑ These are formed in intestine from primary bile acids by the bacterial action. ❑ These are directly formed into bile salts in the liver. ❑ Example: Deoxycholic acid and lithocholic acid.
Cholerectics	**Cholagogues**
❑ The agents (e.g. bile salts) which stimulate the secretion of bile from liver is referred to as cholerectics. ❑ Example: bile salts, secretin, vagal stimulation.	❑ Any substances that increase the bile flow from gall bladder is known as cholagogue. ❑ Example: cholecystokinin, fatty acids.

Pendular movements	Peristaltic movements
❑ This is the mixing type of movement seen in small intestine.	❑ This is the propulsive type of movement seen in small intestine.
❑ This is the side-to-side swaying movements produced due to contraction and relaxation of longitudinal muscle layers.	❑ Example: This is defined as a passing of wave of contraction preceded by a wave of relaxation.
❑ It is responsible for to-and-fro movements of contents.	❑ It propels the intestinal contents into aboral direction.

Micelles	Chylomicron
❑ In the intestine about 20-30 molecules of bile salts aggregate to form a micelle which helps in ferrying the fat digestion products from the intestinal lumen to the intestinal cells.	❑ This is a reformed lipids that is covered with a layer of B-lipoprotein which are released from the intestinal cell by exocytosis.

Pancreatic amylase	Salivary amylase
❑ It acts both on boiled and unboiled starch and related polysaccharides to convert it into maltose, maltriose and alpha dextrin.	❑ It acts only on boiled starch to convert it into maltose, and alpha dextrin.

Kwashiorkor	Marasmus
❑ It is usually seen in recently weaned infants.	❑ It is usually seen in infants who have weaned early or have never breast fed.
❑ Edema is present.	❑ Edema is absent.
❑ Body weight remains normal.	❑ Body weight is reduced.
❑ It is characterised by impaired appetite.	❑ It is characterised by voracious appetite.
❑ Serum albumin is reduced.	❑ Serum albumin is normal or slightly reduced.
❑ It is characterised by puffy and moon shaped face.	❑ It is characterised by shriveled and monkey like face.

D. Short answer type:

1. What will happen if lower esophageal sphincter fails to relax?

In this case food is accumulated in the oesophagus leading to dilatation of proximal oesophagus. This condition is known as Achalasia cardia.

2. What will happen if we do not chew the food properly before swallowing?

In this case (i) larger food particles can cause strong and painful contractions of oesophagial mucosa (ii) there will be no digestion of fruit and raw vegetables because of non-breakage of undigestible cellulose membrane around these substances.

3. How regurgitation from duodenum is normally prevented?

It is normally prevented by the constriction of pyloric sphincter due to stimulating action of CCK and secretin.

4. Explain: Alcohol intoxication can be avoided if it is consumed after ingestion of a drink rich in fat?

Fat rich fluid results very low gastric emptying leading slow rate of entry of alcohol in the intestine for absorption. Thus there is low absorption rate of alcohol inside the body which avoids alcohol intoxication.

5. How gastric mucosa is resistant to autodigestion?

The presence of mucosal-bicarbonate barrier outside gastric mucosal cell prevents the acid or peptic digestion of its mucosal cells,

6. What will happen if total gastrectomy is done?

It results:

- Pernicious anemia
- Predisposes iron deficiency anemia as conversion of iron from ferric to ferrous form requires HCl.
- Dumping syndrome i.e. development of weakness, dizziness and sweating after meal.

7. What will happen to BER after vagotomy?

It will be irregular and disorganized.

8. What will happen and why if acid chyme entering the duodenum fails to get neutralized?

In this case the acid in the duodenum causes (i) more release of secretin which leads secretion of alkaline watery pancreatic juice with poor enzyme content (ii) feeble stimulation of CCK-PZ. Both these effects delay gastric emptying.

9. What will happen if phopholipase A_2 gets activated in the pancreatic ducts?

In this case (happens usually in acute pancreatitis) there is disruption of pancreatic tissue and necrosis of surrounding fat which may be fatal.

10. Why anemia is associated with liver disorder?

It is because liver is the site of RBC formation.

11. How gall stones are formed?

Cholesterol gallstones are formed when cholesterol concentration of bile exceeds the solubilizing capacity of bile whereas pigment gall stones are formed by the precipitation of calcium salts of unconjugated bilirubin.

12. Defecation after meals is the rule in children — justify.

It is due to gastrocolic reflex with the absence of voluntary control of defection.

13. A child passes stools only once in 3 weeks. What is the likely diagnosis? Explain.

It is Aganglionic megacolon (Hirschsprung's disease) which is characterised by blockade of both peristalsis and mass contraction in distal colon and pelvic-rectal junction due to congenital absence of plexus or due to degeneration of myenteric plexus.

14. Why the focal fat content in an infant is more than of adult?

It is because the fat absorption process is not matured in infants.

15. Why the loss of fluid from colon in chronic diarrhoea results in severe hypokalemia?

In chronic diarrhoea there may be severe hypokalemia due to loss of excess K^+ due to high electrochemical potential difference between blood and intestinal lumen (ileum and colon).

16. What will happen if Na^+ – glucose carrier becomes defective?

In this case there will be loss of Na^+ and glucose resulting severe dehydration during diarrhoea.

E. MCQ:

1. The oxyntic glands of stomach has all the cells except (i) mucous neck cells (ii) peptic cell (iii) oxyntic cells (iv) G cell. (iv)

2. The daily secretion of saliva in normal person is (i) 1500 ml/day (ii) 2500 ml/day (iii) 500 ml/day (iv) 5 L/day. (i)

3. Hypersalivation does not occur in (i) pregnancy (ii) parkinsonism (iii) fever (iv) neoplasm of mouth. (iii)

4. The oxyntic cells secrete (i) HCl (ii) intrinsic factor (iii) both (iv) none of the above. (iii)

5. The water content in gall bladder bile is (i) 98% (ii) 89% (iii) 2% (iv) 11%. (ii)

6. The amount of bile salts in liver bile is (i) 0.9% (ii) 6% (iii) 42% (iv) 24% (i)

7. The carbohydrate splitting enzyme in saliva is (i) alpha amylase (ii) elastase (iii) maltase (iv) lipase. (i)

8. Pancreatic bicarbonate secretion is mainly stimulated by (i) Gastrin (ii) VIP (iii) CCK-PZ (iv) Secretin. (iv)

9. The BER in G-I tract is generated by (i) Myenteric plexus (ii) Meissner's plexus (iii) Interstitial cell of Cajal (iv) longitudinal muscle. (iii)

10. Secondary bile acids are formed in (i) intestine (ii) liver (iii) pancreas (iv) gall bladder. (i)

11. The maximum amount of pancreatic secretion is produced during (i) gastric phase (ii) cephalic phase (iii) intestinal phase (iv) intergasric phase. (i)

12. Mass peristalsis is seen in (i) colon (ii) rectum (iii) small intestine (iv) stomach. (i)

13. The vagotomy affects the HCl secretion in (i) Gastric phase (ii) Cephalic (iii) Both i and ii (iv) none. (iii)

14. Peristalsis in GIT is initiated by (i) sympathetic nerve (ii) parasympathetic nerve (iii) Myenteric plexus (iv) Meisner's plexus. (iii)

15. All are the functions of gall bladder except (i) absorption of water (ii) absorption of bicarbonate (iii) storage of bile (iv) secretion of bile salts. (iv)

16. Entry of acid chyme into duodenum mainly causes (i) release of secretin (ii) release of CCK (iii) inhibition of G-I motility (iv) secretion of enzyme rich pancreatic juice. (i)

17. Lipid solule bilirubin is converted to water soluble bilirubin by (i) liver (ii) kidney (iii) small intestine (iv) stomach. (i)

18. Achalasia is a condition characterised by (i) persistent opening of LES (ii) excessive tone of LES (iii) pyloric stenosis (iv) incompetence of LES. (ii)

19. Gastro-esophagial relux is a condition occurs due to (i) persistent opening of LES (ii) excessive tone of LES (iii) pyloric stenosis (iv) incompetence of LES. (iv)

20. The entry of carbohydrate rich food into the duodenum mainly stimulates the prodction of one of the following hormones from GIT (i) GIP (ii) VIP (iii) secretin (iv) somatostatin. (i)

21. The best stimulus for pancreatic enzyme secretion is (i) gastrin (ii) secretin (iii) CCK-PZ (iv) somatostatin. (i)

22. MMC is seen during (i) cephalic phase (ii) intestinal phase (iii) gastric phase (iv) interdigestive phase. (iv)

23. MMC is initiated during interdigestive phase by (i) somatostatin (ii) motilin (iii) ACh (iv) noradrenalin. (ii)

24. Vagal stimulation cause stimulation of following cell of stomach (i) chief cell (ii) G cell (iii) ECL (iv) all of the above. (iv)

25. Parietal cell is stimulated by (i) ACh (ii) gastrin (iii) histamin (iv) all of the above (iv)

26. Fatty food (i) stimulates HCl secretion (ii) inhibits HCl secretion (iii) not related with HCl secretion. (ii)

27. Bile acids are synthesised from (i) cholesterol (ii) triglycerides (iii) both (iv) none of the above. (i)

28. In lithogenic bile the chances of development of gall stone is (i) increases (ii) decreases (iii) remain unaltered. (i)

29. End products of pancreatic lipase digestion is (i) monoglycerides (ii) fatty acids (iii) glycerol (iv) all of the above. (iv)

30. In the normal person the large intestine undergoes mass peristalsis at the rate of (i) once or twice/ day (ii) 15-20 times/day (iii) 50 times/day (iv) 7 times/day. (i)

8 Excretory System

A. Long type:

1. Define GFR. What is it's normal value? What do you mean by net filtration pressure with special reference to different forces that affect NFP? Enumerate the factors regulating GFR.

Definition: It is the amount of plasma filtered by all the nephrons of both the kidneys in unit time i.e. per min, or per day.

Normal value:

- 125 ml/min
- 180 lit/day

Dynamics of filtration through glomerular membrane: The forces which cause filtration of fluid through the glomerular capillary membrane is known as **Net filtration force (NFP) or Filtration Pressure** which is determined by following pressures:

- **The force which allows filtration:**
  - Glomerular capillary hydrostatic pressure (P_G):
    - It is the hydrostatic pressure of blood present in glomerular capillaries.
    - Normal value-60 mm Hg.
  - Colloidal osmotic pressure in Bowman's Capsule (π_B)
    - It is the oncotic pressure of proteins present in the filtrate of Bowmans capsule.
    - Normally it's value is 0 mm Hg as in normal condition almost no plasma proteins are filtered through glomerular membrane.
- **The force which opposes filtration:**
  - Glomerular capillary oncotic pressure (π_G):
    - It is the colloidal osmotic pressure exerted by he plasma proteins present in glomerular capillary blood.
    - It's average normal value is 32 mm Hg.
  - Bowmans capsular hydrostatic pressure (P_B):
    - It is the hydrostatic pressure exerted by the filtrate present in Bowman's capsule.
    - It's normal value is 18 mm Hg.

So, the net filtration pressure or effective filtration pressure that allows filtration is

NFP= $P_G + \pi_B - \pi_G - P_B$
$= 60 + 0 - 32 - 18$
$= 60 - 32 - 18$
$=$ 10 mm Hg.

Factors affecting GRF: Glomerular filtration rate (GFR) is directly determined by ***Net filtraton pressure*** and ***Filtration coefficient*** (Kf) as follows:

GFR= Kf X NFP
$=$ Kf X $(P_G + \pi_B - \pi_G - P_B)$
$=$ 12.5 ml/min/mmHg X 10 mmHg
$=$ 125 ml/min.

Thus the factors affecting the GFR are:

1. **Bowman's capsular hydrostatic pressure (P_B):** As this pressure opposes the filtration, GFR is inversely related to this P_B. However, any changes of this pressure do not normally serve as a primary mechanism for regulating GFR. Though in certain pathological conditions in which urinary flow is obstructed (e.g. Stone in urethra or kidney) → the P_B increases → reduces GFR.

2. **Glomerular capillary hydrostatic pressure (P_G):**

- GFR is directly proportionate with P_G i.e. Rise of P_G results in increase in GFR and vice versa. This pressure serves an important role to regulate GFR.
- It is further determined by — (i) Arterial pressure (ii) Renal blood flow (iii) Afferent arteriolar resistance and (iv) Efferent arteriolar resistance.

Thus all these factors affect the GFR by affecting P_G by the mechanism discussed below:

(i) Arterial B.P.: Within the range of 60 mm Hg to 180 mm Hg of arterial BP, GFR remains constant in spite of any change of arterial BP because of autoregulatory mechanisms operated in the kidney. But any fall of BP below 60 mm Hg and rise of BP above 180 mm Hg has direct relationship with the GFR.

(ii) Renal blood flow: GFR is directly related with RBF i.e. increase in RBF tends to raise GFR by increasing PG and vice versa.

(iii) Afferent arteriolar resistance: Constriction of afferent arterioles reduces the P_G and thereby GFR i.e. afferent arteriolar resistance is inversely proportionate to P_G and thereby to GFR.

(iv) Efferent arteriolar resistance: It has biphasic effect depending on the extent of vasoconstriction as follows:

- Mild to moderate efferent arteriolar constriction without affecting normal RBF → ↑ P_G → ↑ resistance to outflow glomerular capillaries → ↑ GFR.
- Whereas severe constriction of efferent arteriole → stagnation of blood in the glomerular capillary tuft → filtration of protein free plasma in large amount due to the long stay of blood in the glomerular capillay tuft →↑ concentration of plasma protein in the blood present in glomerular capillary tuft →↑ colloidal oncotic pressure in the glomerular capillary →↓ GFR.

3. Glomerular capillary oncotic pressure (π_G):

- It is inversely related with GFR i.e. any increase in π_G results decrease in GFR and vice versa.
- It is further directly determined by (a) arterial plasma oncotic pressure (b) filtration fraction and thus rise in arterial plasma oncotic pressure and also rise in filtration fraction results rise in π_G and thus reduction of GFR.
- In dehydration there is hemoconcentration → increase in plasma protein concentration →↑ π_G →↓ GFR.

- Similarly in case of hemodilution or hypoproteinemia →↓ plasma protein concentration →↓ π_G →↑ GFR.

4. Bowman's Capsular oncotic pressure:

- It is directly related with GFR. However in normal condition it has negligible influence on GFR as normally no filtration of plasma proteins take place to be entered into Bowman's capsule.
- In case of glomerulonephritis etc. there is filtration of plasma proteins due to damage of glomerular membrane →↑ π_B →↑ GFR.

5. Filtration coefficient (Kf):

- It is directly related with GFR however in normal kidney it has no significant role in glomerular filtration.
- It is further determined by permeability of the glomerular capillary membrane and surface area and thus both these factors determine GFR by influencing Kf.
- Permeability of glomerular membrane is directly related with Kf and thus GFR. This permeability of glomerular membrane inturn depends on (I) number of glomerulus, (II) thickness of glomerular membrane.

  (I) Number of glomerulus: Any disease affecting glomeruli of the kidney results damage of glomerulus → decrease in number of glomerulus →↓ in permeability →↓ in Kf →↓ GFR.

  (II) Thickness of glomerular membrane: It is inversely related with permeability and thus GFR. For example: In some diseases e.g. chronic uncontrolled hypertension and DM →↑ thickness of glomerular membrane →↓ in permeability →↓ in Kf →↓ GFR.
- Surface area of capillary bed: It is directly related with the permeability and thus with the GFR. If the number of functional glomerular capillary membrane is decreased (in some renal diseases) there is reduction of surface area of capillary bed → results decrease in permeability →↓ in Kf →↓ GFR.

6. Other factors (indirect):

- **Age**: GFR decreases with advanced age due to fall in RBF and cardiac output.
- **Sympathetic stimulation**:
  - **Mild to moderate** sympathetic stimulation → constriction of both afferent and efferent arterioles → No significant change of RBF → No significant change of GFR.
  - **Severe** sympathetic stimulation → more severe constriction in efferent arteriole →↓ RBF →↓ GFR.

2. What is JGA? Describe it's role in regulating GFR. How GFR is measured with special reference to the substance used?

***Juxtaglomerulus apparatus (JGA)*:**

- It is defined as the specialised organ of the kidney situated near the glomerulus of the nephron.
- It consists of Macula densa cells, Juxtaglomerular cells and Lacis cells.
- It is responsible for secretion of renin into the blood which not only controls the GFR and renal blood flow but also systemic blood pressure through angiotensins and aldosterone.

***Regulation of GFR by JGA:* Autoregulation:**

This is the local feedback mechanism in the kidney by which the JGA of the kidney keeps the glomerular filtration rate at a constant level which is known as autoregulation of GFR and renal blood flow. The autoregulation of RBF and thus GFR is mediated by:

(i) Myogenic activity of afferent arteriole (**Myogenic theory**)

(ii) **Tubuloglomerular feedback** mechanism which is constituted again by two mechanisms:

a. **Afferent arteriolar feedback** mechanism

b. **Efferent arteriolar feedback** mechanism.

Out of those mechanisms myogenic theory and afferent arteriolar feedback mechanism are the main mechanisms by which autoregulation of GFR is maintained by auto regulating RBF. Whereas efferent anteriolar mechanism helps to regular GFR upto certain extent without regulating RBF. The detail of these mechanisms are illustrated with flow chart FC 8A and 8B. Similarly in response to fall of GFR just opposite evens take place to regulate GFR (Fig. FC 8B).

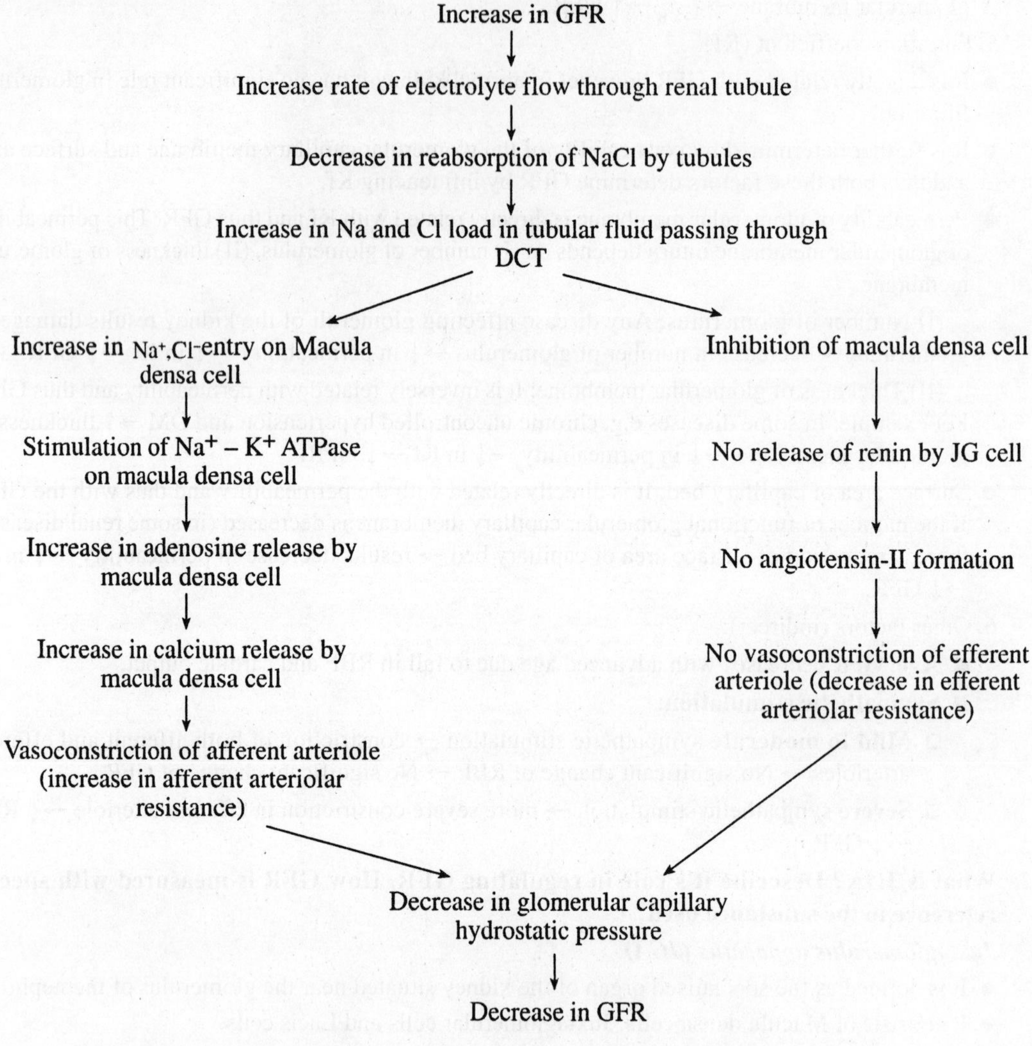

Fig. FC. 8.A : Afferent arteriolar feedback theory

***Measurement of GFR*:**

- **Principle:** The GFR can be measured by following principle:

If a substance (X) present in plasma is freely filtered at glomerulus and neither reabsorbed, nor secreted into the tubule then the amount of that substance excreted per minute will be equal to the amount of substance filtered i.e.

Amount of substance excreted = Amount of that substance filtered

or, Urinary concentration of 'X' (Ux) x Urine volume/min (V) = Plasma concentration of 'X' (Px) **X** GFR.

or, Ux **X** V = Px **X** GFR

or, GFR = Ux **X** V/Px

- **On the basis of this principle some chemical substances (e.g. Inulin) are injected into the body and concentration of that substances in plasma and urine is measured to obtain GFR. On the basis of the substance injected the GFR can be determined by two methods:**

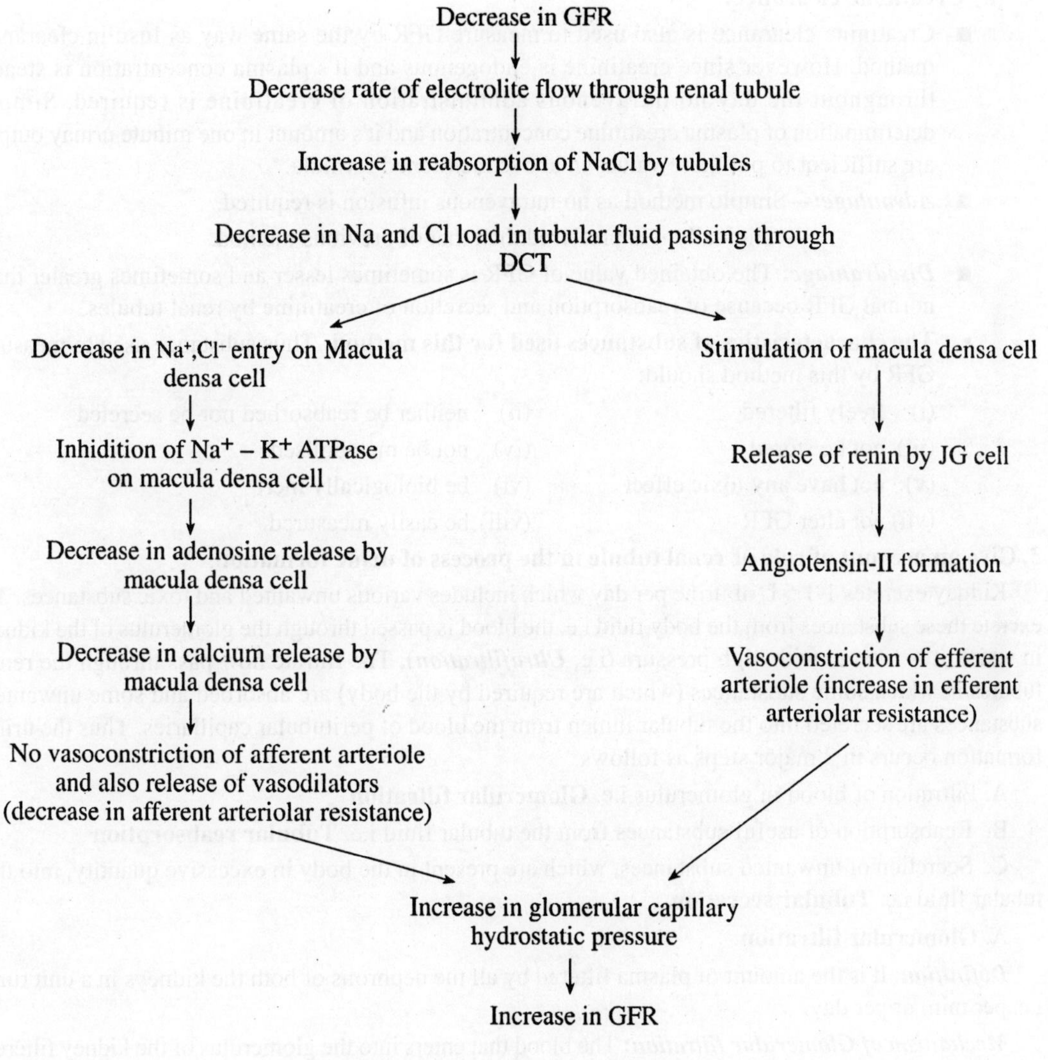

FC 8B: Efferent arteriolar feedback theory

(i) Inulin clearance method:

■ ***Procedure***

❑ Intravenous administration of large dose of insulin followed by continuous infusion of insulin (to compensate it's loss through urine) to maintain it's plasma level at constant.

- Urinary concentration of Inulin (Ux) and volume of urine excreted per minute (V) are determined after collecting urine sample.
- Plasma sample is collected and it's Inulin concentration is measured.
- Inulin clearance is thus calculated by the formula:

Inulin clearance = Vx **X** V/Px

- ***Advantage***: It is the most accurate method.
- ***Disadvantage***: It requires continuous infusion of inulin.

(ii) **Creatinine clearance:**

- Creatinine clearance is also used to measure GFR by the same way as Insulin clearance method. However since creatinine is endogenous and it's plasma concentration is steady throughout the day no intravenous administration of creatinine is required. Simple determination of plasma creatinine concentration and it's amount in one minute urinay output are sufficient to put these values in above mentioned formula.
- ***Advantage***:—Simple method as no intravenous infusion is required.
  — Clinically it is preferred than that of previous method.
- ***Disadvantage***: The obtained value of GFR is sometimes lesser and sometimes greater than normal GFR because of reabsorption and secretion of creatinine by renal tubules.
- **The characteristics of substances used for this method:** Thus substance used to measure GFR by this method should:

(i) freely filtered
(ii) neither be reabsorbed nor be secreted
(iii) not be stored
(iv) not be metabolised
(v) not have any toxic effect
(vi) be biologically inert
(vii) not alter GFR
(viii) be easily measured.

3. Give an account of role of renal tubule in the process of urine formation.

Kidney excretes 1-1.5 L of urine per day which includes various unwanted and toxic substances. To excrete these substances from the body fluid i.e. the blood is passed through the glomerulus of the kidney in which it is filtered with high pressure (i.e. ***Ultrafiltration***). The filtrate now pass through the renal tubules in which some substances (which are required by the body) are absorbed and some unwanted substances are secreted into the tubular lumen from the blood of peritubular capillaries. Thus the urine formation occurs in 3 major steps as follows:

A. Filtration of blood in glomerulus i.e. **Glomerular filtration**

B. Reabsorption of useful substances from the tubular fluid i.e. **Tubular reabsorption**

C. Secretion of unwanted substances, which are present in the body in excessive quantity, into the tubular fluid i.e. **Tubular secretion.**

A. **Glomerular filtration:**

Definition: It is the amount of plasma filtered by all the nephrons of both the kidneys in a unit time i.e. per min. or per day.

Mechanism of Glomerular filtration: The blood that enters into the glomerulus of the kidney filtered through the glomerular capillary membrane (known as ***glomerular membrane***) by the process of bulk transport of fluid which is facilitated by the high pressure within glomerular capillary tuft and requisite structural features of glomerular membrane as follows:

It consists of 3 major layers as follows:

(i) **Glomerular capillary endothelial cell layer:** It is constituted by flat and thin cell layer having pore of 50-100 mm diameter called ***fenestrae*** through which blood cells can not pass, thereby allowing retention of blood cells and also plasma proteins.

(ii) **Basement membrane of capillary endothelial cell layer and Bowman's capsular cell layer:** These are composed of proteoglycans and collagens which are negatively charged thereby opposes the filtration of mainly plasma proteins.

(iii) **Epithelial cell layer of visceral layer of Bowman's capsule:**

- It gives out series of foot processes called ***podocytes.***
- The spaces in between the podocytes are having diameter of 25 nm which is known as ***Filtration slit*** which allows the filtrate to come across Bowman's Capsule.

Dynamics of filtration through glomerular membrane: The forces which cause filtration of fluid through the glomerular capillary membrane is known as **Net filtration force (NEF)** or **Filtration Pressure** which is determined by following pressures:

- **The force which allows filtration:**
  - Glomerular capillary hydrostatic pressure (P_G):
    - It is the hydrostatic pressure of blood present in glomerular capillaries.
    - Normal value - 60 mm Hg.
  - Colloidal osmotic pressure in Bowmans Capsule (π_B).
    - It is the oncotic pressure of proteins present in the filtrate of Bowmans capsule.
    - Normally it's value is 0 mm Hg as in normal condition almost no plasma proteins are filtered through glomerular membrane.
- **The force which opposes filtration:**
  - Glomerular capillary oncotic pressure (π_G):
    - It is the colloidal osmotic pressure exerted by the plasma proteins present in glomerular capillary blood.
    - It's average normal value is 32 mm Hg.
  - Bowmans capsular hydrostatic pressure (P_B):
    - It is the hydrostatic pressure exerted by the filtrate present in Bowman's capsule.
    - It's normal value is 18 mm Hg.

So, The net filtration pressure or effective filtration pressure that allow filtration is

$$\begin{aligned} NFP &= P_G + \pi_B - \pi_G - P_B \\ &= 60 + 0 - 32 - 18 \\ &= 60 - 32 - 18 \\ &= 10 \text{ mm Hg.} \end{aligned}$$

B. ***Tubular reabsorption*:**

a. *General considerations*:

- After the formation of glomerular filtrates by glomerular filtration it is moved through the renal tubules. During it's movement through the renal tubules large quantity of water, electrolytes and other useful substances are reabsorbed by the tubular epithelial cells which inturn diffuses to peritubular capillary supplied to the epithelial cells of renal tubules. This transport of solutes from the tubular fluid into the peritubular capillary is known as tubular reabsorption.
- All the substances reabsorbed in the renal tubules are not in same quantity. Depending on the degree of reabsorptions these substances are classified into 3 groups:

  (i) **High threshold substances:** The substances which are completely reabsorbed and therefore not appear in the urine normally are known as high threshold substances e.g. glucose, amino acids, vitamins etc.

  (ii) **Low threshold substances:** The substances, which are not reabsorbed completely and therefore appear in the urine normally if the plasma levels of such substances is slightly more, are termed as low threshold substance e.g. urea, uric acid, phosphate etc.

(iii) **Non-threshold substances:** The substances which are not at all reabsorbed rather secreted in urine irrespective of their plasma level are known as non-threshold substances. Example: creatinine

b. *Substances reabsorbed by renal tubules:*

- Actively reabsorbed: Na^+, K^+, Ca^{2+}, $PO_4^=$ $SO_4^=$, HCO_3^-, glucose, amino acids, ascorbic acid, ketone body, uric acid.
- Passively reabsorbed: Water, Cl^-, urea.

c. *Site of reabsorption:*

- PCT: Glucose, amino acids, Na^+, K^+, Ca^{2+}, HCO_3^-, Cl^-, $PO_4^=$, water, uric acid.
- Loop of Henlee : Na^+ and Cl^-,
- DCT and CT: Water, Na^+, HCO_3^-

d. *Mechanism of reabsorption:*

I. ***Active transport process:*** Reabsorption of Na^+, glucose and amino acids, chloride, bicarbonate, K^+ etc. take place by the different parts of renal tubule occurs by both primary active and secondary active transport.

- Primary active transport: In the basolateral surface of PCT epithelium there are $Na^+ - K^+$ pump which pumps out Na^+ from epithelial cell interior to renal interstitial fluid thence to blood of peritubular capillary. This mechanism requires the help of $Na^+ - K^+$ ATPase enzyme.
- Secondary active transport: This mechanism is operated in between tubular lumen and tubular epithelial cell along the concentration or electrical gradient derived due to operation of primary active transport i.e. because of the running of primary active transport at the basolateral surface Na^+ is pumped out of the cell creating electrical and concentration gradient which drives Na^+ from lumen to cell interior by carrier mediated process as follows:

  (i) Na^+ - Solute Symport mechanism: When Na^+ is pumped out from cell to peritubular capillary by primary active transport, there is a establishment of concentration and electrical gradient that results binding of Na^+ (along with glucose / amino acids / phosphates) to the carrier protein present in brush border of luminal surface. This results entry of Na^+ coupled with other solute which is again pumped out from cell to peritubular capillaries (Fig. 8.1).

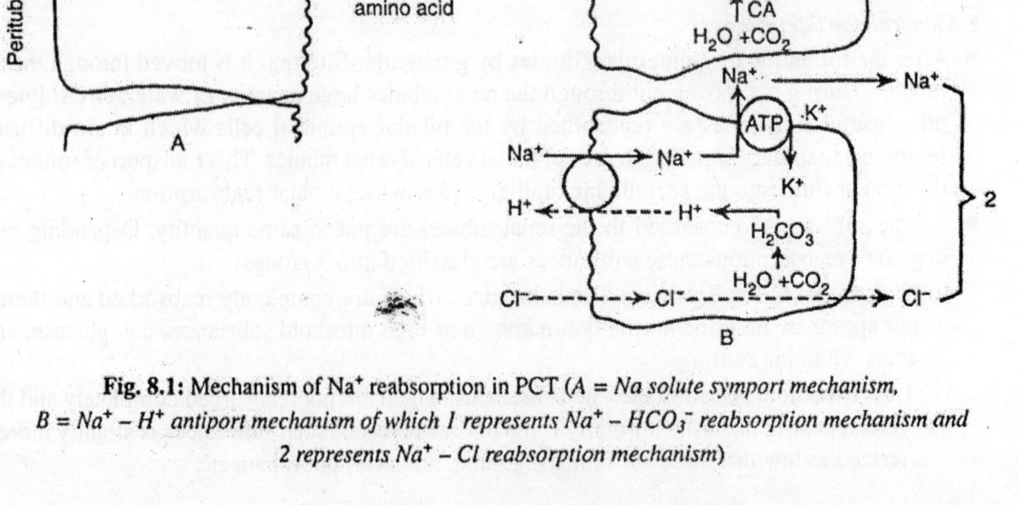

Fig. 8.1: Mechanism of Na^+ reabsorption in PCT (*A = Na solute symport mechanism, B = $Na^+ - H^+$ antiport mechanism of which 1 represents $Na^+ - HCO_3^-$ reabsorption mechanism and 2 represents $Na^+ - Cl$ reabsorption mechanism*)

(ii) $Na^+ - H^+$ Antiport system: Primary active transport of Na^+ from cells interior to peritubular capillary also results apical entry of Na^+ associated with secretion of H^+ into the tubular fluid. The H^+ secreted in this process may be derived either from H_2CO_3 or from formic acid. In the former case the net result is $Na^+ - HCO_3^-$ reabsorption and in the later case the net result is $Na^+ - Cl-$ reabsorption (Fig. 8.1).

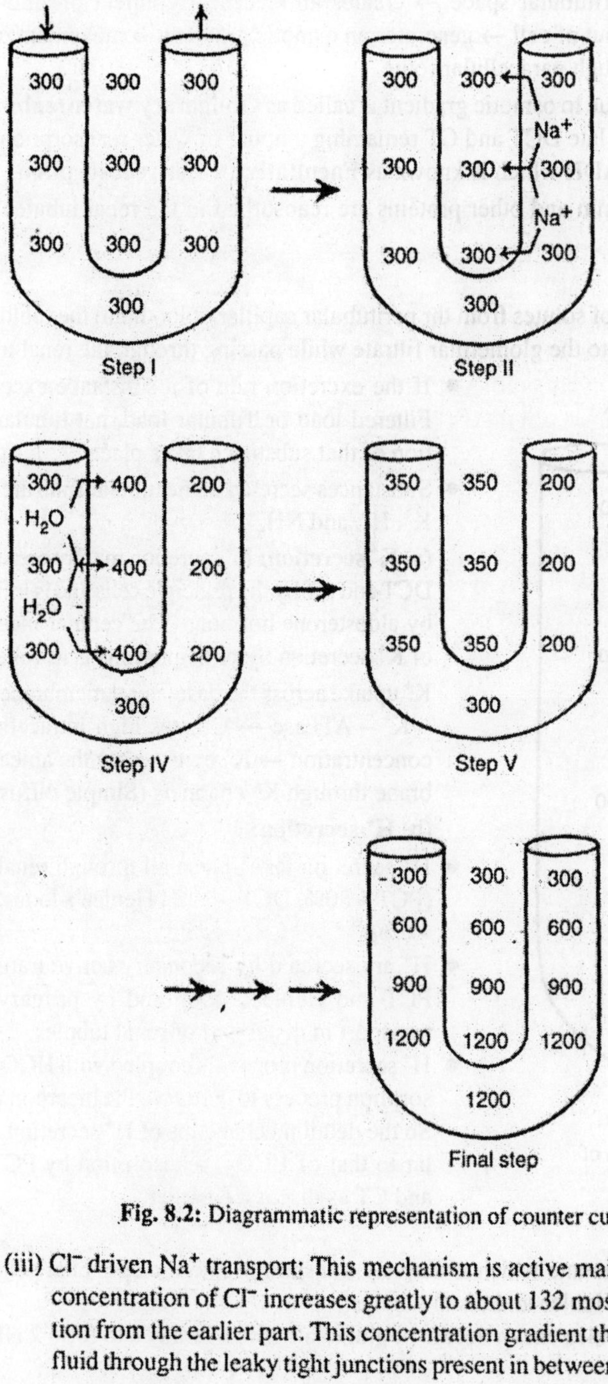

Fig. 8.2: Diagrammatic representation of counter current multiplier system

(iii) Cl^- driven Na^+ transport: This mechanism is active mainly in lower end of PCT where tubular concentration of Cl^- increases greatly to about 132 mosmol / lit because of only Na^+ reabsorption from the earlier part. This concentration gradient thus drives Cl^- from lumen to peritubular fluid through the leaky tight junctions present in between the epithelial cells (Paracellular route).

This reabsorption of Cl^- generates potential difference in later segment which results the passage of Na^+ from lumen to peritubular capillary through the paracellular route.

II. ***Passive transport*** process e.g.: Solvent drag mechanism (33%): The remaining of Na^+ (33%) along with some amount of urea and other ions are reabsorbed passively and through paracellular route by solvent drag which is as follows:

Efflux of Na^+ from cell into peritubular space → creates an electrical gradient of anions (Cl^-, HCO_3^-)→ efflux of Cl^- and HCO_3^- out of cell → generates an osmotic gradient → movement of water containing Na^+, Cl^-, HCO_3^- etc. through paracellular route.

This way of water reabsorption due to osmotic gradient is called as **Obligatory water reabsorption** which takes place mainly in PCT. In late DCT and CT remaining amount of water reabsorption occurs under the influence of the hormone ADH which is known as **Facultative water reabsorption.**

III. ***Pinocytosis*:** Traces of albumin and other proteins are reabsorbed in the renal tubules by this process.

C. ***Tubular secretion*:**

- Secretion means the transport of solutes from thr peritubular capillary blood into the tubular fluid i.e. addition of the substances to the glomerular filtrate while passing through the renal tubule.

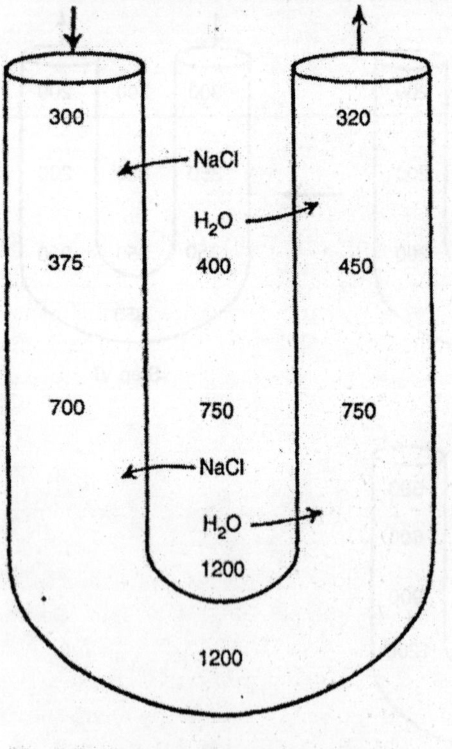

Fig. 8.3: Diagrammatic representation of counter current exchanger system

- If the excretion rate of a substance exceeds the Filtered load or Tubular load, net tubular secretion of that substance takes place.
- Substances secreted in the tubular fluid are mainly K^+, H^+, and NH_4^+.

(a) **K^+ secretion:** K^+ secretion mainly occurs in the DCT and CT by the principle cells and is influenced by aldosterone hormone. The cellular mechanism of K^+ secretion by principle cells is as follows:

K^+ uptake across the basolateral membrane by $Na^+ - K^+$ – ATPase → Creates high intracellular K^+ concentration → K^+ exits across the apical membrane through K^+ channels (Simple diffusion).

(b) **H^+ secretion:**

- H^+ secretion takes place all through renal tubule (PCT – 80%, DCT – 10%, Henlee's loop-5%, CT – 5%).
- H^+ are secreted by secondary active transport in PCT and Henlee's loop and by primary active transport in distal part of renal tubules.
- H^+ secretion process is coupled with HCO_3^- reabsorption process to conserve the bicarbonate ions. So the detail mechanisms of H^+ secretion is similar to that of HCO_3^- reabsorption by PCT, DCT and CT as discussed earlier.

(c) **NH_4^+secretion:**

- NH_4^+ is synthesised from glutamate which is actively transported into the epithelial cells of the PCT, thick ascending loop of Henlee and distal tubules.
- Inside the cells of the renal tubules one molecule of glutamate is metabolised to form 2 NH_4^+ and two HCO_3^-.

- The NH_4^+ is secreted into the tubular lumen by $Na^+ - NH_4^+$ antiport system whereas 2 HCO_3^- moves along the basolateral surface and diffused to the peritubular capillary along with Na^+ by carrier proteins (Fig. 8.6).
- Thus the secretion of two molecule of NH_4^+ in the urine results the generation of two new HCO_3^- which are reabsorbed to plasma to increase the plasma bicarbonate buffer.

4. Describe the mechanism involved in concentration and dilution of urine.

The concentrating mechanism of urine in the renal tubule not only depends on the function of ADH but also depends on the specific osmotic gradient within the peritubular spaces of the medulla (medullary interstitium). In the corticomedullary junction of the medullary interstitium the osmolality of the fluid is 300 to 600 mosm/kg. Further deep into the medulla, the osmolality rises more and more till it becomes maximum at the level of the tip of the medulla (U turn) where it becomes nearly 1200 mosmol/kg. Thus the medullary osmolality continuously rises from the outermost zone to the deeper zone i.e. an osmotic gradient is produced in between the corticomedullary junction and the tip of the medulla. The factors that build up this gradient is as follows:

A. Counter current (opposite) flow of fluid across the Henlee's Loop.
B. Active transport of Na^+ and Co-transport of Cl^- through ascending limb of Henlee's loop.
C. Passive diffusion of water through descending limb of Henlee's loop.
D. Active transport of ions and urea from collecting duct.

The process in which all of these factors help in establishing this osmotic gradient is known as ***Counter current multiplier mechanism*** and once established this medullary osmotic gradient is maintained by the mechanism known as ***Counter current exchanger mechanism***.

Counter current multiplier mechanism:

(1) Let us consider that the loop of Henlee is filled with fluid of osmolality 300 mosm/kg (step-I of Fig. 8.2). Now it is assumed that the flow of fluid is momentarily stopped (step II). As the ascending limb is impermeable to water and active pump within the ascending limb pumps the Na^+ from the tubular fluid to the medullary interstitium and because of co-transport of Cl^- from tubular fluid to the medulla interstitium, the concentration of solutes is decreased from the tubular fluid of initial part of ascending limb and osmolality within the medullary interstitium is increased from 300 to 400 mosl/kg due to entry of solutes from tubular fluid to tip of the medullary interstitium (Step-III). Now as the descending limb of Henlee's loop is permeable to water and impermeable to solutes the tubular fluid near the U turn of descending limb quickly reaches osmotic equilibrium because of passive absorption of water from tubular fluid i.e. at the level of U turn. The tubular fluid in the descending limb adopts the same osmolality (350 mosm/kg) to that of nearby medullary interstitium (Step-IV).

(2) Now again it is considered that the fluid in the descending limb resumes movement and moves forward and another small quantity of isotonic fluid is delivered into the descending limb from the proximal tubule. Due to the fresh entry of isotonic fluid (300 mosml/kg) some portion of fluid having 350 mosml/kg osmolality will move from descending limb to the level of U turn of ascending limb (step-V). This forward movement of fluid is again stopped momentarily. So due to active pumping activity solutes from the fresh fluid at the ascending limb will loose the solutes to the medullary interstitium resulting decreased concentration of solutes at the level of descending limb and increased concentration of solutes in the nearby medullary ascending limb which will be 500 mosml/kg. Same process will be continued in the upper part of the ascending limb resulting low osmolality within the upper part of the ascending limb and higher osmolality in the nearby region of medullary osmolality. Now due to higher osmolality within the medullary interstitium water will move from descending limb to medullary interstitium and fluid within the descending limb will quickly reach same osmolality with that of nearby zone of medullary interstitium.

(3) Now again the fresh isotonic fluid is entered into the descending limb and the process of concentration is repeated. By repeatitions (4-6 times) of the whole process an osmotic gradient will be established within the corticomedullary junction and tip of the medulla. At the corticomedullary junction it will be little bit more than 300 mosml/kg which will go on increasing with depth of the corticomedullary junction and at the tip of the medulla it will be approximately 1200 mosml/kg osmolalily (Final step).

Thus the repeated flow of iso osmotic (isotonic) fluid from proximal tubule to Henlee's loop helps in establishing the osmotic gradient of increasing solute concentration from corticomedullary junction to tip of the medullary interstitium due to the counter current (opposite) flow of urine through 'U' tubule of Henlee's loop and differential reabsorptive properties of solutes through the ascending and descending limb. This procedure for establishing the osmotic gradient within the medullary interstitium is known as ***Counter current multiplier system.***

Counter current exchanger system:

A. *Significance*: Blood flow must be provided to the renal medulla to supply the metabolic needs of the cells in this part of the kidney. Without a special medullary blood flow system, the solutes pumped into the renal medulla by the counter-current multiplier system would be rapidly dissipated. There are two special features of the renal mudullary blood flow that contribute to the preservation of the high osmotic gradient within the medullary interstitium. First feature is the low medullary blood flow to this region helps to minimize solute loss from the medullary interstitium and the 2nd and most important factor is that the vasa recta serves as counter-current exchanger system which minimizes the washout of the solutes from the medullary interstitium and maintains the osmotic gradient once developed by counter-current multiplier mechanism.

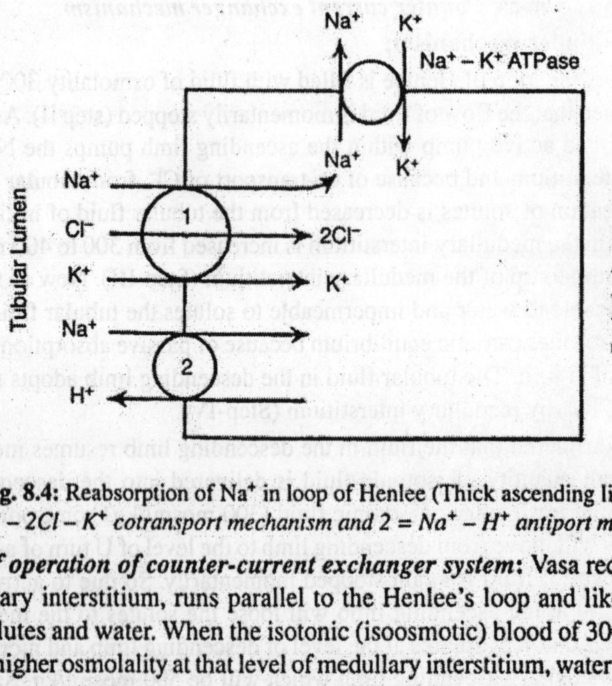

Fig. 8.4: Reabsorption of Na^+ in loop of Henlee (Thick ascending limb)
1 = Na^+ – 2Cl – K^+ cotransport mechanism and 2 = Na^+ – H^+ antiport mechanism

B. *Mechanism of operation of counter-current exchanger system*: Vasa recta that gives the blood supply to the medullary interstitium, runs parallel to the Henlee's loop and like other capillaries it is permeable to both solutes and water. When the isotonic (isoosmotic) blood of 300 mosml/kg enters into the vasa recta, due to higher osmolality at that level of medullary interstitium, water is passively reabsorbed from blood of vasa recta and solutes go to the blood within the vasa recta from medullary interstitium resulting higher solute concentration of blood that flows deep to the medulla. In the next layer, blood is again hypoosmotic than the nearby fluid of the medullary interstitium. So again water is absorbed passively from blood within vasa recta from medulla resulting higher osmolality of the blood in that region. Thus as the blood descends towards tip of the medulla, it becomes progressively more concentrated and when it reaches to the tip of the medulla, the osmolality of the blood becomes same to that of tip of the medulla which is about 1200 mosm/kg. Now as blood ascends back towards the cortex it becomes less concentrated as solutes diffuse back to medullary interstitium and water moves into the vasa recta. This exchange mechanism is reverse because now the blood has to flow through from higher osmolality to lower osmolality. Thus when the blood leaves the cortex it's osmolality becomes a little bit more than 300 mosml/kg H_2O. Diagrammatic representation of the counter-current exchanger system is illustrated in (Fig. 8.3).

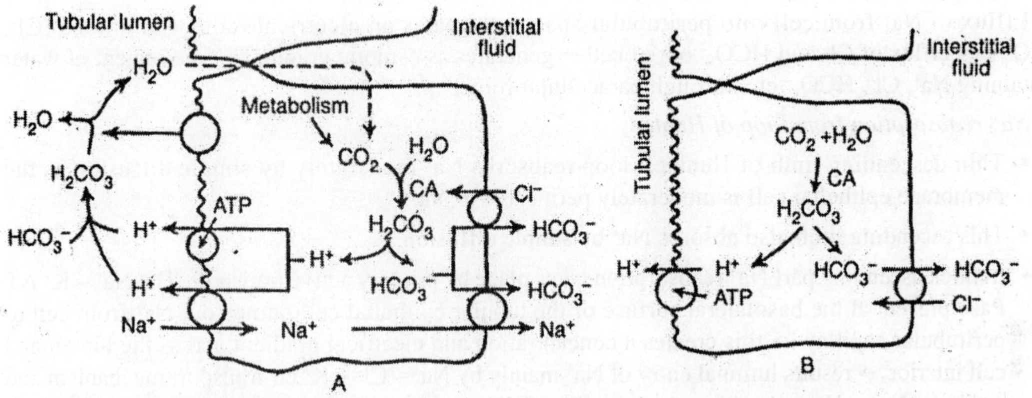

Fig. 8.5: Reabsorption of bicarbonate ions in PCT (A) and in distal nephrons (B)

5. Describe the mechanism of Na^+ reabsorption by renal tubules. How it is regulated?

Allmost entire amount of Na^+ filtered at the glomerulus are reabsorbed by the different parts of renal tubules, however the maximum amount in reabsorbed by PCT.

Reabsorption of Na^+ in PCT :

I. Active transport process (67%): Reabsorption of Na^+ by PCT occurs by both primary active and secondary active transport.

- Primary active transport: In the basolateral surface of PCT epithelium there are $Na^+ - K^+$ pump which pumps out Na^+ from epithelial cell interior to renal interstitial fluid thence to blood of peritubular capillary. This mechanism requires the help of $Na^+ - K^+$ ATPase enzyme.
- Secondary active transport: This mechanism is operated in between tubular lumen and tubular epithelial cell along the concentration or electrical gradient derived due to operation of primary active transport i.e. because of the running of primary active transport at the basolateral surface Na^+ is pumped out of the cell creating electrical and concentration gradient which drives Na^+ from lumen to cell interior by carrier mediated process as follows:
  (i) Na^+ – Solute Symport mechanism: When Na^+ is pumped out from cell to peritubular capillary by primary active transport, there is an establishment of concentration and electrical gradient that results binding of Na^+ (along with glucose / amino acids / phosphates) to the carrier protein present in brush border of luminal surface. This results entry of Na^+ coupled with other solute which is again pumped out from cell to peritubular capillaries (Fig. 8.1A).
  (ii) $Na^+ - H^+$ Antiport system: Primary active transport of Na^+ from cells interior to peritubular capillary also results apical entry of Na^+ associated with secretion of H^+ into the tubular fluid. The H^+ secreted in this process may be derived either from H_2CO_3 or from formic acid. In the former case the net result is $Na^+ - HCO_3^-$ reabsorption and in the later case the net result is $Na^+ - Cl^-$ reabsorption (Fig. 8.1B).

(iii) Cl^- driven Na^+ transport: This mechanism is active mainly in lower end of PCT where tubular concentration of Cl^- increases greatly to about 132 mosmol/lit because of only Na^+ reabsorption from the earlier part. This concentration gradient thus drive Cl^- from lumen to peritubular fluid through the leaky tight junctions present in between the epithelial cells (Paracellular route). This reabsorption of Cl^- generates potential difference in later segment which results the passage of Na^+ from lumen to peritubular capillary through the paracellular route.

II. Solvent drag mechanism (33%): The remaining of Na^+ (33%) is reabsorbed passively and through paracelluar route by solvent drag which is as follows:

Efflux of Na^+ from cell into peritubular space → creates an electrical radient of anions (Cl^-, HCO_3^-) → efflux of Cl^- and HCO_3^- out of cell→ generates as osmotic gradient → movement of water containing Na^+, Cl^-, HCO_3^- etc. through paracellular route.

Na^+ reabsorption from loop of Henlee:

- Thin descending limb of Henlee's loop reabsorbs Na^+ moderately by simple diffusion as the membrane epithelial cell is moderately permeable to Na^+.
- This ascending limb also absorbs Na^+ by simple diffusion.
- In thick ascending part Na^+ reabsorption takes place by primary active transport. The $Na^+ - K^+$ AT Pase present at the basolateral surface of the tubular epithelial cell pumps out Na^+ from cell to peritubular capillay → this creates a concentration and electrical gradient across the lumen and cell interior → results luminal entry of Na^+ mainly by $Na^+ - Cl^- - K^+$ co-transport mechanism and partly by $Na^+ - H^+$ antiport mechanism (Fig. 8.4).

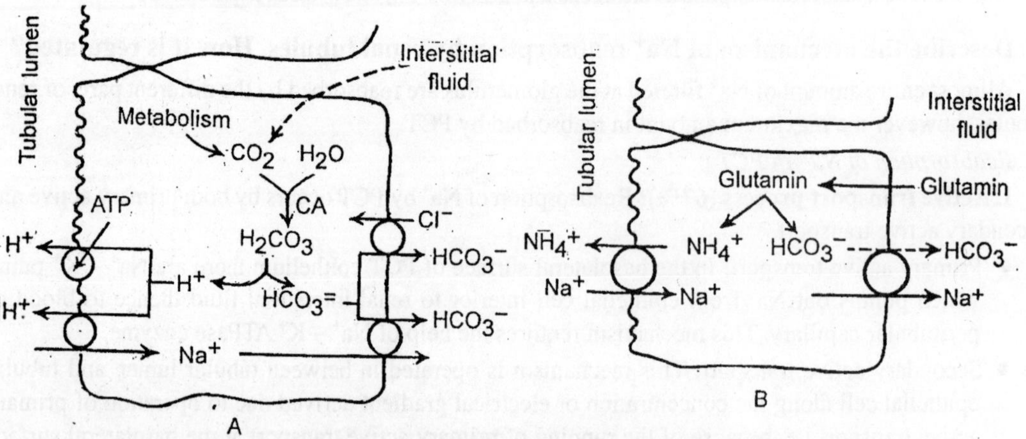

Fig. 8.6: Generation of new HCO_3^- *(A = H_2CO_3 derived H^+ secretion process and B = Glutamine derived NH_4^+ secretion process)*

Na^+ reabsorption through late distal tubule and cortical collecting duct:

- Histologically these parts of renal tubule are composed of 2 types of cells—principle cells and intercalated cells. The principle cells reabsorbs Na^+ and water from lumen and secrete K^+ into the lumen whereas the intercalated cells reabsorbs K^+ ions and secretes H^+ into the tubular fluid.
- The Na^+ reabsorption by the principal cells is mediated through the $Na^+ - K^+$ pump present at basolateral surface. Pumping out of Na^+ from cell to peritubular capillary creates concentration gradient of Na^+ (Na^+ deficiency inside the cell) that results reabsorption of Na^+ from tubular fluid to cell interior through luminal surface by:

(I) Mostly Cl^- driven Na^+ transport. (II) Partly $Na^+ - H^+$ or $Na^+ - K^+$ Antiport mechanism.

Regulation of Na^+ reabsorption: Different neural and hormonal factors regulate renal reabsorption (thereby renal excretion) of salt and water by influencing GFR and tubular reabsorption process. However both these processes act in concert with the pressure natriuresis and pressure diuresis mechanism making the regulatory mechanism more effective. The mechanisms by which Na^+ reabsorption is controlled by the kidney is as follows:

(i) ***Arterial baroreceptor and Low pressure stretch receptor mechanism*** (pressure natriuresis system):

In response to any alteration of blood volume these mechanisms are activated or inactivated to regulate the Na^+ reabsorption by the renal tubules and thus maintain the constancy of the ECF or blood volume. The detail of these mechanisms are illustrated under question number 8 of chapter 4.

In case of rise of blood volume or ECF volume opposite response takes place to reduce Na^+ reabsorption and thereby Na^+ excretion is increased.

(ii) ***Renin–angiotensin–aldosterone mechanism*:** By this mechanism also Na^+ reabsorption through renal tubule is regulated. The detailed mechanism is illustrated under question number 8 of chapter 4.

(iii) ***Atrial natriuretic peptide system*:** This system becomes active only when the blood volume is excessively raised. The detail of this mechanism is illustrated under question number 8 of chapter 4.

6. Describe the role of kidneys in maintaining acid base balance.

The normal pH of arterial blood is 7.40 + 0.02. The pH must remain within this narrow normal range as the functions of many vital proteins of our body are strongly dependant on the pH. So if the pH changes beyond the normal range there will be deterioration of enzymatic actions leading to devastating changes in our body like loss of myocardial activity that leads to cardiac failure, loss of vascular tone leading hypotension, alteration of CNS function and etc. This pH is maintained within the normal range by means of 3 defense mechanisms.

1. ***Buffering action of physiological buffers*:** Any addition of acids or alkalies in the body fluid is immediately buffered by different physiological buffers present in the blood or ECF (bicarbonate, proteins and phosphate buffers).

2. ***By adjusting pulmonary ventilation*:** Any moderate disturbances in acid base balance mainly by volatile acids (CO_2) is corrected within minutes by appropriate adjustments of pulmonary ventilation.

3. ***By adjusting renal function*:** Disturbances in acid base balance specially by the fixed acids or nonvolatile acids (sulphuric acid, phosphoric acid) or organic acids (like lactic acid, acetoacetic acid, β-OH-butyric acid) are also compensated by appropriate adjustment of renal function which takes hours to days to be effective and provides long term regulation.

Role of Kidney:

- Metabolism of different food product within the cell produces different acidic by-product like—
  1. CO_2 (carbonic acid by product) – which is eliminated by respiratory adjustment.
  2. Non carbonic acid byproduct – which is eliminated or buffered in which kidney has important role.
- Kidney helps in pH regulation by following ways:

  ***A. Reabsorption of filtered bicarbonate*:** The renal glomeruli filters more than 4000 mosm of bicarbonate/day. This loss of bicarbonate can never be compensated only by generating new bicarbonates by the kidney. So the reabsorption of this filtered bicarbonate is very much essential. Fortunately the filtered HCO_3^- is reabsorbed by renal tubules almost completely. This is why in renal diseases, in which kidney is unable to absorb all the filtered bicarbonate, urinary loss of bicarbonate may lead to acidosis. HCO_3^- reabsorption occurs throughout the renal tubules except in the descending limb of Henlee's loop, however maximum reabsorption takes place in PCT, DCT and CT. The mechanism by which HCO_3^- is reabsorbed is as follows (Fig. 8.5).

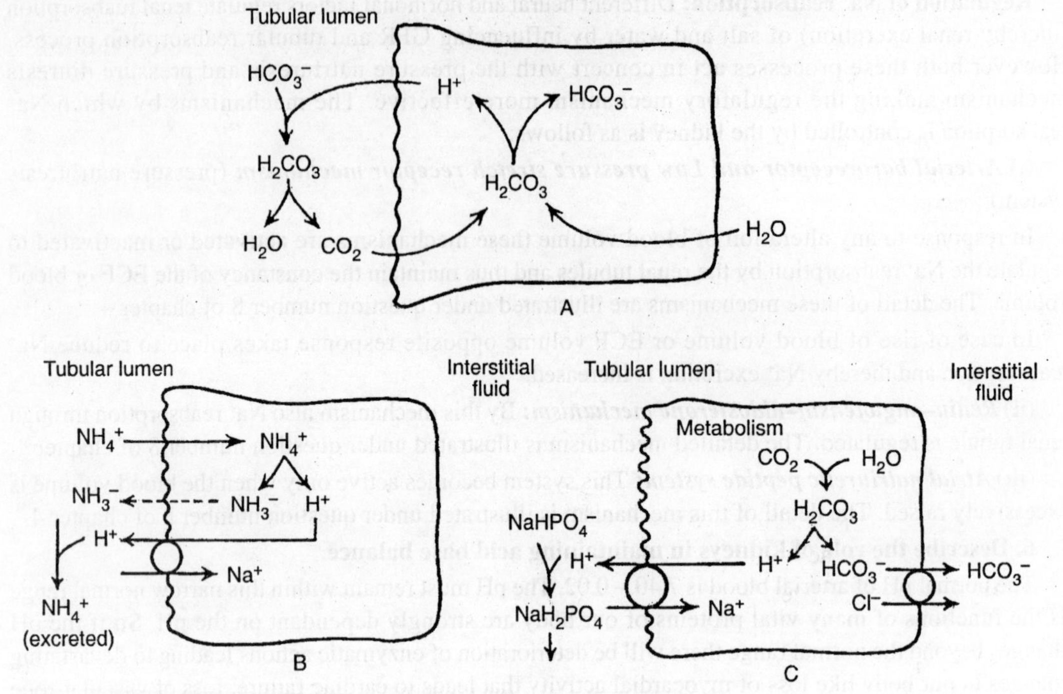

Fig. 8.7: Elimination of secreted H^+ *(A = buffering of HCO_3^-, B = buffering action of NH_3 and C = buffering of PO_4^-)*

(i) ***Reabsorption in PCT*: 90% of the filtered HCO_3 is reabsorbed in the PCT by secondary active** transport via Na^+/H^+ antiport system as described in fig. 8.5A.

(ii) ***Reabsorption in DCT and CT***: Remaining 10-15% of filtered HCO_3^- is reabsorbed by the DCT and CT via $K^+ - H^+$ exchanger or H^+ – ATPase mechanism.

B. *Generation of new HCO_3– coupled with H^+/NH_4^+ secretion*:

- This is to compensate the loss of physiological buffers from the body due to—
  (i) buffering action of nonvolatile acids, phosphoric acids added in the blood.
  (ii) Conversion nonvolatile acids into CO_2.
- The maximum amount of bicarbonate generated in the kidney is 500 mosmol/day.
- There are 2 mechanisms by which HCO_3^- is generated by the kidney:
  (a) ***H_2CO_3 derived H^+ secretion process*:**
  This occurs specially in the intercalated cells of collecting ducts (Fig. 8.6A). In this process CO_2, either derived from metabolism of epithelium cell or entered from peritubular capillary blood reacts with H_2O to form H_2CO_3 by the enzyme, carbonic anhydrase. This H_2CO_3 is rapidly ionised to form H^+ and HCO_3^-. HCO_3^- is transported to peritubular space by $Na^+ - HCO_3^-$ symport and $Cl^- - HCO_3^-$ antiport mechanism. Whereas the H^+ is—
  (i) actively pumped out in tubular fluid and
  (ii) transported out in carrier mediated process in exchange of Na^+.

(b) ***Glutamine derived NH_4^+ secretion process***: This occurs mainly in proximal tubule. In this process glutamine is metabolised to form NH_4^+ and HCO_3^-. The bicarbonate is diffused into peritubular capillary due to concentration gradient and NH_4^+ is secreted in tubular fluid in exchange of Na^+ (Fig. 8.6B).

C. ***Elimination (excretion) of secreted H^+***: As seen above the generation of new HCO_3^- and reabsorption of filtered HCO_3^- is accomplished by secretion of H^+ into the tubular fluid. If the secreted H^+ allowed to stay back freely in the lumen, the pH of tubular fluid will rapidly fall to a level which is too corrosive for any living tissue. So to prevent this, the secreted H^+ are buffered in the tubular lumen by two buffer systems—**ammonia buffer** and **phosphate buffer.** The major sites of urine acidification is in DCT and CT.

(a) ***Buffering action by HCO_3^-***: This occurs mainly in PCT. In this mechanism the bicarbonate buffers present in tubular lumen reacts with secreted hydrogen ion to form H_2CO_3 which then rapidly ionizes to H_2O and CO_2 (Fig. 8.7A).

(b) ***Buffering action of NH_3***:

- NH_3 present in epithelial cells of mainly PCT and DCT either enters the tubular cell by secretion or synthesises in th cell itself by deamination of glutamine, and glutamic acid and other amino acids like aspargine, glycine etc.
- This NH_3 passively diffuses (Non ionic diffusion) to tubular lumen along it's concentration gradient due to its lipid solubility.
- In the lumen NH_3 reacts with secreted H^+ form NH_4^+ which is relatively lipid insoluble and thus can not enter the epithelial cell again (Fig. 8.7B).
- This NH_4^+ is eliminated through urine.
- Thus the secreted H^+ is buffered in urine as NH_4^+ which do not cause the pH of urine to fall.

(c) ***Buffering action of phosphate***:

- The buffering action of phosphate mainly occurs in DCT and partly in collecting duct (Fig. 8.7C).
- Out of the total amount of phosphate filtered in glomerulus only 25% is available for buffering action as 75% is reabsorbed by the renal tubules.
- The (Fig. 8.7C) illustrates the detail mechanism in which the H^+ secreted in the tubular lumen thus reacts with HPO_4^- (dibasic phosphate ions) to form acidic sodium dihydrogen phosphate (NaH_2PO_4) which is termed as ***Titrable acid.*** This titrable acid is excreted through the urine.

8. What is micturition? Discuss it's mechanism. How micturition reflex is controlled?

The process of emptying of the bladder and evacuation of the urine out of the body after the bladder becomes filled is known as ***Micturition.***

Mechanism of Micturition:

(A) *Filling of bladder*:

- When the urine is collected in the pelvis of ureter. The pelvis starts contracting and this contraction is transmitted through the ureter as peristaltic wave which drives the urine towards urinary bladder through the ureters.
- As the urine is collected by the bladder drop by drop intravesicular pressure gradually rises upto 5-10 cm of water.
- Further addition of urine up to 200-300 ml into the bladder do not cause any rise of intravesicular pressure due to intrinsic tone of the bladder wall (i.e. relaxation of detrusor muscle) that obeys **Laplace's law**.

- When the amount of urine collection becomes more than 300-400 ml there is sudden rise in intravesicular pressure which initiates-micturition reflex i.e. urge for micturition is started. However, the micturition becomes voluntarily inhibited by the higher centers until a suitable opportunity for emptying the bladder comes. This inhibition is mediated by contraction of external urethral sphincters and perineal muscles and relaxation of detrusor and contraction of internal sphincter.
- When the pressure to 100 cm of H_2O due to collection of 700-800 ml of urine the micturition follows involuntarily due to powerful contraction of detrusor muscle and reciprocal relaxation of internal and external urethral sphincter.
- This relationship between intravesical pressure changes with changes in volume of urine collected in the bladder can be plotted in a graph paper. Such a record is known as ***Cystometrogram*** (Fig. 8.8).

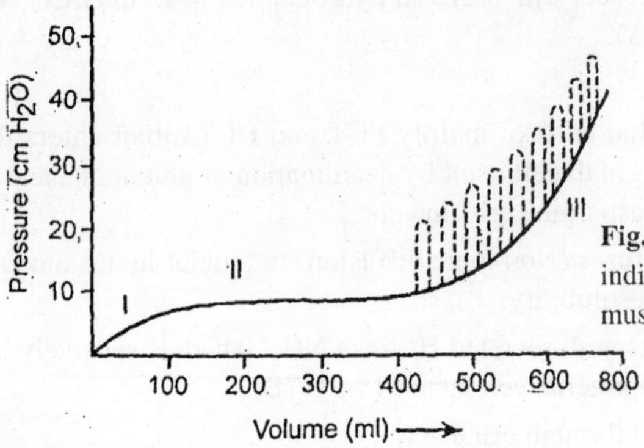

Fig. 8.8: Cystometrogram (dotted line indicates the contraction of detrusor muscle)

Emptying of bladder:

- The act of micturition is essentially a reflex though it is usually inhibited voluntarily and also can be initiated voluntarily at any stage. However, when the anatomical capacity of bladder exceeds then it is initiated involuntarily.
- As urine accumulates, the bladder gets distended and the intravesicular pressure rises. When the pressure in the bladder rises to 15-20 cm of water the stretch receptors, present in the wall of bladder are stimulated. The afferent impulse now is conducted to the spinal cord (sacral segments) through the pelvic nerves. The efferent impulse from spinal cord is then transmitted to the bladder to cause contraction of detrusor muscle and thus micturition reflex is initiated.
- Once micturition reflex is initiated, it is self regenerative i.e. the initial contraction of bladder wall further stimulates the receptors to initite more powerful contraction of detrusor muscle (powerful micturition reflex).
- This cycle repeat again and again until bladder undergoes strong contraction.
- If this micturition reflex is not succeeded in emptying the bladder due to strong contraction of external and internal urethral sphincter this regenerative cycle ceases and the reflex remains in inhibited state for maximum an hour till another micturition reflex starts.
- Once the micturition reflex becomes powerful enough it initiates another reflex that passes through pudendal nerves to external urethral sphincter. This leads the relaxation of external sphincter and thus urethral opening is opened to alllow the urine to pass out due to strong pressure inside the bladder.
- The whole phenomenon is represented in detail by following flow chart.

  Collection of urine by urinary bladder → increase in intravesicular pressure → stimulation of stretch receptors present the wall of urinary bladder → transmission of sensory impulses to sacral segments of spinal cord via pelvic nerve → transmission of efferent impulses to urinary bladder via pelvic nerve → contraction of detrusor muscle and relaxation of internal urethral sphincter → passing of urine through urethra → stimulation of stretch receptors present in the wall of urethra → transmission of impulses through pelvic nerve to spinal cord → inhibition of pudendal nerve → relaxation of external urethral sphincter → voiding of urine

Control of micturition:

Micturition reflex is a purely spinal cord reflex but it can be inhibited or facilitated by supraspinal centers as follows:

1. Strong facilitatory and inhibitory centers in the brain stem.
2. Facilitatory and inhibitory centers in the hypothalamus.
3. Some centers in the cerebral cortex are mainly inhibitory but at times become facilitatory. These cortical centers normally keep the micturition reflex partially inhibited all the time except when micturition is desired. Even if micturition reflex occurs, the voiding of urine is kept prevented by the higher centers due to it's inhibition to spinal centers until an opportunity to empty the bladder is found.

When convenient opportunity comes cortical centers facilitate sacral micturition centers to initiate micturition reflex along with inhibition of external urethral sphincter so that urine is passed out.

B. Short Notes:

1. Juxta glomerular apparatus:

- It is defined as the specialised organ of the kidney situated near the glomerulus of the nephron.
- It consists of:

(a) Macula densa cells:

- The initial part of distal tubule is passed through the angle between afferent and efferent arterioles of the glomerulus. At this part of distal tubule the epithelial cells are specialised and are known as ***macula densa cells*** (Fig. 8.9).

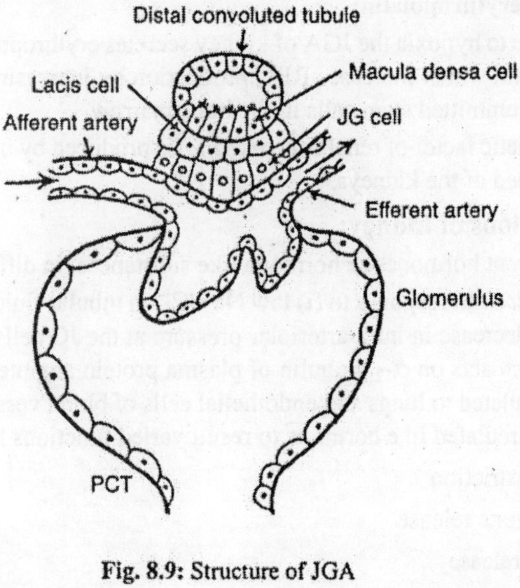

Fig. 8.9: Structure of JGA

- These cells act as a sensor of a tubular fluid flow and composition. These are activated by low content of Na^+ in the tubular fluid and regulate renin secretion by the kidney and also help in autoregulation of GFR by tubulo-glomerular feedback.

(b) Extraglomerular messangial cells (Lacis cell):

- These cells are located in the triangular area surrounded by afferent arteriole, efferent arteriole and macula densa cells.
- These are supporting cells of JGA and contractile in nature by which it plays an important role in regulation of glomerular filtration.

(c) Juxtaglomerular (JG) cells (Granular cell, Polkissen cell):

- These are the modified smooth muscular cells present in the wall of the afferent and efferent arterioles before entering the glomerulus.
- These are granular cells which synthesise, store and release renin in response to sustained hypotension and also in Na^+ deficiency in tubular fluid.
- These also act as baroreceptors and gives response to changes in the transmural pressure gradient between the afferent arteriole and the interstitium.

- **Function:**

a. Secretion of renin: JG cells of JGA secrete renin into the blood in response to reduction of blood pressure, reduction of ECF volume, increase in sympathetic activity, decreased Na^+ load in tubular fluid, increase in circulatory catecholamines, PGs. This renin, once secreted, acts on plasma protein angiotensinogen of blood to form angiotensin-I which inturn is converted to angiotensin-II in the lungs which has following effects:

- constriction of systemic arteries $\rightarrow\uparrow$ BP
- maintenance of GFR and renal blood flow (autoregulation of GFR and RBF).
- stimulation of adrenal cortex to release aldosterone $\rightarrow\uparrow$ Na^+ and H_2O reabsorption by distal nephrons of the kidney.
- stimulation of neurohypophysis to secrete more ADH
- acts on hypothalamus and increases thirst sensation.

b. Secretion of erythropoietin:

- In response to hypoxia the JGA of kidney secretes erythropoietic factor which helps to form erthropoietin which increases RBC production by increasing the number of erythropoietin sensitive committed stem cells in the bone marrow.
- Erythropoietic factor of renal source (85%) is produced by interstitial cells in the peritubular capillary bed of the kidneys.

2. Endocrine functions of kidney:

- It secretes different hormones or hormone like substances in different condition e.g.
  - ***Renin secretion***: In response to (i) low Na^+/Cl^- in tubular fluid (ii) stimulation of sympathetic system (iii) decrease in intra-arteriolar pressure at the JG cells, there is release of renin from JG cells which acts on α-$_2$ globulin of plasma protein angiotensinogen to from angiotensin-I which is circulated to lungs and endothelial cells of blood vessels to convert it as angiotensin-II which is circulated like hormone to result varied functions like:
    - ☐ Vasoconstriction
    - ☐ Aldosterone release
    - ☐ ACTH release
    - ☐ ADH release
    - ☐ Na^+/Cl^- absorption through PCT
    - ☐ Stimulation of thirst center by acting on subfornical organs.

- ***Erythropoietin*:** In response to hypoxia peritubular capillary interstitial cells produce erythropoietin which acts on erythropoietin sensitive stem cells CFU (E) in the bone marrow and thus increases RBC production.
- ***Medullipin*:** Mudullipin is secreted from renal papilla and acts in opposite to renin-angiotensin mechanism to regulate arterial B.P.
- Conversion of Cholecalciferol (Vit D_3) to 1-25 Dihydroxy cholecalciferol which helps in regulation of Ca^{2+} concentration in body fluids.
- ***Prostaglandins*:** PGI_2 and PGE_2 produced by the interstitial cells in the renal papilla in response to rise in medullary blood flow results vasodilatation and thus reduces blood pressure.
- ***Kallikrein–Bradykinin System*:** Kallikrein enzyme produces by renal parenchyma acts on plasma protein kininogen to convert it as bradykinin which is potent vasodilator and also produces diuresis and natriuresis.

3. Barrington reflex:

Barrington described six integrated reflexes which is responsible for act of micturition in the cat. These micturition reflexes are collectively known as ***Barrington reflex.***

(1) Contraction of the detrusor and reciprocal relaxation of internal sphincter evoked by distension of bladder.

(2) Contraction of the detrusor evoked by urine passage through the urethra.

(3) Transient and weak contraction of the detrusor due to distension of the proximal urethra.

(4) Relaxation of external sphnicter when urine passes through the urethra.

(5) Relaxation of external sphnicter due to distension of bladder.

(6) Relaxation of the external sphincter, bladder and urethra caused by the distension of the bladder.

Center, Afferent and Efferent pathway of Barrington reflex

Barrington's reflex no.	Afferent	Efferent	Higher Center
1.	Pelvic	Pelvic	Hindbrain
2.	Pudendal	Pelvic	Hindbrain
3.	Hypogastric	Hypogastric	Spinal cord
4.	Pudendal	Pudendal	—do—
5.	Pelvic	Pudendal	—do—
6.	Pelvic	Pelvic	—do—

4. Peculiarities of renal circulation:

These are as follows:

1. All the blood entering the kidney has to pass through the glomerulus to facilitate the proper and complete filtration of all blood entering the kidney.

2. It is a type of ***portal circulation*** as two set of capillary plexus—glomerular capillary tuft and peritubular capillary plexus, are present in kidney.

3. Renal glomerular capillaries have high pressure due to—

(i) Presence of short and wide renal artery directly arised from aorta.

(ii) Efferent arteriolar diameter is less than the afferent arteriolar diameter.

This high pressure in the glomerular capillaries is helpful for effective glomerular filtration.

4. The rate of renal blood flow is comparatively high so that all blood is filtered within 4-5 mins in order to excrete the metabolic by products (urea, uric acid, creatinine etc.) quickly.

5. There are two types of blood circulation in kidney:
   (i) ***Greater circulation***—The blood supply to the cortex is more (85-86%)
   (ii) ***Lesser circulation***—The blood supply to the medulla is less (14-15%) to maintain the osmotic gradient present in the medullary interstitium which is required for concentrating or diluting the urine.

6. The existence of ***Ludig shunt*** helps the kidney to maintain it's normal function even during chronic kidney disease in which glomerulus are blocked.

7. ***Autoregulation of renal blood flow*** (In cortex): In between 90-220 mm Hg of arterial B.P. the renal blood supply remains constant.The kidney has got this capacity to maintain this constant blood supply, by tubulo glomerular feedback mechanism even if the arterial pressure varies significantly.

8. The A-V difference of O_2 is minimum in kidney.

9. O_2 consumption in kidney is quite large i.e. 6ml /100 gm /min.

5. Tubuloglomerular feedback:

- Signals originating from renal tubules controls the glomerular filtration by feedback mechanism which is called as ***Tubuloglomerular feedback***.
- In this process the rate of flow of fluid and concentration of NaCl in tubular fluid in distal tubule provides the feedback information to the glomerulus to control the rate of filtration by two mechanisms—
  - Afferent arteriolar feedback mechanism
  - Efferent arteriolar feedback mechanism

  Out of those mechanisms afferent arteriolar feedback mechanism are the main mechanisms by which autoregulation of GFR is maintained by auto regulating RBF. Whereas efferent arteriolar mechanism helps to regulate GFR upto certain extent without regulating RBF. The detail of these mechanisms are illustrated with flow chart FC 8.A and 8.B. Similarly in response to fall of GFR just opposite events take place to regulate GFR.

6. Glomerular membrane: It consists of 3 major layers (Fig. 8.10) as follows:

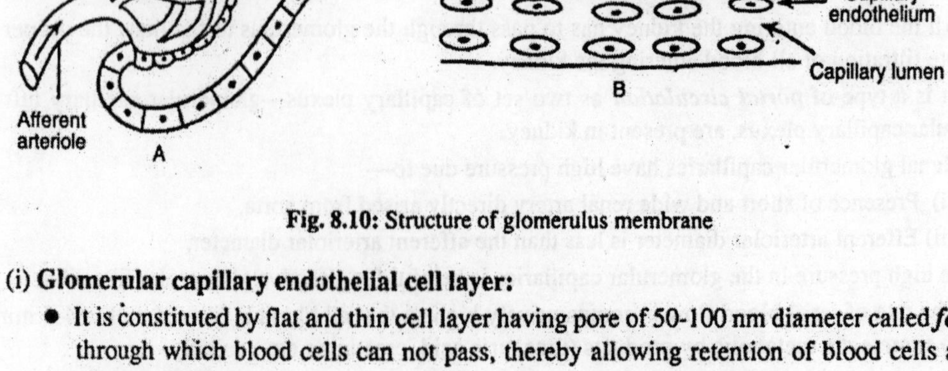

Fig. 8.10: Structure of glomerulus membrane

(i) Glomerular capillary endothelial cell layer:

- It is constituted by flat and thin cell layer having pore of 50-100 nm diameter called ***fenestrae*** through which blood cells can not pass, thereby allowing retention of blood cells and also plasma proteins.

(ii) **Basement membrane of capillary endothelial cell layer and Bowman's capsular cell layer:**

- These are composed of proteoglycans and collagens which are negatively charged thereby opposes the filtration of mainly plasma proteins.

(iii) **Epithelial cell layer of visceral layer of Bowman's capsule:**

- It gives out series of foot processes called ***podocytes.***
- The spaces in between the podocytes are having diameter of 25 nm which is known as ***Filtration slit*** which allows the filtrate to come across Bowman's Capsule.

7. Filtration fraction:

- It is the ratio of GFR to renal plasma flow.
- Normal range is 0.16 to 0.20.
- It is a better index of glomerular activity e.g. decreased BP increases filtration fraction without much change in GFR.
- In glomerulonephritis and ureteral obstruction by renal stones the filtration fraction is reduced or GFR is reduced.

8. TmG and Splay:

- TmG is the maximum amount of substance that is absorbed by renal tubules in one minute.
- It refers to the limitations of tubular capacity of a substance to transport or reabsorb.
- Normal TmG is 375 mg/min in male and 300mg/min in a female.
- When the blood sugar level exceeds the TmG value it is excreted into urine but practically glucose appears in urine when blood sugar concentration (venous blood) exceeds 180 mg /100ml. This anomaly between the predicted value and practical value is called as ***Splay***.

9. PAH clearance:

- PAH clearance test is based on the Fick's principle and helps to measure the renal blood flow. Procedural protocol are as follows:
  - To measure the RPF by this test the para aminohippuric acid is intravenously injected continuously to maintain a very low and constant plasma level (0.02 mg / ml).
  - The urine sample is collected by catheterisation.
  - The concentration of PAH in urine is also measured.
  - Now the RPF is calculated by:

    $$RPF = U_{PAH} \times V / P_{PAH} = 630 \text{ ml/min}$$

  - This is called as ***effective renal plasma flow*** (ERPF) as some blood bypasses the nephrons. So the total plasma flow can be calculated by applying extraction ratio of PAH which is about 0.9. So,

    $$RPF = ERPF/\text{Extraction ratio} = 630 \text{ ml}/0.9 = 700 \text{ ml.}$$

  - Now with the help of haematocrit value (Hct) the whole blood flow (RBF) can also be calculated as follows:

    $$RBF = RPF \times 1/1\text{-Hct} = 700 \times 1/1\text{-}0.45 = 700/0.55 = 1273 \text{ ml / min}$$

- In this method RPF is measured by injecting Para-amino hippuric acid (PAH) and then determining the concentration of PAH in urine and plasma. The extraction ratio (i.e. arterial concentration minus renal venous concentration divided by arterial concentration) for PAH is high because PAH is filtered from glomerulus and secreted by tubular cells. The renal plasma flow usually is calculated by dividing the amount of PAH in urine by the plasma level of PAH ignoring the concentration of PAH in renal venous blood.

- This test is also used clinically to estimate the tubular secretory capacity. Any decrease in maximum secretory capacity of the tubules for PAH value indicates the tubular damage.

10. Creatinine clearance:

- This is the method to measure the GFR based on Fick's principle.
- Creatinine clearance is also used to measure GFR by the same way as Inulin clearance method. However since creatinine is endogenous and it's plasma concentration is steady throughout the day no intravenous administration of creatinine is required. Simple determination of plasma creatinine concentration and it's amount in one minute urinary output are sufficient to put these values in above mentioned formula.
- *Advantage*:
  - Simple method as no intravenous infusion is required.
  - Clinically it is preferred than that of previous method.
- *Disadvantage*: The obtained value of GFR is sometimes lesser and sometimes greater than normal GFR because of reabsorption and secretion of creatinine by renal tubules.

11. Inulin clearance:

- This is the method to measure the GFR based on the Fick's principle.
- Procedure—
  - Intravenous administration of large dose of Inulin followed by continuous infusion of inulin (to compensate it's loss through urine) to maintain it's plasma level at constant.
  - Urinary concentration of Inulin (Ux) and volume of urine excreted per minute (V) are determined after collecting urine sample.
  - Plasma sample is collected and it's Inulin concentration is measured.
  - Inulin clearence is thus calculated by the formula:

$$\textbf{Inulin clearance} = \frac{U_x XV}{P_x}$$

- *Advantage*: It is the most accurate method.
- *Disadvantage*: It requires continuous infusion of inulin.

12. Urea clearance:

- This test is used to measure the rate of excretion of waste products.
- It can be done by collecting urine samples of one hours for twice and collecting blood at the end of 1st hour to determine it's urea content. Urine samples are then measured and their urea contents are determined separately. Minute output of urine is calculated.
- The urea clearance is now calculated as follows:
  - If the minute output of urine is 2ml or more the maximum urea clearance (C_m) is calculated as per following formula:

$$\textbf{Urea clearance} = \frac{U_u XV}{P_u}$$

Where U_u = urea in mg/ml of urine, V = Volume of urine (ml / min) and P_u = Urea in mg / ml of plasma. **The normal value of C_m is 60-90 ml/min**

  - If the minute output of urine is less than 2 ml the standard urea clearance (C_s) is calculated as per following formula:

$$\text{Urea clearance} = \frac{U_u X\sqrt{V}}{P_u}$$

13. Role of urea in counter current system:

- Collecting duct acts as osmotic equilibrating device to contribute urinary concentration which is facilitated by the urea cycle in between ascending limb of loop of Henlee and collecting duct.
- Urea is absorbed by facilitated diffusion from the inner medullary collecting duct which enters the medullary interstitium and from there into the ascending limb of loop of Henlee. When it reaches the collecting duct it is absorbed again. This is known as Urea cycle in between ascending limb of loop of Henlee and collecting duct.
- When urea is reabsorbed from tubular fluid to medullary interstitium water moves out of tubular fluid to maintain osmotic balance. Thus urine is more concentrated. Water that enters the interstitium is taken up by vasa recta and consequently osmolar dilution of interstitium is prevented.

14. Loop Diuretics:

- These help to result diuresis by inhibiting Na^+, K^+, and Cl^- reabsorption in the thick ascending limb of loop of Henlee and thus there is loss of these electrolytes along the water.
- Example: Furosemide and ethacrynic acid which inhibits $Na^+ - K^+ - 2Cl^-$ co-transporter in the thick ascending limb of loop of Henlee.

15. Buffer systems in the kidney:

- There are 3 buffer systems in the kidney namely—
  1. Bicarbonate buffer in PCT
  2. Phosphate buffer in PCT and CD
  3. Ammonia buffer in PCT and DCT.
- *Bicarbonate buffer in PCT*: Bicarbonate ion after filtration into tubular fluid reaches a concentration about 24 mili moles. At this concentration it is an effective buffer for the tubular acids. It binds with H^+ to form carbonic acid which rapidly breaks down to form CO_2 and water by the action of carbonic anhydrase enzyme present at the brush border of PCT. The CO_2 diffuses to tubular cell and react with water to resecrete acid into tubule and absorb bicarbonate into interstitium (Fig. 8.7A).
- *Phosphate buffer*: Secreted acids react with phosphate buffer to burn monobasic phosphates which gets excreted when sodium gets reabsorbed (Fig. 8.7C).
- *Ammonia* buffer: Soluble ammonia diffuses through cell membrane into tubular fluid which then reacts with acid to form ammonium ion that subsequently gets excreted (Fig. 8.7B).

16. Tests for glomerular function: The main tests for determining the glomerular function are Inulin clearance test and Creatinine clearance test. For detail see the short note on Inuline clearance and Creatine clearance methods.

17. Test for tubular function: The main tests to assess the tubular function are PAH clearance test and Urea clearance test. For detail see the short note on PAH clearance and Urea clearance methods.

18. Acidosis and alkalosis: Decrease of pH of blood below it's normal range is known as ***acidosis*** and increase in pH of blood above it's normal range is termed as ***alkalosis***. It is of two types:

- **Respiratory acidosis and respiratory alkalosis:**
  - Acidosis or alkalosis caused due to decreased or increased pulmonary ventilation resulting decreased or increased CO_2 loss respectively is known as respiratory acidosis or alkalosis.
  - Respiratory acidosis occurs in pathological conditions causing reduced breathing capacity e.g. obstruction in respiratory passage, pneumonia etc.
  - Respiratory alkalosis is caused due to increased pulmonary ventilation which is seen in high altitude.

- **Metabolic acidosis and metabolic alkalosis:**
  - **Metabolic acidosis is defined as the fall of blood pH below the normal range due to bicarbonate depletion in the body where as metabolic alkalosis is referred to as the rise of blood pH above the normal value due to increased bicarbonate concentration of CO_2 in the body.**
  - **The causes of metabolic acidosis are:**

    (a) Failure of kidney to excrete acids normally formed in the kidney.

    (b) Formation of excess metabolic acids by the body.

    (c) Addition of metabolic acids by G-I absorption or by intravenous administration.

    (d) Loss of base from the body.
  - **The causes of metabolic alkalosis are:**

    (a) Loss of Cl^- from the body due to excessive vomiting (mainly gastric content)

    (b) Excessive aldosterone secretion

    (c) Excessive ingestion of alkaline drugs

    (d) Administration of diuretics

19. Cystometrogram:

- The relationship between intravesicular pressure changes with changes in volume of urine collected in the bladder can be plotted in a graph paper. Such a record is called as ***cystometrogram*** (Fig. 8.8).
- It consists of 3 segments—I, II, and III.

  i. Phase I : This sudden initial rise is due to accumulation of urine upto 150 ml which stretches the bladder wall → contraction of bladder wall → rise in intravesicular pressure.

  ii. Phase II : In this phase no change of intravesicular pressure inspite of further accumulation of urine in bladder up to 400 ml which is due to—
  - Laplace law.
  - Plasticity of smooth muscle.

  iii. Phase III : Steep rise of intravesicular pressure due to sudden reduction of volume of urinary bladder due to contraction of detrussor muscle.

20. Micturition reflex:

- The act of micturition is essentially a reflex though it is usually inhibited voluntarily and also can be initiated voluntarily at any stage. However, when the anatomical capacity of bladder exceeds then it is initiated involuntarily.
- As urine accumulates, the bladder gets distended and the intravesicular pressure rises. When the pressure in the bladder rises to 15-20 cm of water the stretch receptors, present in the wall of bladder are stimulated. The afferent impulse now is conducted to the spinal cord (sacral segments) through the pelvic nerves. The efferent impulse from spinal cord is then transmitted to the bladder to cause contraction of detrusor muscle and thus micturition reflex is initiated.
- The whole phenomenon is represented in detail by following flow chart:

  Collection of urine by urinary bladder → increase in intravesicular pressure → stimulation of stretch receptors present in the wall of urinary bladder → transmission of sensory impulses to sacral segments of spinal cord via pelvic nerve → transmission of efferent impulses to urinary bladder via pelvic nerve → contraction of detrusor muscle and relaxation of internal urethral sphincter → passing of urine through urethra → stimulation of stretch receptors present in the wall of urethra → transmission of impulses through pelvic nerve to spinal cord → inhibition of pudendal nerve → relaxation of external urethral sphincter → voiding of urine.

21. Sweat gland:

- In the deep layer of the skin there are sweat glands that secrete the sweat.
- Sweat glands are of two types (A) Ecrine and (B) Apocrine

A. Ecrine (Merocrine) sweat glands:

a. *Distribution*—It is present all over the body but more on palm, soles, head, trunk and extremities.

b. *Structure*—It consists of 2 parts (i) **Body or fundus** (ii) **Duct**—It is a long tube originated from coiled structure and opens into the skin surface.

c. *Secretions*—The secretion of this gland is known as sweat which consists of mainly water (99.5%) and solids (0.5%) like Na^+, Cl^-, K^+, Ca^{2+}, urea, lactic acids etc. The cubical or polygonal epithelial cells of the body of sweat gland secretes these substances from plasma into the tubular lumen known as ***primary secretion*** or ***precursor secretion***. While passing through the duct of the gland Na^+, Cl^- and water are reabsorbed from the primary secretion by the epithelial cell lining of the duct. This results excretion of **hypotonic** sweat secretion at skin surface normally.

d. *Innervations*—Cholinergic sympathetic fibers.

e. *Type of sweating*—Thermal sweating.

B. Apocrine sweat glands:

a. *Distribution*—Found mainly in axilla, around the nipples, and in female in labia majora and mons pubis.

b. *Structure*—These are comparatively larger and developed from hair follicle and fully developed after puberty. It has also (i) highly coiled tubular structure present at about the junction of epidermis and dermis (ii) a very short duct that opens into the hair follicle but not on skin surface.

c. *Secretion*—

- The secretion is similar to that of ecrine gland though it is thick, milky and odourless (The odour arising out of axilla is due to bacterial action on the secretions at axillary surface).
- The secretion is stimulated by epinephrine.
- The ceruminous gland of external auditory meatus and cilliary glands of eyelids are modified apocrine glands.

d. *Innervations*—No nerve supply to these glands.

e. *Type of sweating*—Non thermal.

The sebaceous gland secretes oil for the hair and skin which is known as ***sebum***. Sebum is rich in triglycerides, fatty acids and cholesterol that have an antifungal action. It not only acts as an lubricant but also as an bacteriostatic agent.

22. Dialysis:

- Removal of waste materials and toxic substances and normalization of body fluid volume and composition by means of artificial kidney is called as dialysis or hemodialysis.
- Principle of this process is diffusion of solutes from an area of higher concentration to the area of lower concentration through a semipermeable membrane.
- The frequency and duration of dialysis depends on the degree of renal disorder, however it is usually done thrice in a week in case of severe uremia.
- Amount of blood in dialysis mechanism is 500 ml at a time and the rate of blood flow is about 200-300 ml/min.
- Complications: The common complications of dialysis are sleep disorder, anxiety, depression etc.

23. Fanconi syndrome:

- It is an autosomal recessive disorder of generalized proximal tubular dysfunction.

- This is characterised by urinary wasting of amino acids, phosphate, glucose, bicarbonate and potassium due to failure of reabsorption in PCT.
- The notable abnormalities are: decrease in blood phosphate and blood uric acid, glucose and amino acids in urine and proximal tubular acidosis.

24. Escape phenomenon:

- A decrease in plasma Na^+ stimulate aldosterone secretion → aldosterone increases tubular reabsorption of Na^+ and water → expansion of ECF volume due to water retention → natriuresis Hence aldosterone by itself is unable to produce significant amount of Na^+ and water retention. This is known as escape phenomenon.
- In the absence of ADH-Thirst mechanism aldosterone is unable to maintain proper Na^+ balance because of escape phenomenon.

C. Differentiate between:

Cortical nephrons	Juxtamedullary nephrons
❑ Located in the superficial region of cortex.	❑ Located in the juxtamedullary region of cortex.
❑ More in number (85%).	❑ Less in number (15%).
❑ Size of glomerulus is small.	❑ Size of glomerulus is larger.
❑ Length of loop of Henlee is shorter.	❑ Length of loop of Henlee is longer.
❑ Rate of filtration is slow.	❑ Rate of filtration is fast.
❑ Blood supply is mediated through peritubular capillaries.	❑ Blood supply is mediated through peritubular capillaries and vasa recta.
❑ Renin content is more.	❑ Renin content is less.
❑ Main function is urine formation and excretion of waste products.	❑ Main function is urine concentration.
❑ Efficiency of concentrating urine is less.	❑ Efficiency of concentrating urine is more.

Peritubular capillary plexus	Vasa recta
❑ Supplies blood to both cortical and juxtamedullary nephrons.	❑ Supplies only to juxtamedullary nephrons.
❑ It is short and branched.	❑ It is straight and long.
❑ It is responsible for reabsorption of mainly electrolytes.	❑ It is responsible for concentration and dilution of urine by counter current mechanism.

Transcellular transport	Paracellular transport
❑ It is the mechanism in which transport of substances take place from tubular lumen to tubular cell through apical (lumen) surface of the cell membrane.	❑ It is the mechanism in which transport of substances take place from tubular lumen into interstitial fluid present in lateral intercellular space through tight junction between the cells.
❑ This is the major route (70%-80%) of transport of all electrolytes.	❑ This is the minor route (20%-30%) of transport of all electrolytes.
❑ This is mediated mainly by energy required and carrier mediated process.	❑ This is mainly dependant on concentration/pressure/electrical gradient.

Glomerular filtration	Systemic filtration
❑ It occurs in glomerulus of kidney. ❑ The pressure gradient responsible for glomerulur filtratiion is considerably high. ❑ Capillary exchange area is less. ❑ Filtration rate is 180 L/day.	❑ It occurs in all systemic arteries at all the tissues. ❑ The pressure gradient responsible for systemic filtration is comparatively less. ❑ Capillary exchange area is enormous (100 m^2). ❑ Filtration rate is 20 L/day.

Obligatory reabsorption	Facultative reabsorption
❑ This type of water reabsorption is secondary to sodium reabsorption. ❑ Water reabsorption takes place through transcellular route via Aquaporin—I water channels and also through para cellular route. ❑ It is not dependant on medullary concentration gradient.	❑ This type of water reabsorption is dependant on ADH hormone. ❑ Water reabsorptioin takes place only through transcellular route via Aquaporin—II water channels. ❑ It is dependant on medullary concentration gradient.

Counter current multiplier system	Counter current exchanger system
❑ It takes place in between Henlee's loop and interstitial fluid surrounding the Henlee's loop in juxtamedullary nephrons. ❑ It is responsible for establishment of osmotic gradient in medullary interstitial fluid. ❑ Urea has no role in this machanism.	❑ It takes place in between interstitial fluid surrounding the Henlee's loop and vasa recta in juxtamedullary nephrons. ❑ It is responsible for maintenance of osmotic gradient once established by CCM System. ❑ Urea has significant role in this mechanism.

Water diuresis	Osmotic diuresis
❑ If water is taken more than the need of the body the excess water is excreted which is known as water diuresis. ❑ It is characterised by diuresis of dilute urine upto a volume of 20 L/day. ❑ Water reabsorption is decreased due to ADH effect. ❑ It inhibits ADH release.	❑ Loss of large amount of urine due to osmotic effect of solutes like glucose is known as osmotic diuresis. ❑ It is characterised by diuresis of isotonic urine with very large urine flow rate > 20 L/day. ❑ Water reabsorption is decreased due to osmotic effect. ❑ It stimulates ADH release.

Renal threshold	TmG
❑ It is the plasma level of glucose and is expressed in mg/100 ml. ❑ It is less stable index of PCT function. ❑ It is affected by 'Splay'.	❑ It is the rate of glucose transport and is expressed in mg/min. ❑ It is more stable index of PCT function. ❑ It is not affected by 'Splay'.

D. Short answer type:

1. Give physiological basis of high pressure in glomerular capillaries.

High pressure in glomerular capillaries is due to the facts that:

- afferent arterioles are short and directly originated from abdominal aorta.
- diameter of efferent arteriole is smaller than afferent arteriole resulting relative high resistance in efferent arteriole.

2. Explain why medullary blood flow does not show autoregulation.

This is to preserve high osmotic gradient present in medullary interstitium which is responsible for concentration and dilution of urine by Henlee's loop.

3. Why renal failure develops in persons with poor renal perfusion?

Renal failure develops in persons with poor renal perfusion as filtration of plasma is the pressure dependant process. If the perfusion pressure becomes less than 50 mmHg the kidney can not filter the blood and thus develops renal failure.

4. Explain: High protein diet increases the ability of kidney to concentrate urine.

High protein diet increases the ability of kidney to concentrate urine by increasing the filtered load of urine derived from high protein substances.

5. Give other examples of counter current systems in our body.

It is also present in skin, arteries and venae commitants of the limb and also in villous blood vessels in the small intestine.

6. What will happen if blood flow in the vasa recta increases?

In this situation the established osmotic gradient in between medullary interstitium and blood within vasa recta will lost.

7. Give the physiological basis of the major site of urine acidification are the DCT and CT.

The major site of urine acidification are the DCT and CT as almost all the H^+ within the tubular lumen is secreted due to tubular secretion of the H^+ from DCT and CT.

8. What will happen if afferent nerve to urinary bladder is sectioned?

It will result automatic bladder which is characterised by:

- Patient is unware of a state of distention of bladder.
- Dribbling of urine.
- Normal voluntary micturition.

9. What will happen if urinary bladder is completely denervated?

It will result:

- Complete loss of voluntary micturition.
- Bladder becomes flaccid and distended called isolated bladder or decentralized bladder.

10. What are the role of urinary buffer?

The urinary buffer systems (i.e) bicarbonate, phosphates and ammonia used to bind free H^+ and thereby prevents the backward leakage of H^+ to the intercellular space and also permitting more acids to be secreted.

E. MCQ:

1. In each kidney there are about (i) 5 million (ii) 10 million (iii) 1 million (iv) 10 lakh nephrons. (ii)
2. Glomerulus is the part of (i) Bowman's capsule (ii) renal corpuscle (iii) renal tubule (iv) JGA. (ii)
3. The function of juxtamedullary nephrons are (i) concentration of urine (ii) reabsorption of ions (iii) secretion (iv) all of the above. (i)
4. Macula densa cells are present in the (i) afferent arteriole (ii) efferent arteriole (iii) PCT (iv) DCT (iv)
5. Total number of cortical nephrons are (i) 85% (ii) 70% (iii) 15% (iv) 30%. (i)
6. Following is not the component of JGA (i) Macula densa cell (ii) Intercalated cells (iii) Lacis cell (iv) JG cells. (ii)
7. JG cells secrete rennin in response to (i) rise of blood pressure (ii) increase of sympathetic activity (iii) rise of Na^+ load (iv) rise of ECF volume. (ii)
8. Erythropoietic factor is mainly released by (i) interstitial cells of peritubular capillary bed (ii) JG cells (iii) Lacis cells (iv) all of the above. (i)
9. Normal blood supply of kidney is (i) 1300 ml/min (ii) 2300 ml/min (iii) 500 ml/min (iv) 100 ml/min. (i)
10. The normal glomerular capillary hydrostatic pressure is (i) 10 mmHg (ii) 0 mmHg (iii) 32 mmHg (iv) 60 mmHg. (iv)
11. The normal Bowman's capsular oncotic pressure is (i) 10 mmHg (ii) 0 mmHg (iii) 32 mmHg (iv) 60 mmHg. (ii)
12. The factors allow filtration are as follows except (i) glomerular capillary hydrostatic pressure (ii) Bowman's capsular oncotic pressure (iii) Bowman's capsular hydrostatic pressure (iv) none of the above. (iii)
13. Filtration coefficient is determined by following factors except (i) number of glomerulus (ii) thickness of glomerulus (iii) arterial BP (iv) surface area of capillary bed. (iii)
14. Following neurohumoral substances increases the GFR except (i) Norepinephrine (ii) Epinephrine (iii) Prostaglandins (iv) all of the above. (iii)
15. The Tm of glucose is (i) 30 mg/min (ii) 30 gm/min (iii) 80 mg/min (iv) 300 mg/min. (iv)
16. Following substances are actively reabsorbed by the renal tubules except (i) sodium (ii) bicarbonate (iii) uric acid (iv) urea. (iv)
17. Following substances are passively reabsorbed by the renal tubules except (i) glucose (ii) water (iii) chloride ion (iv) urea. (i)
18. In presence of maximum ADH the water is reabsorbed by the renal tubule is (i) 88% (ii) 99% (iii) 1% (iv) 12%. (ii)
19. Following substances are secreted by the renal tubules except (i) K^+ (ii) H^+ (iii) NH_4^+ (iv) urea. (iv)
20. The normal value of urea clearence is (i) 60-90 ml/min (ii) 120-150 ml/min (iii) 300-320 ml/min (iv) none of the above. (i)
21. The renal threshold of glucose is (i) 100 mg (ii) 200 mg (iii) 400 mg (iv) 80 mg. (ii)
22. The normal pH of urine is (i) 4-8 (ii) 1-3 (iii) 6-9 (iv) none of the above. (i)
23. Renal plasma flow is determined by (i) PAH clearance (ii) Inulin clearance (iii) Urea clearance (iv) Thermal dilution method. (i)

24. Diluting segment of nephron is (i) ascending segment of Henlee's loop (ii) descending segment of Henlee's loop (iii) early DCT (iv) collecting duct. (iii)
25. Following is the sensitive marker of renal function (i) plasma glucose level (ii) plasma creatinine level (iii) blood urea level (iv) plasma amino acid level. (ii)
26. Glucose reabsorption mostly occurs in the (i) PCT (ii) Loop of Henlee (iii) DCT (iv) collecting duct. (i)
27. The part of the nephron impermeable to water is (i) PCT (ii) Ascending limb of Loop of Henlee (iii) DCT (iv) collecting duct. (ii)
28. Facultative reabsorption of water from DCT is influenced by (i) cortisol (ii) Aldosterone (iii) ADH (iv) Adrenalin. (iii)
29. In the absence of ADH the maximum amount of filtered water is absorbed in the (i) PCT (ii) CT (iii) DCT (iv) Henlee's loop. (i)
30. After ingestion of 1 litre of water there is increase in urine formation which is due to (i) increased glucose in urine (ii) increase in electrolytes in urine (iii) increase in GFR and decrease in ADH release (iv) increase in GFR and increase in ADH release. (iii)
31. Nocturnal enuresis in children occurs due to (i) increase in ADH release (ii) increase in aldosterone release (iii) increase in ANP release (iv) decrease in ADH release. (iv)
32. In the PCT the H^+ secreted mainly buffered by (i) Protein (ii) NH_3 (iii) Na_2HPO_4 (iv) HCO_3^-. (iv)
33. Angiotensin –II causes the following effects except (i) inhibition of thirst sensation (ii) stimulation of ADH release (iii) stimulation of aldosterone release (iv) vasoconstriction. (i)
34. The normal daily urinary output in normal healthy person is (i) 500 ml (ii) 1500 ml (iii) 5000 ml (iv) 50 ml. (ii)
35. The normal filtered load of sodium in kidneys is about (i) 1 kg /day (ii) 2 kg /day (iii) 5 kg /day (iv) 0.5 kg/day. (iv)
36. The acidity of urine is chiefly due to the presence of (i) bicarbonate (ii) phosphoric acid (iii) acetoacetic acid (iv) lactic acid. (iv)
37. Goldblatt kidney (i) is an ischemic kidney (ii) produces renin (iii) both (iv) none of the above. (iii)
38. Alkali reserve of blood means (i) blood bicarbonate (ii) blood phosphate (iii) all of the buffers of blood taken together (iv) only I and ii. (iii)
39. The urinary bladder is innervated by (i) sympathetic (ii) parasympathetic (iii) somatic nerves (iv) all of the above. (iii)
40. The physiological capacity of urinary bladder is (i) 100 ml (ii) 200 ml (iii) 250-450 ml (iv) 500-750 ml. (ii)

9 Endocrinal System

A. Long type:

1. Enumerate the hormones secreted by pituitary gland. Describe the function, mode of action and regulation of GH. Write in brief about the effects of hypersecretion of anterior pituitary hormones.

Different hormones secreted by the anterior pituitary gland are:

I. Growth hormone (GH)
II. Prolactin (PRL)
III. Thyroid stimulating hormone (TSH)
IV. Adreno cortico stimulating (trophic) hormone (ACTH)
V. Follicle stimulating hormone (FSH)
VI. Leutinising hormone (LH)

Growth hormone (GH):

- **Plasma GH level** 5-8 ng/ml in children
  2-4 ng/ml in adult.
- **Function:** The functions of GH are as follows:

1. On Growth:
   - It increases the number and size of the cell of almost all the tissues.
   - It increases the growth of long bone at epiphyseal cartilage till the fusion between shaft and each end of epiphysis (i.e. before adolescence).
   - It also promotes periosteal growth by stimulating osteoblasts and thus is responsible for increasing thickness of the bone (after adolescence).
2. On protein metabolism: **Anabolic effect**
   - It increases protein synthesis by—
     (i) increasing amino acid transport through cell membrane → increasing amino acid level in cells.
     (ii) RNA translation and DNA transcription.
   - It decreases protein and amino acid catabolism by increasing fat catabolism. This is why it is known as ***"protein sparer"***.

3. On Fat metabolism: **Catabolic effect.**
   - It increases mobilisation of fatty acids (FA) from adipose tissue → Increased triglyceride content in adipose tissue and increase in FA level in blood.
   - It promotes conversion of FA to acetyl CoA which is utilised by TCA cycle to obtain energy.
   - It increases hepatic oxidation of FA to ketone bodies, acetoacetic and β-OH-butyric acid (ketogenic effect).
   - It also causes release of ketone bodies from liver into the blood.
4. On carbohydrate metabolism: **Hyperglycemic effect.**
   - It reduces the peripheral utilisation of glucose by the cells → increase in blood sugar level (Pituitary diabetes).
   - It increases glycogen formation and deposition in the cell.
   - It stimulates insulin secretion directly and also by indirectly through blood glucose level → continuous secretion results burning out of the β cells of pancreas → development of diabetes mellitus.
5. Growth hormone induces growth of thymus gland.
6. It also increases milk production in lactating women.

- **Mode of action of GH:** Action of GH on tissue and metabolism is mediated both by directly and indirectly.

I. Indirect action (Growth Promoting action): It is mediated through a family of polypeptides called **Somatomedins.** GH stimulates liver to synthesize and release somatomedin (mainly 'C' type) which binds with a carrier protein in blood and slowly enters into the tissue to promote prolong growth promoting action in skeletal and extra skeletal tissues like bone growth, protein synthesis and cell proliferation.

II. Direct (Anti insulin) action: GH directly influences fat and carbohydrate metabolism to increase lipolysis and blood sugar level.

- **Control of GH secretion:** Secretion of GH is mainly regulated by hypothalamo-hypophyseal target organ axis as illustrated by diagram (Fig. 9.1).

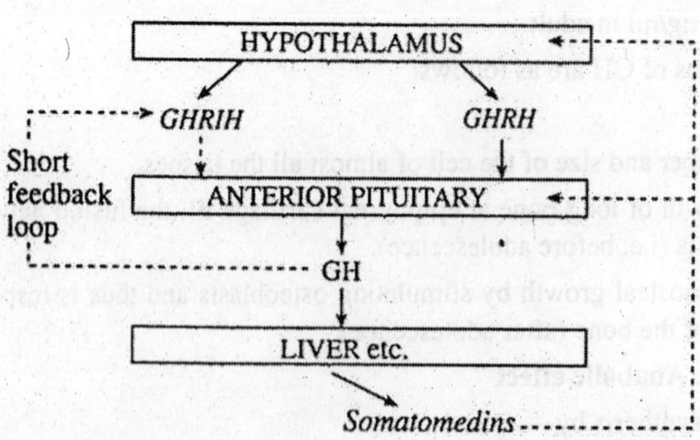

Fig. 9.1: Schematic diagram showing control of GH secretion (Solid line indicates stimulation and dotted line indicates inhibition

Under different conditions like under nutrition and stress, different stimulus like starvation, hypoglycemia, low FA level in blood, exercise, emotion, excitement, trauma can stimulate the hypothalamus to secrete GHRH which acts on anterior pituitary to secrete GH. GH inturn is responsible for release of somatomedins from liver, pancreas etc. Increase of blood level of somatomedins inhibits further secretion of GH by directly acting on pituitary and indirectly by inhibiting GHRH release from hypothalamus. Growth hormone can also inhibit it's own secretion via a short feedback loop by releasing GHRIH (somatostatins) which inturn inhibits synthesis and release of GH

Hypersecretion of GH: It results—

a. **Gigantism:** In children

- Cause: Excessive increase in length of long bone due to oversecretion of GH before adolescence.
- Characteristics: — 8-9 feet height
  — Hyperglycemia

b. **Acromegaly:** In adult

- Cause: Excessive growth of membranous bones (e.g. cranium, nose, supraorbital ridge, lower jaw etc.) as their growth is not ceased even after adolescence.
- Features:
  - Normal height as long bone can not grow after adolescence due to fusion of epiphysis of long bones with the shafts.
  - ***Prominent brow*** due to enlargement of the frontal, mastoid, ethmoid and maxillary sinuses.
  - ***Prognathism*** i.e. elongation and widening of the mandible.
  - ***Acral parts*** due to periosteal growth of metacarpals and metatarsals.
  - ***Acromegalic facies*** i.e. thickening of the skin and coarsening of facial features.
  - Enlargement of heart (caridomegaly), liver (hepatomegaly), spleen (spleenomegaly) and kidney (renomegaly).

2. Name the hormones of posterior pituitary. Discuss the source, function, regulation and disorders of ADH.

Hormones of posterior pituitary: Two hormones are secreted from this lobe, these are antidiuretic hormone (ADH) and oxytocin.

ADH:

- **Source:** Supraoptic nucleus of hypothalamus.
- **Function:**
  1. It increases water permeability of distal convoluted tubules (mild action) and collecting duct (mainly) → increases water reabsorption → decreases urinary output.
  2. It also stimulates ACTH release from anterior pituitary → increases aldosterone secretion.
  3. It decreases medullary blood flow.
  4. In excessive doses it causes peripheral vasoconstriction → increases BP.
- **Control of ADH secretion:** ADH secretion is regulated by hypothalamus in response to different stimuli like hyperosmolality, hypovoluemia, stress.

  (I) **Hyperosmolality:** Increase osmolality in body fluids stimulates hypothalamic osmoreceptor which inturn intiates action potential to stimulate release of ADH from posterior pituitary. The detail mechanism is as follows:

  Any increase in osmolality of body fluid → increase in osmolality of ECF in brain tissue → water moves out from osmoreceptor → shrinkage of osmoreceptor → generation and conduction of impulse down the Hypothalamo-Hypophyseal tract → secretion of ADH → drainage to general circulation → increase in water permeability in renal tubules → increase water volume in ECF → **Correts the osmolality.**

(II) **Hypovolemia:** It is by following mechanism:

Hypovolemia → Stimulation of venous low pressure baroreceptor → stimulation of supraoptic nucleus of hypothalamus via vagus nerve → increase in ADH release → increase water reabsorption → **normalcy** of body fluid volume.

(III) **Stress:** Different stressful conditions like exercise, pain, fear etc. can stimulate ADH release directly by stimulating supraoptic nucleus or hypothalamus.

- ***Disorders of ADH:***

A. Disorders of hyposecretion of ADH: Diabetes insipidus.

■ Cause:

(I) Neurogenic: Failure of ADH secretion due to genetic defect or destruction or damage of hypothalamus or posterior pituitary resulted from head injury, tumour, surgery, encephalitis etc.

(II) Nephrogenic: Failure of renal response to ADH

■ Features:

❑ Polyuria due to decreased water reabsorption by kidney.

❑ Polydipsia due to thirst sensation.

B. Disorders of Hypersecretion of ADH: SIADH (Syndrome of inappropriate secretion of ADH). See under short note.

3. Name the thyroid hormones with their source. Describe the synthesis, storage, release and transport, functions and regulation of thyroid follicular hormones.

The thyroid hormones are:

1. Thyroxine (90%) and Tri-iodothyronine (10%): synthesised by thyroid follicular cells.
2. Thyrocalcitonin or calcitonin: synthesised by parafollicular cells of thyroid gland.

Thyroid follicular (T_3 and T_4) hormones:

- ***Biosynthesis:***

Step 1: *Absorption of dietary iodine* in GI tract and subsequent conversion to reduced form i.e. iodide (KI).

Step 2: *Iodide trapping* (Iodide pump): The active transport of iodide by the thyroid follicular cell from the circulation is energy requiring process which is primarily dependant on Na^+-K^+ pump present in basolateral surface of follicular cell membrane. The outward movement of Na results uptake of Na along with Iodine by the carrier protein called **Na-I-symporter (NIS)** by the thyroid follicular cell from ECF. This results rise of concentration of iodine inside the cell from which it is again pumped to colloid by the help of another carrier protein called **Pendrin**. This mechanism is called as **Iodide trapping.**

Step 3: *Oxidation of Iodide* by the follicular cell to either nascent iodine (Io) or I_3^- by the enzyme peroxidase in presence of H_2O_2.

Step 4: *Organification of thyroglobulin*: The protein forming mechanism within the epithelial cell synthesises the protein thyroglobulin and is released through the apical cell membrane into the colloid matter. Seconds to minutes after it's secretion the oxidised iodine binds with the thyrosin amino acid of thyroglobulin molecule to first from monoiodotyrosins (MIT) and then diodotyrosine (DIT) by the enzyme iodinase.

Step 5: *Coupling*: One MIT and DIT are formed then one molecule of MIT – couples with one molecule of DIT to form T_3 and 2 molecules of DIT fuse together via an either bridge to form T_4.

Step 6: *Storage*: After synthesis each thyroglobulin molecule contains 5-6 molecule of thyroxin T_4, and an average of 1 T_3 molecule for every 14 molecules of T_4. In this form thyroid hormones are stored in the follicule in an amount sufficient to supply the body with its normal thyroid hormone requirement, for 2-3 months.

Step 7: *Release*: When necessary the apical portion of the thyroid cell engulfs little thyroglobulin containing thyroid hormones from the colloid of the acinus by the process of endocylosis. The engulfed thyroglobulin now fuses with the lysosomes of the follicular cells resulting proteolysis of thyroglobulin by the enzyme protease to release, T_3 and T_4 into the venous blood draining the thyroid.

1 ***Transport of thyroid hormone*:** T_4 and T_3 combine with plasma protein and is circulated via blood.

- 80% of T_3 and T_4 bind with thyroxine binding globuline (TBG)
- 10-20% of T3 and T4 bind with thyroxine binding prealbumin (TBPA)
- Remaining percentage of hormones bind with albumin.

1 ***Function of T_4 and T_3*:** The function of thyroid hormone (T_4 and T_3) can be divided into 3 major groups as follows:

(a) On growth and development: T_4 and T_3 affect in all aspects of growth i.e. physical (skeletal, muscular, visceral), mental and sexual. The general effect is to cause nuclear transcription of large number of genes. Therefore all cells of body, enzymes, proteins and other substances increase that help in overall growth. An important effect of thyroid hormones is to promote growth and development of brain during fetal life and for the first few years of postnatal life. If the fetus does not secrete sufficient thyroid hormones there is poor brain development resulting mental retardation. This type of child is known as ***Idiot child.***

(b) On metabolism:

(i) **General metabolism**—Increase in BMR as much as 60-100% by increasing $Na^+ - K^+$ ATPase activity.

(ii) **Carbohydrate metabolism**—stimulates almost all aspects of carbohydrate metabolism indirectly may be by enhancing the activity of adrenaline and insulin. The effects are :

- Gluconeogenesis
- Glycogenolysis
- Increased rate of glucose absorption from GI tract.

(iii) **Fat metabolism:** All aspects of fat metabolism are enhanced by the thyroid hormones. These effects are:

- $\downarrow$ the quantity of cholesterol, phospholipids and triglycerides in the plasma
- $\uparrow$ free fatty acid level in the blood
- $\uparrow$ oxidation of FFA by the cells
- mobilisation of fat from adipose tissue.

(iv) **Protein metabolism:** In moderate concentration thyroid hormones have anabolic effect causing increase in RNA and protein synthesis and in high concentration of hormones there is catabolic effect on proteins.

(v) **Vitamin metabolism:** It increases the need of the vitamin which are essential part of enymes and coenzymes.

(vi) **Mineral metabolism:** It increases loss of Ca^{++} and thus causes osteoporosis.

(c) On individual organ system:

(i) **Cardiovascular system:** It has following effects:

- Vasodilation and increase in blood flow to the tissue to facilitate rapid utilisation of O_2.
- Increase in cardiac output to facilitate increase of blood flow to the tissue.
- Increase in the excitability of heart to cause increase in heat rate.
- Increase in strength of heart beat.
- Increase in circulatory blood volume due to vasodilatation.
- Increase in systolic BP and decrease in diastolic BP → pulse pressure and no change of mean pressure.

(ii) **On respiratory system:** It increases both the rate and depth of respiration.

(iii) **On Gastrointestinal system:** It increases:

- appetite → increase in food intake
- rate of secretion of digestive juices
- motility of the GI tract. (Thus **lack of thyroid hormone results constipation**).

(iv) **On central nervous system:** It promotes the development of brain during fetal life and also in early years of post natal life.

(v) **On sleep**: In case of hyperthyroidism there is a feeling of constant tiredness but difficult to sleep.

(vi) **On muscular system:** Normal level of thyroid hormones is required for normal activity of muscle. Excessive thyroid hormones results weakness of muscle and lack of thyroid hormones result sluggishness of muscle.

(vii) **On reproductive system**: Normal level of thyroid hormone is required for normal activity of reproductive system. Lack of thyroid hormones in male causes complete loss of libido and excess of thyroid hormones causes impotence. In female lack of thyroid hormone results menorrhagia, polymenorrhoea and irregular menstrual cycle.

1 ***Regulation of T_3 and T_4 secretion***: There are 3 major mechanisms by which thyroid hormone secretion is controlled. These are:

(a) ***Hypothalamic—pituitary—thyroid axis***: Thyroid stimulating hormone (TSH) is the major regulator of the thyroid hormone secretion.

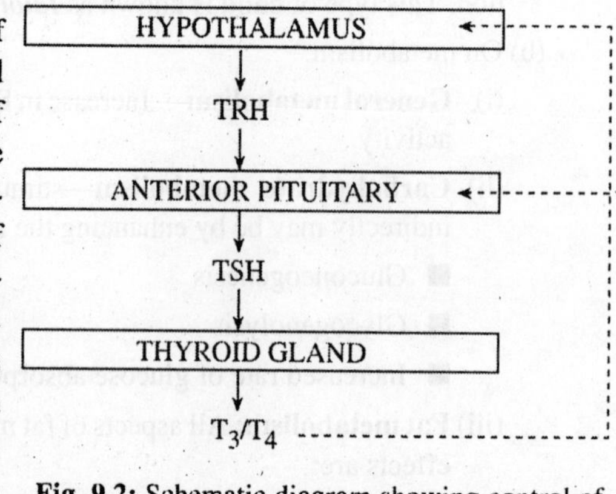

Fig. 9.2: Schematic diagram showing control of thyroid secretion (Solid line indicates stimulation and dotted line indicates inhibition)

In response to different neurogenic stimulation and also cold, hypothalamus secretes TRH which binds with the specific cell surface receptors on pituitary thyrotropes to stimulate TSH synthesis and secretion. TSH inturn increases the secretion of T_3 and T_4 by the thyroid gland as illustrated by following (Fig. 9.2).

TSH increases the thyroid hormone secretion by following ways:

(i) Increased proteolysis of thyroglobulin → increased release of thyroid hormones.
(ii) Increasing activity of Iodide pump.
(iii) Increasing iodination and coupling reaction
(iv) Increasing size and secretory activity of thyrosis cells
(v) Increasing number of thyroid cells.

(b) ***Feedback regulation of thyroid secretion***: Increased level of T_3 and T_4 hormone in blood exerts a negative feedback control on mainly pituitary and partly hypothalamus to secrete TSH and TRH respectively as shown in above mentioned block diagram. Thus secretion of T_3 and T_4 is reduced by the low level of TSH from anterior pituitary.

(c) ***Autoregulation***: Up to a certain limit availability of iodine for synthesis of thyroid hormones remains constant by this process even though there is a wide fluctuation of food iodine. For example:

Deficiency of dietary iodine → Iodine trapping mechanism becomes super efficient → more utilisation of I_2 from blood → more synthesis of T_3 and T_4.

Similarly if dietary iodine intake becomes high iodine trapping mechanism becomes less effective and thus less amount of I_2 is absorbed by the thyroid follicular cell resulting fall of thyroid hormone secretion.

4. Describe the functions of PTH. How PTH, Vit D_3 and Calcitonin helps in Ca^{+2} regulation.

Parathormone (PTH): *Function*:

1. *It causes rise of serum Ca^{2+} level by—*

(a) Promoting ***bone resorption*** i.e. mobilisation of Ca^{2+} from bone to ECF in two phases as follows:

(i) Immediate phase: Within a few minutes to 2 hours after PTH release, there is an increase mobilisation of Ca^{2+} from bony fluid to ECF and thereby to plasma due to activation of osteocytic activity (osteocytic pump activity) present within the osteocytic membrane system. This effect is known as ***osteolysis***.

(ii) Slow or delayed phase: After about 12 hours of PTH administration again hypercalcemia is seen which is due to activation of osteoclastic activity by the PTH. Though PTH can not directly influence the osteoclastic activity, the receptors present on the osteoblast when get bound with PTH not only the Ca^{2+} pump is activated but also the osteoblast sends the signal to osteoclast to activate it. This activation of osteoclast occurs in two stages:

– Immediate activation of osteoclasts that are already formed.
– Formation of new osteoclastic system.

Once activated these osteoclast secretes proteolytic enymes, acids (citric and lactic acid) which causes digestion and desolution of organic matrix of bone and eventually releases Ca^{2+} to blood.

(b) *acting on kidney in the following manner*:

(i) PTH increases Ca^{2+} reabsorption in the distal tubule, collecting tubule and collecting duct and thereby increases plasma Ca^{2+} level.
(ii) It converts Vit-D to active 1-25 dihydroxycholecalciferol in the kidney which increases Ca^{2+} absorption by the GIT.

(c) *acting on GIT*: PTH greatly enhances both calcium and $PO_4^{=}$absorption from the duodenum by increasing 1-25 – Vit. D_3.

2. It decreases serum $PO_4^{=}$ level by inhibiting $PO_4^{=}$ reabsorption in the proximal tubule of the kidney allowing excretion of more PO_4^{-} in urine.
3. It also increases urinary excretion of Na^+, K^+ and HCO_3^- and decreases urinary excretion of NH_4^{2+} and H^+ ions.

Integrated role of PTH, Calcitonin and Vitamin D_3 in bone metabolism (Ca^{2+} regulation):

Normal level of plasma calcium varrics from 9-11 mg%. This level of calcium is required to be maintained because of it's effect on neuromuscular and cardiac excitability and also proper bone mineralisation and maintenance of cell membrane integrity. Mainly three hormones namely PTH, calcitonin and vit-D_3 are responsible for regulation of the plasma calcium level. However in humans calcitonin has minimal role in rugulating the plasma calcium level except in some pathological cases like Paget's disease and osteosclerosis.

In response to fall of plasma calcium level there is increase in PTH release which increases the plasma calcium level by acting on bone, kidney and also in GIT as illustrated by flow chart FC 9A, whereas in response to any rise of plasma calcium level beyond the normal range there is decreased release in PTH which results withdrawl of its above mentioned affect to minimise the plasma calcium level (FC 9B).

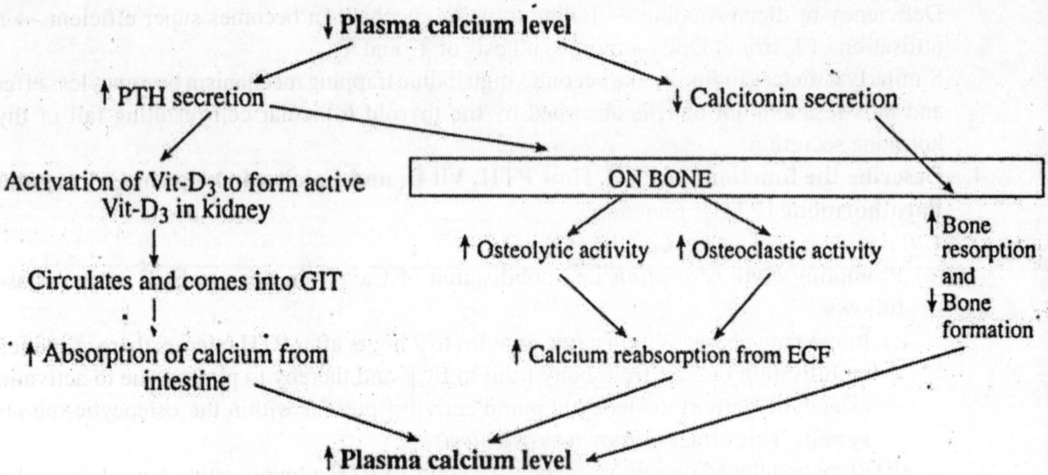

FC 9A: Schematic diagram showing integrative action of PTH, Calcitonin and Vit-D_3

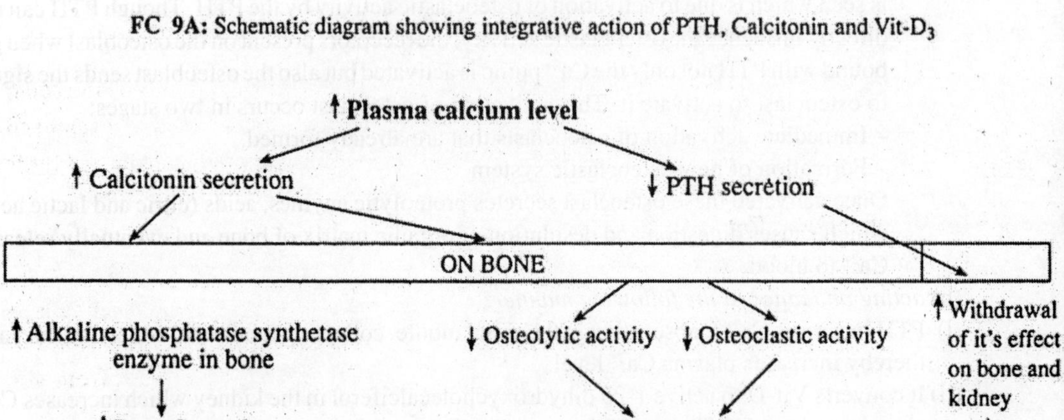

FC 9B: Schematic diagram showing integrative action of PTH, Calcitonin and Vit-D_3

5. Enlist the hormones secreted from pancreas. Explain the functions and regulation of Insulin secretion.

The Pancreatic hormones are:

(a) Insulin:

- **Source:** β cells of islets of Langerhans of pancreas

(b) Glucagon:

- **Source:** α cells of islets of Langerhans of pancreas

(c) Somatostatin:

- **Source:** D cells of islets of pancreas.

(d) Pancreatic polypeptide:

- **Source:** F Cells of islets of Langarhans.

Function of Insulin: Insulin reduces the blood glucose level by affecting carbohydrate, fat and protein metabolism.

(a) *Carbohydrate metabolism*: It increases—

(i) Glucose uptake by most of the tissues by increasing glucose permeability through plasma membrane and thus increases peripheral utilisation of glucose.

(ii) Glycogenesis in liver, muscle, etc. by:

- inhibiting phosphorylase enzymes which causes splitting of liver glycogen to glucose.
- increasing activity of glucokinase which converts glucose to glucose $-6\text{-}PO_4^{=}$ which can not cross the cell membrane.
- increasing activity of glycogen synthetic enzymes like phosphofructokinase, glycogen synthetase etc.

(iii) It decreases glucose formation by inhibiting glucose synthetic enzyme i.e. carboxylase and PEP carboxykinase to inhibit gluconeogenesis.

(iv) It promotes conversion of all excess glucose into fatty acids in adipose tissue.

(b) *Protein matabolism*: **Protein synthetic action**

(i) It increases transport of amino acids into the cells.

(ii) It inhibits catabolism of proteins and decreases rate of release of amino acids by the cells.

(iii) In liver it decreases gluconeogenesis and thus conserves amino acids for protein synthesis.

(iv) It also increases translation of mRNA and transcription of selected DNA aiding synthesis of more enzymes that promote carbohydrate, protein and fat storage.

(c) *On fat metabolism*: **Fat storage and synthesis**

(i) It increases synthesis of FFA and triglycerides in muscles, adipose tissue and liver by:

- stimulating lipoprotein lipase which causes breakdown of triglycerides in other cells → ↑ FFA in blood →↑ FFA in adipose tissue →↑ triglycerides formation.
- inhibiting hormone sensitive lipase in adipose tissue →↓ release of FFA from stored triglycerides.

(ii) It increases fat storage in adipose tissue by activating lipoprotein lipase in the capillary wall of adipose tissue → splits triglyceride into FA → absorption of fatty acids by fat cell → conversion to triglycerides.

Thus insulin is *glycogenic, anti gluconeogenic, antilipolytic* and antikitotic. Because of these qualities it favours storage of absorbed nutrients and thus is known as *Hormone of Energy storage* or *Hormone of abundance.*

Regulation of insulin secretion:

(a) *Negative feedback* control by blood glucose and amino acid level (**Substrate control**): Insulin secretion is mainly controlled by level of blood glucose and also by amino acids. Acute elevation of glucose causes increase in concentration of insulin in two phases (Fig. 9.3).

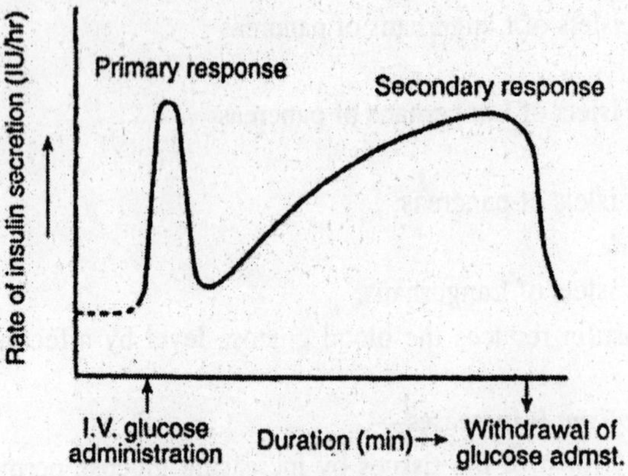

Fig. 9.3: Regulation of insulin secretion

(i) Rapid phase (Primary secretion): Within 3-5 mins of glucose administration insulin secretion increases 10 times due to release of **preformed (Labile pool)** insulin which returns to normal in another 5-10 mins.

(ii) Slow phase (Secondary secretion): Again after 15 minutes insulin secretion rises for 2-3 hours due to release of **newly synthesised** insulin. The rise of level is also greater than the initial phase.

(b) *Neural Control*:

(i) Control by ANS:

- Stimulation of splanchnic (sympathetic adrenergic) nerves → release of catecholamines → stimulation of α adrenergic receptors → decrease insulin secretion.
- Whereas stimulation of vagus → ACh release → increase in insulin secretion.

(ii) Control by CNS: Hypothalamus by controlling ANS regulates insulin secretion in following ways:

- Feeding → absorption of food stuffs from GIT → stimulation of vagus via hypothalamus → increase insulin secretion.
- Starvation → sympathetic activation via hypothalamus → decrease in insulin secretion.

(c) *Hormonal control*: Different hormones also regulate secretion of insulin. **For example:**

- GI hormones like Gastric Inhibitory Peptide (GIP), gastrin, secretin, CCK-PZ etc. increase insulin secretion.
- GH increases insulin secretion directly by stimulating β cell. GHIH has reverse action.
- Glucagon suppresses insulin secretion by paracrine effect on β cells.

6. Discuss the function and regulation of glucagon secretion. Add a note on diabetes mellitus.

***Glucagon*:**

- **Function:**

(a) Glucagon **increases blood sugar** level by—

(i) promoting glycogenolysis in liver by facilitating conversion of glycogen to glucose -1- PO_4* and thence glucose.

(ii) increasing gluconeogenic action by—

- activating enzymes of gluconeogenic pathway.
- activating enzymes required for amino acid transport to the liver.

(b) Beyond physiological limit of glucogon concentration in the blood it also—

(i) activates adipose cell lipase to increase lipolysis and thus increase FFA level in blood.

(ii) inhibits storage of triglycerides in the liver and prevents the uptake of FA by the hepatocyte. This increases the availability of FA in blood.

So glucagon is anti insulin i.e. gluconeogenic, glycogenolytic and lipolytic and thereby called as *Hormone of energy release.*

- **Regulation:**
  - Decrease in blood glucose level by **negative feedback** way increase glucagon secretion and vice versa. Though this effect is **dependant on insulin.**
  - Amino acids (specially gluconeogenic) increase glucagon secretion **(This action is not antagonist to insulin action).**
  - Insulin inhibits the glucagon release by paracrine control on α cells.
  - Both sympathetic and vagus stimulation increases glucagon secretion.
  - Some GI hormones like CCK, gastrin, somatostatin, secretin etc. inhibit glucagon secretion.
  - Exaustive exercise increases glucagon secretion upto 5 times without fall of blood glucose level.

Diabetes mellitus:

- **Definition:** It is defined as the clinical condition which is characterised by **"flow of sugar"** in urine.
- **Cause:** Decreased secretion of insulin resulted either from hereditary defect or obesity in which condition β cells becomes unresponsive and also decreases it's number.
- **Characteristics:**
  - *General:*

— Hyperglycemia	— Glycosuria
— Polyuria	— Polydipsia
— Polyphagia	— Loss of weight
— Hypovolemia	— Hypotension
— Nausea	— Hypokalemia
— Ketosis, fatty liver	— Muscle wasting

  - *Long term complications:*
    - ❑ Atherosclerosis due to deposition of LDL which can lead angina, MI and cerebro vascular disorder.
    - ❑ Microangiopathy i.e. thickening of capillary wall due to deposition of oxidised product of glucose 'Sorbitol' which can block renal arterial capillary (***diabetic nephropathy***) and retinal arterial capillary (***diabetic retinopathy***).
    - ❑ Neuropathy due to degeneration of peripheral nerve fiber.
- **Types:** 2 types:

(a) Insulin dependant diabetes mellitus (IDDM) or Type-I or Juvenile diabetes:

- occurs due to autoimmuno disease
- appears below age of 40

- loss of β cell and deficiency of insulin
- not associated with obesity

(b) Noninsulin dependent diabetes mellitus (NIDDM) or Type II diabetes:

- occurs due to pancreatic disease or Cushing's syndrome or Acromegaly
- appears after age of 40
- total loss of insulin secretion
- rarely associated with ketosis

7. Describe in brief the regulation of blood sugar level. What is glucose tolerance test?

Regulation of blood glucose: Regulation of plasma glucose within the normal range is very critical for survival because plasma glucose is the main fuel of the nervous tissue. The plasma glucose level is regulated basically by the level of plasma glucose by regulating the secretion of different hormones like insulin, glucagon, epinephrine, growth hormone, thyroid hormones and cortisol. After a meal when the absorption of end products of digestion results an increase in blood glucose level there is increased secretion of insulin and inhibition of glucagon release. Consequently glucose is metabolised to yield energy in the liver and skeletal muscle as well as stored as glycogen. When the glycogen stores are saturated all the extra glucose is converted to fatty acids in the liver which are stored as triglycerides in the adipose tissue. This results in decrease in blood glucose level to the normal level.

Whereas about 6 hours after food intake when glucose delivery to the circulation stops resulting fall of glucose level in the blood, the glucagon secretion is increased and insulin secretion is decreased. If fasting condition is further continued there are recruitment of epinephrine and then GH and other hormones which ultimately increases blood glucose level by gluconeogenesis, lipolysis, increased ketosis as well as decreasing glucose utilization by peripheral tissues. The detail mechanism is illustrated by the flow chart (Fig. FC 9C).

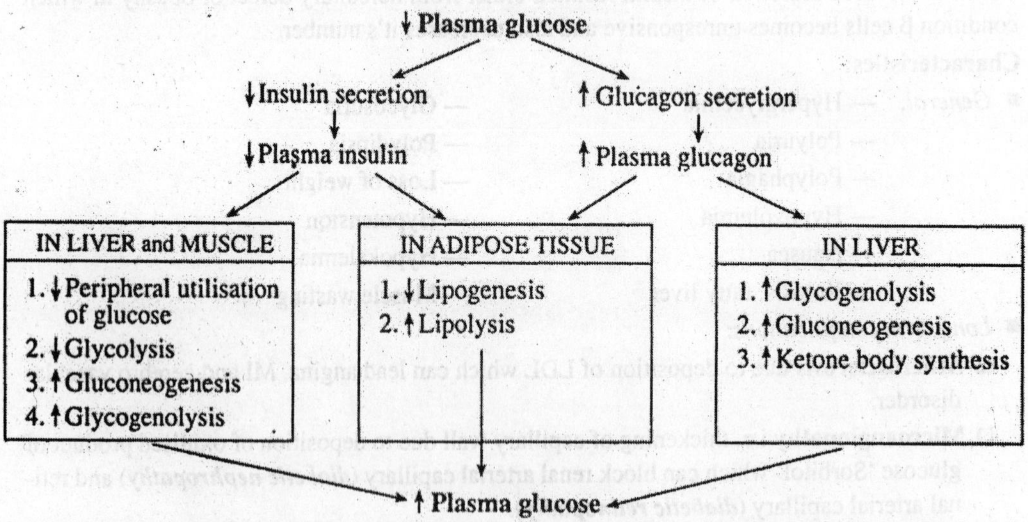

FC 9C: Integrative role of insulin and glucagon in regulating blood glucose

- **Glucose tolerance test (GTT):** This is the test by which the diabetes mellitus is diagnosed. For this test fasting blood glucose level of the person is measured and then glucose is fed to him orally at a dose of 1G/Kg body weight and post prandial (after glucose administration) blood glucose level is measured from the blood samples collected at least upto 2 hr with half an hour intervals. The values are plotted in a graph which is known as ***glucose tolerance chart*** (Fig. 9.4).

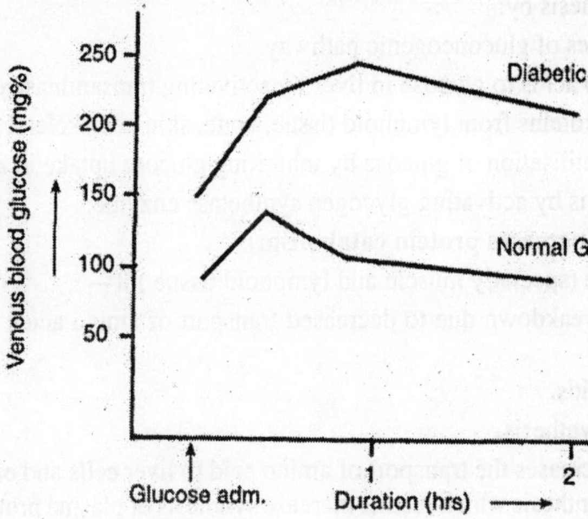

Fig. 9.4: Graphical representation of glucose tolerance test in normal and diabetic person

- **Analysis of data:**

(i) The person is **normal** if—

- his fasting blood glucose is < 80 mg%
- post prandial (PP) value is < 140 mg%
- Post prandial value returns to fasting level after 2 hours

(ii) The person is **diabetic** if

- his fasting blood glucose level is > 120 mg%
- his PP value is > 200 mg%
- PP value does not return to fasting level even after 2 hr.
- at least 2 PP value as high as 200 mg% or more

8. Classify the hormones secreted by adrenal cortex with the example. Explain the source, actions and regulation of secretion of cortisol.

There are 3 major types of adrenocortical hormones-mineralocorticoids, glucocorticoids and sex steroids.

A. Mineralocorticoids:

- Example: Aldosterone, Deoxycorticosterone

B. Glucocorticoids:

- Example:
  - Natural form-Cortisol (mainly), corticosterone, cortisone
  - Synthetic form-prednisone, cortisone, methylprednisolone, dexamethasone.

C. Adrenal androgens:

- Example: Androstenidione, Dehydroandrostenidione (DHEA), oestrogen and progesteron and testosterone in small amount.

Cortisols:

- Source: Mainly zona fasiculata and partly zona reticularis.

- Function:

(i) On carbohydrate metabolism: **(Increases blood glucose level)**: It increases blood glucose level by:

I. increasing gluconeogenesis by:
- activating all enzymes of gluconeogenic pathway.
- by converting amino acids to glucose in liver by activating transaminase enzyme.
- by breaking down proteins from lymphoid tissue, bone, skin and skeletal muscle.

II. decreasing peripheral utilisation of glucose by inhibiting glucose uptake in adipose tissue.

III. increasing glycogenesis by activating glycogen synthetase enzyme.

(ii) On protein metabolism **(Increases protein catabolism)**:

I. **In extrahepatic tissue** (specially muscle and lymphoid tissue) it—
- increases protein breakdown due to decreased transport of amino acids and formation of RNA.
- mobilises amino acids.
- decreases protein synthesis.

II. **In hepatic tissue** it increases the transport of amino acid to liver cells and enhances enzymes required for protein synthesis which results increase synthesis of plasma proteins and increase conversion of amino acids to glucose.

(iii) On fat metabolism: **(Increases FA level in blood and ketosis)**:
- Glucocorticoids increases fatty acid level in blood by promoting mobilisation of fatty acids from the adipose tissues.
- Glucocorticoids increases ketone body formation (ketosis) by increasing utilisation of fatty acids for energy (secondarily due to reduction of glucose availability in the cell by cortisol). However this effect occurs only if insulin secretion is less.
- It promotes deposition of fat in unusual sites on the body to result ***moon like face*** and ***buffalo hump***.

(iv) Mineral metabolism: **(Mild aldosterone like activity)**: It—
- increases Na^+ reabsorption by renal tubules.
- decreases K^+ reabsorption by renal tubules.
- decreases Ca^{+2} reabsorption by renal tubules.
- decreases Ca^{+2} absorption in GIT.

(v) On nucleic acid metabolism: It decreases nucleic acid synthesis except in liver.

(vi) Non metabolic effects:

(I) ***Anti-inflammatory effects***: In response to any tissue injury by trauma or infection they become inflammated because of increased blood flow, leakage of large quantities of plasma out of capillaries and infiltration of leucocytes for healing. Cortisol blocks the early stages of inflammation and rapid resolution of the healing by:
- stabilising lysosomal membrane to prevent rupture of lysosomes and release of proteolytic enzymes from damaged tissue.
- decreasing leucocyte margination, emigration, chemotaxis, phagocytosis of bacteria.
- reducing release of histamin and interleukin-1 which causes rise of body temperature.
- decreasing capillary permeability to prevent loss of plasma into tissues.
- suppressing lymphoid tissue to reduce lymphocyte and antibody formation.
- healing process is enhanced by increasing mobilisation of amino acids for repair and increasing amount of FA and glucose for cellular energy.

(II) ***Anti-stress effect*:** The exact mechanism by which glucocorticoid combats the manifestations of stress is not known but it is presumed that in stressful condition it helps the tissues to get more fatty acids for energy and more blood supply to meet the increased demand of O_2 and washing out of CO_2.

(vii) On individual organ system:

I. ***On CVS*:** It helps to maintain normal blood pressure due to it's mild aldosterone like activity that is why in deficiency state (Hyposecretion of glucocorticoids e.g. in Addison's disease) hypotension is resulted due to:

- $\downarrow Na^+$ retention
- $\downarrow$capillary permeability $\rightarrow$ exodous of fluid from blood to tissues
- vasospasm by norepinephrine and epinephrine.

Similarly during over secretion of glucocorticoids (in Cushing syndrome) there is hypertension due to opposite phenomenon.

II. ***On CNS*:** It regulates the mood and behavior of a person e.g.

- In deficiency state-there is depression and irritability.
- In excess state-euphoria occurs.

III. ***On digestive system*:** It increases HCl secretion. This is why in excess state of glucocorticoids peptic ulcer occurs.

IV. ***On Blood*:** (i) It increases RBC count and Hb% by inhibiting phagocytosis of old RBC. (ii) It also increases WBC count.

V. ***On skeletal muscle*:** Normal activity of muscle requires the normal level of glucocorticoids. If there is any change of glucocorticoid level beyond normal there is muscle weakness.

VI. ***On bone*:** It—

- increases Ca^{+2} drainage from body.
- increases osteoclastic activity.
- both the response are responsible for osteoporosis.

- ***Regulation of glucocorticoid secretion*:** Glucocorticoid secretion from adrenal cortex is regulated by hypothalamo-hypophyseal adrenal axis. In response to demand of glucocorticoids hypothalamic neurones once stimulated which release CRH into anterior pituitary to secrete ACTH which in turn stimulates secretion of glucocorticoids from adrenal cortex (Fig. 9.5). Increased blood level

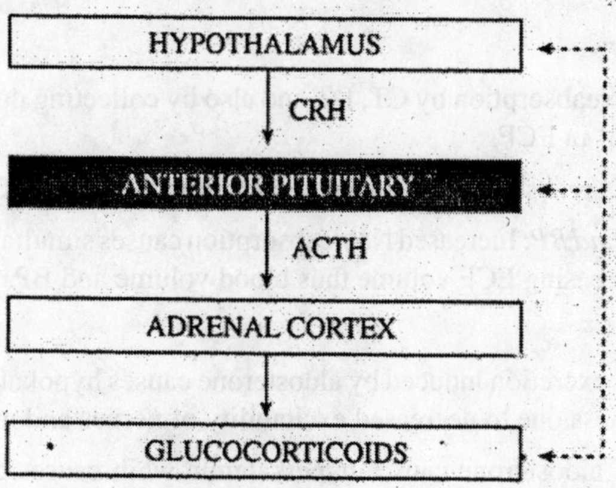

Fig. 9.5: Regulation of glucocorticoid secretion (pathway in dotted line represents negative feedback)

of glucocorticoids inturn by negative feedback way controls the further secretion of ACTH from pituitary and CRH from hypothalamus and thus glucocorticoid secretion is controlled.

This hypothalamo-hypophyseal-adrenal axis is under the influence of 2 factors — **Stress and Circadian rhythm** i.e. stress and circadian rhythm regulate the glucocorticoid secretion by regulating Hypothalamo-hypophyseal-adrenal axis.

(A) ***Stress***: Stress of any kind stimulates hypothalamus and thus acts on hypothalamo-hypophyseal adrenal axis by acting through either limbic system system or reticular formation as explained by following block diagram:

(B) ***Circadian rhythm***: There is diurnal variations of ACTH secretion which results diurnal variation of glucocorticoids secretion, which is maximum in between 6-9 AM. This diurnal variation of ACTH secretion is controlled by a **biological clock** situated either in ***limbic system*** and or in ***suprachiasmatic nucleus***.

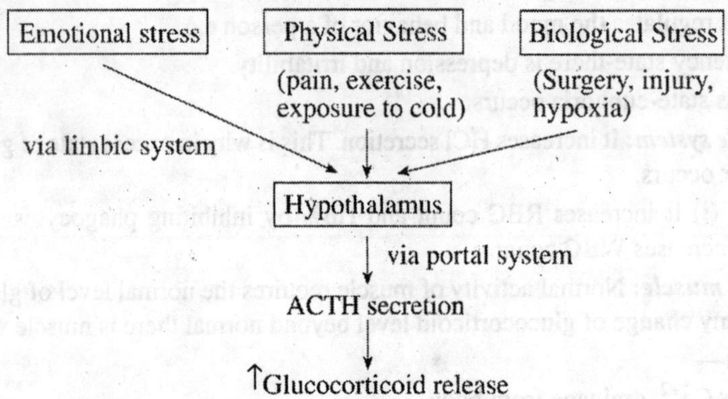

9. Describe the source, daily secretion, actions and regulation of aldosterone.

- Source: Zona glomerulosa
- Daily secretion – 150-300 μg/day
- Function: Mineralocorticoids are essential for life as absence of mineralocorticoids will result death of the person due to **'shock'** resulted from hypovolemia. The function of aldosterone are a follows:

(i) *On Renal tubules*:

- Increases Na^+ reabsorption by CT, DT and also by collecting duct thereby increases total quantity of Na^+ in ECF.
- It decreases K^+ reabsorption by renal tubules thus increasing K^+ excretion.

(ii) *On ECF volume and BP*: Increased Na^+ reabsorption causes simultaneous osmotic absorption of water thus increasing ECF volume thus blood volume and BP.

(iii) *On muscles*:

- Increase in K^+ excretion induced by aldosterone causes hypokalemia which inturn results muscle weakness due to decreased excitability of nerves and muscles.
- Deficiency of aldosterone causes hyperkalemia whih causes cardiac toxicity and even death due to cardiac failure.

(iv) *On pH of blood*: It causes secretion of K^+ and also H^+ ions which results mild degree of alkalosis i.e. rise in pH of blood.

(v) *On sweat glands and salivary glands*:

n It increases the Na^+ and Cl^- absorption from the ducts of these glands.

n It secretes K^+ and HCO_3^- through this ducts.

(vi) *On Intestine*: It increases absorption of Na^+ by the colon of GI tract.

1 Regulation of aldosterone secretion:

(i) *Renal regulation*: Secretion of aldosterone is primarily controlled by the ***renin—angiotensin system*** as illustrated by flow chart FC 9D.

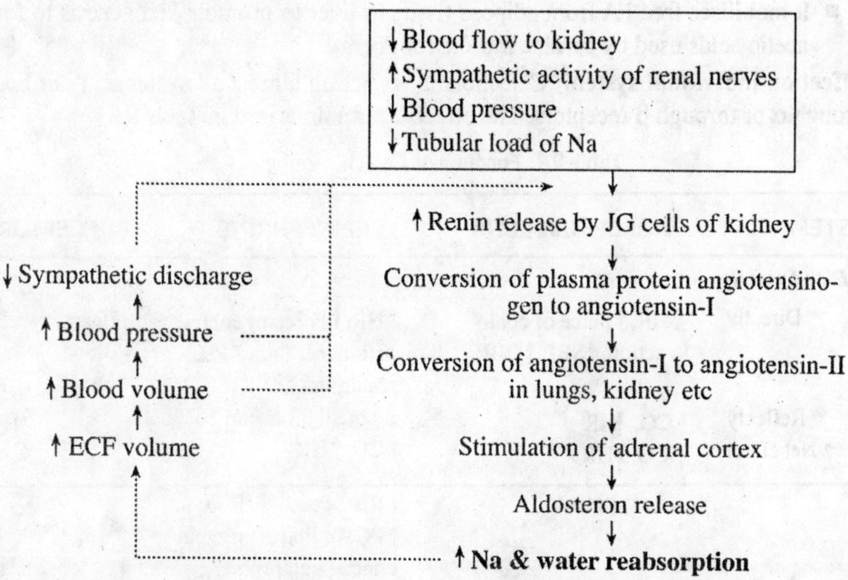

FC 9D: Schematic diagram showing regulation of aldosterone secretion (pathway indicating in dotted line represents negative feedback regulation)

(ii) *Negative feedback regulation*: Rise of ECF volume due to water and Na^+ reabsoption by aldosterone inhibits the further release of renin to control the secretion of aldosterone as shown by dotted lines of previous flow chart.

(iii) *Direct regulation*: Different factors like hyponatremia, hyper kalemla, circadian rhythm, atrial matriuretic peptide and the stress of any kind also stimulate adrenal cortex directly and also through hypothalamo-hypophysial-adrenal axis (i.e. through ACTH, though it's potency is very less) to increase aldoserone secretion.

10. Define catecholamines. Explain the metabolic action and regulation of secretion of catecholamines. How it helps in Fight and Flight reaction?

1 Adrenal medullary hormones i.e. adrenalin or epinephrine (80% in human) and nor adrenalin or nor epinephrine (20% in human) are chemically dihydroxylated phenolic amines which are collectvely known as ***catecholamines***.

1 Functions of catecholamines:

(a) **Metabolic effect:** The metabolic effects of catecholamines are mainly through epinephrine (EP). Nor epinephrine (NE) has little effect. The effect of catecholamines are as follows:

(i) ***On carbohydrate metabolism* (↑Blood sugar level):**

Epinephrine increases blood glucose level by acting on both liver and muscles:

- In liver: It increases glycogenolysis by—
  - activating glycogen phosphorylase enzyme
  - inhibiting glycogen synthetase enzyme
- In muscles: It increases muscle glycogenolysis by activating adenylate cyclase and thus cAMP induced glycogen phosphorylase.

(ii) *On fat metabolism*: lipolytic and ketogenic

- It stimulates lipolysis by activating triglyceride lipase.
- It mobilises free FA from adipose tissue to liver to promote ketogenesis to form aceto acetic acids used by cardiac muscle for energy.

(b) Effect on individual system: Catecholamines act on almost all systems in our body either through α or through β receptors. The effects are summarised in Table 9A.

Table 9A: Function of Catecholamines

SYSTEM	NOREPINEPHRINE	EPINEPHRINE	RECEPTOR INV.
1. Heart & Blood vessels			
* Directly	$\uparrow$HR, $\uparrow$Force of contraction, $\uparrow$SBP, $\uparrow$DBP	$\uparrow$HR, $\uparrow$Force of contraction, net fall of PR resulting $\uparrow$DBP	Heart — Beta Blood vessels — Alpha
* Reflexly	$\uparrow$CO, $\uparrow$HR	no or slight rise of BP	
* Net effect	$\uparrow$CO, $\uparrow$HR	$\uparrow$CO, $\uparrow$HR	
2. Blood	Less potent	$\uparrow$RBC count, $\uparrow$Hb% $\uparrow$PCV, $\uparrow$Plasma protein conc., $\uparrow$neutrophil count, $\downarrow$CT	
3. CNS	stimulation resulting anxiety, hyperventilation coarse tremor	same as NE	
4. GIT	same as EP with less potency	$\downarrow$tone and motility constriction of sphinctors	Alpha and Beta
5. Skin	contraction of pilomotor muscle, localised sweating	same as NE	Alpha
6. Urinary bladder	same as EP with less potency	relaxation of detrusor contraction of trigone and sphinctor resulting retention of urine	Alpha and Beta
7. SK Muscle	same as EP	$\uparrow$blood supply and force of contraction	Beta
8. Smooth muscle	same as EP with less potency	relaxation of stomach and intestinal muscle $\uparrow$intestinal motility constriction of sphinctor	Alpha and Beta

- *Regulation of hormone secretion*:

(a) **Nervous control:** It is the main regulatory mechanism by which catecholamine secretion is regulated by spinal sympathetic (Splanchnic) nerves originated from T_5-T_9 segments of spinal cord. The detail mechanism is as follows:

Stimulus
↓ +
Reticular formation and Hypothalamus
↓ +
Splanchnic nerves to release of ACh
↓ +
Medullary chromaffin cells
↓
Secretion of EP and NE

(b) **Stress induced secretion:** Different stressful condition like fear, anxiety, pain, trauma, hemorrhage, hypoxia, severe hypotension and hypoglycemia stimulate the sympathetic nervous system and thus control adrenal medullary hormone secretion.

The general adaptation syndrome is contributed by sympatho—adrenal medullary system in which adrenal medullary hormones contribute to the ***Fight or Flight response*** by following ways:

(i) allow more light to enter into eye by relaxing accommodation and producing pupillary dilatation.
(ii) provides better perfusion of vital organs and muscles.
(iii) shortends the bleeding time (if wounded).
(iv) reinforcing the alert and arousal state by decreasing the threshold in reticular formation.
(v) Increasing glycogenolysis in liver and lipolysis in adipose tissue to increase energy supply.

B. Short Notes:

1. Hypothalamo-Hypophyseal System:

- Hypothalamus is connected with pituitary gland both anatomically and functionally. This connection between the hypothalamus and pituitary is called as hypothalamo-hypophyseal axis or system.
- The connection with anterior pituitary is mediated through portal blood vessels which is known as hypothalamo-hypophyseal portal system, whereas the connection between hypothalamus and posterior pituitary is mediated through neurons known as hypothalamo-hypophyseal tract.
  - Hypothalamus controls the anterior pituitary via a special route known as ***hypothalamo-hypophyseal portal system***. Different Hypothalamic neurones synthesise different releasing and releasing inhibitory hormones which are remain stored in their synaptic knob present in the region of median eminence and close to the capillary loops. In response to appropriate stimulus there is stimulation of these neurones which ultimately control the release of pituitary hormones as illustrated by following flow chart:

    Stimulation of hypothalamic neurones synthesing releasing and releasing inhibitory hormones→ passing of action potential to their synaptic knob close to capillary blood → release of neuro secretory materials (RH and RIH) into the tissue fluid in close proximity to the capillary blood of hypothalamo–hypophyseal portal vessels → absorption of RH and RIH into capillary blood of portal vessels → drainage to anterior pituitary → stimulation of appropriate pituitary cell to release tropic hormones → drainage of tropic hormone from anterior pituitary via general circulation → control the function of different target endocrine gland.

- ***Hypothalamo-hypophyseal tract:*** This nerve tract originates from the cell bodies of supraoptic and paraventricular nuclei of hypothalamus. Their axons descend into the pituitary stalk and end in the posterior pituitary. Neuro secretory materials synthesised by these neurones are transported by the carrier protein **Neurophysin–I** and **Neurophysin–II** along the axons and stored in their axon terminals. In response to appropriate stimulus when the action potential is transported through these axons and reaches their axon terminal these neurosecretory materials (Hormones) are released which inturn is absorbed within the blood vessels and ultimately circulated throughout the body via general circulation.

2. Feedback control:

- When the rate of secretion of a hormone is controlled by the plasma level of that particular peripheral gland hormones or of substances (e.g. glucose, fatty acids etc.) arising from the tissue metabolism influenced by that particular hormone is called as feedback control.
- It can be two types:

A. *Negative feedback:*

- When increased concentration of a hormone and it's metabolites decrease the rate of further secretion of that hormone it is called as negative feedback which is of 3 types-long loop, short loop and ultra short loop.
- Virtually all the tropic hormones secreted from the anterior pituitary cause the changes in either of the concentration of peripheral gland hormones (like thyroid, adrenal and gonadal hormones) or of substances e.g. glucose, free fatty acids etc. These peripheral gland hormones or substances arising from the tissue metabolism can exert negative feedback control (occasionally positive) on both hypothalamus and pituitary (Fig. 9.6) known as ***long-loop feedback inhibition***. The tropic hormones can also exert negative feedback control over the secretion of hypothalamic releasing hormones (Fig. 9.6) which is known as ***short-loop***

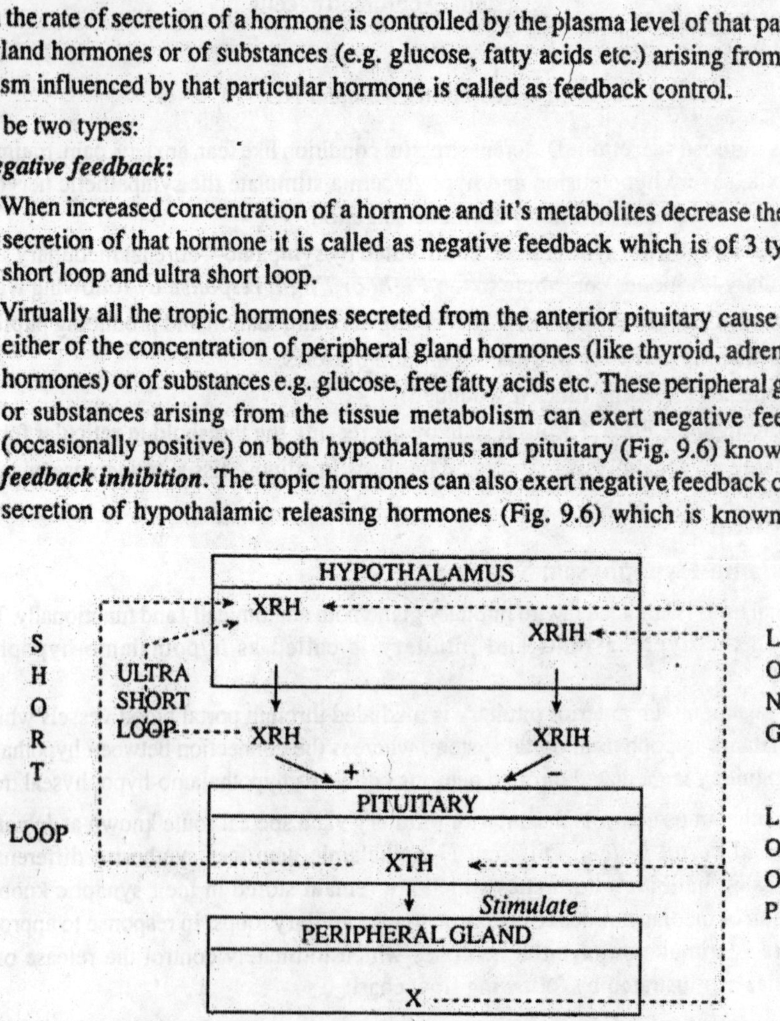

Fig. 9.6: Schematic diagram showing overall control of hypothalamo-hypophyseal-target organ axis (Solid line indicates stimulation and dotted line indicates inhibition)

feedback mechanism. Finally hypothalamic releasing hormones can even inhibit their own synthesis and release of releasing hormones and stimulate the release of releasing inhibitory hormones (Fig. 9.6) which is known as ***ultra-short-loop*** feedback.

B. Positive feedback:

- When increased concentration of a hormone and it's metabolites increase the rate of further secretion of that hormone it is called as positive feedback.
- The example is LH surge that occurs just before ovulation under the control of estrogen level in blood.

3. Neuroendocrine transducer:

- Hypothalamus acts as neuroendocrine transducer as it converts the neural signal to release the hormones from different endocrine glands and thereby controls different bodily functions.
- The hypothalamus can be considered as a central relay station for collecting and integrating signals from diverse sources and funneling them to the pituitary. Through the multisynaptic input the pain, sleep, wakefulness, emotion, rage, olfactory sensations, light, thought, thirst, appetite, temperature all these sensations ultimately reach to the hypothalamus via Thalamus, RAS, Limbic system, Neocortex, Eye, etc. which inturn control different body functions by controlling both anterior and posterior pituitary gland as shown by following block diagram:

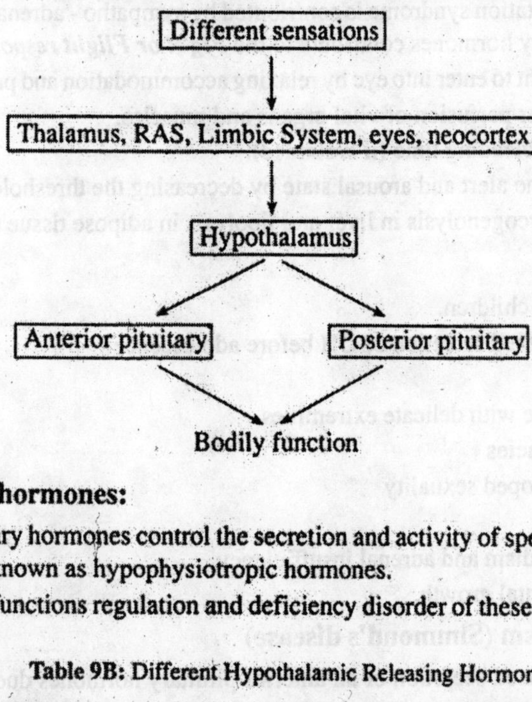

4. Hypophysiotropic hormones:

- The anterior pituitary hormones control the secretion and activity of specific peripheral endocrine glands which are known as hypophysiotropic hormones.
- The name source, functions regulation and deficiency disorder of these hormones are tabulated in table 9B.

Table 9B: Different Hypothalamic Releasing Hormone

Hormones	Source	Target cell	Function
1. GHRH	Arcuate Nucle	Somatotropes	Stimulate GH secretion by anterior pituitary
2. GHRIH	Anterior Paraventricular Nucleus	-do	inhibit GH secretion
3. CRH	Paraventricular Nucleus	Corticotropes	ACTH release

Contd.

Hormones	Source	Target cell	Function
4. GnRH	Arcuate Nucleus and Preoptic nucleus	Gonadotropes	Gonadotropin secretion
5. TRH	Paraventricular nucleus	Thyrotropes	TSH secretion
6. PIH	Arcuate nucleus	Lactotropes	Prolactin secretion

5. Stress:

- As per Selye (1955): "Stress is the sum of all nonspecific changes caused by function or damage".
- It is fundamentally a physiological response, the primary object of which is to maintain life and reestablish the normal state.
- The general manifestation of stress are called the ***general adaptation syndrome*** which occurs into 3 stages as follows:
  - **(i) The alarm reaction—occurs before adaptation.**
  - **(ii) The stage of Resistance—optimal adaptation occurs.**
  - **(iii) The stage of exhaustion—adaptation is lost.**
- The general adaptation syndrome is contributed by sympatho - adrenal medullary system in which adrenal medullary hormones contribute to the ***Fight or Flight response*** by following ways:
  - (i) allow more light to enter into eye by relaxing accommodation and producing pupillary dilatation.
  - (ii) provides better perfusion of vital organs and muscles.
  - (iii) shortens the bleeding time (if wounded).
  - (iv) reinforcing the alert and arousal state by decreasing the threshold in reticular formation.
  - (v) increasing glycogenolysis in liver and lipolysis in adipose tissue to increase energy supply.

6. Dwarfism:

- This occurs in children.
- **Cause:** Decreased secretion of GH before adolescence.
- **Features:**
  - Short stature with delicate extremities
  - Immature facies
  - Underdeveloped sexuality
  - Fatness
  - Hypothyroidism and adrenal insufficiency
  - Normal mental growth.

7. Panhypopituitarism (Simmond's disease)

- **Cause:** Decreased secretion of all anterior pituitary hormones due to degeneration or atrophy of anterior lobe.
- **Features:**

⇒ In childhood
  - Dwarfism
  - No pubertal changes
  - No sexual functions

⇒ In adult
  - Normal height

- ☐ Premature senility
- ☐ atrophy of thyroid, adrenal and gonads.

8. Adiposo-genital syndrome:

- **Cause:** Lesion of anterior pituitary (which accounts for sexual immaturity and dwarfism) and of hypothalamus.
- **Features:** Obesity, sexual infantilism and dwarfism subnormal intelligence, lethargic, polyurla, feminine distribution in male (in adult).

9. SIADH:

- **Cause:** Excessive secretion of ADH
- **Features:**
  - ■ Increase in ECF volume due to water retention.
  - ■ Hypernatriuria due to decrease secretion of aldosterone resulted from expansion of ECF volume.
  - ■ Water intoxication (over hydration syndrome). This is due to: ↑ Water retention →↑ movement of water into interstitial space (Edema) →↓ osmolality within interstitial space → water shift within ICF → dilution of cellular enzymes → dilution or over hydration syndrome.
- It is seen in head injury, ectopic production of ADH as occurs in carcinoma of lungs, pancreas, ovary etc., neurogenic disorders like meningitis, encephalitis, multiple sclerosis, Guilian Berre syndrome etc.

10. Endemic goiter:

- This is due to lack of iodine in soil that is seen in some parts of the world.
- **Cause:** Lack of Iodine → decrease in production of T_3 and T_4 → decrease in T_3 / T_4 level in blood → no inhibition of TSH release → more TSH release → increase in size of thyroid gland and synthesis of thyroglobulin. In case of moderate deficiency there is hyperplasia of the gland without sign and symptoms of excess thyroid hormone secretion which is known as **Simple Goiter.**
- **Features:**
  - ■ Increase size of the gland results swelling in the throat
  - ■ decreased T_3 and T_4 level in plasma
  - ■ increase in TSH level in plasma.

11. Graves disease:

- **Cause:** Hypersecretion of thyroid hormones due to action of LATS produced in the body
- **Features:** (i) **General symptoms** e.g.
  - ■ Loss of weight
  - ■ Fine tremor
  - ■ Anxiety
  - ■ Feeling of excessive heat
  - ■ Tachycardia, palpitation
  - ■ High systolic B.P.

(ii) **Toxic goiter**—Swelling of gland with sign and symptom of over secretion of thyroid hormones.

(iii) **Exopthalmos**—Protrusion of the eyeballs due to oedematus swelling of the retroorbital tissues and degenerative changes in the extra ocular muscles.

- Medical treatment includes antithyroid drugs, iodine therapy, etc. and surgical treatment is done by subtotal or total thyroidectomy.

12. Tetany:

- **Cause:** The exact physiological reason behind occurrence of tetany is illustrated by following flow chart.
  Accidental damage or removal of parathyroid gland during surgery of thyroid or in cancer in larynx → ↓ serum Ca^{2+} level rapidly within 2-3 days. → increase irritability of nerves as well as neuromuscular junctions → contraction of muscle in response to subthreshold stimulus and even spontaneous contraction of muscle → uncontrolled, painful, prolonged contraction of voluntory muscle which is characterised as tetany.
- **Features:**
  - General convulsion (in children).
  - **Carpopedal syndrome** or **Accoucher's hand**—This is due to muscular spasm leading to uncontrolled prolonged flexion of the metacarpophalangeal joints while the fingers remain extended.
  - **Laryngeal strider**—Due to spasm in laryngeal smooth muscle breathing can stop. So the patient tries to inspire voluntarily which results entry of air through larynx with an crowing sound which is known as laryngeal stridor. In extreme cases the patient can die as breathing totally stops. This is the reason the PTH hormone is called as **essential hormone.**
  - **Chvostek's sign**—Taping of the facial nerve at the ramus of mandibol in front of ear of this types of patient produces painful spasm of facial muscle which is known as Chvostek's sign.
  - **Trousseau's sign**—Slight pressure on the limbs causes development of Carpopedal syndrome like posture of upper limbs which is known as Trousseau's sign.
  - ECG changes - prolonged ST segment with abnormal T wave
  - Clotting defects.
  - Tingling and numbness in extremities (paraesthesia).
  - Stiffness of hands and feet due to increased contractility of skeletal muscle.
  - Facilitates cataract formation.
- Sometimes the subject will not show the symptoms unless elicited which is known as subclinical or *latent tetany.*

13. Conn's syndrome:

- **Cause:** Excess aldosterone secretion due to tumor or hyperplasia of Z. Glomelulosa of adrenal cortex.
- **Features:**
  - Muscular weakness (due to prolonged hypokalemia).
  - Hypokalemic nephropathy.
  - ↑Plasma Na^+.
  - ↑Plasma aldosterone level without oedama due to aldosterone escape.
  - ↑Urinary aldosterone level.
  - ↓In plasma K^+.
  - ↓Plasma renin.
  - Albuninuria.
  - Polyurea due to high GFR.
  - Polydipsia due to loss of water through urine.
  - Alkalosis due to more loss of H^+ ion in urine.
  - Hypertension due to increased blood volume.

14. Adrenal diabetes:

- Diabetes mellitus due to hyperfunction of adrenal cortex is known as adrenal diabetes.

- It increases blood glucose level by:
  (I) increasing gluconeogenesis by:
  - activating all enzymes of gluconeogenic pathway.
  - by converting amino acids to glucose in liver by activating transaminase enzyme.
  - by breaking down proteins from lymphoid tissue, bone, skin and skeletal muscle.

  (II) decreasing peripheral utilisation of glucose by inhibiting glucose uptake in adipose tissue.

  (III) increasing glycogenesis by activating glycogen synthetase enzyme.

  (IV) by increasing protein catabolism in extrahepatic tissue and **in hepatic tissue** it increases the transport of amino acid to liver cells and enhances enzymes required for protein synthesis which results increase synthesis of plasma proteins and increase conversion of amino acids to glucose.

  (V) It inhibits the insulin stimulated glucose uptake in skeletal muscle and adipose tissue.

15. Somatomedins:

- The effects of GH on growth, cartilage and protein metabolism depends partly on the production of insulin like growth factors which are earlier known as somatomedins.
- The principal circulating somatomedins are IGF-1 or somatomedins –C and IGF-II.
- The somatomedin-C is alpha peptide produced by the liver and the kidney in response to GH.
- It is polypeptide containing 70 amino acids.
- Plasma concentration is 10-700 ng/ml which peaks at the puberty.
- It mainly causes skeletal and cartilage growth.

16. Gigantism:

- The excessive increasing in height due to oversecretion of GH before adolescence is known as gigantism.
- **Causes:** Pituitary or hypothalamus tumor causing excess secretion of GH or GHRH respectively.
- **Features:**
  - 8 –9 ft height
  - hyperglycemia.

17. Growth spurt:

- Though the growth rate of human beings is different at different stages of life, there are two periods of rapid growth. The period of rapid growth is called as ***growth spurt.***

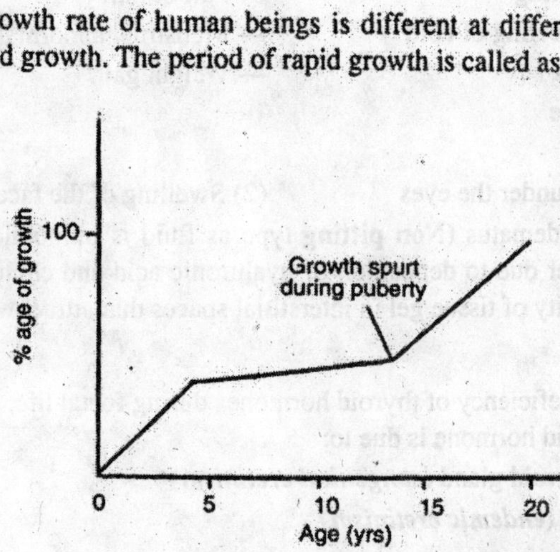

Fig. 9.7: Graphical representation showing growth spurt

- It is of two types (Fig. 9.7).
  - Infantile that occurs during infancy.
  - Pubertal that occurs during late puberty.
- Growth spurt appears 2-3 years earlier in girls than boys.

18. Stress and Catecholamines:

- The general adaptation syndrome of stress is contributed by sympatho - adrenal medullary system in which adrenal medullary hormones contribute to the ***Fight or Flight response*** by following ways:
  (i) allow more light to enter into eye by relaxing accommodation and producing pupillary dilatation.
  (ii) provides better perfusion of vital organs and muscles.
  (iii) shortends the bleeding time (if wounded).
  (iv) reinforcing the alert and arousal state by decreasing the threshold in reticular formation.
  (v) increasing glycogenolysis in liver and lipolysis in adipose tissue to increase energy supply.
- These physiological process to protect the body to counteract the stress is as follows: Stress → CRH release and increase in ADH release → increase in adrenergic discharge → increase in (i) plasma catecholamines concentration which thereby increases glycogenolysis and (ii) cortisol concentration that promotes gluconeogenesis. Plasma catecholamines also increase the supply of FFA to heart and also increases cardiac output and blood pressure and promotes supply of substrate to the tissues.
- In acute stage of stress a general state of arousal and vigilance is maintained by catecholamines.
- In chronic stage reproductive functions, sexual activity and feeding are suppressed which are also mediated by catecholamines.

19. Myxoedema:

- **Cause:** Due to extreme deficiency of thyroid hormones in adult life due to:
  - Autoimmuno disease of thyroid (Hashimoto's disease) where specific immunoglobin destroys thyroid gland.
  - Hypo function of anterior pituitary or hypothalamus.
- **Features:**

— Mental slowing	— Fall of hair
— Excessive feeling of cold	— Menstrual abnormality (In women)
— Bradycardia	— Weight gain
— Husky voice	

In advanced age:

(1) Bagginess under the eyes (2) Swelling of the face

- This is due to the oedematus (**Non pitting** type as fluid is immobile) swelling because of accumulation of water due to deposition of hyaluronic acid and chondroitin sulphate which form excessive quantity of tissue gel in interstitial spaces that attract water.

20. Cretinism:

- **Cause:** due to extreme deficiency of thyroid hormones during foetal life, infancy and childhood. This deficiency of thyroid hormone is due to:
  - Congenital lack of thyroid gland (***congenital cretinism***)
  - Iodine lack in the diet (***endemic cretinism***)
- **Features:**
  - Physical, sexual and mental retardation

- Short stature with short club like fingers, deformed bones and teeth.
- Rough, thick, dry and wrinkled skin with scanty hairs.
- Pot bellied abdomen with protruding umbilicus.
- Idotic look.
- Susceptibility to cold.
- Fall in blood sugar, high cholesterol, low blood iodine, high blood TSH level.

This type of child is known as *cretin*.

21. LATS:

- **Long acting thyroid stimulating antibody (LATS) are the types of thyroid stimulating antibodies which bind with the same membrane receptor of thyroid follicular cells that binds TSH. These antibodies induce continual activation of the cAMP system with resultant development of hyperthyroidism known as *Grave's Disease*.**
- These are the IgG type of immunoglobins.

22. Antithyroid drugs:

- The clinical manifestations of hyperthyroidism are due to an excess of circulating thyroid hormones. So reduction of thyroid acitivity and hormonal effects can be minimized by some drugs known as antithyroid drugs.
- These drugs exert their effect by interfering (i) with the production (ii) releasing (iii) action of thyroid hormones.
- All such drugs can be classified physiologically as follows:
  - Drugs which affect active transport of iodide e.g.percholate.
  - Drugs which affect iodination of thyroglobulins e.g. thioamides, iodide.
  - Drugs which affect coupling reaction e.g. thioamides, sulfonamides.
  - Drugs which affect hormonal release e.g. iodide.
  - Drugs which affect peripheral deiodination of T_4 to T_3 e.g. thiouracils.
  - Drugs which affect hormonal transport or action e.g. cholestyramines.
  - Drugs which affect hormone excretion.

23. Cushing syndrome:

- Causes: Hyper secretion of cortisol due to—
  - excessive ACTH secretion resulted from tumor of corticotroph of anterior pituitary or ectopic ACTH secreting tumor e.g. in lungs.
  - tumor in the adrenal cortex.
- Features:
  - Retardation of growth
  - Thinning of skin and subcutaneous tissue
  - Wasting of muscle (***Steroid Myopathy***)
  - Osteoporosis due to decrease protein deposition in bone

  These are due to increase protein catabolism.
  - Hyperglycemia, glycosuria (which is known as ***adrenal diabetes***) due to increase carbohydrate metabolism.
  - ***Pendular abdomen*** with ***Purple Striae***
  - Moon like face and buffalo hump.

  These are due to centrepetal distribution of fat.

- Increased facial hairs (***Hirsutism***) and development of acne.

These are due to increased adrenal androgen.

24. Addison's disease:

- **Cause:** Due to bilateral destruction of adrenal cortex due to TB, autoimmuno disorder or fungal infection.
- **Features:**
  - Hypotension
  - Anorexia, nausea, vomiting, diarrhoea which results dehydration, loss of weight and decrease in blood volume.
  - Muscular weakness.
  - Pigmentation of skin, mucous membrane.
  - ↓ Ability to tolerate stress.
  - Excess ACTH level due to absence of negative feedback.
- Addison's disease in which failure of glucocorticoid release in response to sudden stress or infection leads severe disability is known as **Addisonian crisis.**

25. Adrenogenital syndrome:

- **Cause:** Excessive secretion of adrenal androgen
- **Features:**
  - *In children*:
    - ☐ Little girl menstruate at age 2
    - ☐ Little boy show early development of testis, penis and other secondary sexual characters.
  - *In adult*: Tendency of conversion to the secondary characters of opposite sex. Thus adult women develop male secondary sex character known as ***adrenal virilism*** and adult male show feminisation called ***adrenal feminisation***.

26. Fight and flight reaction: See under the short note 'stress and catecholamines'.

27. Phaeochromocytoma:

- **Cause:** Hypersecretion of adrenal medullary hormone due to tumor of chromaffin cell in adrenal medulla.
- **Features:**
  - — Sustained hypertension upto even 300/200 mmHg
  - — Headache, sweating (adrenergic sweating)
  - — severe palpitation,
  - — Anxiety, weakness, dizziness
  - — Pale, cold and moist skin.
  - — Blurred vision
  - —↑Bleeding time.
  - — Increased Blood glucose, BMR
  - —↑ Urinary excretion of glucose.

28. Diabetes mellitus and its complication: See under Q. 6.

29. Physiologic gut factor:

- There are more than 100 active peptides which make the G-I tract as the largest endocrine gland. Previously it was suggested that it acts locally thereby named as ***Local hormones or physiologic gut factor***.

- Recently it is found that it's action is not limited to GIT. Instead they act as multifunctional intra-cellular regulators e.g. growth factors, neurotransmitters, cytokines and fertility factor. Thereby the hormone of GIT are no more local hormones but may be viewed as ***intracellular messengers.***
- The main GI hormones, their source and function are summarised in Table 9C:

Table 9C: Major Hormones in G-I-tract

NAME	SOURCE	STIMULUS	FUNCTION
Gastrin	1. G cells of antrum of stomach 2. upper part of small intestine	1. Vagal stimulation 2. Peptide in stomach	Increases HCl secretion Decreases insulin secretion Increases G I mucosal growth Helps in Constriction of LES
Secretin	S cells in duodenum	acidity in chyme	Decreases gastric secretion Decreases gastric emptying Increases pancreatic bicarbonate secretion
CCK-PZ	I cells of upper small intestinal mucosa	peptides & long chain fatty acids	Increases pancreatic enzyme secretion Increases Gall bladder contraction
VIP	1. Gut endocrine cells 2. Nerves of GIT	vagal stimulation	Increases insulin secretions Decreases gastric secretions Decreases gastric motility Increases pancreatic bicarbonate secretion Increases intestinal water and electrolytes secretion Induces vasodilation of salivary glands
GIP	K cells of duoneum	fatty food	Increases insulin secretion Decreases HCl secretion Increases gastric motility
Motillin	1. M cells of upper small intestine 2. Enterochromaffin cells	not known	Increases gastric motility
Somato-statin	D cells of pancreas, Gastric antral mucosa	very low pH in stomach	Inhibits G cells Decreases HCl secretion.

30. Pineal gland:

- **Location:** Lies between the superior colliculi of brain. It acts as ***neuroendocrine transducer.***
- **Hormone:** Melatonin, serotonin, pineal polypeptide
- Functions of melatonin:
  - It is concerned with regulation of onset of puberty. It secretes some gonadotrophin inhibitory substance which delays puberty.
  - It increases the secretion of serotonin in CNS.
  - It has anti aggressive action.
  - It enhances the growth hormone level.
  - In amphibians it is responsible for skin colour.

31. GTT:

- This is the test to diagnose the diabetes mellitus.
- For this test fasting blood glucose level of the person is measured and then glucose is fed to him orally at a dose of 1G/Kg body weight and post prandial (after glucose administration) blood

glucose level is measured from the blood samples collected at least upto 2 hr with $\frac{1}{2}$ an hour intervals. The values are plotted in a graph which is known as ***glucose tolerance chart*** (Fig. 9.4).

- **Analysis of data:**
  - The person is **normal** if—
    - his fasting blood glucose is < 80 mg%
    - post prandial (PP) value is < 140 mg%
    - post prandial value returns to fasting level after 2 hours
  - The person is **diabetic** if—
    - his fasting blood glucose level is > 120 mg%
    - his PP value is > 200 mg%
    - PP value does not return to fasting level even after 2 hr
    - at least 2 PP value as high as 200 mg% or more.

32. ADH:

- **Source:** Supraoptic nucleus of hypothalamus.
- **Function:**
  - It increases water permeability of distal convoluted tubules (mild action) and collecting duct (mainly) → increases water reabsorption → decreases urinary output.
  - It also stimulates ACTH release from anterior pituitary → increases aldosterone secretion.
  - It decreases medullary blood flow.
  - In excessive doses it causes peripheral vasoconstriction → increases BP.
- **Control of ADH secretion:** ADH secretion is regulated by hypothalamus in response to different stimuli like hyperosmolality, hypovoluemia, stress.
  - **Hyperosmolality:** Increase osmolality in body fluids stimulate hypothalamic osmoreceptor which inturn intiates action potential to stimulate release of ADH from posterior pituitary. The detail mechanism is as follows:

    Any increase in osmolality of body fluid → increase in osmolality of ECF in brain tissue → water moves out from osmoreceptor → shrinkage of osmoreceptor → generation and conduction of impulse down the Hypothalamo-Hypophyseal tract → secretion of ADH → drainage to general circulation → increase in water permeability in renal tubules → increase water volume in ECF → **Corrects the osmolality.**
  - **Hypovolemia:** It is by following mechanism:

    Hypovolemia → stimulation of venous low pressure baroreceptor → stimulation of supraoptic nucleus of hypothalamus via vagus nerve → increase in ADH release → increase water reabsorption → **normalacy** of body fluid volume.
  - **Stress:** Different stressful condition like exercise, pain, fear etc. can stimulate ADH release directly by stimulating supraoptic nucleus of hypothalamus.
- Due to ADH deficiency there is increased urinary output which is known as Diabetes Insipidus.

33. Functions of thymus:

- The main role of thymus gland is to produce lymphocytes which take part in immunity. Besides this it also produces a substance which circulate through blood to act on peripheral lymphoid tissue thereby considered as a hormone.
- Function: stimulates production of T- lymphocytes both in thymus and peripheral lymphoid tissue.

34. Kinins:

- These are the peptide hormones cleaved from their precursors which are of two types—high molecular weight (HMW) kininogen and low molecular weight (LMW) kininogen. The cleavage of kinins from their precursor is done by protease called ***Kallikreins.***

- In humans two types of kinins are identified –bradykinin from HMW kininogen and Kallidin from LMW Kininogen.
- Along with other proteins of their family these form the ***Kinin-Kallikrein system.***
- The general functions of Kinin-Kallikrein System are:
  - Vasodilatation.
  - Contraction of extravascular smooth muscles especially smooth muscle of intestine.
  - Stimulation of pain fibers.
  - Increases capillary permeability.

35. Simmond's disease:

- It is a rare pituitary disease in which secretion of all anterior pituitary hormones is decreased.
- It occurs due to either atrophy or degeneration of anterior pituitary.
- It is characterised by—
  - Rapidly developing senile decay i.e. 30 years old person look like 60 years old.
  - Loss of body hair and teeth.
  - Dry and wrinkled skin.

36. Frohlich's disease:

- It is a pituitary disease mainly in adolescence boys.
- It occurs due to hypoactivity of anterior and posterior pituitary due to (i) tumor (ii) injury (iii) atrophy of pituitary gland and hypothalamic region which is concerned with food intake and and gonadal development.
- It is characterised by obesity and hypogonadism and dwarfism if the disease starts in growing age.
- It also occurs in adults which is known as adult type Frohlich's syndrome.

C. Differentiate between:

Pituitary dwarfism	Hypothyroid dwarfism
❑ This is due to hypo function of pituitary gland.	❑ This is due to hypo function of thyroid gland.
❑ It is characterised by stunted growth.	❑ It is characterised by stunted growth with bloated body.
❑ Mental retardation is absent.	❑ Mental retardation is present.
❑ Growth of different parts of the body is proportionate.	❑ Growth of different parts of the body is not proportionate.
❑ Reproduction may be normal (except in panhypopituitarism).	❑ Reproduction is affected.

Somatomedins	Direct effect of GH
❑ Growth promoting action of GH is mediated through somatomedins.	❑ It has anti insulin like action.
❑ Acts on skeletal and extra skeletal like protein synthesis and cell proliferation.	❑ It acts on carbohydrate metabolism to increase lipolysis and blood sugar level.

T_3	T_4
❑ It is only 9%-10% of total secretion.	❑ It is 90% of total secretion.
❑ Potency of T_3 is much more (4 times).	❑ Potency of T_4 is less.
❑ Duration of action of T_3 is less.	❑ Duration of action of T_4 is more.
❑ T_3 acts on the target cells immediately.	❑ It acts on the target cells slowly.
❑ Rate of secretion is 4-5 μg/day.	❑ Rate of secretion is 80-90 μg/day.
❑ Normal plasma level is 0.12 μg/dl.	❑ Normal plasma level is 8 μg/dl.
❑ T_3 is found freely in the plasma.	❑ T_4 is usually bound with plasma protein for transportation.
❑ It is the true and principal intracellular hormone as after entering the peripheral tissues most of T_4 is deiodinated to form T_3.	❑ It is metabolised to form T_3 in peripheral tissues.

Carotinemia	Jaundice
❑ In both the cases there is yellowish coloration of skin but carotinemia is due to increase of plasma level of β-carotins.	❑ It is due to increase in plasma bilirubin level (more than 2 mg%).

Non pitting oedema	Pitting oedema
❑ When edema develops due to swelling of the cells or clotting of interstitial fluid in the presence of fibrinogen, it is called as non pitting edema.	❑ When the intracellular fluid volume increases enormously it flows freely through the tissue spaces due to pressure gradient which is known as pitting edema because when this area is pressed with the finger displacement of fluid occurs producing a depression or pit.
❑ It is hard and a pit is not formed by pressing.	❑ Pit is formed.
❑ Example: seen during myxoedema.	❑ Example: Hypervolemia, renal failure etc.

Endemic goiter	Exopthalmic goiter
❑ It is due to hypothyroidism.	❑ It is due to hyperthyroidism.
❑ In this case there is enlargement of thyroid gland due to lack of iodine.	❑ In this case there is enlargement of thyroid gland due to action of Thyroid Stimulating Immunoglobin.
❑ There is decrease in T_3/T_4 secretion.	❑ There is increase in T_3/T_4 secretion.
❑ It is also characterised by increase in TSH level.	❑ It is also characterised by decrease in TSH level.
❑ It is a type of nontoxic goiter.	❑ It is a type of toxic goiter.

Primary adreno-cortical insufficiency	Secondary adreno-cortical insufficiency
❑ It is due to hypofunction of adrenal cortex.	❑ It is due to hypofunction of pituitary or hypothalamic disease that affect CRH release.
❑ ACTH level becomes high in this case.	❑ ACTH level is low in this case.
❑ It is associated with aldosterone deficiency.	❑ It is not associated with aldosterone deficiency.
❑ It is associated with skin pigmentation due to high ACTH level.	❑ Skin pigmentation is not seen.

Primary aldosteronism	Secondary aldosteronism
❑ It is due to excessive aldosterone secretion due to tumour/hyperplasia of zona glomerulosa of adrenal cortex.	❑ It is due to excessive accumulation of aldosterone due to activation of rennin-angiotensin aldosterone system in case of cirrhosis of liver and cardiac failure.
❑ It is characterised by decrease in plasma rennin level.	❑ It is characterised by increase in plasma rennin level.
❑ Edema is usually not seen.	❑ Edema is usually seen.

Primary hyper thyroidism	Secondary hyper thyroidism
❑ It is due to defect in thyroid gland.	❑ It is due to defect outside the thyroid gland e.g. pituitary or extra thyroidal tissues.
❑ Example: adenoma of thyroid, goiter, carcinoma, Grave's disease, iodine excess.	❑ Example: tumour in pituitary and extra thyroidal tissues.

Osteosclerosis	Osteoporosis
❑ There is increased calcified bone in patient with metastatic tumour, lead poisoning and hypothyroidism.	❑ It is a bone disease characterised by the loss of bone matrix and minerals due to execessive bone resorption and decreased bone formation.
❑ Bone is very hard and not fragile.	❑ Bone is very hard and not fragile.

Osteocytes	Osteoclasts
❑ These are responsible for maintenance of bone.	❑ These are responsible for bone resorption.
❑ It is derived from mature osteoblast cells.	❑ It is derived from hemopoietic stem cells via monocytes (CFU-M).

Ricket	Adult ricket
❑ It is the bone disease in children characterised by inadequate mineralisation of bone matrix.	❑ It is the bone disease in adults also known as osteomalacia.
❑ It is characterised by bowing of long bones of lower limbs.	❑ It is not characterised by bowing of long bones of lower limbs.

D. Short answer type:

1. What will happen if pituitary dwarf is treated with testosterone and why?

If pituitary dwarf is treated with testosterone there is initial growth of few inches followed by stoppage of growth as testosterone terminates growth by causing epiphyseal closure.

2. What will happen if whole pituitary gland is removed in a person?

Removal of whole pituitary gland is not fatal provided glucocorticoids are administered regularly.

3. What will happen if one year old child suffers from hypothyroidism?

He will suffer from cretinism.

4. What will happen if T_4 is administered to a normal person?

If T_4 is administered to a normal person radioactive iodine uptake will be decreased because of T_3 suppression.

5. What will happen if TSH is administered in an individual with I_2 deficiency?

If TSH is administered in an individual with I_2 deficiency it will result enlargement of thyroid gland i.e. goiter.

6. What will happen to serum cholesterol level in myxoedema?

In myxoedema serum cholesterol level will be decreased as T_4 increases serum cholesterol level.

7. What will happen to T_4 secretion if I_2 is ingested in large amount?

In this situation T_4 secretion will be decreased (Wolf Charikoff effect) due to:

1. Prevention of incorporation of iodine to tyrosin
2. Decreasing in proteolysis of thyroglobulins
3. Decrease in blood flow to thyroid → decrease in metabolism.
4. Decrease in TSH effect on thyroid gland.

8. What will happen to T_3, T_4, and TSH levels in Graves disease?

In Grave's disease there is increase in T_3 and T_4 level and normal or decrease in TSH level.

9. What will happen to functional state of thyroid gland if intake of vegetables of Brassicaceae family is increased?

Though Brassicaceae family contain goitrogenic agents yet increase intake of these usually not harmful.

10. What will happen if corticoids are given in an individual suffering from epilepsy?

In epileptic patients glucocorticoid is not administered as excess of glucocorticoids stimulate the activity of brain excitability producing convulsions.

11. What will happen if prolonged treatment with glucocorticoids is stopped suddenly?

Prolonged treatment with glucocorticoids produces adrenocortical atrophy. So sudden stoppage of such therapy may cause death of that person due to circulatory collapse which is known as ***adrenal crisis***. It can be avoided by slowly decreasing the glucocorticoids dose over a long period.

12. Give physiological basis of Acromegaly.

Acromegaly means enlargement of peripheral organs due to excessive secretion of GH during adulthood after the closure of epiphyseal end plate of long bones. Thereby the growth occurs only those areas where cartilage persists.

13. Give physiological basis of African Pigmies.

It is a clinical condition in which growth is retarded due to decrease in cellular receptors on the cell on which GH acts, in spite of normal level of GH and somatomedins.

14. Give physiological basis of diabetogenic action of GH.

GH is diabetogenic i.e. it increases blood sugar level by increasing release of glucose from liver and decreases glucose uptake by adipose tissue and skeletal muscle by antagonizing the insulin.

15. Give physiological basis of ketogenic action of GH.

GH is ketogenic i.e. it increases hepatic oxidation of fatty acids to ketone bodies, acetoacetic acid and beta-hydroxybutyric acid.

16. Give physiological basis of non pitting edema in myxoedema.

In myxoedema → low thyroid hormone secretion → decrease in catabolism of mucopolysaccharides, hyaluronic acid and chondroitin sulphate → deposition of these substances under the skin and subcutaneous tissue → increase in osmotic pressure → increase in water and NaCl retention → dry, coarse and puffy appearance of skin (non pitting edema).

17. Give physiological basis of amenorrhoea during post patrum period.

High serum level of prolactin inhibits LH secretion which is responsible for ovulation and thereby menstruation. During post patrum lactation PRL level is high → inhibition of LH secretion → decrease in LH level → no ovulation → no menstruation i.e. amenorrhoea.

18. Give physiological basis of high sleeping pulse rate in hyperthyroidism.

It is because of increased sympathetic activity on beta receptors by T4 and catecholamines.

19. Give physiological basis of DM in hypothyroid patients.

It is due to dominating action of T_4 on following:

- Increased glucose absorption from intestine by T_4.
- Increase in glycogenolysis in liver, heart, skeletal muscle by T_4.
- Increase in gluconeogenesis in liver by T_4.
- Increase breakdown of insulin.
- Decrease rate of secretion of insulin.

20. Give physiological basis of use of T_4 metabolites as cholesterol lowering agents.

T_4 metobolites have greater cholesterol lowering activity than natural occuring form of T_4 whereas other activity of thyroid is less.

21. Give physiological basis of impaired fertility in women in alteration of thyroid activity.

Alteration of thyroid activity impairs fertility in women as normal level of T_4 is essential for normal menstruation and fertility.

22. Why glucocorticoids when used in patients with bacterial infection must be used along with antibiotics?

This is because glucocorticoids will minimize the sign and symptoms of bacterial infection without much minimization of harmful effect of bacteria. Thus there may be delay in diagnosis and starting of antibiotic treatment → fatal to the person.

23. Why glucocorticoids do not produce mineralcorticoids effect on the kidneys?

It is due to presence of 11 β-hydroxycorticoids type-2 enzyme which converts glucocorticoids to their 11-oxy derivatives → prevention of binding of glucocoritcoids to mineralocorticoids receptors in kidney → no mineralocorticoids effect on kidney.

24. Why in DM glucocorticoids should not be administered?

In DM, glucocorticoids increase plasma lipid level and increase ketone body formation thus diabetic becomes worse.

25. Give physiological basis of a person suffering from hypothyroidism is advised to avoid cabbage in his diet.

Cabbage contain progoitrin and progoitrin activator which converts progoitrin into goitrin which is an active antithyroid agent that results incorporation of iodine with tyrosin thereby less thyroid hormone production. This is why a person suffering from hypothyroidism is advised to avoid cabbage in his diet.

26. Give physiological basis of higher incidences of fractures after 40 years of age.

After 40 years of age there is normally progressive loss of bone mass (osteoporosis) due to increased osteoclastic activity that increases bone resorption. This is why fractures are more common in old age.

27. Give physiological basis of chronic renal disease may produce secondary hyperparathyroidism.

In chronic renal disease → decrease formation of 1-25 DHCC formation by diseased kidney → prolonged decrease in serum calcium → to compensate this low serum calcium there is hypertrophy of parathyroid known as secondary hyperparathyroidism by feedback stimulation.

28. Give physiological basis of pregnant women have higher total plasma 17-hydroxycorticoids levels without symptoms of glucocorticoids excess.

In case of pregnancy there is high synthesis of corticosteroid binding globulins by increased level of oestrogen → increase in protein bound cortisol and decrease in free cortisol → stimulation of ACTH secretion → increase in plasma cortisol to a level which saturates the CBG and free cortisol level returns to normal → bound cortisol concentration remains increased but ACTH secretion comes back to normal → no glucocorticoids excess.

29. Give physiological basis of anemia in chronic adrenal insufficiency.

It leads to moderate anemia because of withdrawal of stimulatory effect of glucocorticoids on erythropoiesis.

30. Give physiological basis of glucocorticoids are used in prevention of rejection of tissue transplant.

Glucocorticoids are used in prevention of rejection of tissue transplant as glucocorticoids reduces or prevents the immunoresponse of the recipient to an organ transplant.

31. Give physiological basis of diabetic patients fail to gain weight inspite of polyphagia.

During diabetic mellitus polyphagia though increases the intake of food, it can not induce weight gain rather there may be weight loss as there is intracellular glucose deficiency → mobilization of fats and breakdown of proteins in the muscles → weight loss.

32. Explain: Glucagon is a hormone of energy release.

Glucagon is anti insulin i.e. gluconeogenic, glycogenolytic and lipolytic and thus favours the energy release and thereby called as ***hormone of energy release.***

33. Explain: Insulin is a hormone of energy storage.

Insulin is *glycogenic*, *anti gluconeogenic*, *antilipolytic* and anti ketotic. Because of these qualities it favours storage of absorbed nutrients and thus is known as *Hormone of Energy storage* or *Hormone of abundance.*

34. Explain that the diabetic patients are given K^+ supplements when treated with insulin.

If diabetic patients are treated with insulin there may be severe hypokalemia which is fatal. Hence in such patients K^+ should also be given.

35. Explain: diabetic ketoacidosis produces marked resistance to insulin.

It is by:

- Producing metabolic acidosis → cellular dehydration
- Producing large amount of free fatty acids
- Increasing the activity of glucagons, GH and glucocorticoids.

36. Explain: Ketoacidosis is more severe in obese compaired to thin persons.

Diabetic Ketoacidosis is more severe in obese persons because it is directly related with the amount of fat stores in the body.

37. Explain: FFA estimation is a better index to asses the severity of DM than the blood sugar.

It is because FFA levels also becomes high in diabetis mellitus as that of glucose.

38. Explain: DM is more a disease due to disturbance of lipids than carbohydrates metabolism.

Disturbances in fat metabolism is so prominent in DM that it has been called more as a disease of lipids.

39. How does histamin produces allergic reactions?

Histamine produces allergic reaction by causing severe bronchoconstriction and profound fall of arterial blood pressure.

40. How do antihistaminic drug act?

Antihistaminic drug acts by following way:

- β adrenergic receptor agonist (isoprenaline, epinephrine etc.) causes relaxation of smooth muscle in the bronchioles and thus counteracts the effect of histamine.
- H_1 receptor antagonists (promethazine) acts as a competitive inhibition to prevent histamin induced contraction of smooth muscles of bronchi and intestine.
- H_2 receptor antagonists (cimetidin) inhibits the histamin induced HCl secretion.

41. Mention the role of PGs in inflammation.

PGs induce inflammation by:

- Increasing the histamin induced vascular permeability.
- Sensitizes cutaneous nerve endings to the bradykinin induced pain sensation.

42. Can Vit. D be called as a hormone?

In PCT of kidney vit. D (25 HCC), obtained from diet or skin, is hydroxylated to form 1-25-DHCC or active vit D_3 which is circulated through the blood to perform varried functions such as:

(i) It increases Ca^{+2} and $PO_4^{=}$ mobilisation from bone.

(ii) It increases Ca^{+2} and $PO_4^{=}$ absorption through GIT.

(iii) It increases reabsorption of Ca^{+2} from DCT and CT and $H\ PO_4^{=}$ from PCT.

Thus as it has the hormone like action it can be referred as hormone.

43. How can cretinism be prevented in the offsprings?

It is by providing the foetus with sufficient iodine to synthesise it's thyroid hormones.

44. Can T_4 be used to promote weight loss?

No, as T_4 is helpful for promoting weight gain as it increases protein synthesis and can cause increase release of GH.

45. Why adrenal cortex is essential for life?

Adrenal cortex secretes mineralocorticoids like aldosterone which is essential for life as absence of mineralocorticoids will result death of the person due to **'shock'** resulted from hypovoluemia. Besides this deficiency of aldosterone causes hyperkalemia which causes cardiac toxicity and even death due to cardiac failure.

46. Justify: The changes in eosinophil levels are used as index of ACTH secretion.

Glucocorticoids excess results decrease in eosinophil count. So low eosinophil count may be considered as the hyperactivity of glucocorticoids which may be due to high level of ACTH.

E. MCQ:

1. Oxytocin release is not regulated by (i) suckling of breast (ii) stretching of uterus (iii) stretching of cervix wall (iv) progesterone. (iv)
2. All but one are secreted by posterior pituitary gland (i) MSH (ii) ADH (iii) Oxytocin (iv) Neurophysin. (i)
3. Prolactin has following function (i) growth of mammary gland (ii) milk secretion from mammary gland (iii) inhibition of ovulation (iv) all of the above. (iv)
4. Melatonin is secreted by (i) Anterior pituitary (ii) Adrenal medulla (iii) Hypothalamus (iv) Pineal gland. (iv)
5. Which one of the following has the greatest effect on plasma osmolarity (i) progesteron (ii) vasopressin (iii) DHEA (iv) cortisol. (ii)
6. The hardest part of our body is (i) Bone (ii) Nails (iii) Dentin (iv) Enamel. (iv)
7. Which of the following in not essential in normal synthesis of thyroid hormones (i) Iodine (ii) Thyroglobulin (iii) TSH (iv) Ferritin. (iv)
8. The thyroid uptake of radio active iodine is not affected by (i) TSH (ii) TRH (iii) T4 (iv) Calcitonin. (iv)
9. The secretion of which hormone would be least affected by a fall in ECF volume (i) vasopressin (ii) aldosterone (iii) CRH (iv) oestrogen. (iv)
10. Total destruction of pancreatic beta cell does not result in (i) a rise in plasma H^+ conc (ii) a fall in plasma amino acid concentration (iii) a rise in plasma glucose concentration (iv) a fall in plasma HCO_3^- conc. (ii)
11. Which has the highest effect in causing osteoporosis (i) Cortisol (ii) Thyroxine (iii) Oestrogen (iv) PTH. (iii)
12. Osteoblasts are concerned with (i) bone resorption (ii) bone accretion (iii) formation of osteoclasts (iv) synthesis of acid phosphate. (ii)
13. All but one does not produce tetany (i) ↑ Mg^{++} level (ii) Alkalosis (iii) EDTA (iv) Low PTH level. (i)
14. The absence of oedema in primary aldosteronism is due to (i) Escape phenomen (ii) release of ANP (iii) both (i) and (ii) (iv) None. (iii)

15. In NIDDM(i) Insulin secretion from beta cells is deficient (ii) demand of insulin by the body rises (iii) none. (iii)
16. Insulin secretion is stimulated by (i) carbohydrate rich meal (ii) protein rich meal (iii) both (iv) none. (iii)
17. Healing of wound is (i) opposed by cortisol (ii) favoured by cortisol (iii) not affected by cortisol. (ii)
18. The receptors of protein hormones are present in the target cell (i) membrane (ii) cytosol (iii) nucleus (iv) DNA. (i)
19. Receptors of estrogen are present in (i) membrane (ii) cytosol (iii) nucleus (iv) none. (iii)
20. Organification of tyrosine molecule is helped by (i) TSH (ii) thyroperoxidase enzyme (iii) both (iv) none. (iii)
21. Daily secretion of GH in (i) 0.2 – 4 mg/day (ii) 4-8 mg/day (iii) 0.5-1.0 mg/day (iv) 104-110 mg/day. (i)
22. All these are functions of GH except (i) increases protein synthesis (ii) increases protein catabolism (iii) increases blood glucose level (iv) increases overall growth of skeletal and extra skeletal tissues. (ii)
23. All are the hypofunction disorder of GH except (i) Adiposogenital syndrome (ii) Simmond's disease (iii) Cushing syndrome (iv) Dwarfism. (iii)
24. The source of ADH is (i) Supraoptic N of hypothalamus (ii) Supraoptic N of thalamus (iii) paraventricular N of hypothalamus (iv) Somatotroph of pituitary. (i)
25. Grave's disease in due to hypersecretion of (i) GH (ii) TSH (iii) Thyroid hormones (iv) Glucocorticoids. (iii)
26. Cretinism occurs in (i) Hyperfunction of thyroids hormones (ii) Hypofunction of thyroids (iii) hyperfunction of glucocorticoids (iv) hypofunction of glucocorticoids. (i)
27. Non pitting oedema is a feature of (i) Grave's disease (ii) Tetany (iii) DM (iv) Myxoedema. (iv)
28. All but one are the thyroids hormones (i) T3 (ii) T4 (iii) Calcitonin (iv) Parathormone. (iv)
29. The major site of action of PTH are as follows expect (i) GIT (ii) Kidney (iii) Liver (iv) Bone. (iii)
30. Normal Serum Ca^{++} level is (i) 9-10 mg/100 ml (ii) 9-10 mg/100 ml (iii) 9-10 μg/100 ml (iv) 0.9-1.0 mg/100 ml. (iii)
31. Tetany is due to (i) Hypofunction of thyroids (ii) Hyperfunction of thyroids (iii) Hypofunction of parathyroid (iv) Hyperfunction of parathyroids. (iii)
32. Laryngeal stridor is clinical feature of (i) Acromegally (ii) Simmond's disease (iii) Grave's disease (iv) Tetany. (iv)
33. Aldosterone is synthesized by (i) Z. *glomerulosa* (ii) Z. *fascicularis* (iii) Z. *reticularis* (iv) Both (i) and (ii). (i)
34. All are the natural form of glucocorticoids except (i) Cortisol (ii) Cortisone (iii) Corticosterone (iv) Dexamethasone. (iv)
35. Cortisol is transported by all except one (i) albumin (ii) cortisol binding globulin (iii) prealbumin (iv) free form. (iii)
36. Following is not the function of glucocorticoid (i) decreased FA level in blood (ii) ketosis (iii) ↑protein catabolism (iv) $\downarrow Ca^{+}$ absorption in GIT. (i)
37. Purple striae is the clinical features of (i) Cretinism (ii) Cushing syndrome (iii) Conn's syndrome (iv) Addison's disease. (ii)

38. Adisonian crisis in due to the failure of (i) glucocorticoid release (ii) mineralocorticoid release (iii) adrenal steroidal release (iv) gonadal steroidal release. (i)

39. All are the functions of catecholamines except (i) glycogenolysis (ii) gluconeogenic (iii) lipolytic (iv) ketogenesis. (ii)

40. Fight or flight response in mediated by the hormone (i) Thyroid Hormone (ii) Steroid Hormone (iii) Parathyroid Hormone (iv) Adrenal medullary hormone. (iv)

41. All are the examples of pancreatic hormone except (i) Insulin (ii) Glucagons (iii) Secretin (iv) Somatostatin. (iii)

42. Insulin has following action except (i) glycogenic (ii) antilipolytic (iii) antiketotic (iv) gluconeogenic. (iv)

Central Nervous System

10

A. Long type:

1. Define neurone. Describe the structure and properties of neurone. How the impulse travels through the nerve fibers?

Neurone is defined as the structural and functional unit of the nervous system.

Structure of neurone:

Like other cells the neurone has also all the organelles in it's cytoplasm except centrosome (therefore unable to divide). However it is different from others because of presence of 2 processes i.e. axon and dendrites. Thus each neurone consists of soma or nerve cell body, dendrites and axon (Fig. 10.1).

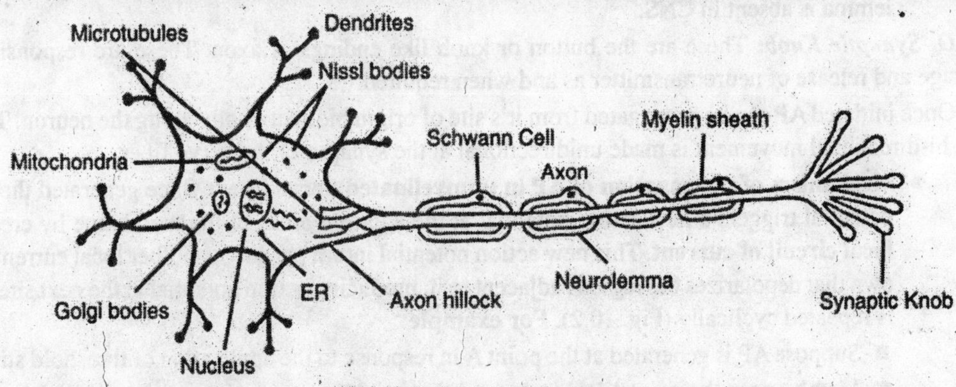

Fig. 10.1: Structure of neurone

A. *Soma or nerve cell body*:

It is irregular shaped and constituted by a mass of cytoplasm called ***neuroplasm*** enclosed by a cell membrane. The cytoplasm of each nerve cell contains:

- a centrally placed nucleus.
- some membranous organelles containing ribosomes present throughout the soma, dendrites but not in the axons. These organelles, responsible for protein synthesis in the neurons are called Nissl bodies.
- some thread like structures present in the form of a network in soma and it's processes called ***neurofibrils*** consisted by microfilaments and microtubules.

- some mitochondria present throughout the soma and axon.
- and also golgi apparatus responsible for packaging of proteins into granules.

B. Dendrite:

- These are 5-7 processes extending out from the soma and are branched repeatedly.
- These transmit impulse towards the cell body.

C. Axon:

- It is the longer process of the nerve cell arised from a broadened area of the cell body known as ***Axon Hillock*** which is characterised by absence of nissl granules.
- In it's center there is a cytoplasmic fluid known as axoplasm which is surrounded by a membrane called ***axolemma.*** The axoplasm along with the axolemma is called as the **axis cylinder of the nerve fiber.**
- Axoplasm contains mitochondria, neurofibrils, axoplasmic vesicles but no Nissl bodies. Therefore the proteins synthesised by the soma are to be transmitted through the axon by axonal flow.
- Most of the axons are insulated by a concentric layer of protein—lipid complexes known as ***Myelin Sheath*** except the initial segment of axon, at it's endings and also at it's periodic constrictions about 1mm apart called ***Nodes of Ranvier.***
- The axon which contains myelin sheath is known as **myelinated nerve fiber** and is responsible for rapid transmission of electrical impulse. Whereas the axon which is not enclosed by myelin sheath is known as **Non myelinated nerve.**
- Surrounding the myelin sheath there is a thin membrane called ***neurolemma*** which contains ***Schwann cells.*** It is necessary for the formation of myelin sheath or myelinogenesis process.
- In non myelinated nerve fiber the neurilemma continuously surrounds axolemma. This neurilemma is absent in CNS.

D. Synaptic Knob: These are the button or knob like endings of axon. These are responsible for storage and release of neurotransmitter as and when required.

Once initiated AP can be propagated from it's site of origin bidirectionally along the neuron. Though this bi-directional movement is made unidirectional at the synapse of the nerve fiber.

- **Mechanism of propagation of AP in unmyelinated nerve fiber:** Once generated the action potential triggers a new action potential at the adjacent areas of the membrane by creating a **local circuit of current.** This new action potential inturn produces another local current of it's own that depolarizes the regions adjacent to it, producing action potential at the next site which is repeated cyclically (Fig. 10.2). **For example:**
  - Suppose AP is generated at the point A in response to the application of threshold stimulus.
  - Membrane at the point A is depolarised (i.e. inside electropositive and outside electronegative), whereas the adjacent areas (B and C) is in resting stage (**resting area**) still maintaining RMP i.e. **inside electronegativity.**
  - This results flow of '+' ions from **depolarised area** (Point A) to **adjacent resting area** (Point B and C) in inside and flow of + ions from resting areas (B and C) to depolarised area (point A) in outside of the membrane. Thereby completing a local circuit.
  - This local circuit of current flow alters the potential difference across the membrane at site B and C that leads sudden opening of voltage gated Na^+ channels at the site B and C.
  - This results rapid entry of Na^+ inside at point B and C making these areas depolarized. In the meantime the previously depolarized area (i.e. point A) repolarised due to exit of K^+ through voltage gated K^+ channels.

- Thus depolarization wave is passed from point A to B and C which is continued resulting bilateral conduction of action potential.

- **Mechanism of propagation of AP in myelinated nerve (Saltatory conduction): In** case of myelinated nerve the myelin sheath acts as a insulator and does not allow the current flow. Therefore the flow of ions and local circuit of current flow occurs only through the **Nodes of Ranvier.** Thus current flows **from depolarised node of Ranvier** to nearby **resting node of Ranvier** which are placed apart resulting jumping of impulse from one node to another node. This type of propagation of action potential is known as ***Saltatory*** or ***Jumping conduction*** which is faster than in unmyelinated nerves.

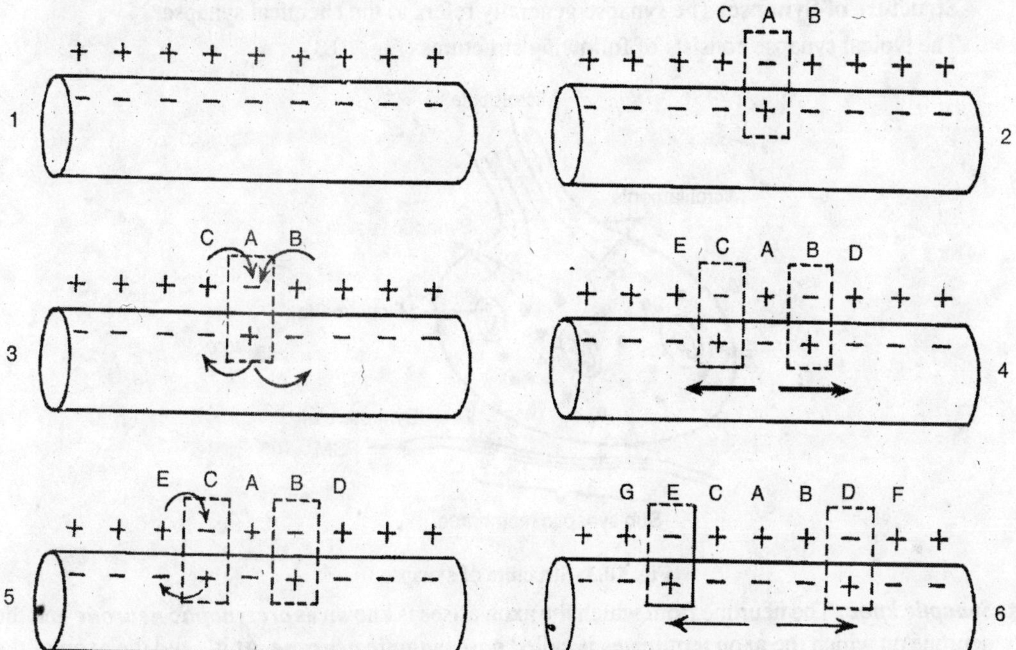

Fig. 10.2: Diagrammatic representation showing nerve conduction in unmyelinated nerve

. Define synapse. Describe its structure and properties.

The synapse is defined as the **junction between the two neurones.**

Types of synapse: Synapse is classified on the basis of anatomical configuration and also on the basis of mode of function.

***A. Anatomical classification*:** As per the anatomical configuration the synapse is of 3 types as follows:

(a) *Axosomatic synapse:* In this type of synapse axon of one neurone terminates at the cell body or soma of another neurone.

(b) *Axodendritic synapse*: In this type of sympse axon of one neurone terminates on dendrite of next neurone.

(c) *Axoaxonic synapse*: In this synapse the axon of one neurone terminates on the axon of another neurone.

***B. Functional classification*:** On the basis of mode of function synapse is again classified as 3 types as follows:

(a) *Chemical synapse*: The synapse through which electrical impulse is propagated from one neurone to next via the release of chemical substances or neurotransmitter is called chemical synapse.

(b) *Electrical synapse*: In this type of synapse the anatomical continuity between the presynaptic and post synaptic neurones is provided by gap junction through which electrical impulse can be transmitted directly without releasing neurotransmitter. This type of synapse is found little extent in nervous system and in some non nervous cells like cardiac muscle, smooth muscle of intestine and the epithelial cells of lens.

(c) *Conjoint Synapse*: The synapses where transmission is both chemical and electrical is known as ***conjoint synapse***.

Structure of Synapse: The synapse generally refers to the chemical synapse.

The typical synapse consists of following structures (Fig. 10.3).

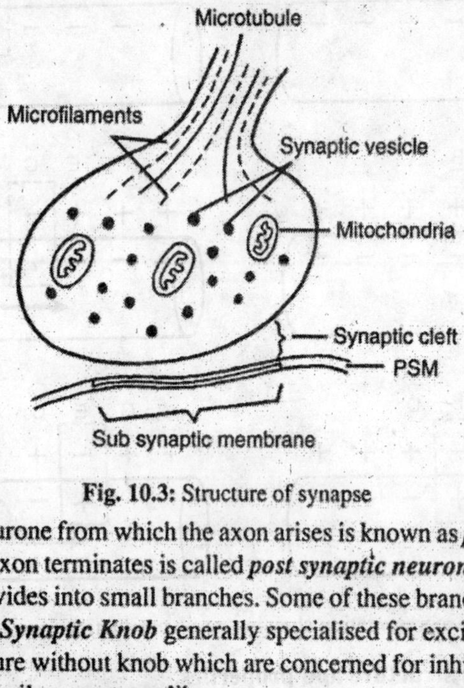

Fig. 10.3: Structure of synapse

A. *Synaptic knob*: The neurone from which the axon arises is known as ***presynaptic neurone*** and the neurone on which the axon terminates is called ***post synaptic neurone***. At it's end the axon of the presynaptic neurone divides into small branches. Some of these branches end as a knob like swollen structure known as ***Synaptic Knob*** generally specialised for excitatory function whereas others end as coiled structure without knob which are concerned for inhibitory action. However both of the ends comprise similar structures like:

(a) *Mitochondria*—helps in synthesising neurotransmitter.

(b) *Synaptic vesicle*—store neurotransmitter substances.

(c) *Microtubules*—helps in the transportation of synaptic vesicles down the axon.

B. *Synaptic cleft*: In between the presynaptic membrane and post synaptic membrane there is a gap of 20-30 nm called ***Synaptic Cleft***. The basal lamina of this cleft contains **cholinesterase enzyme** which destroys acetyl choline.

C. *Post synaptic membrane*: The membrane of the post synaptic neurone which involves in forming synapse is called ***subsynaptic membrane*** and the remainder of membrane of post synaptic neurone is called post synaptic membrane. Usually the receptors are located on the subsynaptic membrane.

Properties of synapse:

A. *Law of forward (one way) conduction*: Synapse allows the conduction of impulses in one direction only i.e. from the presynaptic neurone to the post synaptic neurone. This direction of propagation of impulse is known as ***Orthrodromic conduction*** and this law is known as **Bell-Magnedie Law** or **law of forward conduction.** The propagation of impulse in reverse direction is known as ***Antidromic conduction*** which is restricted by the synapse due to the inability of releasing NT from the dendrites of presynaptic membrane.

B. *Law of convergence and divergence*: In some synapses (e.g. in spinal motor neurons) many presynaptic neurones terminate on a single post synaptic neurone known as ***Convergence*** (Fig. 10.4A). In other cases in most of the synapses, one presynaptic neurone terminates on many post synaptic neurones (Fig. 10.4B) known as ***Divergence.***

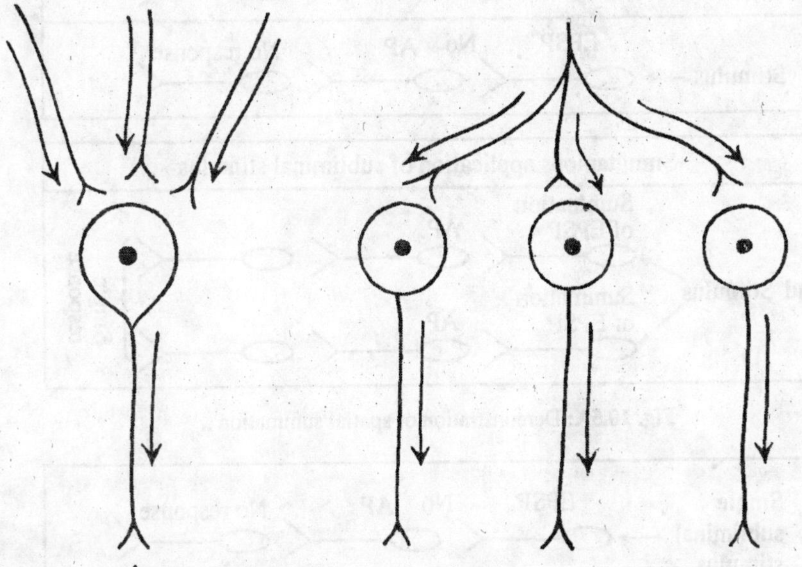

Fig. 10.4: Properties of synapse (A = law of convergence and B = law of divergence

C. *Presence of synaptic delay*: There is a delay of about **0.5 m sec** during the transmission of impulse from one neurone to another via a single synapse. This is known as ***Synaptic delay*** which is due to:

- time taken for release of NT.
- time taken for movement of NT from presynaptic membrane to post synaptic membrane (PSM) via ECF of synaptic cleft.
- time taken to open the ligand gated channels and entry of ions inside the cell membrane of PSM in response to binding of NT to receptor protein.

D. *Presence of fatigueness*: Repeated stimulation of presynaptic neurone leads to gradual decrease and finally disappearance of postsynaptic response, This is known as ***Synaptic fatigue*** or ***Habituation*** which is due to:

- exhaustion of neurotransmitters from the synaptic knob.
- decreased release of NT from the synaptic knob due to inactivation of voltage gated Ca^{++} channels.

E. *Ability to summate the response*: When a number of presynaptic excitatory terminals are stimulated simultaneously (***spatial summation***) or when a single presynaptic terminal is stimulated repeatedly (***temporal summation***), there is gradual increase of excitatory post synaptic potential or EPSP (Fig. 10.5). This property of synapse is known as ***Summation.***

F. *Occlusion and Subliminal fringe*: When two afferent excitatory nerves (i and ii) are stimulated simultaneously (Fig. 3.7) the sum total responses obtained is lesser than the responses obtained by the individual nerve. This property is known as Occlusion.

On the other hand when two afferent excitatory nerves are stimulated simultaneously the sum total responses obtained is greater than the responses obtained by the individual nerve. This phenomenon is known as ***Subliminal Fringe.***

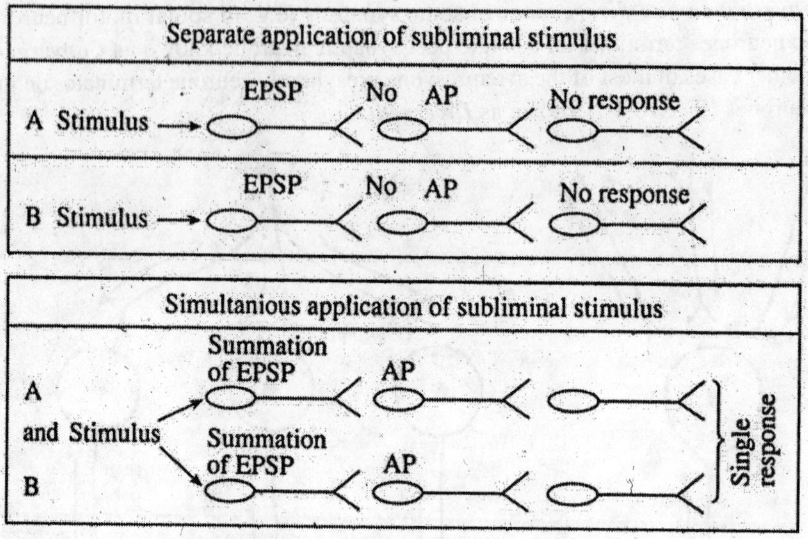

Fig. 10.5A: Demonstration of spatial summation

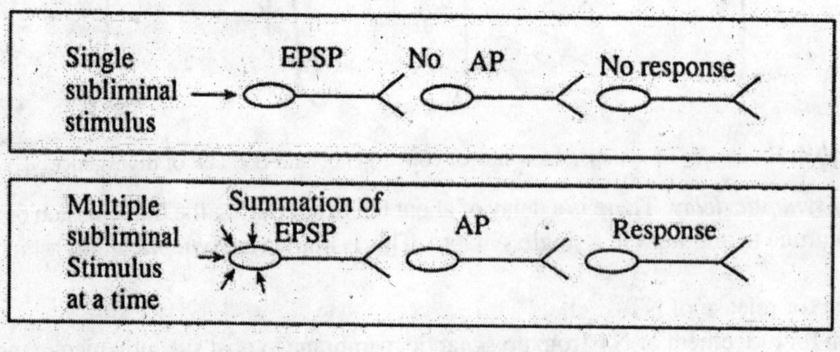

Fig. 10.5B: Demonstration of temporal summation

G. ***Synaptic plasticity*****:** Synaptic transmission can be increased or decreased on the basis of past experience. This property is known as ***Synaptic plasticity*** which plays an important role in learning and memory.

3. Describe the sequence of events of synaptic transmisson. How inhibition at synapse is achieved? Give its physiological significance.

Mechanism of synaptic transmission: The main function of the synapse is to transmit the electrical impulses from one neurone to next though some synapse is inhibitory to the transmission of electrical impulses. The sequence of events of both the function is represented by flow chart FC 10A (next page).

Physiological significance of synaptic inhibition: Vasodilatation of the blood vessels and relaxation of the muscles are important physiological functions on which the homeostatic functions of the body solely depends. These are purely due to the synaptic inhibition. Besides this synaptic inhibition is responsible for efficacy of neuronal and muscular tissue.

Spread of action potential down the axon and reaches to presynaptic membrane of axon terminal

↓

Opening of voltage gated calcium channels present in presynaptic membrane

↓

Influx of calcium ion from ECF into the synaptic knob

↙ ↘

Attraction of negatively charged synaptic vesicles from cytoplasm of synaptic knob

Phosphorylation of proteins that binds synaptic vesicles to the cytoskeleton inside the synaptic knob

↘ ↙

Synaptic vesicles are lined interior to the presynaptic membrane

↓

Release of neurotransmitter to the synaptic cleft by exocytosis

↓

Binding of these neurotransmitters to the receptors present in subsynaptic membrane

EITHER

Opening of ligand gated Na^+ channels in post synaptic and subsynaptic membrane

↓

Entry of Na^+ inside the post synaptic membrane

↓

Slight depolarisation of PSM known as excitatory post synaptic potential (EPSP)

↓

Summation of EPSP due to the simultaneous discharge of many terminals

↓

Initiation of action potential which now propagates down the post synaptic neurone to reach another synapse (i.e. **Excitation of post synaptic neurone**)

OR

Opening of ligand gated Cl^- and K^+ channels in response to release of inhibitory neurotransmitter

↓

Entry of Cl^- inside and/or exit of K^+ out of PSM

↓

Hyperpolarisation of PSM known as inhibitory post synaptic potential (IPSP)

↓

Increases the threshold value for initiating the AP by any stimulus

↓

No passing of electrical impulse towards the post synaptic neurone (i.e. **inhibition of post synaptic neurone**)

FC 10A: Schematic diagram showing mechanism of synaptic transmission

4. With suitable diagram describe neuromuscular junction. Discuss in brief the mechanism of neuromuscular transmission.

The junction between the terminal branch of the motor nerve fiber and the muscle fiber is known as ***Neuromuscular Junction*** or ***Myo-Neural Junction***.

Structure: Both the light and E/M structure is represented by (Fig. 10.6).

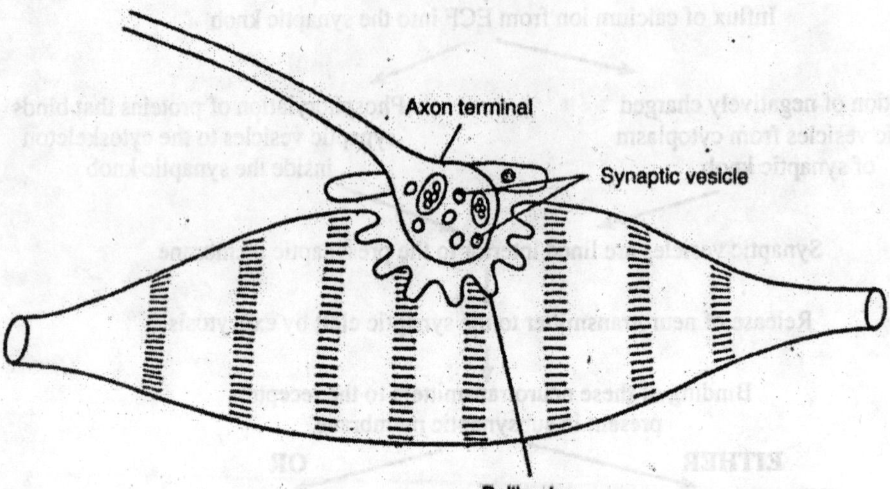

Fig. 10.6: EM structure of neuromuscular junction

- ***Light microscopic:*** While approaching to the muscle fiber each terminal branch of the motor nerve fiber looses it's myelin sheath close to the muscle and divides into a number of terminal buttons or end feet. Each of these terminal buttons invaginates inside the muscle fiber and makes a close and intensive contact with a specialised part of muscle sarcoplasm known as ***Motor end plate***.
- ***Electron microscopic:*** The membrane of the nerve ending close to the muscle is called ***pre synaptic membrane*** whereas the muscle membrane is known as ***post synaptic membrane***. The space between these two membranes is called as ***synaptic cleft***. At the terminal buttons there are many mitochondria and synaptic vesicles which contain the neurotransmitter substances Acetyl Choline (ACh). Mitochondria on the other hand contains ATP which provides the energy for the synthesis of ACh. Whereas the synaptic cleft contains basal lamina the matrix of which contains large quantity of enzyme acetyl cholinesterase which hydrolyses the ACh once it's action is over.

  Underneath the nerve endings, the muscle membrane of motor end plate is thrown into a number of folds called ***Palisades*** which increase the surface area on which ACh can act. Moreover on the post synaptic membrane there are some receptors which are stimulated by both ACh and Nicotine. These receptors are called as Nicotinic ACh receptors.

Mechanism of neuromuscular transmission: The mechanism of neuromuscular transmission is represented sequentially by the following flow chart:

Propagation of action potential to presynaptic membrane of motor nerve ending → opening of voltage gated Ca^{++} channels of presynaptic membrane of motor nerve terminal → entry of Ca^{++} from ECF to terminal button → release of ACh from terminal button to the synaptic cleft by exocytosis → ACh diffuses quickly (within few hundred microseconds) to the post synaptic membrane → binding of ACh to the nicotinic ACh receptor present on the post synaptic membrane → opening of ligand gated Na^{+} channels *present on the post synaptic membrane → entry of Na^+ ions from ECF to muscle inside → depolarisation of post synaptic membrane to develop local potential called* ***End Plate Potential (EPP)*** *which is not propagatory in nature → When this EPP reaches to a threshold of –40 to –50 mv it causes generation of action (spike) potential which propagate all through the muscle to initiate muscular contraction.*

5. Define reflex. Describe a reflex arc with the help of suitable diagram. Classify reflexes. What is mass reflex?

It is the involuntary or autonomic response elicited by specific stimulus of threshold intensity with the involvement of CNS.

Reflex are:

- It is the pathway through which any reflex action is mediated.
- The **Components** of reflex arc are (Fig. 10.7) as follows:

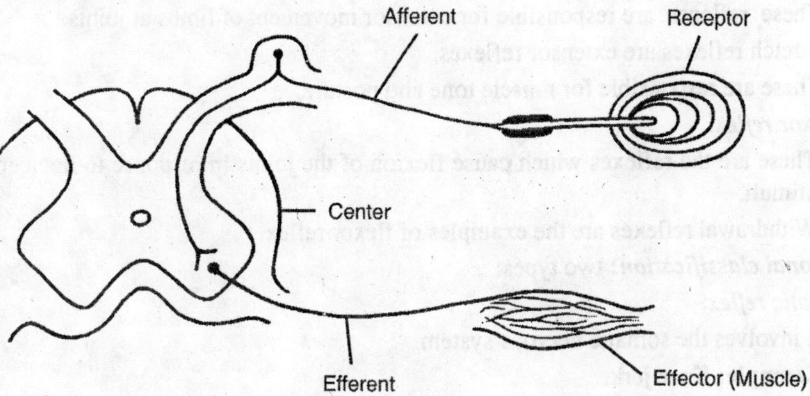

Fig. 10.7: Diagrammatic representation of a reflex arc

(i) ***Receptor***—This detects the change of internal or external environment and transmits the impulse to center.

(ii) ***Afferent (sensory) nerve***— It carries the impulse from receptor to center.

(iii) ***Higher centers***—It is the part of CNS where afferent limb ends and either synapses directly with efferent motor neurone or establish connection with the efferent neurone via interneurones.

(iv) ***Efferent (Motor) nerve***—It carries the efferent impulses from the center to the effector organ.

(v) ***Effector organ***—These are basically muscles or glands which shows the reflex action.

Classification of reflex:

A. Depending on inborn or acquired: It is of 2 types—

(a) *Unconditioned reflex*:

- These reflexes are present since birth i.e. inborn.
- **Example**: Salivation after taking food, knee jerk etc.

(b) *Conditioned reflex*:

- These are not present from birth but acquired in later life on the bass of past experiences through conditioning and learning.
- **Example:** Salivation by seeing tasty food the taste of which is known.

B. Depending on he number of synapses present in the reflex arc: It is of 2 types:

(i) Monosynaptic reflex:

- When there is only one synapse present in the reflex arc it is known as monosynaptic reflex.

- **Example:** Knee jerk, Ankle jerk etc.

(ii) Polysynaptic reflex:

- When more than one synapse is present in the reflex arc it is known as polysynaptic reflex.
- **Example:**
    - Withdrawl reflex i.e. protective reflex e.g. automatic withdrawl of limb if it comes in contact with hot object.
    - Plantar reflex i.e. scratching the outer border of the sole of foots by blunt object results **dorsiflexon of toes.**

***C. Physiological classification*:** It is of 2 types:

(i) Extensor reflex:

- These reflexes are responsible for extensor movement of limbs at joints.
- Stretch reflexes are extensor reflexes.
- These are responsible for muscle tone and posture.

(ii) Flexor reflex:

- These are the reflexes which cause flexion of the joints in response to nociceptive (pain) stimuli.
- Withdrawal reflexes are the examples of flexor reflex.

***D. Functional classification*:** two types:

(i) Somatic reflex:

- It involves the somatic nervous system.
- **Example:** Knee jerk.

(ii) Autonomic reflex:

- It involves the autonomic nervous system.
- **Example:** Sino-aortic reflex, Gastro-colic reflex, etc.

***E. Clinical classification*:** It is of 4 types:

(i) Superficial reflexes:

- These are initiated by stimulating appropriate receptors of skin and mucus membrane.
- These are usually polysynaptic.
- **Example:** Planter reflex, Corneal reflex, Conjuctival reflex, Cremasteric reflex, etc.

(ii) Deep reflexes:

- These are elicited on stroking the tendon.
- These are basically stretch reflexes.
- **Example:** knee jerk, ankle jerk etc

(iii) Visceral reflexes:

- These are the reflexes in which part of the reflex arc is formed by autonomic nervous system.
- **Example:** Pupillary reflex, Carotid sinus reflex etc.

(iv) Pathological reflexes:

- These are not found normally.
- Elicited in case of diseased state.

Mass reflex:

- In the recovery stage of reflex activity after complete transaction of spinal cord, sometimes a widespread reaction can be elicited by scratching the skin over the lower limbs or the anterior abdominal wall depending upon the level of lesion. This is known as Mass reflex.

- This is characterized by spasm in flexor muscle of both lower limb, evacuation of bladder with profuse sweating.

6. Define receptors. Classify it. Why it is called as biotransducer? Enumerate its properties.

Definition: The receptor is a modified and specialised sensory or afferent nerve ending which undergoes rapid depolarisation in response to a specific stimulus of a threshold intensity and ultimately sends the information to the CNS.

Classification: Receptors are generally classified into two types—

A. *Exteroceptors*: This gives response to stimuli arising from **outside the body**. These are further subdivided into 3 groups.

a. **Cutaneous:** These are mechanoreceptors present in the skin and are of 4 types as per the nature of stimulus.

i. *Touch receptors*—like **Meissner's corpuscle** and **Merkel's disc.**

ii. *Pressure receptors*—like **Pacinian corpuscle.**

iii. *Thermo receptors*—like **Krause's end bulb** for cold and **Ruffini's end organ** for warm temperature.

iv. Pain receptors—like free nerve endings.

b. **Chemoreceptors:** These give response to chemical stimuli. **Example:** Taste buds for taste sensation and olfactory cells for smell sensation.

c. **Telereceptors:** These are stimulated in response to the stimuli arising away from the body like hair cells of ***Organ of Corti*** for hearing and ***rods and cones*** in retina for vision.

B. *Interoceptors*: These give response to stimuli arising **within the body**. These are of two types.

a. **Viscero receptors:** Present in viscera and are stimulated either—by stretch (stretch receptor) or pressure (baroreceptor), or chemicals (chemoreceptor) or osmolarity of body fluid (osmo receptors).

b. **Proprioceptors:** These are stimulated in response to the change in position of different body parts. These include receptor in labyrinth apparatus, and muscle spindle, golgi tendon, pacinian corpuscle etc. in muscle, ligament, joint, tendon etc.

Receptors are known as ***bio transducer*** i.e. it acts as a transducer which converts any form of energy (touch, pressure, temperature, etc.) into electrical energy and transmit this electrical energy to higher centers.

Properties:

a. It obeys the ***Law of Adequate Stimulus***: Each type of receptor gives maximum response to a particular or specific stimulus. However it can give incomplete response to other type of stimulus provided the intensity of stimulus is higher. **For example** warm water stimulates Ruffini's receptor at lower intensity of stimulus producing a specific response though it also stimulates the free nerve endings of pain at high intensity of stimulus and this response is incomplete. This property of the receptor is known as Law of Adequate Stimulus or ***Specificity of Response.***

b. It obeys ***Muller's Doctrine of specific nerve energy***: Sensation produced by the impulses generated in a receptor depends on the specific part of the brain that they ultimately activate. This principle as per the name of Muller is known as **Muller's Doctrine of specific nerve energy.** This property explains why stimulation of a touch receptor causes sensation of touch not cold.

c. It obeys ***Law of Projection***: Stimulation of any part of sensory pathway i.e. from sense organ to cortex results the conscious sensation which is referred only to the location of the receptor of that specific sensory pathway. **For example** if a limb is lost by amputation or accident the patient feels intense pain and proprioceptive sensations in that particular non existing limb which is amputed, due to the irritation of the damaged nociceptive and proprioceptive afferents at the stump of the removed limb. This type of sensation of pain in non existing limb is called ***Phantom limb*** and as the sensations are referred to the absent limb where receptors used to be located it is known as **Law of projection.**

d. It obeys ***Law of Intensity Discriminations***: The information about the intensity of stimulus is perceived by the sensory cortex through two mechanisms as follows:
   - by variating the frequency of the action potential generated by the given receptor in response to a stimulus.
   - by altering the number of receptors involvement to transmit the impulse i.e. the more the strength of stimulus, the more the number of receptors activated (**Recruitment of sensory units**). This property explains how it is possible to tell whether the pain is mild, moderate or severe; touch is crude or fine.

e. It has got the property of adaptation: If a receptor is stimulated by a stimulus of constant strength over a long period, the frequency of the action potential generated by that receptor gradually decreases due to **accommodation** of sensory nerve fiber to the generator potential. This phenomenon is known as ***adaptation***. The degree of adaptation varies with the type of receptors and on this basis receptors are of two types:
   - ***Phasic receptors***—Get adapted rapidly and transmit impulses only when the strength of stimulus is changed e.g. touch, pressure and olfactory receptors.
   - ***Tonic receptors***—These are poorly, slowly and incompletely adapting receptors therefore they can transmit the impulse for long period even if the intensity of stimulus remains constant. e.g. pain and cold receptors.

f. It also obeys ***Weber Fechner's law***: The intensity of stimulus is directly proportional to the magnitude of generator potential (G.P.) which inturn is directly proportional to the frequency of action potential. This relationship between intensity of stimulus, size of G.P. and frequency of action potential in the receptor (afferent nerve) is known as **Weber Fechner's law.**

g. **Electrical properties:** When a receptor is stimulated a nonpropagatory, monophasic depolarisation occurs which is similar to EPSP in synapse, EPP in neuromuscular junction or electrotonic potential in nerve fiber. This monophasic, non propagatory depolarising wave is known as ***Receptor Potential*** or ***Graded Potential*** which does not obey all or none law. When this GP becomes strong enough action potential is initiated.

7. Draw a well lebelled diagram of cross section of the spinal cord showing location and functions of major ascending tracts. Describe the spino cerebellar tract.

Structure of spinal cord:

In histological study of cross sectioning, spinal cord has following structures (Fig. 10.8):

A. Fissure: On the anterior surface there is a deep furrow known as ***anterior median fissure or septum*** and on the posterior surface there is less prominent furrow known as ***posterior median fissure*** or ***sulcus.***

B. Central canal: Between these fissures there is central canal which contains cerebro spinal fluid or CSF.

C. Gray matter: This is 'H' shaped, and contains cell body of nerve fibers. It is comprised of 3 columns or ***Horns*** as follows:

(a) **Dorsal gray horn:**
   - It is narrow, sensory.
   - Cell body of these neurones are in dorsal root ganglia that is present outside the horn.

- It contains different nerve cell groups as follows—

  (a) *Nucleus proprius*: Present at the tip of the posterior gray horn and receives sensory information like sense of position, movement and two point discrimination.

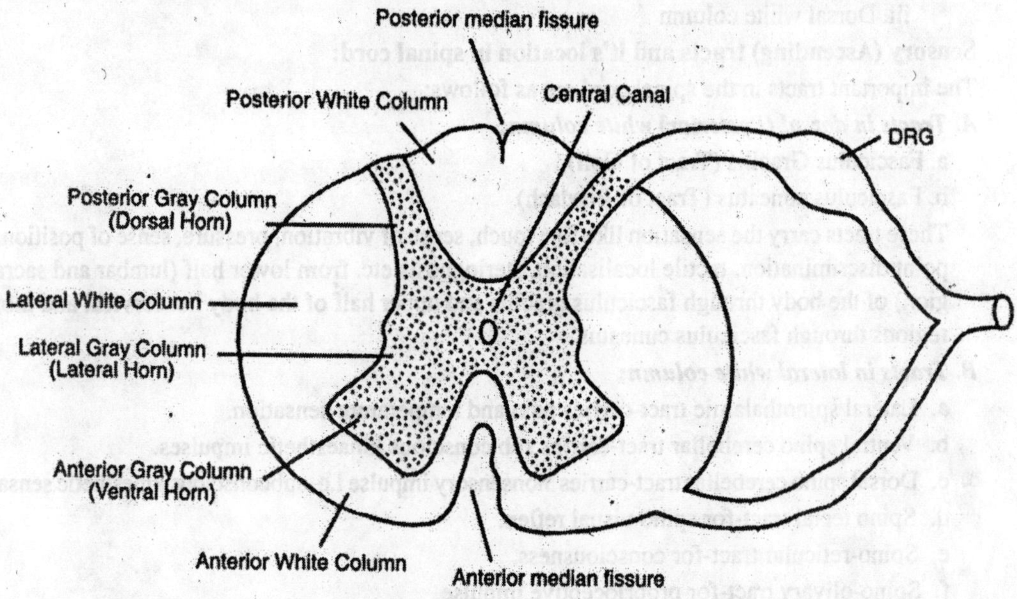

Fig. 10.8: Cross section of spinal cord

  (b) *Substantia gelatinosa of Rolando* (golgi type II neurones): It receives afferent fibers concerned with pain, temperature, touch etc. from dorsal root.

  (c) *Nucleus dorsalis* (Clarke's column): It receives proprioceptive information.

  (d) *Visceral afferent Nucleus*: It receives visceral afferent information.

(b) **Ventral gray horn:**

- It is broad, motor in function.
- Mostly golgi type-I cells are present.
- It's cell body is present within the horn.
- It contains ventral horn cells which is connected with alpha (α) and gamma (γ) motor neurones which innervate the muscles.
- The different ventral horn cells present in gray matter are—

  (i) *Medial group of ventral gray neurones* e.g. Dorso medial (DMN) and ventromedial nucleus (VMN)

  (ii) *Lateral group of ventral gray neurone* e.g. Retrodorso-lateral nucleus (RDLN), Dorso-lateral (DLN) and Ventrolateral (VLN) nucleus.

  (iii) *Central group of ventral gray neurones* e.g. Phrenic and accessory nucleus.

(c) **Intermediolateral horn:**

- This is present only in the thoracic and in first two lumbar segments only.
- Cell body of sympathetic neurones are located in this horn.

D. White matter:

- It is the outermost layer and contains axons of ascending and descending tracts.

- It is of again 3 types:
  - i. Anterior white column
  - ii. Lateral white column
  - iii. Dorsal white column

Sensory (Ascending) tracts and it's location in spinal cord:

The important tracts in the spinal cord are as follows:

A. Tracts in dorsal (Posterior) white column:

a. Fasciculus Gracilis (Tract of Goll)

b. Fasciculus cuneatus (Tract of Burdach)

These tracts carry the sensation like fine touch, sense of vibration, pressure, sense of position, two point discrimination, tactile localisation, steriognosis etc. from lower half (lumbar and sacral region) of the body through fasciculus gracilis and upper half of the body i.e. cervical and thoracic regions through fasciculus cuneatus.

B. Tracts in lateral white column:

a. Lateral spinothalamic tract-carries pain and temperature sensation.

b. Ventral spino cerebellar tract-carries sub conscious kinaesthetic impulses.

c. Dorsal spino cerebellar tract-carries nonsensory impulse i.e. subconscious kinesthetic sensation.

d. Spino tectal tract-for spino visual reflex.

e. Spino-reticular tract-for consciousness.

f. Spino-olivary tract-for proprioceptive impulse.

C. Tracts in ventral white column:

Ventral spinothalamic tract-carries crude touch sensation.

Detail pathway of spinocerebellar tract: The subconscious kinaesthetic sensation is carried by dorsal and ventral spinocerebellar tract which is described by the help of flow chart FC 10B.

Fibers from neurones of dorsal root ganglia reaches the **marginal cells** of dorsal horn cell of gray matter of spinal cord
→ Majority fibers cross the midline → Ascend through lateral white column of opposite side of spinal cord → Ascend up and terminate in the cortex of anterior lobe of cerebellum
→ Some fibers do not cross the midline → Ascend through lateral white column of same side of spinal cord → Ascend up and terminate in the cortex of anterior love of cerebellum of same side

Fibers from neurones of dorsal root ganglia reaches the **Clarke's column** of dorsal gray matter of spinal cord → 2nd order neurones orginate and reach lateral white column of same side → Ascend up and reaches medulla → Enter cerebellum to terminate in the cortex of anterior lobe of cerebellum

FC 10B: Flow chart describing dorsal and ventral spinocerebellar tract

8. Name the receptors and tract carrying touch and pressure sensation. Briefly discuss the pathway of touch sensation.

Touch and pressure sensation:

Receptors: Meissner's corpuscle, Merkels disc, Pacinian corpuscle (pressure) and also Rufini's end organs.

***Nerves*:**

(i) **For fine touch:**

1. Fasciculus gracilis (receives afferent from lower half) i.e. lumbar and sacral segment of the body.
2. Fasciculus cuneatus (receives afferent from upper half) i.e. cervical and thoracic regions of the body.

(ii)For crude touch-Ventral spinothalamic tract.

***Pathway*:**

(i) **For fine touch** (Dorsal column pathway, Fig. 10.9): Detail of this pathway is presented by following flow chart (FC 10C). The sensory input **to sensory cortex** is responsible for **perception of touch sensation.**

(ii) **For crude touch:** The pathway is known as ***Anterolateral pathway*** (Fig. 10.10) and the sensory tract is ***Ventral spinothalamic tract*** (VSTT). The detail course and termination is described in flow chart (FC 10D).

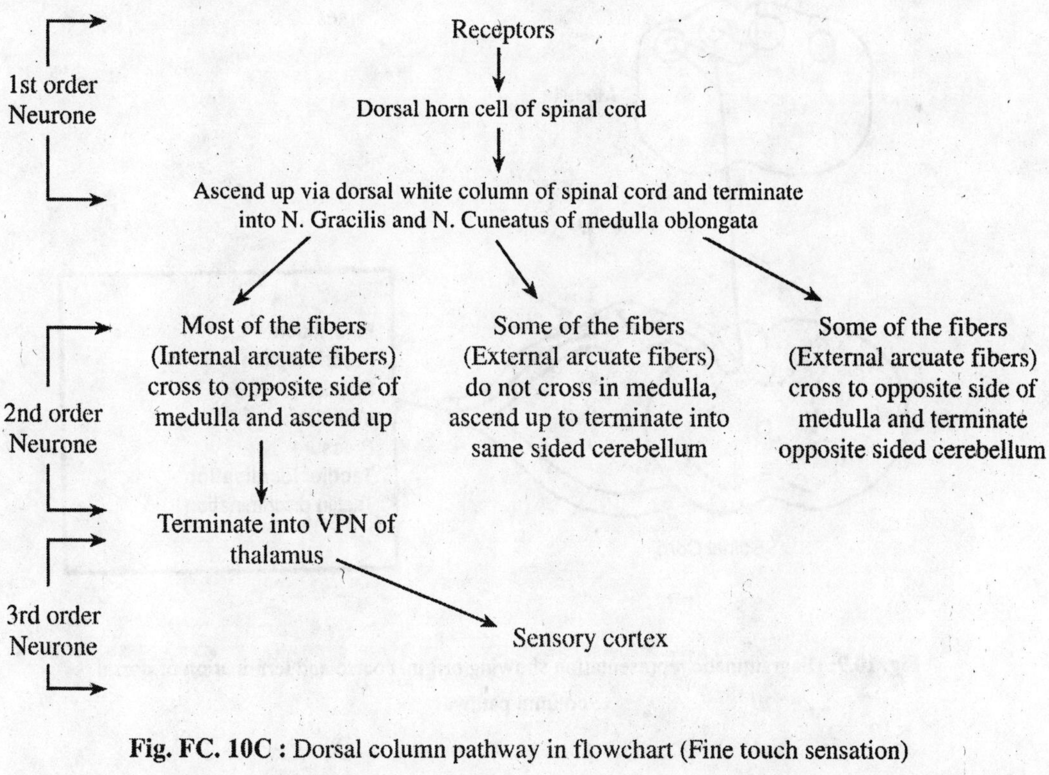

Fig. FC. 10C : Dorsal column pathway in flowchart (Fine touch sensation)

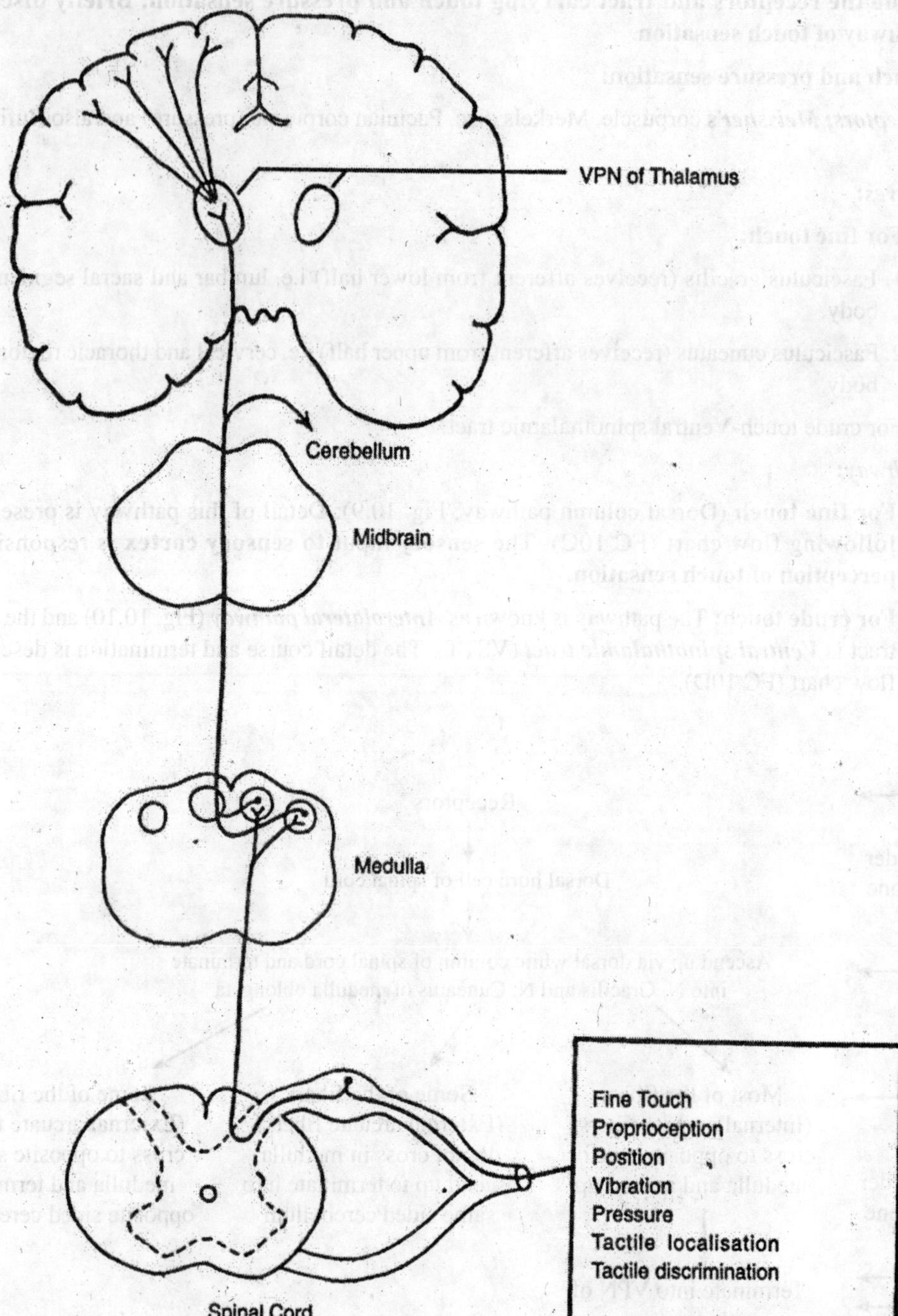

Fig. 10.9: Diagrammatic representation showing origin, coarse and termination of dorsal column pathway

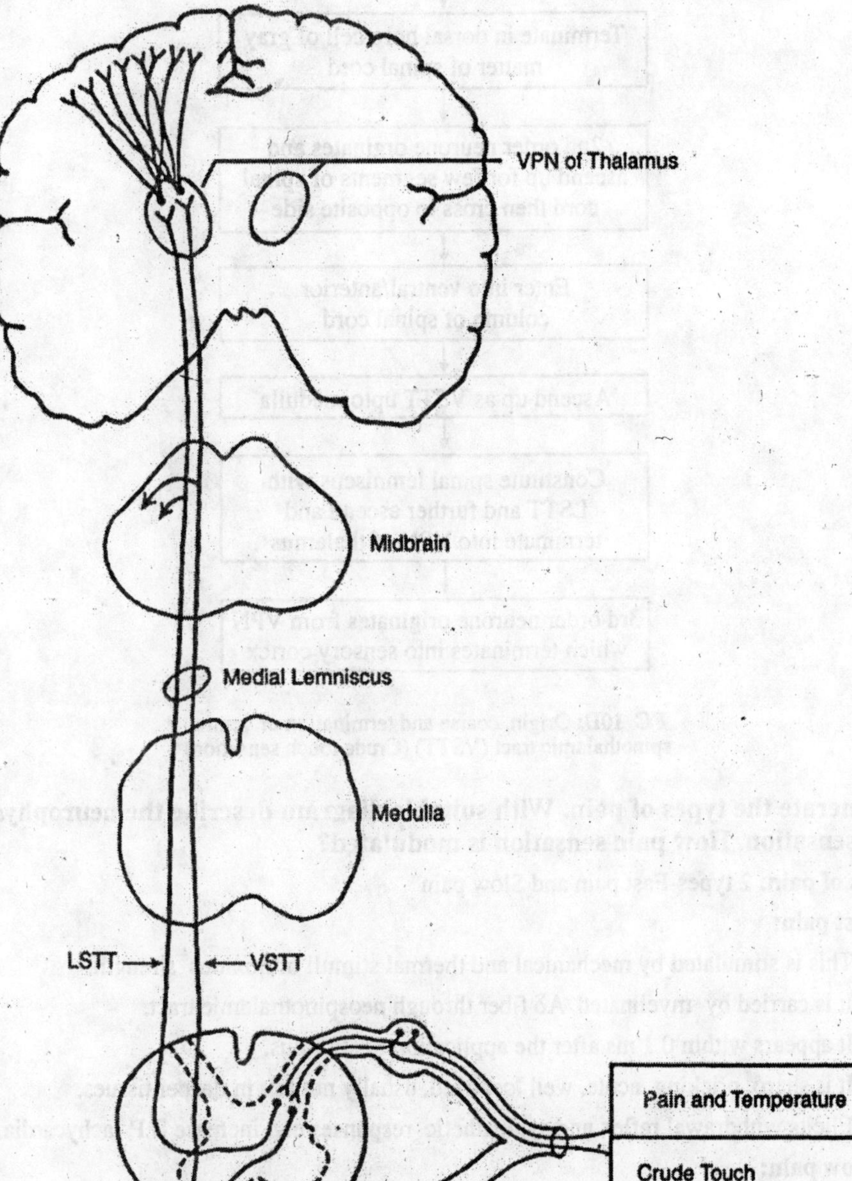

Fig. 10.10: Diagrammatic representation showing origin, coarse and termination of ventral spinothalamic tract (VSTT) and lateral spinothalamic tract (LSTT)

Receptors

↓

Terminate in dorsal horn cell of gray matter of spinal cord

↓

2nd order neurone orginates and ascend up for few segments of spinal cord then cross to opposite side

↓

Enter into ventral/anterior column of spinal cord

↓

Ascend up as VSTT upto medulla

↓

Constitute spinal lemniscus with LSTT and further ascend and terminate into VPN of thalamus

↓

3rd order neurone originates from VPN which terminates into sensory cortex

FC 10D: Origin, coarse and termination of ventral spinothalamic tract (VSTT) (Crude touch sensation)

9. Enumerate the types of pain. With suitable diagram describe the neurophysiology of pain sensation. How pain sensation is modulated?

Types of pain: 2 types-Fast pain and Slow pain

(i) Fast pain:

- This is stimulated by mechanical and thermal stimuli of noxious strength.
- It is carried by myelinated Aδ fiber through neospinothalamic tract.
- It appears within 0.1 ms after the application of stimulus.
- It is sharp, pricking, acute, well localized, usually not felt in deeper tissues.
- Elicits withdrawal reflex and sympathetic responses e.g. increase B.P, tachycardia.

(ii) Slow pain:

- This is initiated by mechanical and thermal stimuli of noxious strength and also chemicals associated with inflammation.
- It is carried by ***unmyelinated C*** fibers through paleospinothalamic tract.
- It appears a few seconds after application of stimulus and it's intensity increases slowly and lasts longer.
- It is burning, throbbing type of pain, poorly localized.
- It elicits emotional perception, nausea, vomiting, fall of BP, reduction in muscle tone.

Neurophysiological basis of pain (Fig. 10.10):

- **For fast pain:**

Impulse from nociceptors are carried by **Aδ fibers** to marginal cells of **posterior horn of spinal cord**

↓

2nd order neurone originates which crosses the midine and reaches **to lateral white column**

↓

ascend up through **anterolateral system** as neospinothalamic tract

↙ ↘

Some fibers terminate into reticular formation of midbrain hypothalamus and PAG neurones

Most fibers terminate in VPN of thalamus

↙

3rd under neurone originates which goes to basal areas of brain and somato-sensory area of **cerebral cortex.**

- **For slow pain**:

Stimulus is carried **by 'C' fiber** which enters into Lamina I and Lamina II (Substantia gelatinosa) cells of posterior horn cell of spinal cord.

↓

2nd order neurone originates which cross the midline to enter lateral white matter of spinal cord

↓

ascend up through **anterolateral system** as paleospinothalamic tract

↙ ↘

Most fibers terminate into one of these areas
(i) tectum
(ii) reticular nuclei of medulla, pons, mesencephalon
(iii) Periaquiductal gray regions

↓

Impulses **to intralaminar nuclei of thalamus**

few fibers terminate into **VPN of thalamus**

↓

different sensory areas of cerebral cortex including limbic cortical areas and hypothalamus

Modulation of pain: Our body has intrinsic capacity to inhibit the pain sensation which is known as modulation of pain or **endogenous pain relieve system.** This is achieved by two systems: ***(a) Gate control theory, (b) Descending pain inhibiting system.***

(a) ***Gate control theory.*** (Operated at spinal cord level): This theory is proposed by **Melzack and Wall** in 1965. As per this theory the dorsal horn acts as a gate. Stimulation of large fibers (i.e.

touch and pressure sensation) along with small fibers (pain fibers i.e. Ad and C fibers) close the gate thereby intensity of pain is less whereas stimulation of only small fiber results more intense feeling of pain. This is because when only pain fibers are stimulated the impulse is transmitted to SGR cells thereby to brain via spinothalamic tract to result pain sensation. Whereas stimulation of tactile receptors (touch and pressure) along with pain receptors results presynaptic inhibition at the SGR level via collaterals of Dorsal column pathway (Fig. 10.11). This results inhibition of pain.

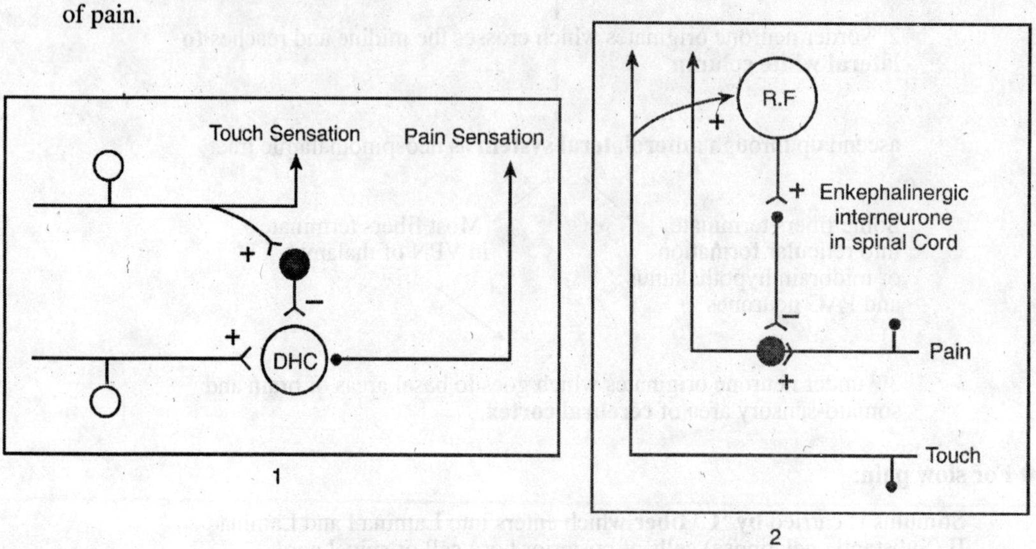

Fig. 10.11: Diagrammatic representation of gate control theory (1 = *Original concept of gate control theory*, 2 = *Recent concept of gate control theory*)

(b) *Descending pain inhibiting (DPI) system*: **Operated at brain level:** Different neurotransmitters like serotonin and opioid peptides like enkephalin, endorphin and dynorphin etc. inhibit the pain pathway before the pain sensation reaches into the brain. The detail mechanism is represented by following flow chart:

Peraqueductal gray area of midbrain and upper pons surrounding the aqueduct of Sylvius → enkephalinergic neurons originate which terminate on nucleus raphe Magnus → serotonergic neurons originate which terminate on spinal cord → enkephalinergic interneurones in the spinal cord inhibits the incoming Type C and Aδ fibers in spinal cord at dorsal horn → thus there is **Pain relief**.

10. Describe the origin, course, termination and functions of pyramidal tracts. Why these are so named?

Pyramidal tracts are those tracts which originate directly from motor cortex to spinal motor neurones. These are of two types—

(i) Corticospinal tract—Motor fibers of cerebral cortex to ventral horn cell of spinal cord constitute **corticospinal tract.** It is of again 2 types:

(1) Lateral corticospinal or crossed/indirect pyramidal tract.

(2) Anterior corticospinal or uncrossed/direct pyramidal tract.

(ii) Corticobulbar tract—Motor fibers originating from cerebral cortex, when terminates in brainstem structure is known as corticobulbar tract.

- ***Origin of corticospinal tract***: Corticospinal tract originates from—

  (i) Primary motor cortex (area 4) — 30% of fibres.

(ii) Premotor area (area 6) and Supplementary motor area (30% fibers)

(iii) Somatic sensory area (area 3,1,2)- 40% fibers.

- *Coarse and termination*: After originating from area 4, area 6, and somatic sensory area of cerebral cortex the motor fibers pass through posterior limb of the internal capsule and then downwards through the brain stem, forming pyramids in the medulla. Majority of the fibers cross to the opposite side and descend as lateral corticospinal tract whereas some fibers do not cross to the opposite side in the medulla but pass down the cord as ventral corticospinal tract (Fig. 10.12). The detail pathway is illustrated by the help of following flow chart:

Motor fibers from area 4, area 6 and parietal lobe

↓

Leave motor cortex and converge in corona radiata

↓

Pass through posterior limb of internal capsule

↓

Pass through basis peduncle of midbrain

↓

Pass through pons

↓

Enters in medulla as a thick bundle of fibers giving a pyramidal shape

↙	↘
Most of the (80-85%) fibers cross the midline in the lower part of medulla and enter into lateral white column of spinal cord	Remaining fibers (15-20%) do not cross the midline in the medulla and enter into anterior or ventral column of spinal cord
↓	↓
Descend down the spinal cord segments as lateral corticospinal tract	Descend down the spinal cord segments as ventral corticospinal tract
↓	↓
Terminate in the anterior gray column of all spinal segments to make synapse with interneurons of spinal cord	At each spinal segments it cross the midline and terminate in anterior gray column of spinal cord of cervical and upper thoracic level
↓	↓
Interneuron then make synapse with α and γ motor neurone	At each spinal cord level ultimately synapse with interneurone which innervate α and γ fibers
↘	↙

Muscle

- *Functions*:

  i. Lateral corticospinal tract: It brings about fine and precise voluntary movements (motor activity) of the body especially fine and precise movements of finger and hand for skilled activity.

ii. Ventral corticospinal tract: It is responsible for voluntary movements mainly for postural adjustments and gross body movement.

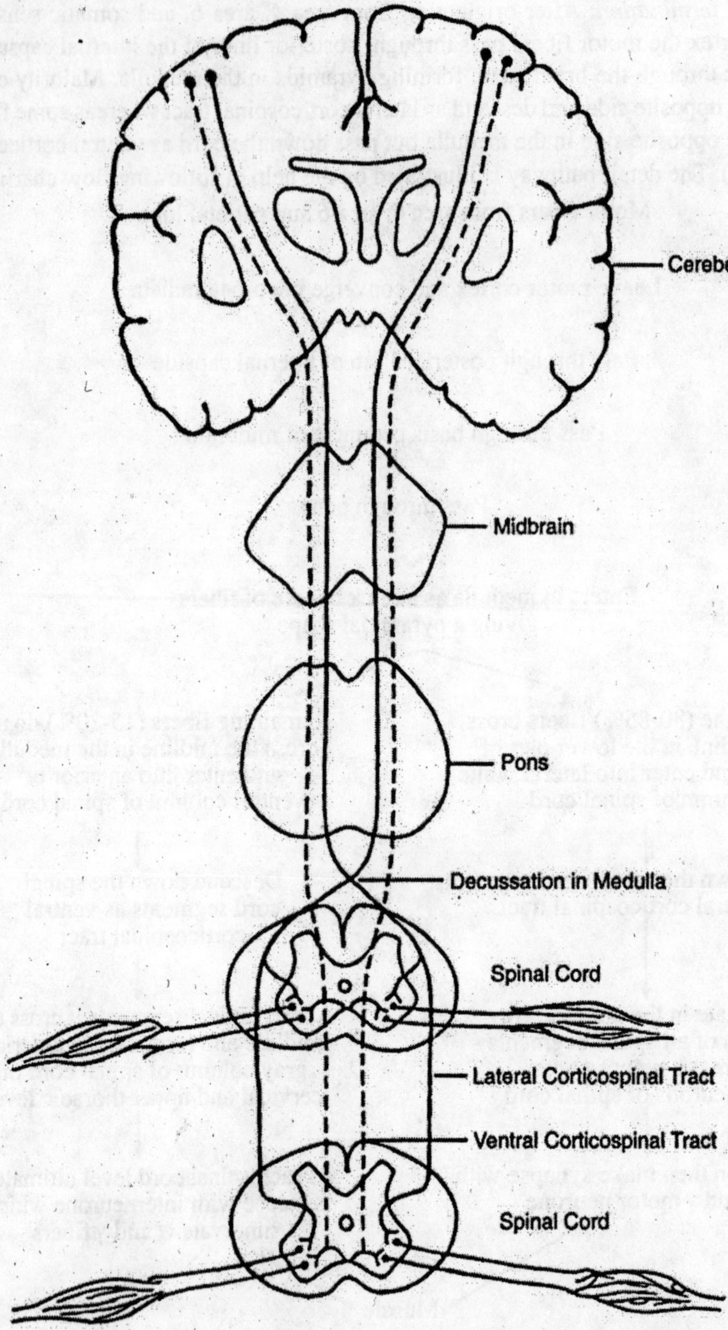

Fig. 10.12: Diagrammatic representation of origin, coarse and termination of pyramidal tracts (Solid line represents lateral corticospinal tracts and dotted line represents ventral corticospinal tracts)

iii. *Corticobulbar tract*: It initiates the voluntary movements of muscles of larynx, pharynx, face, jaw, eye, palate etc.

- *Why pyramidal tracts are so named?*

Pyramidal tracts are so named because—

(i) They are originated from **Pyramidal** or **Betz** (Giant) cells in precentral gyrus of the motor cortex.

(ii) While coming out of pons the scattered corticospinal fibers are grouped and entered the medulla as a thick bundle forming ***Pyramid*** shape.

11. Enumerate the phylogenetic division of cerebellum. Explain how a normal man is comfortably balanced in the upright position.

Phylogenetic division: 3 divisions:

(i) Archeo cerebellum: It includes floculo nodular lobe.

(ii) Paleo cerebellum: includes lingula, central lobe, culmen, lobulus simplex, ovula, pyramid and para floculi.

(iii) Neo cerebellum: includes decline, tuber and lateral hemispheres.

Human beings are comfortably balanced in upright positions by mainly controlling body posture by following ways:

- The muscles that maintain upright posture are controlled by the brain and by reflex pathways that are passed into the neural networks of the brain stem and spinal cord to variate the threshold of the spinal stretch reflex i.e. the basic reflex involved in the maintenance of posture is the stretch reflex which is modulated by different supra spinal centers to maintain muscle posture.
- The afferent impulses for the maintenance of posture (muscle tone also) arise from kinesthetic receptors, vestibular apparatus and retina of the eye. The centers which maintain the posture are at cerebral cortex, cerebellum, brain stem and spinal cord. The efferent pathways are the α motor neurones to the skeletal muscles and all those reflexes which take part in the maintenance of posture are known as **Postural reflexes** (Fig. 10.13).
- The postural reflexes not only maintain the body in an upright balanced position but also provide constant adjustments necessary to maintain a stable possible background for voluntary activity. This adjustment is done by two reflexes:

(a) Static reflexes—in which sustained contraction of muscle take place at rest.

(b) Phasic or Statokinetic reflex—in which adjustment takes place during movements.

(a) Static reflexes: It is of 4 types:

(i) **General static reflexes or *righting reflexes*:** This maintains an upright position of the body by a chain of reactions following one another in an orderly sequence as follows:

(I) Labyrinthine righting reflexes acting upon the neck muscles.

(II) Neck righting reflexes acting upon the body.

(III) Body righting reflexes acting upon the head.

(IV) Body righting reflexes acting upon the body.

(V) Optical righting reflexes.

All these reflexes except last one can be studied in ***thalamic*** or ***blind folded normal animal***.

(ii) **Local static reflexes:** These help to support the body in different position against the gravity. These can be studied in decorticate animals.

(iii) **Segmental static reflexes:** These help during walking and is basically mediated by crossed extensor reflex and can be studied experimentally by spinal animal.

(iv) **Statotonic or altitudinal reflexes:** These decrease or increase the tone of the skeletal muscle of the limb in accordance to the altitude or position of the head. These reflexes are best studied in decerebrate preparation.

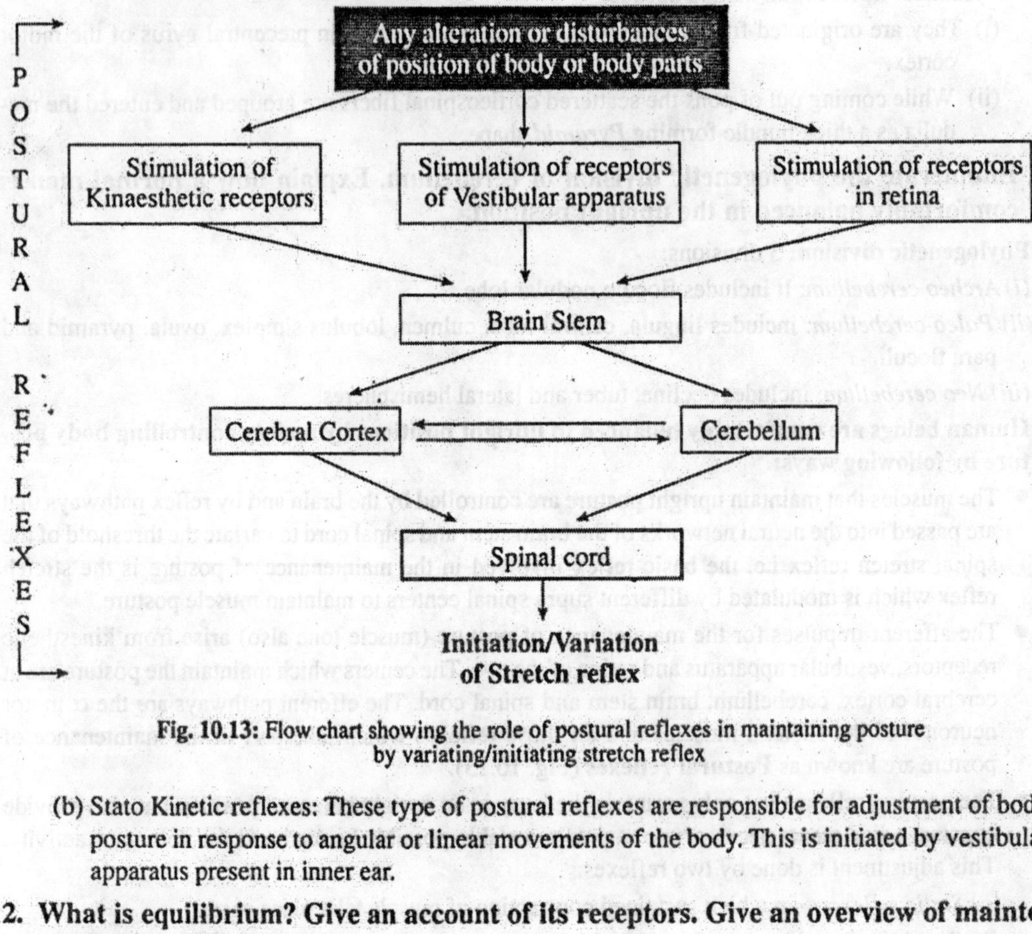

Fig. 10.13: Flow chart showing the role of postural reflexes in maintaining posture by variating/initiating stretch reflex

(b) **Stato Kinetic reflexes: These type of postural reflexes are responsible for adjustment of body posture in response to angular or linear movements of the body. This is initiated by vestibular apparatus present in inner ear.**

12. What is equilibrium? Give an account of its receptors. Give an overview of maintenance of equilibrium.

***Definition*: Equilibrium is the maintenance of line of gravity constant at rest and during movement by adjusting the tone in different muscles.**

***Receptors*:**

- **The receptor organ for maintenance of equilibrium is vestibular apparatus present in membranous labyrinth of internal ear.**
- **Vestibular apparatus consists of**
  (i) ***Three Semicircular canals* namely:**
    (a) Anterior or Superior canal
    (b) Posterior canal
    (c) Lateral / Horizontal / External canal
  (ii) ***Vestibule or Otolith organs* consisting of:**
    (a) Utricle
    (b) Saccule

- Among the two ends of each semicircular canal one end is narrow and another one is enlarged. This enlarged end is known as ***Ampulla*** which contains the receptor organ known as ***Crista Ampullaris*** which is formed by neuroepithelial cells named ***hair cells*** that function as receptor cell. These hair cells are stimulated by the movement of endolymph at the beginning and end of rotary movement. So these are termed as ***Rotary receptors***.
- Whereas the receptor organs ***Utricle*** and ***Saccule*** are called as ***Maculae*** which is also formed by neuroepithelial cells or hair cells like crista ampullaris and also some supporting cells. These hair cells of maculae are sensitive to:

  1. *effect of change of gravity*—this is why known as ***Gravity receptors***.

  2. *movement of endolymph*.
- Besides these receptors of vestibular apparatus, the visual receptors, proprioceptors in muscle and joints and body surface receptors also have role in maintaining equilibrium.

Maintenance of equilibrium: In response to any change of body part or body from its line of gravity the body/body parts restore its original position (line of gravity) by the mechanism illustrated by flow chart (FC 10E).

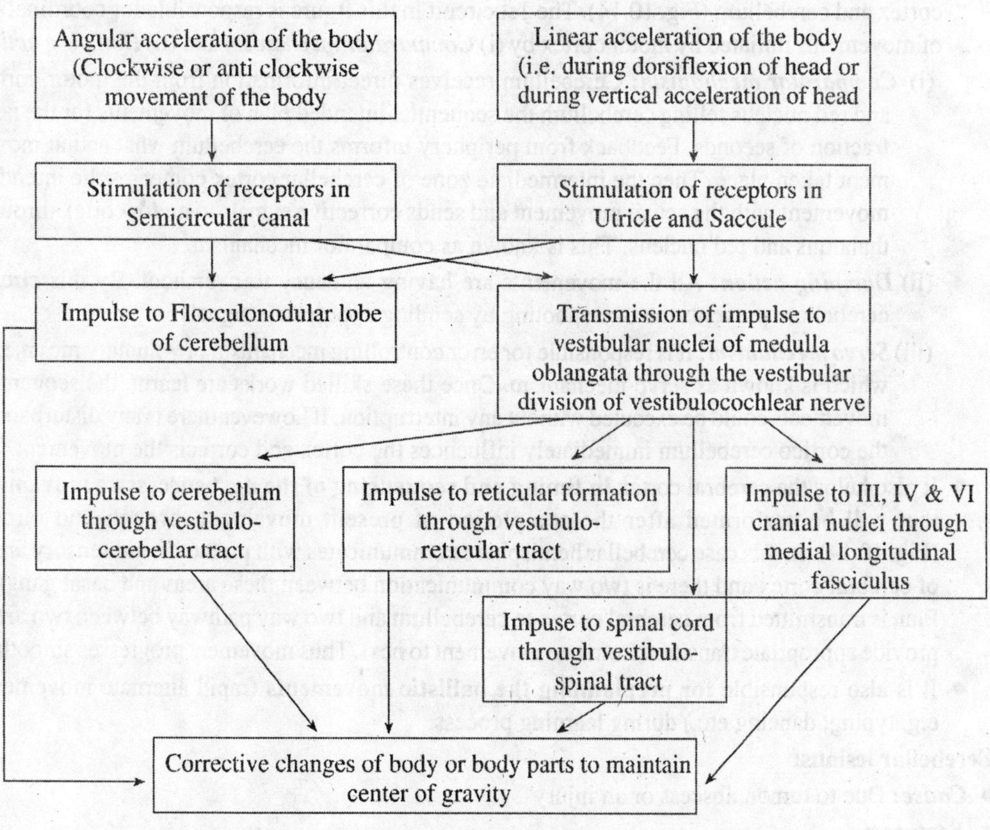

FC. 10E : Integrative mechanism of maintenance of equilibrium

13. Describe in brief the function of cerebellum. Add a note on cerebellar lesions.

Functions of cerebellum: Cerebellum is **not able to initiate** any **motor activity** but **assists the action** initiated from any other region of CNS specially cerebral cortex. It regulates both voluntary as well as non voluntary motor activity (tone, posture and equilibrium). **Cortico cerebellum mainly regulates voluntary activity whereas vestibulo-cerebellum and spino-cerebellum control non voluntary activity.**

a. ***Function of Vestibulo cerebellum*:** It plays an important role in maintenance of tone, posture and equilibrium by following pathway:

Information regarding gravity, linear and angular movement → through vestibulo cerebellar tract impulse goes to vestibulo cerebellum → through vestibulospinal / reticulospinal tract impulse goes to spinal cord → through α and γ motor neurons impulse goes to muscles → correction of posture and equilibrium if altered.

b. ***Functions of Spino cerebellum*:**

- It is a receiving area for tactile, proprioceptive, auditory and visual impulses.
- It regulates postural reflexes by modifying muscle tone by facilitatory gamma motor neurones which inturn reflexly modify the activity of alpha motor neurone.

c. ***Functions of corticocerebellum*:**

- It mainly controls over voluntary movements. There is feedback circuit between the periphery (muscle, joints etc.) and the cerebellum and also independant feedback circuit between motor cortex and cerebellum (Fig. 10.14). The 1st circuit in this figure is responsible for coordination of movements initiated by motor cortex by (i) *Comparator mechanism* and (ii) *Damping action*
    (i) ***Comparator mechanism*:** Cerebellum receives direct information from the motor cortex and red nucleus telling cerebellum the sequential intended plan of movements for the next fraction of seconds. Feedback from periphery informs the cerebellum what actual movement taken place. Then the intermediate zone of cerebellar cortex compares the intended movement with the actual movement and sends corrective signals to motor cortex through thalamus and red nucleus. This is known as comparator mechanism.

    (ii) ***Damping action*:** All the movements are having tendency to overshoot. By this circuit cerebellum prevents the overshooting by sending appropriate signals.

    (iii) ***Servo mechanism*:** It is responsible for error controlling mechanism of voluntary movments which is known as servo mechanism. Once these skilled works are learnt, the sequential movements could be executed without any interruption. If however there is any disturbances the cortico cerebellum immediately influences the cortex and corrects the movement.
- It also helps the cerebral cortex **in timing and sequencing of the next successive movement** that will be performed after the completion of present movement through 2nd circuit (Fig. 10.14). In this case cerebellar hemisphere communicates with premotor and sensory areas of cerebral cortex and there is two way communication between these areas and basal ganglia. Plan is transmitted from cerebral cortex to cerebellum and two way pathway between two areas provide appropriate transition from one movement to next. Thus movement progresses smoothly.
- It is also responsible **for preplanning the ballistic movements** (rapid alternate movements e.g. typing, dancing etc.) during learning process.

Cerebellar lesions:

- ***Cause*:** Due to tumor, abscess or an injury
- ***Features*:**

    (i) *Disturbances in tone and posture*:
    - Atonia or hypotonia which results disturbances in maintaining postural reflex.
    - Slow oscillatory movements in deep reflex instead of brisk movement.

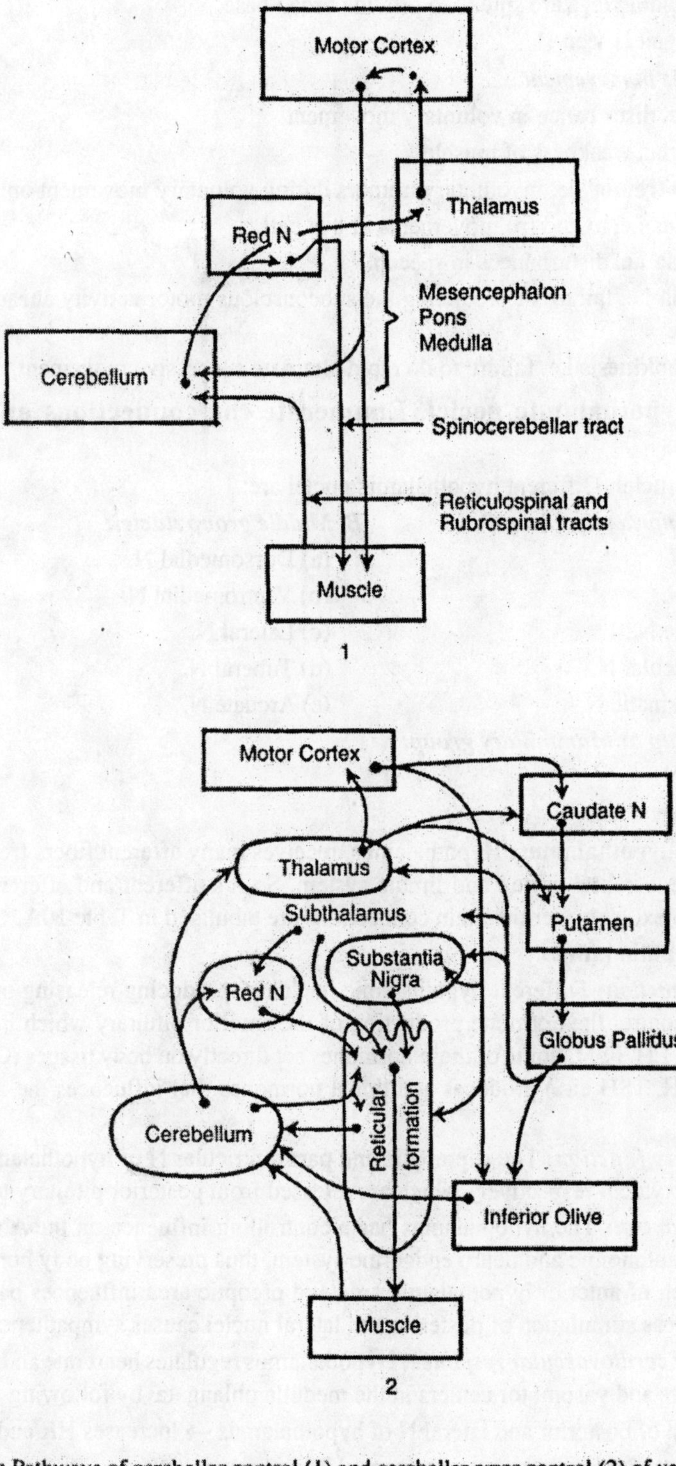

Fig. 10.14: Pathways of cerebellar control (1) and cerebellar error control (2) of voluntary movements

(ii) *Disturbances in equilibrium*:

- While standing legs are spread to provide broad base.
- Drunken gait is seen.

(iii) *Disturbances in movement*:

- **Ataxia** i.e. disturbance in voluntary movement.
- **Asthenia** i.e. weakness of muscle.
- **Intention tremor** i.e. involuntary tremors during voluntary movement only.
- **Nystagmus** i.e. to and fro movements of eye ball.
- **Dysarthria** i.e. disturbances in speech.
- **Dysmetria** i.e. failure of predicting the subconscious motor activity ahead of time resulting overshoot.
- **Adiadochokinesis** i.e. failure to do rapid alternate successive movement.

14. Name the hypothalamic neclei. Enumerate the connections and functions of hypothalamus.

Hypothalamic nuclei: Different hypothalamic nuclei are:

A. Anterior or Supraoptic group:

(a) Preoptic N.
(b) Anterior N.
(c) Supra optic N.
(d) Paraventricular N.
(e) Suprachiasmatic N.

B. Middle group nuclei:

(a) Dorsomedial N.
(b) Ventromedial N.
(c) Lateral N.
(d) Tuberal N.
(e) Arcuate N.

C. Posterior group or Mammillary group:

(a) Posterior N.
(b) Mammillary body.

Connections of hypothalamus: Hypothalamus, receives many afferent fibers from the viscera, the olfactory membrane, cerebral cortex and limbic system. So it's afferent and efferent connections are numerous and complex. However the main connections are tabulated in Table 10A.

Functions of hypothalamus:

A. Endocrine function: Different hypothalamic nuclei by producing releasing or releasing inhibitory factors control the hormone production of the anterior pituitary which includes GH, PRL, ACTH, TSH, LH, FSH. Some of these hormones act directly on body tissues (GH, PRL) whereas others (ACTH, TSH etc.) produces additional hormones that influences the activity of general body tissues.

B. Neurosecretory function: The supraoptic and paraventricular N of hypothalamus secretes vasopressin and oxytocin respectively which are released from posterior pituitary to exert it's action.

C. Autonomic control: The hypothalamus has a controlling influence on the ANS and appears to integrate the autonomic and neuro endocrine system, thus preserving body homeostasis. Electrical stimulation of anterior hypothalamic area and preoptic area influences parasympathetic responses whereas stimulation of posterior and lateral nuclei causes sympathetic responses.

D. Regulation of cardiovascular response: Hypothalamus regulates heart rate and BP by controlling cardiac centers and vasomotor centers in the medulla oblangata by following way:

(i) Stimulation of posterior and lateral N of hypothalamus $\rightarrow$ increases HR and arterial BP.
(ii) Stimulation of preoptic area $\rightarrow$ decreases HR and arterial BP.

Pathway	Origin	Destination
1. ***Afferent***		
i. Medial and Spinal lemniscus	Visceral and somatic structure	Hypothalamic N
ii. Tractus solitarious	Visceral and somatic structure	Hypothalamic N
iii. Reticular formation	Visceral and somatic structure	Hypothalamic N
iv. Visual fibers	Retina	Suprachiasmatic N
v. Auditory fibers	Inner ear	Hypothalamic N
vi. Medial forebrain bundle	Olfactory mucosa	Hypothalamic N
vii. Hippocampo-hypothalamic fibers	Hippocampus	N of Mammillary body
viii. Tegmental fibers	Tegmentun	Hypothalamic N
ix. Amygdaloid-hypothalamic fibers	Amygdala	Hypothalamic N
x. Thalamo-hypothalamic fibers	Dorsomedial and Midline N of thalamus	Hypothalamic N
2. ***Efferent***		
i. Descending fibers in RF, Brainstem and spinalcord	Preoptic, Anterior, Posterior and Lateral N of thalamus	Cranio-sacral and thoraco-lumbar outflows
ii. Mammillo-thalamic tract	Mammilari body	Anterior N of thalamus

Table 10A: Main afferent and efferent connection of hypothalamus

E. Regulation of body temperature*:** Normally the hypothalamus sets the body temperature at 98°F - 98.6°F (orally). When the temperature set point is altered in response to extremes in environmental temperatures or infection, hypothalamus plays an important role to normalise the set point. In this relation **Anterior hypothalamus** acts as ***Heat Loss Center and **Posterior hypothalamus** acts as ***Heat Gain Center*** and **Preoptic area** acts as ***Central Thermo receptors.***

In response to any alteration of the body temperature these centers normalise the body temperature by following mechanism:

Rise of Body temperature

↓

Stimulation of central thermoreceptors i.e. preoptic area of hypothalamus

Stimulates heat loss centre i.e. Ant. hypothalamic nuclei → **Stimulation of sweat glands to secrete sweat** → **Heat loss from body surface by evaporating sweat** → **Normalise BT**

Inhibition of posterior hypothalamus → **Inhibit vasomotor center** → **Cutaneous vasodilatation** → **Heat loss** → **Normalise BT**

Normalise BT

F. Regulation of food intake*:** Hypothalamus also regulates the food intake. **Lateral hypothalamus** acts as a ***Hunger or Feeding center*, Ventromedial N** acts as a ***Satiety center and **glucose sensitive receptors present in ventromedial nucleus** serves as a ***Glucoreceptors***. So after food when blood glucose level increases it inhibits the feeding center to stop intake of food by following mechanism:

After meal → increase in blood glucose level → stimulation of glucostat (Glucorceptors) → stimulation of satiety centre → stop taking food further. In response to starvation opposite mechanism follows to inhibit satiety center and thus stimulation of feeding center to initiate urge of taking food.

G. ***Regulation of water balance: Hypothalamus*** also regulates the body water volume and **Lateral nucleus of hypothalamus** acts as a ***Thirst Center***. Increase in osmolarity of the body stimulates hypothalamus which inturn increases water intake. The detail mechanism is as follows:

↑ Osmolarity of the body fluid

↙	↘
Stimulation of osmoreceptors close to lateral N. of hypothalamus	Stimulation of supraoptic N.
↓	↓
Stimulation of thirst center	ADH release
↓	↓
Rise of water intake	Water retention
↘	↙

Normalisation of body water volume and osmolarity

H. ***Regulation of sleep and wakefulness***: Sleep is a negative phenomenon due to inhibition of Wakefulness center present in mammillary body of hypothalamus by anterior hypothalamus i.e. stimulation of **anterior hypothalamus** induces sleep by inhibiting the wakefulness center present in mammillary body.

I. ***Control of circadian rhythm***: The hypothalamus controls many circadian rhythms e.g. body temperature, adrenocortical activity, eosinophil counts, renal secretion etc. The **supra chiasmatic nucleus of hypothalamus** acts as a ***Biological Clock*** which receives afferent fibes from the retina and sends the signal to many hypothalamic nuclei to control these activity. Thus suprachiasmatic nucleus synchronizes the various body rhythms in response to 24 hr. light dark cycle.

J. ***Control of emotional behaviour***: Emotion and behaviours are the function of the hypothalamus, limbic system and the prefrontal cortex. The hypothalamus is believed to act as an integrator of afferent information received from other areas of CNS and brings about the physical expression of emotion like increase of HR, increase of BP, dryness of mouth, sweating etc.

There are two centers in hypothalamus which are involved in the behavioural and emotional changes. These two centers are:

(i) *Median forebrain bundle and Ventromedial N of hypothalamus* as a ***Reward center.***

(ii) *Posterior and lateral nucleus of hypothalamus* as a ***Punishment center.***

Stimulation of punishment center results pain, fear, defense reaction and other elements of punishment whereas stimulation of reward center satisfies the person and persons becomes pleasant.

15. Define learning. What are the types of learning? What are its neurophysiological basis? Describe in brief the classical conditioning of learning. What is its difference with instrumental conditioning of learning?

***Definition*:** Learning is a neural mechanism by which the individual changes his/her behaviour as the result of his/her past experiences.

***Types of learning*:** There are two forms of learning.

(A) Non associative learning and (B) Associative learning

A. Non associative Learning: In this type of learning the learning process does not depend on a particular relationship between what is learnt and some other stimulus. It is of 2 types:

(a) **Habituation**—It occurs when a neutral stimulus is repeatedly applied. For the 1st time when it is applied it evokes a novel reaction which is called as 'Orientation reflex' or 'What is it ?' response. On repeated application of the same stimulus, the lesser response is evoked and ultimately subject totally ignores the stimulus as he gets habituated to it.

Example: The ticking noise of a new clock may be annoying and cause difficulty in sleeping. However after several nights the clock is no longer noticed.

(b) **Sensitization**—It is opposite to habituation where repeated stimulus evoke greater and greater response gradually.

Example: The mother used to sleep through many kinds of noise but wakes promptly when her baby cries.

B. Associative Learning: It occurs when learning involves some relationship between two or more stimuli at a time. It is of 3 types:

(a) Classical conditioning of learning (Classical Conditioned reflex)

(b) Instrumental conditioning

(c) Discriminative conditioning.

Neural basis of learning: The learning is due to some changes in the neuronal circuit through which the response is performed in response to a specific stimulus. These changes are:

(i) increase in number of functional synaptic terminals involved in this process.

(ii) expansion of the post synaptic neurones.

(iii) increase in synaptic efficacy.

Classical conditioning of learning: It is based on the temporal association between a neutral conditioned stimulus and an unconditioned (inborn) stimulus that elicits an unlearned response, provided that the timing relationship is maintained. This is first experimented by Pavlov in dog. So this is also termed as **Pavlovian conditioning of learning.** The experimental protocol of this experiment which is responsible for learning a new thing is as follows:

i. Food only to the dog ⟶ results salivation
(unconditioned stimulus)

ii. Ringing of bell only ⟶ results no salivation

iii. Food + Ringing of bell ⟶ results salivation

iv. Ringing of bell only ⟶ results salivation
after repeating step iii for some days *(conditioned response is learnt)*

Instrumental conditioning of learning:

- **Konorski and Skinner** applied different term in conditioning of learning in which they used a instrument known as ***'Skinner Box'***.

- In this Skinner box the hungry animal like rat is kept and the animal suddenly gets the food pellet for the 1st time by pressing of the liver by chance. Once he gets the food next time he tries to get the food by pressing the liver after trial and error. After some days/times he ultimately learns to get the food by pressing the liver as and when required.
- In this case **food is the unconditioned response** and **pushing of the lever** is the **conditioned response.**

16. Define memory. Enumerate its type with special reference to its neurophysiological basis.

Definition: It is defined as the storage mechanism of which is learnt and recalling it as and when required.

Types of memory: It is of 3 types:

(A) Short term memory

(B) Intermediate long term memory

(C) Long term memory.

(A) Short term memory:

- It is the memory that lasts for seconds to minutes.
- Example—remembering the new phone number for as long as the number is being dialled.
- It is due to:
  - (a) continual neuronal activity due to travelling of signal through a circuit of reverberating neurones (***Reverberating circuit theory***).
  - (b) prolonged facilitation or inhibition of presynaptic neurone terminals by facilitatory inhibitor terminal (Fig. 10.15) which is known as ***presynaptic facilitation or inhibition***.
  - (c) ***Post tetanic potentiation*** of presynaptic terminals i.e. after repeated stimulus (tetanisation) the neurones get fatigued and stop working to recover. However after recovery they show increased activity.

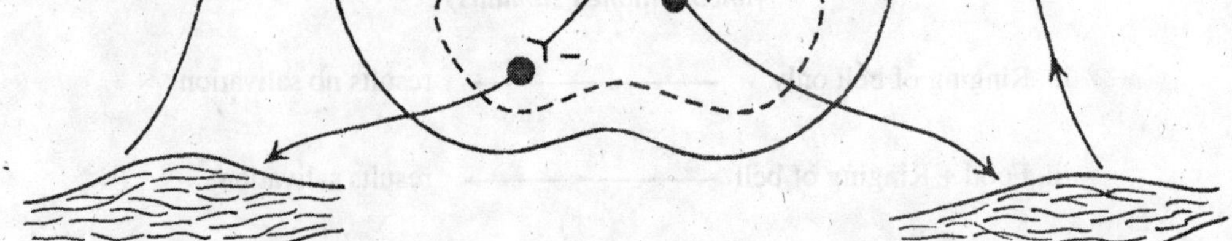

Fig. 10.15: Presynaptic inhibition and presynaptic facilitation of short term memory

(B) Intermediate long term memory:

- It lasts for days to weeks but eventually is lost unless they are converted to long term memory.
- This results from temporary physical or chemical changes or both at the presynaptic terminal.

- It is due to:
  - (a) presynaptic facilitation or inhibition.
  - (b) long term changes in the membrane properties of the entire post synaptic neurone in response to two stimulus acting simultaneously at two separate site on a single sensory neurone.

(C) Long term memory:

- It is stored in brain as **'memory engram'** or ***'memory trace'*** and can be recalled up to years or even after a long time.
- It is due to structural changes at the synapse that enhance or suppress signal conduction.
- It is due to—
  - (a) Increase in area of neurotransmitter release site in the presynaptic terminal during development of long term memory traces due to continual passage of impulse for long time.
  - (b) Increased number of neurotransmitter vesicles in the presynaptic terminal.
  - (c) Increase in number of functional synaptic terminals.
- Site of memory storage:
  - ❑ It is randomly stored in the brain.
  - ❑ However important sites are:
    - — Hippocampus of limbic system
    - — Wernick's area of cerebral cortex.

17. What are the thalamic nuclei? Describe the connections, functions and effects of lesions of thalamus.

Nucleus of thalamus: The main nuclear masses in the thalamus are:

A. Anterior parts: Anterior thalamic nuclei

B. Medial part: Dorsomedial nucleus

C. Lateral part: divided into two groups:

(a) *Dorsal group of lateral mass*: 2 nuclei—

- (i) Dorsolateral nucleus
- (ii) Posterolateral nucleus

(b) *Ventral group of lateral mass*: 3 nuclei—

- (i) Anteroventral nucleus
- (ii) Lateral-ventral nucleus
- (iii) Posteroventral nucleus which includes—
  - Ventral posterolateral N.
  - Ventral posteromedial N.

D. Posterior group of thalamus: 2 parts—

(a) *Pulvinar*

(b) *Metathalamus*—which includes:

- Medial geniculate body (MGB)
- Lateral geniculate body (LGB)

E. Other nuclei of the thalamus:

(a) Intralaminar nuclei

(b) Midline nuclei

(c) Reticular nucleus

Connections of Thalamus: There are 2 important functional connections present between the thalamic nuclei and other areas of CNS.

A. Every thalamic nuclei (except the reticular nucleus) sends axons to different parts of cerebral cortex and every part of the cerebral cortex gives reciprocal fibers to the thalamic nuclei.

B. It is an relay station for two sensory motor axonal loops involving the cerebellum and basal nuclei.

The summary of neural connection of different thalamic nuclei is represented by Table: 10.b

Functions: Thalamus is primarily concerned with somatic functions which includes:

1. It acts as a major sensory relay station.
2. It is a center for integration of sensory impulses and is responsible for—
   (a) **integration and modifications** of peripheral sensory input before sending cerebral cortex.
   (b) **determination** of the quality of crude sensations i.e. affective nature of the sensation.
3. It is responsible for perception of sexual sensation.
4. It plays important role in arousal and alertness reaction due to its connection with RAS.
5. It serves as a center for integration of motor functions due to it's connection with basal ganglia, cerebellum and motor cortex.
6. It is an integrating center for sleep.
7. It is also responsible for recent memory, speech and emotion.
8. It plays an important role in genesis of electrical activity of the brain i.e. EEG.

Thalamic lesion leads ***Thalamic syndrome*:**

- ***Causes*:** Mostly due to blockade of one of the arteries supplying thalamus.
- ***Symptoms / Features*:**
  - ***Thalamic pain*:** spontaneous and often excessive pain on opposite side of the body which may be aroused by simply light touch or by cold.
  - Loss of all sensations.
  - ***Asteriognosis*** i.e. inability to recognise a known object by handling with closed eyes.
  - ***Ataxia*:** Incoordination of voluntary movement due to loss of kinesthetic sensation.
  - ***Thalamic phantom limb*** i.e. inability to locate the position of limb with closed eyes.
  - ***Thalamic hand***—In some patients the contralateral hand is held in an abnormal posture i.e. moderate flexion at wrist joint with hyper extension of all fingers.
  - Abnormal involuntary motor movements like—
    - ***Chorea*** i.e. quick jerky movements
    - Intention tremor
    - ***Athetosis*** i.e. slow writhing and twisting movements.

B. Short Notes:

1. Muscle spindle:

- Muscle spindles are spindle shaped stretch receptors embedded within the skeletal muscles.
- Each muscle spindle is attached to the endomysium of the muscle at it's tapering end.
- Each muscle spindle is made up of 2-12 muscle fibers called ***Intrafusal Muscle fiber*** which lies parallel to the extrafusal muscle fibers in the muscle.
- Ends of these muscle fibers do not contain contractile proteins, therefore are **noncontractile.** This portion is the **sensory portion** of the intrafusal fibers.
- Depending on the arrangement of nuclei in it's central portion it is of two types—
  1. Nuclear Bag fiber, 2. Nuclear Chain fiber.

Table 10B: Thalamic nuclei, the connection and their function

Thalamic N	Afferent connection	Efferent connection	Function
1. Anterior Thalamic N	Mammilothalamic tract, Cingulate Gyrus, Hypothalamus	Cingulate Gyrus, Hypothalamus	Emotion and recent memory
2. Dorsomedial N	Prefrontal cortex, Hypothalamus and other thalamic N	Prefrontal cortex, Hypothalamus and other thalamic N	Integration of somatic, visceral and olfactory information in relation to emotional feeling and subjective states
3. Latero-Dorsal, Latero-Posterior, Pulvinor N	Cerebral cortex and other thalamic Nuclei	Cerebral cortex and other thalamic Nuclei	Unknown
4. Ventral anterior N	R.F., S.N., C.P., Premotor cortex, Corpus Striatum, other thalamic N	R.F., S.N., C.P., Premotor cortex, Corpus Striatum, other thalamic N	Influences activity of motor cortex
5. Ventral lateral N	Same as above	Same as above	Same as above
6. Ventral posteromedial N	Trigeminal lemniscus, Gastatory fibers	Area 3, 1, 2 of cerebral cortex	Relays common sensations to consciousness
7. Ventral posterolateral N	Medial and Spinal lemniscus	Area 3, 1, 2 of cerebral cortex	Relays common sensations to consciousness
8. Intralaminar N	RF, Sponothalamic and Trigeminal, Hypothalamic	Cerebral cortex via thalamic N and Corpus Striatum	Influences level of consciousness and alertness
9. Midline N	R.F.	Unknown	Unknown
10. MGB	Inferior colliculus, Lateral lemniscus from both the ears	Auditory radiation to superior temporal gyrus	Hearing
11. LGB	Optic tract	Visual cortex	Visual information

- Portions of either sides of the intrafusal fibers are striated (striated poles) because of presence of actin and myosin.
- Functions:
  - Takes part in initiating stretch reflex.
  - Participates in regulating muscle tone and posture.
  - Concerned with conscious perception of joint movement and position of the body.
  - Monitors the velocity of muscle contraction, change of velocity of muscle contraction and also length of the extrafusal muscle fiber.

2. Stretch reflex:

- ***Definition*:** When a skeletal muscle with an intact nerve supply is stretched it contracts. This response is known as ***stretch reflex***.
- ***Examples*:**
  - **Knee jerk** (When patellar tendon is struck by a knee hammer it stretches the quadriceps muscles that results contraction of quadriceps muscles causing the elevation of leg).
  - **Ankle jerk**
- ***Characteristics*:**
  - It is highly developed in antigravity muscles i.e. the muscles which oppose the force of gravity (e.g. extensor group of muscles of legs and flexor group of muscles of arms).
  - The receptor involved in this reflex is known as **muscle spindle.**
  - It becomes **hypoactive** due to:
    - destruction of afferent / efferent nerves.
    - stimulation of inhibitory areas in the brain (e.g. Motor cortex, Basal ganglia, Inhibitory reticular formation etc).
    - inhibition of facilitatory areas in the brain (e.g. vestibular nucleus, facilitatory reticular formation etc.).
    - hypothyroidism.
  - Stretch reflex becomes **hyperactive** due to:
    - destruction / inhibition of inhibitory areas in brain.
    - stimulation of facilitatory areas in brain.
    - any factor (e.g. reinforcement or ***Jendrassik's manoeuvre***) which increases the efferent discharge.
    - hyperthyroidism.
- These are of two types:
  - Dynamic or phasic:
    - It helps in movement.
    - Usually white muscle fibers participate in this type of reflex.
  - Static or tonic:
    - It helps in maintaining muscle tone and posture.
    - Usually red muscles participate in this type of reflex.
- ***Functions*:** (i) It maintains the muscle tone.
  (ii) It helps to maintain muscle posture.

3. Steriognosis:

- It is the ability of the subject to identify the texture, size, shape and weight of a familiar object with closed eyes.
- It is a synthetic sensation and is due to stimulation of different types of receptors e.g. touch, pressure, temperature etc.
- The pathway involved is dorsal column pathway.
- The center responsible for this sensation is area-5, 7 of parietal lobe and area-40 of the supramarginal gyrus of cerebral cortex.
- In lesion of dorsal columns and thalamic syndrome this ability is lost which is known as ***asteriognosis.***

4. Two-point discrimination:

- When two stimulus are applied simultaneously on two separate point of the skin beyond a minimal distance only two touch point is perceived as a single stimulus. The minimal distance that permits two touch stimulus to be perceived as two separate points is known as two-point discrimination.
- The receptors involved are fine touch receptors.
- The pathway is dorsal colomn pathway.
- Any abnormality of this sensation indicates the cortical lesion as this is one of the cortical sensation (others are tactile localisation and steriognosis).

5. Dermatomal rule:

- Pain is referred to a structure which is developed from the same embryonic segment or dermatome. This is known as dermatomal rule.
- The example: The heart and the inner aspect of left arm are having same embryonic origin.

6. Gait:

- It is a pattern of walking of a person.
- This pattern is generated in the cervical and lumber region of the spinal cord which are dependant on the mesencephalic locomotor region.
- The normal gait of human is walking straight along a straight line with a crossed extensor pattern of the limb.
- Any abnormality of this pattern is known as abnormal gait which are mainly due to: motor deficiency, lack of proper feedback to higher center and structural malformation.
- The examples of abnormal gait are:
  - (i) **Spastic Gait:** The subject walks on a narrow base, has difficulty in bending his knees and drags his feet along. The foot is raised from the ground by tilting the pelvis and the leg is then swung forward so that the foot tends to make an arc (circumduction of the leg). A spastic gait is a feature of **corticospinal lesion.**
  - (ii) **Stamping Gait:** This type of gait is seen in sensory ataxia. The feet is raised very suddenly and moved forwards in a jerk and then brought to the ground like stamping. This gait is best seen in **tabes dorsalis.**
  - (iii) **Drunken or Reeling Gait:** The person walks on a broad base and the feet are planted widely apart and placed irregularly. Such gait is seen in **cerebeller ataxia.**
  - (iv) **Festinant Gait:** The person walks with his body bent forwards and moves with rapid, short, shuffling steps, so that he appears to be trying to catch up with the centre of gravity. The arms

do not swing during walking. This gait is a characteristic feature of **Parkinson's disease** (resulting from a lesion of substantia nigra).

(v) **High stepping Gait:** The person walks lifting his foot higher than normal in order to avoid the toes from catching the ground. Such gait is seen when there is weakness of the extensor muscle of the feet, e.g. **common peroneal nerve palsy.**

(vi) **Waddling gait:** It is an abnormal gait like walking of duck. It is seen in myopathies and muscular dystrophies affecting the trunchal pelvic and thigh muscle. In this case the hips are not properly fixed by the proximal muscle (gluteal muscle) and the trunk movements are exaggerated producing a Rolling or Waddling gait.

7. Spinal shock:

- Complete division of spinal cord or complete transection of spinal cord which occurs due to automobile accidents or gunshot injury results either **Quadriplegia** (paralysis of all 4 limbs) and immediate death due to paralysis of respiratory muscles if transection occurs in cervical segments or **Paraplegia** (paralysis of 2 lower limbs) with survival if transection occurs at thoracic and lumbar segments. This occurs in three stages as follows:

  (i) Stage of spinal shock

  (ii) Stage of reflex activity

  (iii) Stage of reflex failure
- Spinal transection causes immediate and permanent loss of sensation and volume more below the level of lesion which is known as spinal shock.
- Duration of shock in humans in 1-4 weeks though it depends on degree of encephalisation of motor function.
- It may be due to immediate abolition of tonic discharges of motor neurons by descending fibers.
- The features are:
  - Complete paralysis of muscles (flaccidity).
  - Abolition of all reflexes (areflexia).
  - Complete loss of all sensations (anesthesia).
  - Paralysis of bladder and rectum.
  - Penis remain flaccid.
  - Gross fall in BP, Cardiac output if section below T_1 level.

8. Decerebrate Rigidity:

- The sectioning at the mid-collicular level results severe spasticity in the extensor group of muscles of the body. This is called as decerebrate rigidity.
- This occurs due to increased activity of motor neurons that facilitates stretch reflexes. Facilitation of stretch reflexes occurs due to two mechanisms:
  - Increased excitability of the motor neurone pool.
  - Increased rate of discharge of motor neurone.
- The increased extensor rigidity in decerebrate preparation indicates that medulla controls the tone of the antigravity muscles that are involved in maintaining posture.

9. Huntington's disease:

- It is a type of hypokinetic disorders of basal ganglia.
- This is due to degeneration of GABAergic striatonigral pathway i.e. loss of GABA and cholinergic neurons in the striatum.

- It is a genetic defect occurs due to defect in chromosome 4 which codes an abnormal protein *Huntington* that is responsible for this disease.
- It is characterized by:
  - Chorea i.e. rapid involuntary and dancing movements known as Huntington's chorea.
  - Dementia.
  - Slurring of speech.
  - It usually starts between the age of 30-40 years and frequency of occurrence is 5-10 per 10,000.

10. Clircadian rhythm:

- In animals as well as in humans certain body functions are regulated by the day night cycle which is referred as diurnal or circadian rhythm.
- In human beings this diurnal variation is controlled by a biological clock situated either in limbic system or in suprachiasmatic nucleus of hypothalamus.
- The examples are:
  - ACTH and cortisol secretion.
  - Body temperature control.
  - Sleep and wakefulness cycle.

11. Dissociated anaesthesia:

- When the sensation of pain and temperature is lost and touch sensation remains normal it is known as dissociated anaesthesia.
- This is seen in case of syringomyelia, intramedullary tumors, brainstem lesions, thrombosis of postero-inferior cerebellar artery.
- It occurs due to damage of gray matter of spinal cord surrounding the central canal through which spinothalamic tract carrying pain and temperature sensation passes whereas dorsal column pathway that cause touch sensation is spared as it passes through the periphery.

12. Semicircular canal:

- The receptor organ for maintenance of equilibrium is vestibular apparatus present in membranous labyrinth of internal ear which consists of (i) *Three Semicircular canals and (ii) Vestibule or Otolith organ.*
- There are three semicircular canal namely—

  (a) Anterior or Superior canal

  (b) Posterior canal

  (c) Lateral / Horizontal / External canal
- The Among the two ends of each semicircular canal one end is narrow and another one is enlarged. This enlarged end is known as ***Ampulla*** which contains the receptor organ known as ***Crista Ampullaris*** which is formed by neuroepithelial cells named ***hair cells*** that function as receptor cell. These hair cells are stimulated by the movement of endolymph at the begining and end of rotatory movement. So these are termed as ***Rotary receptors.***
- The functions are:
  - Gives information about rotational movements of head to maintain equilibrium during such movements.
  - It also helps in visual fixation during angular rotation of head through initiating vestibulo-ocular reflex.

13. Otolith organ:

- The receptor organ for maintenance of equilibrium is vestibular apparatus present in membranous labyrinth of internal ear which consists of (i) Three Semicircular canals and (ii) vestibule or otolith organ, which consists of utricle and saccule.
- The receptor organs *Utricle* and *Saccule* are collectively called as *Maculae* which is also formed by neuroepithelial cells or hair cells like crista ampullaris and also some supporting cells. These hair cells of maculae are sensitive to *effect of change of gravity* (this is why known as *Gravity receptors)* and *movement of endolymph*.
- The functions are:
  - It gives information about static position of head.
  - Utricle helps in controlling linear acceleration in horizontal direction whereas the sacule respond to linear acceleration of head in vertical direction like tilting or bending of head.

14. Motion sickness:

- It is defined as the syndrome of physiological response during the rapid movement (during travelling) to which the person is not adapted.
- It is due to the excessive stimulation of vestibular apparatus.
- The symptoms are: Nausea, vomiting, sweating, salivation, headache, discomfort etc.
- It is avoided by taking anti emetic drug and avoiding greasy and bulky food before travelling.
- Closing the eye helps in reducing the symptoms.

15. Righting reflexes:

- This is one of the postural reflexes not only maintain the body in an upright balanced position but also provide constant adjustments necessary to maintain a stable possible background for voluntary activity.
- This maintains an upright position of the body by a chain of reactions following one another in an orderly sequence as follows:

  (I) Labyrinthine righting reflexes acting upon the neck muscles.
  (II) Neck righting reflexes acting upon the body.
  (III) Body righting reflexes acting upon the head.
  (IV) Body righting reflexes acting upon the body.
  (V) Optical righting reflexes.

  All these reflexes except last one can be studied in *thalamic* or *blind folded normal animal.*
- These reflexes are useful in correcting the posture of the entire body.
- These reflexes still occur after cerebellectomy but are imperfectly executed.

16. Operant conditioning:

- In this type of instrumental conditioning animal is trained to carry out a task for either to receive a reward or to avoid a punishment.
- In such learning instrumental learning procedure is used but here two stimulus is used-one for correct response and another for incorrect.
- The animals choose between two stimulus and receive a reward for making a correct choice and punishment for making an incorrect choice.
- After sometime he learns to choose the correct choice for getting reward.
- Aversion conditioning or conditioned avoidance reflex occurs in human beings which helps in avoiding ingestion of poisonous foods.

17. Pavlovian conditioning:

- It is based on the temporal association between a neutral conditioned stimulus and an unconditioned (inborn) stimulus that elicits an unlearned response, provided that the timing relationship is maintained.
- This is first experimented by Pavlov in dog. So this is also termed as **Pavlovian conditioning of learning.**
- The experimental protocol of this experiment which is responsible for learning a new things is as follows:

i. Food only to the dog ⟶ results salivation
(unconditioned stimulus)

ii. Ringing of bell only ⟶ results no salivation

iii. Food + Ringing of bell ⟶ results salivation

iv. Ringing of bell only ⟶ results salivation
after repeating step iii for some days *(conditioned response is learnt)*

- It is difficult to maintain conditioned reflex indefinitely, however if conditioned stimulus is paired repeatedly with unconditioned stimulus from time to time condition reflex becomes permanent which is known as reinforcement of conditioned reflex.
- *Physiological utility*: A number of autonomic changes can be achieved by conditioning. For example heart and blood pressure can be decreased by appropriate conditioning.

18. Expression of spoken and written speech:

- There are two parallel systems of speech. One is for understanding the spoken words and producing speech and the other for understanding written word and producing writing.
- The Wernick's rea (area-22) along with area-41 and 42 are the major association area for processing sensory information from the somatic, sensory, visual and auditory cortices and thus responsible for comprehension, recognition and construction of words and language. Whereas the Broca's area (area-44 and 45) located in the prefrontal association cortex adjacent to the motor cortex is concerned with motor aspects of speech hence called as ***motor speech area.***
- On the other hand Exner writing area located in the posterior part of frontal lobe helps the visually perceived words to give expression in writing.

19. OVLT:

This is one of the hypothalamic area present outside the blood brain barrier named as organum vasculosum of lamina terminalis.

20. Wernick's area:

- Posterior most part of the area 22 is called as sensory speech area or Wernick's area. In addition some part of areas 40 and 39 may also form a part of Wernick's area.
- It is responsible for comprehension of both spoken and written speech and meaningful word formation during articulation of speech. So lession of this area results absence of comprehension of sounds and thus person speak without meaning. This is known as sensory Aphasia.
- Area 22 receives input from pre-striate visual areas and projects to frontal lobe, parietal lobe and cingulated gyrus.

21. Amnesia and memory trace:

- It is defined as the inability to recall the memories.
- There are different forms of amnesia:
  - Retrograde amnesia—It is the inability to recall the memories of recent events.
  - Anterograde amnesia—It is the inability of the person to establish new long term memories of those type of information which are basis of intelligence.
  - Hysterical amnesia-loss of permanent memory due to mental disturbances.
  - Alzheimer's disease-loss of recent memory due to damage of cholinergic neurons of brain.
  - Karasakoff's syndrome-memory defects in alcoholic person due to thiamin deficiency.
- Memory trace or ***memory engram*** is referred as a storage of long term memory in brain which can be recalled up to years or even after a long time.
- It is due to following structural changes at the synapse that enhance or suppress signal conduction.
  (a) Increase in area of vesicular release site in the presynaptic terminal during development of long term memory traces due to continual passage of impulse for long time.
  (b) Increase number of neurotransmitter vesicles in the presynaptic terminal.
  (c) Increase in number of functional synaptic terminals.
- Site of memory storage:
  - It is randomly stored in the brain.
  - However important sites are:
    - Hippocampus of limbic system
    - Wernick's area of cerebral cortex

22. Alzheimer's disease:

- It is a degenerative disease of the brain characterized by premature and progressive loss of memory usually in old age.
- It is due to severe loss of cholinergic neurons projecting from basal forebrain to neocortex, amygdala and hippocampus.
- This disease usually starts with loss of short term memory followed by loss of other cognitive functions.
- Cerebral vasodilators, stimulants and high dose of vitamin-B, C, E have beneficial effects in this disease.

23. Broca's area:

- This area is present in the frontal lobe, which is located in the prefrontal association cortex near the motor cortex.
- This was first described by Paul Broca in 1865.
- It is concerned with motor speech area and hence called as motor speech area (area 45 and 44).
- It regulates functions of muscles of lips, tongue, pharynx and larynx.
- Patients with lesion of Broca's area are capable for comprehending a spoken or written word but they are not able to say the word.

24. Opioid peptides:

- There are many opioid peptides (morphin like substances) synthesized endogenously in our body which are collectively known as endorphins.
- The important endorphins are α–enkephalins, β-endorphins, γ-endorphins, dynorphins and etc.

- These substances usually act pre and post synaptically to inhibit the transmission of impulses from Aδ and C fibers and thus acts as analgesic peptides.
- Repeated use of opioid analgesics results in addiction and tolerance mechanisms of which is not clearly known.

25. Sensory honunculus:

- The sensory cortex receives general sensation from all parts of the body. However the various parts of the body have a cortical representation proportionate not to their extensiveness but to their sensory acuity. When the cortical areas are charted out for their peripheral connections and depicted diagrammatically the distorted shape of a ***little man*** emerges. This is called as sensory honunculus.
- Briefly it is the diagrammatic representation of peripheral connections of the sensory cortex.

26. Saltatory conduction:

In case of myelinated nerve the myeline sheath acts as a insulator and does not allow the current flow. Therefore the flow of ions and local circuit of current flow occurs only through the **Nodes of Ranvier**. Thus current flows **from depolarised node of Ranvier** to nearby **resting node of Ranvier** which are placed apart resulting jumping of impulse from one node to another node. This type of propagation of action potential is known as ***Saltatory*** or ***Jumping conduction***.

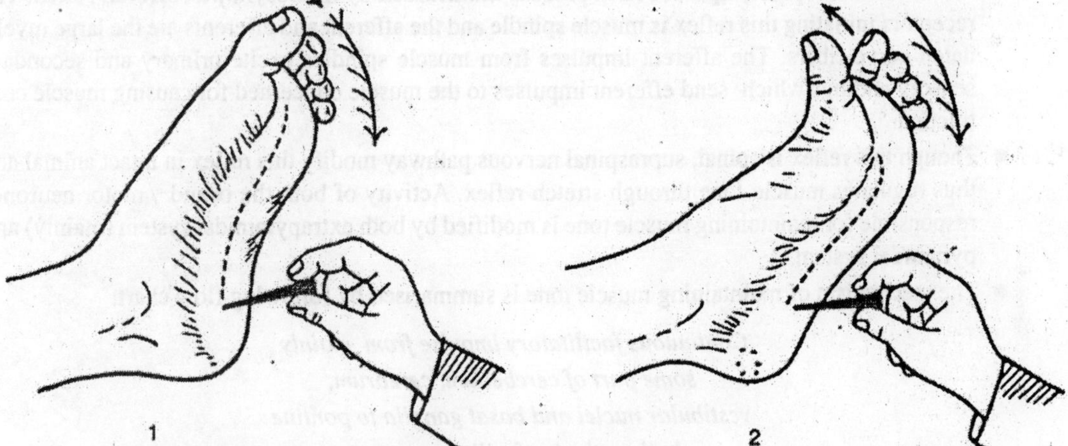

Fig. 10.16: Diagrammatic representation of plantar reflex (*1 = Normal plantar reflex, 2 = Babinski's plantar reflex*)

Mechanism of conduction:

- Suppose AP is generated at the point A in response to the application of threshold stimulus.
- Membrane at the point A is depolarised (i.e. inside electropositive and outside electronegative, whereas the adjacent areas (B and C) is in resting stage (**resting Node of ranvier**) still maintaining RMP i.e. **inside electronegativity**.
- This results flow of '+' ions from **depolarised Node of ranvier** (Point A) to **adjacent resting Node of ranvier** (Point B and C) in inside and flow of + ions from resting **Node of ranvier** (B and C) to depolarised **Node of ranvier** (point A) in outside of the membrane. Thereby completing a local circuit.
- This local circuit of current flow alters the potential difference across the membrane at site B and C that leads sudden opening of voltage gated Na^+ channels at the site B and C.

- This results rapid entry of Na^+ inside at point B and C making these **Node of ranviers** depolarized. In the meantime the previously depolarized **Node of ranvier** (i.e. point A) repolarised due to exit of K^+ through voltage gated K^+ channels.
- Thus depolarization wave is passed from point A to B and C which is continued resulting bilateral conduction of Action potential.

Advantages:

1. It is faster in rate
2. It requires lesser energy.

27. Law of adequate stimulus: Vide under properties of receptors.

28. Adaptation of receptors: Vide under properties of receptors.

29. Muller's Doctrine od specific nerve energy: Vide under properties of receptors.

30. Phantom limb: Vide under properties of receptors.

31. Muscle tone:

Definition: It is defined as the **continuous state of partial tetanus (contraction)** of the muscle maintained by asynchronous discharge of impulses in motor nerves supplying the muscle.

Maintenance of muscle tone:

- Muscle tone is a purely **spinal reflex** process **maintained by monosynaptic stretch reflex**. The receptors initiating this reflex is muscle spindle and the afferent and efferents are the large myelinated nerve fibers. The afferent impulses from muscle spindles excite primary and secondary sensory endings which send efferent impulses to the muscle concerned for causing muscle contraction.
- Though this reflex is spinal, supraspinal nervous pathway modify this reflex in intact animal and thus regulates muscle tone through stretch reflex. Activity of both the α and γ motor neurones responsible for maintaining muscle tone is modified by both extrapyramidal system (mainly) and pyramidal system.
- The mechanism of maintaining muscle tone is summarised by following flow chart:

Continuous facilitatory impulse from mainly some part of cerebellum, cerebrum, vestibular nuclei and basal ganglia to pontine bulboreticular facilitatory areas.

↓

Continuous discharge from bulboreticular facilitatory areas of pons.

↓

Transmission of impulse to γ motor neurone via extrapyramidal tract (mainly) supplying the muscle

↓

Stimulation of muscle spindle due to stretching of central portion of intrafusal fibers of muscle spindle resulted from contraction of muscle fibers in end position of intrafusal muscles of muscle spindle.

↓

impulse goes to spinal cord through primary and secondary sensory nerve endings.

↓

stimulation of α motor neurone

↓

contraction of extrafusal muscle fibers (partial) to maintain muscle tone.

Applied aspect:

- **Abnormal increase of muscle tone (contractile state) is known as hypertonia. It results spasticity or rigidity of the muscle to lead spastic paralysis.**
- **Whereas decrease in muscle tone due to mainly cerebellar disease, disorders of α motor neurones, neuromuscular junctions and muscles is known as hypotonia. It results flaccidity of muscle that leads to flaccid paralysis.**

32. Tabes dorsalis:

- **It is a disease in which degeneration of dorsal nerve root takes place.**
- **Cause: Syphilis.**
- **Features:**
  - **loss of pain, muscle tone, superficial and deep reflexes and micturition reflex**
  - **swollen painless knee joint known as *Charcot's joint*.**
  - **disturbed equilibrium**
  - ***Rhomberg sign* positive**
  - ***stamping gait* is seen**

33. Syringomyelia:

- **It is a disease in which fluid filled cavities are appeared in the spinal cord.**
- **Cause: Due to overgrowth of neuroglial cells in spinal cord accompanied by cavity formation and accumulation of fluid in the cavities.**
- **Features:**
  - **early loss of pain, temperature, crude touch sensation**
  - **flaccid type of paralysis if anterior gray horn is affected**
  - **complete paralysis of 4 limbs if white matter is affected. This is due to damage of pyramidal and extrapyramidal fibers present in spinal cord.**

34. Brown Sequard syndrome:

When there is a partial transection or damage in only one half of the spinal cord, typical motor and sensory changes develop after recovering from the spinal shock which are collectively known as *Brown-Sequard syndrome*. The changes are:

a. **Changes at the level of lesion:**
   - **Complete loss of all sensation due to destruction of dorsal horn cell on the same side.**
   - **Complete lower motor types of paralysis occurs on the same side due to destruction of ventral horn cell.**

b. **Changes below the Level:**
   - **Dissociated sensory loss – i.e.**

- On the same side: Vibration, position, joint, fine touch, deep pressure sensations are lost and crude touch, pain, temperature sensations persist.
- On the opposite side: Crude touch, pain, temperature sensation are lost, others remain intact

- **Upper motor neurone type muscular paralysis** on the same side.

c. **Changes above the level:**

- Part of skin area innervated by the nerves from one or two segments above the level of lesion on the same side becomes hypersensitive to touch and pain.
- Twitching of muscles in upper one or two segments on the same side.

35. Nitric oxide:

- It is a neurotransmitter in CNS and also in NM junctions between the inhibitory motor fibers of intrinsic nerve plexus and smooth muscles of GI tract.
- It exerts vasodilatory effect of ACh on small arteries. Other functions are penile erection, activation of macrophages in brain, destruction of cancer cells, bronchodilation, learning and memory and etc.
- It is produced by non neuronal cells like the endothelial cells of blood vessels from amino acid arginine.
- It's production is activated by ACh, bradykinin, VIP, Substance-P etc.
- It's mode of action is: activation of guanylyl cyclase which results formation of cGMP that ultimately causes relaxation of smooth muscles and thereby vasodilation of small arteries.

36. Postural reflexes: Vide the answer of Q. No. 11.

37. EEG:

Definition: It is the graphic record of electrical activity of the brain recorded from the surface of the scalp.

Waves: Normally 4 waves are seen:

- ***Alpha (α) waves***:
  - It is seen when a person is awake but relaxed with eyes closed. When he opens his eyes or his attention is drawn to any stimulus this alpha rhythm disappears and replaced by faster waves. This is called α blocking.
  - It's frequency is 8-13 cycles / sec.
  - It's amplitude is 50-100 mv.
  - It is mainly recorded from parieto-occipital area.
- ***Beta (β) waves***:
  - It is seen in alert state.
  - It's frequency is > 20-30 cycles / sec.
  - Amplitude: 25-30 mv.
  - It is recorded from frontal and temporal areas.
- ***Theta (θ) waves***:
  - It is seen in infants and children during wakefulness. It is also seen during early stages of slow waves sleep.
  - Frequency: 3-10 cycles /sec.
  - Amplitude: 50-100 mv
  - It is recorded from hippocampus.

- *Delta (δ) waves:*
  - It is seen in stage III and IV of slow wave (deep) sleep.
  - Frequency: < 3 cycles / sec
  - Amplitude: 20-200 mv.

Significance of EEG: EEG is a diagnostic measure of some neurological and sleep disorders e.g.

(i) Epilepsy—presence of (δ) waves in adult during conditions other than sleep
(ii) disorders of midbrain affecting ARAS
(iii) subdural hematoma.

38. Sleep:

Definition: Periodical, reversible and physiological reduction in brain excitablity and body activity is termed as sleep.

Duration: Average duration In adults - > 6 to 8 hr/ day
In children : more than adult.

Neurophysiological basis: The exact cause or neural mechanism of sleep is not fully known. Though there are some theories which explain the physiological reasons of sleep.

(i) *Howell's metabolic theory*: It states that sleep is due to depression of cortical center by acid accumulated during working hours.

(ii) *Cerebral ischemia*: As per this theory during waking hours physical effort is more which leads more blood flow to the skeletal muscle and consequent reduction of blood flow in brain. Continuous reduction of blood flow to brain for prolonged period ultimately induces sleep.

(iii) *Pieron's hypnotoxic theory*: Pieron's theory states that sleep is due to the production of chemicals like hypnotoxin in the brain which suppresses brain activity and thus induces sleep.

(iv) *Pavlov's theory of conditioned inhibition*: Rhythmical alteration of cortical excitation and inhibition conditioned to an environmental factor determines sleep or wakefulness.

(v) *Modern theory*: Sleep is due to the absence of adequate drives of impulses in reticular formation resulting no impulse to cerebral cortex to initiate any motor activity or alertness.

Phases of sleep: sleep is of two types:

1. Slow wave sleep or Orthodox or Non rapid eye movement (NREM) sleep:

- It occupies 70% of sleep period.
- Lasts for every 70-90 min and interrupted by 10-20 mins of REM sleep.
- Produced by absence of desynchronising activity via RAS.
- EEG shows slow, synchronised theta and delta waves.

2. Rapid eye movement (REM) or Paradoxical or fast wave or dream sleep:

- Rapid to and fro movement of eye ball occurs.
- HR and Respiratory rate becomes irregular.
- Occassional muscle twitch can take place.
- Difficult to wake an individual if he is in this phase of sleep.
- Dreams are more vivid.
- Shows fast desynchronised waves.

39. Reticular activating system:

Definition: The term ***'Reticular formation'*** is used for those parts of brain stem (medulla, pons and midbrain) which are characterised by an **interlacing network of nerve fibers.**

Physiological anatomy:

- The reticular formation (RF) consists of deeply placed continuous network of nerve cells and fibers that extend from the spinal cord, through medulla, pons, midbrain, sub thalamus, hypothalamus and thalamus.
- It's components are:

  (i) a central core in the brain stem named ***Brain stem reticular formation (BSRF).***

  (ii) ***Ascending Reticular activating system (ARAS).***

  (iii) ***Descending Reticular components or Pontine / Medullary Reticular spinal fibers (DRAS).***
- Inferiorly the reticular formation is continuous with the interneurones of the gray matter of spinal cord while superiorly impulses are relayed to the cerebal cortex, and cerebellum.

Function:

- It is the neural substrate of consciousness and sleep wake fulness cycle. Multiple ascending pathways carrying continuous sensory information to higher centers are channelled through the reticular formation which inturn projects this information to different parts of the cerebral cortex causing a sleeping person to awake. Absence of transmission of impulse on the other hand is responsible for sleep.
- It is responsible for selective attention or conscious alert state that make perception possible.
- It is an integral part of neural substrates for conditioning and learning.
- Through the Reticulospinal and Reticulobulbar tract it can influence the activity of α and γ motor neurones of spinal cord and thus modulates tone, posture and also postural reflex activity.
- Visceral regulating centers e.g. cardio-vascular, respiratory, swallowing etc. are an integral part of RF and thus very essential for life.
- RF projection controls neuroendocrine system in the hypothalamus.

40. Adiadochokinesis:

- It is the failure to do rapid alternate successive movement.
- This is due to cerebellar lesion.

41. Thalamic syndrome: See the answer of Q. No. 17.

42. Functions of basal ganglia:

These are—

i. Control of voluntary motor activity: In association with the corticospinal system it controls the complex pattern of voluntary motor activity. e.g.

(a) *Cognitive control of motor activity* - Most of the motor activity occurs as a consequence of thoughts generated in mind. This process is known as cognitive control of motor activity. Because of it's feedback and reversible connections with cerebral cortex it plays an important role in cognitive control of motor activity.

(b) It plays important role in—

(i) determining how rapidly a motor activity is to be performed (timing).

(ii) controlling how large the movements will be (scaling).

(c) *Semiautomatic movements*: Semiautomatic functions like swinging of arms while walking etc. are subconsciously controlled by the basal ganglia.

ii. Control of reflex muscular activity: It exerts inhibitory effect on spinal reflexes and regulate activity of muscles to maintain posture.

*iii. **Control of muscle tone:*** Muscle tone is also controlled by basal ganglia especially Substantia Nigra which normally has inhibitory influence to muscle tone.

*iv. **Regulation of sleep and wakefulness:*** Globus Pallidus and Red Nucleus are involved in wakefulness because of their connections with reticular formation.

*v. **It (Globus Pallidus) provides background of muscle tone for the performance of voluntary activity:*** In order to perform the usefull skilled voluntary movements the body and proximal of the limbs have to attain appropriate positions. These associated tonic contraction are initiated by basal ganglia reflexly.

43. Parkinsonism:

- ***This is the hypokinetic syndrome due to lesion of Substantia Nigra resulted from*** decreased secretion of dopamin which results abnormal excitation of basal ganglia.
- **Physiological basis:** Dopamin secreted in caudate nucleus and putamen by substantia nigra is inhibitory. Therefore, destruction of substantia nigra causes withdrawal of inhibition of these structures which inturn become overactive and cause continuous output of excitatory signal to the corticospinal motor system.
- **Features:**
  - ***Lead pipe or Cogwheel rigidity***—due to increase in muscle tone.
  - ***Static tremors***—tremor at rest and disappears during voluntary activity due to oscillatory continuous discharge of pyramidal system by a closed circuit through basal ganglia
  - ***Akinesis***—It is difficulty in initiation or starting movement due to rigidity of the muscles so the automatic associated movements do not occur resulting:
    - *Mask like face* (no facial expression)
    - *Statue like posture.*
    - *Festinant Gait*—The person walks with short quick steps with the body bent forwards as if the person is trying to prevent himself from falling.

44. Papez circuit: Prefrontal lobe forms a closed circuit connecting with thalamus, hypothalamus and hippocampus called as Papez circuit which is responsible for resting EEG, genesis and control of emotion and memory. The detailed cercuit is as follows:

Hippocampus → fornix → mammillary body → mammillary thalamic tract → anterior nuclei of thalamus → cingulate cortex → cingulum → hippocampus.

45. Frontal lobe syndrome: Injury or ablation of frontal lobe results following symptoms:

- lack of concentration and lack of fixing attention
- person loses the ability to solve problem
- lack of initiation and difficulty in planning
- emotional instability
- loss of moral and social sense
- loss of recent memory
- hyperphagia, slight tremor etc.

46. Kluver Bucy syndrome:

- **Cause:** Bilateral destruction of temporal lobe (in animal) along with amygdaloid nucleus and uncus (in human).

- **Features:** — Speech disturbances (Aphasia)
  — Auditory disturbances.
  — Disturbances in smell and taste
  — Dreamy state
  — Visual hallucination

47. Rage and sham rage:

- **Rage:** Stimulation of punishment center by major irritants results aggressive emotional state which is known as Rage.
- **Sham rage:** Stimulation of punishment center by minor irritants when evokes aggressive emotional state then it is known as Sham rage.

48. Bell and Megendie law:

Synapse allows the conduction of impulses in one direction only i.e. from the presynaptic neurone to the post synaptic neurone. This direction of propagation of impulse is known as ***Orthrodromic conduction*** and this law is known as **Bell - Megendie Law or law of forward conduction.** The propagation of impulse in reverse direction is known as ***Antidromic conduction*** which is restricted by the synapse due to the inability of releasing NT from the dendrites of presynaptic membrane.

49. Weber Fechner law: Vide under properties of receptors.

50. Rhomberg's sign:

- In this test the subject is asked to close his or her eyes and stand with the feet close together. If the subject sway or even fall down as soon as he or she closes his or her eyes it is known as Rhomberg's test positive, otherwise it is known as Rhomberg's sign negative.
- It ocurrs in cerebellar disease and also sometimes in tabes dorsalis in which degeneration of dorsal nerve root of spinal cord takes place.
- This is due to sensory ataxia that display the lack of sense of position in both the legs.

51. Wallerian degeneration:

If a nerve fiber is injured either due to obstruction of blood flow or transection of nerve or local administration of toxic chemicals, various changes occur in the nerve fiber and cell body. All these changes are collectively called as **degenerative changes** which are of two types—

(a) Wallerian degeneration: The degenerative changes takes place in the part of the nerve fiber distal to the injury is named as ***Wallerian degeneration*** which occurs within 24 hours of injury. The changes are as follows:

- Swelling of axis cylinder followed by breaking up into smaller pieces.
- Degeneration of myelin sheath into fat droplets occur from 8th to 35th day.
- Multiplication of Schwann cell.
- Removal of debris of axis cylinder and fat droplets by invading macrophages without affecting neurolemmal sheath. So, the **neurolemmal tube** becomes empty and filled by cytoplasm of Schwann cells. These changes take place for about 2 months.

(b) Retrograde degeneration: When the degenerative changes are seen in the part of the axon proximal to the site of injury along with degeneration of cell body, it is known as ***Retrograde degeneration***. These changes occur **only up to the 1st node of Ranvier** near the injury.

52. Epilepsy:

- It is the brain disorder characterized by sudden uncontrolled involuntary muscle contraction (convulsive seizures) or loss of consciousness or both.

- **It occurs due to paroxysmal uncontrolled discharge of impulses from neurons of brain especially cerebral cortex.**
- **It develops only when the excitability of the neurons is increased causing excessive neuronal discharge. The person with epilepsy remains normal in between seizures.**
- **It is of two types: Generalised and localized.**

53. CSF:

Introduction: **The brain is very important but delicate organ. So it needs some extra protection which is also afforded by CSF which fills the space in between the arachnoid and piamatter and acts as a water cushion.**

Properties and composition:

- **Total quantity—150 ml**
- **Pressure—100-200 mm H_2O (Avg.—130 mm H_2O)**
- **Rate of formation—500-800 ml/day**
- **Osmolality—289 mosm / kg / water**
- **Reaction—alkaline**
- **pH - 7.33**
- **Composition:**
  - a. Water—99.13%
  - b. Solids—0.87%
    - i. Na^+—147 m eq /lit
    - ii. K^+—2-9 m eq /lit
    - iii. Ca^{2+}—2.3 m eq /lit
    - iv. Cl^-—110-130 m eq /lit
    - v. HCO_3^-—25.1 m eq /lit
    - vi. Protein—20-30 mg%
    - vii. Glucose—50-85 mg%
    - viii. Cells: CSF Contains 5-6 lymphocytes / cu mm

Location: **It is present in the central canal of spinal cord, subarachnoid space of brain and cerebral ventricles.**

Functions:

(i) **Protective function:** **It covers the brain from inside and acts as a cushion. If there is any injury to head the impact is distributed all over the brain by CSF and thus no single area of brain has to bear high degree of impact. Thus damage to the brain is prevented.**

(ii) **Reservoir of fluid:** **It acts as a reservoir of fluid and during brain odema, resulted either due to brain injury or inflammation, CSF is escaped from the subarachnoid space into the venous sinuses and provides some space so that brain is not pressed.**

(iii) **It also carries nutritive substances to the brain tissue.**

(iv) **It also helps to excrete out waste products of CNS into blood.**

54. Blood brain barrier:

Definition: **The entry of some substances from the blood to the brain ECF is restricted due to barrier offered by the walls of the capillaries supplying the brain. This barrier is known as *Blood-Brain barrier*.**

Structure: It is formed:

- **Mainly** by the **tight junctions** in between the endothelial cell layer of capillaries in the brain.
- **Partly** by foot process of **astrocytes** (glial cells) covering the capillaries in the brain.

Characteristic features:

- It is highly permeable to water, O_2, CO_2, sulfa drugs and erythromycin,
- It is slightly permeable to electrolytes e.g. Na^+, K^+, Mg^{2+}, Cl^-, HCO_3^-, $HPO_4^=$, glucose and drugs like penicillin, chloromycetene and tetracycline.
- It is almost impermeable to H^+, arsenic, gold, serum urea, catecholamines, proteins and bile salts.

Function:

- It maintains the constancy of environment in CNS.
- It protects the brain from endogenous and exogenous toxins in the blood.
- It prevents the escape of neurotransmitters in the general circulation.

55. Babinski's Sign (Plantar reflex):

- This is an important **superficial** reflex.
- Stimulation of the outer edge of the sole of the foot by gentle scratching from the heel towards the little toe and then medially upto the base of the big toe, results **plantar flexion (downward movement) of the great toe and drawing together of other toes. This is known as Babinski's sign negative** or ***plantar reflex*** (Fig. 10.16).
- This type of response appears with the development of pyramidal tracts and thus is seen in normal healthy individuals but in case of **upper motor neurone lesion** there is **dorsiflexon (upward movement) of the great toe and fanning out (abduction) of small toes. This is known as Babinski's sign positive** or ***Babinski's response*** or ***plantar extension***. This type of response is seen in infants (< 1 year old) due to **incomplete development of pyramidal tracts** or during sleep or Cheyne-Stoke's breathing due to hypoxia.

56. Reinforcement or Jendrassik's manoeuvre: Sometimes the reflexes (like ankle jerk or plantar reflex etc.) can not be elicited even in normal person if the person is too conscious about it. In such cases to elicit those reflexes attention of the subject is diverted by asking him **clenching the teeth** or **pulling the locked and flexed fingers** etc. while demonstrating those reflexes. This technique is known as **Reinforcement.**

C. Differentiate between:

Chemical synapse	Electrical synapse
❑ Passage of impulse is through neurotransmitter.	❑ Passage of impulse is not through neurotransmitter but direct.
❑ Anatomical continuity is absent in this type of synapse.	❑ Anatomical continuity is present in this type of synapse.
❑ Gap junction is absent.	❑ Gap junction is present.
❑ Synaptic delay is present.	❑ Synaptic delay is absent.
❑ Transmission of impulse is unidirectional.	❑ Transmission of impulse is bidirectional.
❑ These are common in the body.	❑ These are present only some restricted part of the body.

Spatial summation	Temporal summation
❑ When a number of presynaptic excitatory terminals are stimulated simultaneously with a subthresold stimulus there is elicitation of response which is known as spatial summation.	❑ When a single presynaptic excitatory terminals are stimulated repeatedly at a rapid rate with a subthreshold stimulus there is elicitation of response which is known as temporal summation.

EPSP	IPSP
❑ When a excitatory neurotransmitter acts on a subsynaptic membrane receptors a local depolarizing current develops which is known as EPSP. ❑ It is due to either Na^+ influx or Ca^{2+} influx or closure of K^+ channels. ❑ Results excitation of PSM ❑ Potential of + 8 mv.	❑ When a inhibitory neurotransmitter acts on a subsynaptic membrane receptors a local hyperpolarizing current develops which is known as IPSP ❑ It is due to either Cl^- influx or K^+ efflux or due to closure of Na^+ or Ca_2^+ channels. ❑ Results inhibition of PSM. ❑ Potential of – 2 mv.

EPSP	AP
❑ When a excitatory neurotransmitter acts on a subsynaptic membrane receptors.a local depolarizing current develops which is known as EPSP. ❑ It can be summated. ❑ It is non propagatory. ❑ It does not obey all or none law. ❑ It is initiated by subthreshold stimulus.	❑ The transient change of membrane potential, in response to a stimulus of threshold intensity, which is propagatory in nature is called action potential or AP. ❑ It can not be summated. ❑ It is propagatory. ❑ It obeys all or none law. ❑ It is initiated by threshold stimulus.

Monosynaptic reflex	Polysynaptic reflex
❑ Only one synapse is involved in between the afferent and efferent nerve. ❑ Exam: deep/tendon reflex, stretch reflex.	❑ Two or more synapses are involved in between the afferent and efferent nerve. ❑ Exam: withdrawal/superficial reflex.

Intrafusal fibers	Extrafusal fibers
❑ It comprises muscle spindle present in skeletal muscles and are noncontractile. ❑ Motor innervation is mediated through gama fibers. ❑ It is responsible for maintenance of muscle tone.	❑ It comprises contractile part of skeletal muscles. ❑ Motor innervation is mediated through alpha fibers. ❑ It is responsible for movement of body and body parts.

Superficial reflexes	Deep reflexes
❑ Receptors are located on the surface of the body. ❑ Receptors are naked nerve endings. ❑ It is polysynaptic. ❑ Supraspinal centers are involved. ❑ Response obtained may be ipsilateral or bilateral. ❑ Mostly protective reflex. ❑ Are abolished in UMNL. ❑ Involve a group of muscle and often more than one joint.	❑ Receptors are located on the deeper region of the body. ❑ Receptors are muscle spindle. ❑ It is monosynaptic. ❑ Spinal cord is the higher center. ❑ Response obtained is unilateral. ❑ Mostly postural reflex. ❑ Are exaggerated in UMNL. ❑ Involve a single muscle and a single joint.

Primary sensory innervation	Secondary sensory innervation
❑ Supply at the center position of all the nuclear bag and chain fiber of muscle spindle which are referred to as annulospiral endings. ❑ Responds to both dynamic and static changes in the length of muscle.	❑ Supply at the trail portion of all the nuclear bag and chain fiber of muscle spindle which are referred to as flower spray endings. ❑ Responds to only static changes in the length of muscle.

Spasticity	Rigidity
❑ Increased muscle tone due to failure of inhibitory impulses from cerebral cortex to spinal cord is known as Spasticity. ❑ Seen in pyramidal tract lesion. ❑ Develops due to increased reflex activity of only antagonistic muscle. ❑ Resistance is absent in later stage. ❑ It is stretch sensitive. ❑ Clasp knife type hypertonia is seen.	❑ Increased muscle tone due to removal of inhibitory impulses on gama motor neuron is known as rigidity. ❑ Seen in extra pyramidal tract lesion. ❑ Develops due to increased reflex activity of both antagonistic and agonist muscle. ❑ Resistance is present throughout the passive movement. ❑ It is not stretch sensitive. ❑ Lead pipe and Cog wheel rigidity is seen.

Conditioned reflex	Unconditioned reflex
❑ These reflexes are present since birth. ❑ Examples: Salivation by seeing tasty food, the tastes of which is known. ❑ It is not dependant on past experience. ❑ It is required to develop learning..	❑ These reflexes are not present since birth but acquired in later life. ❑ Examples: Salivation after taking food, knee jerk. ❑ It is dependant on past experience. ❑ To elicit, it requires already existing learning and memory.

Fine touch	Crude touch
❑ Receptors are Meissners's corpuscle, Merkel's disc and nerve endings around hair follicle, Krause's end bulb.	❑ Receptors are Ruffini's end organ.
❑ Receptors are rapidly adapting or slow adapting (Merkel's disc).	❑ Receptors are always slow adapting.
❑ Afferent nerve is Fasciculus gracilis and F. cuneatus.	❑ Afferent nerve is ventral spinothalamic tract.
❑ Pathway is known as dorsal culumn pathway.	❑ Pathway is known as anterolateral pathway.

Lateral spinothalamic tract	Anterior spinothalamic tract
❑ Carries pain and temperature sensation.	❑ Carries crude touch sensation.
❑ 2nd order neurone crosses to the opposite side of same segment in which it enters.	❑ 2nd order neurone ascends up to few segments and then crosses to the opposite side of same segment in which it enters.
❑ Passes through lateral white column of spinal cord.	❑ Passes through anterior or ventral column of spinal cord.
❑ 1st order neurone terminate on a group of cells present in lamina I, II and V.	❑ 1st order neurone terminate on a group of cells present in lamina III and IV.

Proprioception	Kinaesthetic sensation
❑ Perception of joint position and joint movement is known as proprioception.	❑ Perception of only joint movement is known as kinaesthetic sensation.

Fast pain	Slow pain
❑ Characterised by bright, sharp and localised pain.	❑ Characterised by dull, intense and diffuse pain.
❑ Carried by A delta fibers.	❑ Carried by C fibers.
❑ Stimulated in response to noxious stimuli.	❑ Stimulated in response to noxious, mechanical and thermal stimuli.
❑ Synaptic neurotransmitter involved is glutamic acid.	❑ Synaptic neurotransmitter involved is substance-P.
❑ Conduction of this type of pain is blocked by pressure.	❑ Conduction of this type of pain is blocked by anaesthetics, kinins, histamin etc.

Referred pain	Radiating pain
❑ When pain originating in visceral organ is felt in somatic structure away from the origin of pain sensation is called as referred pain.	❑ When visceral pain originating in visceral organ is felt in both somatic and visceral structure and also at distant point, is called as radiating pain.

Referred pain	Radiating pain
❑ Example: cardiac pain in inner part of upper portions of left arm and left shoulder.	❑ Example: Appendicitis pain which starts in the right iliac fossa and radiated towards center of abdoben.

Itch	Pain
❑ Receptors are superficial free nerve endings, 'C' fibers.	❑ Receptors are superficial free nerve endings, 'C' fibers and A fibers.
❑ Evoked by low intensity stimulus.	❑ Evoked by high intensity stimulus.
❑ It induces scratching.	❑ Produced by scratching which subserves the itching.
❑ Morphine makes it worst.	❑ Morphine relieves pain.

Cerebellar ataxia	Sensory ataxia
❑ It is the incoordinated voluntary movement due to cerebellar lesion.	❑ It is the incoordinated voluntary movement due to loss of conscious proprioception.
❑ It is due to lack of motor coordination between agonists, antagonist and synergists muscles that participate in movement.	❑ It is due to lack of sensory coordination between agonists, antagonist and synergists muscles that participate in movement.
❑ Results dysmetria, intention tremor rebound phenomenon, disdidochokinesis.	❑ Results incoordinated, slow and clumsy voluntary movements.

Intention tremor	Resting tremor
❑ Tremor that develops during movement.	❑ Tremor present in resting condition and disappears during sleep and during work.
❑ It is due to lesion either in neocerebellum or in the intermediate zone of cerebellum.	❑ It is due to loss of serotonergic input in basal ganglia.

Parkinson's tremor	Cerebellar tremor
❑ It is fine tremor.	❑ It is coarse tremor.
❑ Frequency is 6-8 Hz.	❑ Frequency is 2-4 Hz.
❑ It occurs at rest.	❑ It occuurs at the end of movement.
❑ It is rhythmic.	❑ It is arrhythmic.

Climbing fiber	Mossy fiber
❑ It is the afferent fiber to cerebellum from neurons of inferior olivary neucleus.	❑ It gives input to cerebellum from other parts.
❑ It constitute olivocerebellar tract.	❑ It constitute spinocerebellar, vestibulo-cerebellar, reticulocerebellar, tecto-cerebellar, cortico-ponto cerebellar tract.

Climbing fiber	Mossy fiber
❑ Relays signal from motor areas of cerebral cortex and proprioceptive impulses from different parts of body.	❑ Relays motor, proprioceptive, exteroceptive, visual and auditory impulses from different parts of body.

NREM sleep	REM sleep
❑ It is associated with rapid to and fro eye movement.	❑ It is not associated with rapid to and fro eye movement.
❑ It shows high voltage waves.	❑ It shows low voltage waves.
❑ It occupies 70% of sleep period.	❑ It occupies 30% of sleep period.
❑ BP, pulse rate, respiration rate are low and regular in this phase.	❑ BP, pulse rate, respiration rate are increased and become irregular in this phase.
❑ Brain activity is less during this phase.	❑ Brain activity is more during this phase.
❑ O_2 consumption is less.	❑ O_2 consumption is more.
❑ Threshold for arousal is less.	❑ Threshold for arousal is more.
❑ Dreams can not be recalled clearly after arousal.	❑ Dreams can be recalled clearly after arousal.
❑ No pontoeniculooccipital spikes (PGO) are present.	❑ Pontoeniculooccipital spikes (PGO) are present.

Cold receptors	Warm receptors
❑ It is thin myelinated A delta fibers.	❑ It is unmyelinated C fibers.
❑ Density is more.	❑ Density is less.
❑ Fire steadily at tissue temperature between 10°C and 35°C.	❑ Fire steadily at tissue temperature between 35°C and 45°C.

Tonic	Phasic
❑ These are poor, slow and incompletely adapting receptors.	❑ These are rapidly adapting receptors.
❑ Example: muscle spindles, baro and chemoreceptors etc.	❑ Example: touch, olfactory receptors.
❑ Transmit signal as long as the stimulus is applied.	❑ Transmit signal only when the strength of stimulus is changed.

Superficial pain	Deep pain
❑ It is sharp and well localised.	❑ It is dull and poorly localised.
❑ It involves the skin and subcutaneous tissue.	❑ It involves the muscle and hollow viscera.
❑ It usually does not radiate.	❑ It usually radiates.
❑ It is associated with reflex withdrawal, increase in heart rate, BP and respiration.	❑ It is associated with decrease in heart rate, BP and respiration.

Pyramidal system	Extra pyramidal system
❑ The spinal motor neurons originate directly from the motor cortex are known as pyramidal system.	❑ The spinal motor neurons via subcortical structures from the motor cortex are known as pyramidal system.
❑ Lesion of this tract produces spasticity in the muscles involved.	❑ Lesion of this tract produces rigidity in the muscles involved.
❑ Descends through the medullary pyramids.	❑ Does not descend through the medullary pyramids.
❑ Originates mostly from area 4 and 6.	❑ Originates mostly from area 6 and subcortical structures.
❑ It is predominantly under cortical control.	❑ It is predominantly under control of basal ganglia and cerebellum.
❑ It controls skilled movements of hands and fingers.	❑ It controls posture and axial movements.

Intracollicular (Classical) decerebration	Ischemic decerebration
❑ Transection between two colliculi is called as Sherrington or Classical decerebration	❑ It is produced by tying both carotid arteries and the basilar artery at the junction of the pons and medulla.
❑ It is fatal.	❑ It is relatively safe.
❑ It is due to gama rigidity.	❑ It is due to alpha rigidity.
❑ It is evident mostly in the extensor antigravity limb muscles.	❑ It results increase in muscle tone that resembles decerebrate rigidity.
❑ Removal of anterior lobe of cerebellum increases the rigidity.	❑ Removal of anterior lobe of cerebellum does not affect the rigidity.

Broca's aphasia	Wernick's aphasia
❑ It is due to lesion in area 44 and 45 (Broca's area).	❑ It is due to lesion in area 22 (Wernick's area).
❑ It is a form of motor aphasia.	❑ It is a form of sensory aphasia.
❑ It is associated with difficulty in speaking (non-fluent aphasia).	❑ It is not associated with difficulty in speaking (fluent aphasia) though speech is often associated with meaningless or incorrect words.
❑ No difficulty in understanding speech.	❑ Difficulty in understanding speech.
❑ Writing is not affected.	❑ Writing is affected.

D. Short answer type:

1. How does Jendrassik's manoeuvre help to elicit deep tendon reflexes?

Sometimes the reflexes (like ankle jerk or plantar reflex etc.) can not be elicited even in normal person if the person is too conscious about it. In such cases to elicit those reflexes attention of the subject is diverted by **clenching his teeth or by pulling his locked and flexed fingers etc. while demonstrating** those reflexes. This technique is known as **Reinforcement**. In this process the stretch reflex becomes **hyperactive** due to increase in efferent discharge.

2. How does pain sensation differs from other sensations?

It differs from other sensations in that:

- It is associated with emotions e.g. fear anxiety etc. and as autonomic functions e.g. increase in heart rate, BP, sweating etc.
- It produces a withdrawal reflex.

3. Give the physiological basis of positive Babinski's sign. Is it a flexor or extensor response?

Stimulation of the outer edge of the sole of the foot by gentle scratching from the heel towards the little toe and then medially upto the base of the big toe, results **plantar flexion (downward movement) of the great toe and drawing together of other toes** (Fig.10.16). This is known as **Babinski's sign negative** or ***plantar reflex***. This type of response appears with the development of pyramidal tracts and thus is seen in normal healthy individuals but in case of **upper motor neurone lesion there is dorsiflexon (upward movement) of the great toe and fanning out (abduction) of small toes. This is known as Babinski's sign positive** or ***Babinski's response*** or ***plantar extension***.

4. List the causes of abnormal Babinski's plantar response. Give it's clinical significance.

This type of response is seen in infants (< 1 year old) due to **incomplete development of pyramidal tracts** or during sleep or Cheyne-Stoke's breathing due to hypoxia.

5. Why is the duration of spinal shock is more in human?

It is because in human beings the entire nervous system works in integrated manner to act as a functional unit. So damage of any part of the nervous system disturbs it's smoothness of workings and thus the functional failure is more severe.

6. Why spinal man cannot stand unsupported?

The limbs of the paraplegic individuals adopt a slight flexon paraplegic. This is why the spinal man can not stand unsupported.

7. Explain why is reading newspaper in a moving bus so difficult?

It is because of excessive stain in the vestibulo-visual fixation mechanism.

8. What will happen if:

- ***Membrane labyrinth is over distended.***

Overdistension of membranous labyrinth results in disorder of vestibular apparatus which is characterised by:

1. Abrupt and often severe dizziness
2. Ringing in the ear
3. Bouts of hearing loss

- ***Otolith reflexes are lacking:***

The otolith reflexes help the muscles in the leg begin to contract before the feet reach the ground in order to cushion the force of impact. This is why the individuals lacking the otolith reflexes are prone to leg injuries while stepping off a bus or walk downstairs.

9. Which will produce greater abnormalities—the lesion in cerebellar cortex or of deep cerebellar nuclei?

Lesion of deep cerebellar neclei will produce greater abnormalities (general defects) because these abnormalities will be persisted life long whereas the lesions of cerebellar cortex cause only movement related abnormalities which gradually disappear because of compensatory changes.

10. What will happen and why to deep reflexes in cerebellar lesion?

Deep reflexes will become weak or pendular e.g. pendular knee jerk due to hypotonia of quadriceps muscle.

11. Give the physiological significance of neural cercuit within the cerebellar cortex.

The cerebellar neural circuit is concerned with modulatory or timing of the excitatory output of the deep cerebellar nuclei to the brain stem and thalamus that helps the cerebellum in coordinating the muscle movements.

12. Why the thalamus is termed as a relay center?

As the thalamus relays the:

- Somesthetic sensations coming from opposite half of body
- Auditory and visual sensation
- Autonomic and emotional reactions
- Impulses from opposite cerebellum on their way to the motor cortex
- Impulses from reticular formation.

13. Give the physiological basis of:

- ***Rigidity***: Rigidity in basal ganglia dysfunction is due to the excessive muscle tone resulted due to—

  A. absence of inhibitory effect on stretch reflex

  B. absence of stimulation of reticular formation → unbalanced activity of inhibitory and facilatatory reticular projection on spinal neurones → excessive muscle tone.

- ***Resting tremor in basal ganglia dysfunction***: During voluntary movements impulses from the motor cortex pass down the descending pathways and stimulate both alpha and gamma motor neurons. The gama efferent stimulate the stretch reflex to stop the involuntary movements which is called as damping effect.

14. What will happen and why if:

- ***Parietal lobe on one side get injured***:

It results:

  - defective response to all stimuli arise in opposite side of the visual /somatic field.
  - loss of finer form of sense perception in the opposite side e.g. tactile localization, tactile discrimination, temperature sense etc.
  - loss of control over the voluntary movements (ataxia).

- ***Inferior parietal lobule is removed***

It results:

  - Asteriognosis
  - Inability to copy designs and objects
  - Patient can not find his way about even in familiar surrounding called spatial discrimination

- ***All connections between prefrontal lobe and thalamus are cut***:

In this case there is no genesis of emotions and resting EEG.

E. MCQ:

1. In a neurone action potential initiates at (i) Node of Ranvier (ii) Dendrites (iii) Synaptic terminals (iv) Initial segmant of axon. (iv)
2. The scavenger of CNS is (i) Schwann cell (ii) Microglia (iii) Neuroglia (iv) Satellite cells. (i)
3. The glial cell that constitute the blood brain barrier is (i) Schwann cell (ii) Microglia (iii) Astrocytes (iv) Oligodendrocytes. (iii)
4. The myelin sheath is formed by (i) satellite cells (ii) oligodendrocytes (iii) astrocytes (iv) schwann cells. (iv)
5. The maximum conduction velocity in nerve fiber is (i) 120 m/sec (ii) 30 m/sec (iii) 12 m/sec (iv) 0.3 m /sec. (i)
6. Which part of the brain is outside the blood brain barrier (i) cerebellum (ii) basal ganglia (iii) hypothalamus (iv) circumventricular organ. (iv)
7. All are the excitatory neurotransmitter except (i) ACh (ii) Serotonin (iii) Glutamin (iv) GABA. (iv)
8. The normal average CSF pressure is (i) 130 mmHg (ii) 13 mmHg (iii) 500 mmHg (iv) 30 mmHg. (i)
9. Spinal cord integrate all of the following action except (i) Stretch reflex (ii) Flexor reflex (iii) Righting reflex (iv) Positive supportive reaction. (iii)
10. The longest neurone present in our body is (i) corticospinal tract (ii) reticulospinal tract (iii) corticobulbar tract (iv) vestibulospinal tract. (i)
11. All are the parts of the midbrain except (i) Substantia nigra (ii) Tegmentum (iii) Hypothalamus (iv) Superior colliculus. (ii)
12. All are the parts of hindbrain except (i) Pons (ii) Pituitary gland (iii) Medulla (iv) Cerebellum. (ii)
13. All are the mixed nerve except (i) oculomotor (ii) glossopharyngeal (iii) vagus (iv) hypoglossal. (iv)
14. Which one is the afferent cranial nerve (i) optic (ii) spinal accessory (iii) trochlear (iv) facial. (i)
15. All are the tracts passing through the lateral white column of spinal cord except (i) lateral spinothalamic tract (ii) dorsal spinocerebellar tract (iii) ventral spinocerebellar tract. (iii)
16. All but one are the type of touch receptors (i) Merkel's disc (ii) Free nerve endings (iii) Meissner's corpuscle (iv) Rufini's end organ. (ii)
17. Fasciculus Gracilis receives input from (i) Lumber and sacral segments of spinal cord (ii) Lumber and thoracic (iii) cervical and thoracic (iv) thoracic and sacral. (i)
18. The nerve for crude touch sensation is (i) lateral spinothalamic tract (ii) ventral spinocerebellar tract (iii) ventral spinothalamic tract (iv) tract of Gall. (iii)
19. The subconscious kinaesthetic sensation is carried by (i) Dorsal spinocerebellar tract (ii) Ventral spinocerebellar tract (iii) both (iv) none of the above. (iii)
20. In case of hemisection of spinal cord following is not true at the level of lesion (i) complete loss of all sensation (ii) complete lower motor neurone types of paralysis (iii) both (iv) none. (iii)
21. Wernick's area is (i) area 41 and 42 (ii) area 21 and 22 (iii) area 4S and 6a (iv) area 19 and 18. (i)
22. All but one are the components of basal ganglia (i) corpus striatum (ii) claustrum (iii) amygdaloid nucleus (iv) thalamic nuclei. (iv)
23. All but one is the features of Parkinsonism (i) mask like face (ii) lead pipe rigidity (iii) drunken gait (iv) statue like posture. (iii)

24. All but one are the normal waves seen in EEG (i) gamma wave (ii) delta wave (iii) beta wave (iv) theta wave. (i)
25. All but one are the brain stem structure (i) cerebellum (ii) pons (iii) midbrain (iv) medulla. (i)
26. Biological clock is present in (i) preoptic nucleus of hypothalamus (ii) suprachiasmatic nucleus of hypothalamus (iii) posterolateral nucleus of thalamus (iv) metathalamus. (ii)
27. All are the clinical features of Kluver Bucy syndrome (i) aphasia (ii) visual hallucination (iii) auditory disturbances (iv) loss of recent memory. (iv)
28. Kluver Bucy syndrome is due to (i) bilateral destruction of temporal lobe of cerebral cortex (ii) bilateral destruction of frontal lobe of cerebral cortex (iii) thalamic lesion (iv) basal ganglia lesion. (i)
29. The number of Broadman's area are (i) 42 (ii) 77 (iii) 72 (iv) 47. (iv)
30. Which are is the primary motor cortex (i) area 4 (ii) area 19 (iii) area 6 (iv) area 22. (i)
31. All but one are the clinical features of Tabes Dorsalis (i) loss of pain sensation (ii) Rhomberg sign negative (iii) stamping gait (iv) loss of micturation reflex. (ii)
32. Syringomyelia is a disease related with (i) basal ganglia (ii) cerebellum (iii) thalamus (iv) spinal cord. (iv)
33. Broca's area is present in the (i) inferior frontal gyrus of left cerebral hemisphere (ii) inferior frontal gyrus of right cerebral hemisphere (iii) parietal lobe of right cerebral hemisphere (iv) post central gyrus. (iii)
34. The natural analgesic substance in our body is (i) glutamate (ii) enkephalin and endorphins (iii) substance-P (iv) histamin. (ii)
35. Visceral pain is caused by all the following stimuli except (i) pressure (ii) stretching (iii) cutting (iv) touch. (iii)
36. Crossed extensor reflex is a (i) monosynaptic reflex (ii) withdrawal reflex (iii) righting reflex (iv) sympathetic reflex. (ii)
37. Hypotonia of skeletal muscle is seen in all the following except (i) thalamic syndrome (ii) cerebellar lesion (iii) tabes dorsalis (iv) pyramidal tract lesion. (iv)
38. All but one of the following are associated with cerebellar lesion (i) spasticity (ii) intention tremor (iii) ataxia (iv) pendular knee jerk. (i)
39. Babinski sign is positive in (i) upper motor neurone lesion (ii) lower motor neurone lesion (iii) cerebellar lesion (iv) thalamic lesion. (i)
40. The function of vestibulocerebellum is (i) initiation of visceral reflexes (ii) planning of movements (iii) co-ordination of movements (iv) maintenance of equilibrium. (iv)

11 Special Senses

A. Long type:

1. Where does taste receptor present? Enumerate the structure of taste buds. Briefly discuss the neurophysiology of taste sensation. What do you mean by modalities of taste sensation?

Location of Taste receptors—

- Taste sensation is perceived by the taste receptors (chemoreceptors) distributed over the surface of the tongue and other regions like mucosa of pharynx, epiglottis and even on the proximal esophagus.
- In the tongue these receptors are clustered in individual taste buds which are located in 3 different types of **tongue papillae:**
  - (i) ***Circumvallate papillae*** —Largest in size, arranged in the form of a 'v' on the surface of posterior part of tongue.
  - (ii) ***Fungi form papillae***—present on the anterior surface of tongue.
  - (iii) ***Filiform papillae***— Smallest, present in the folds along the lateral surface of the tongue. These do not have taste buds.
  - (iv) ***Foliate papillae*** — Absent in adult human beings.

***Structure of taste buds*:**

- The taste bud is composed of about 40 modified epithelial cells (taste cells) which are of principally two types (Fig. 11.1)—
  - ■ ***Gustatory receptor cells*** which has got cilia in one side (Taste pore) and nerves in other side.
  - ■ ***Supporting*** or sustentacular cells which has cilia on taste pore.

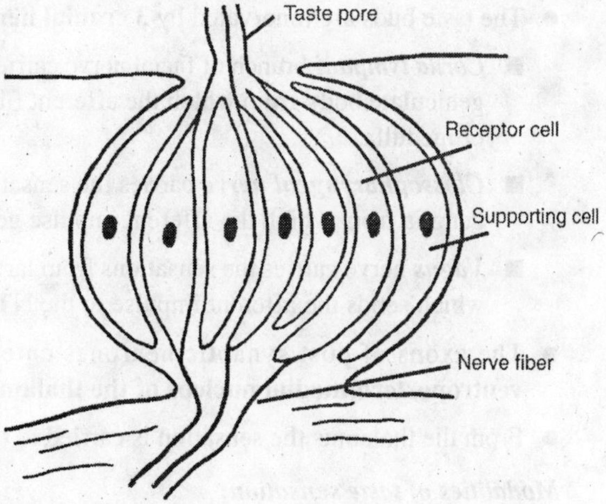

FIG. 11.1: Structure of taste buds

- The outer tip of the taste cells are arranged around a minute pore opening on the tongue surface. This pore is called *taste pores*. From tip of the taste cells several hairs or cilia originate and project through the taste pore to the mouth cavity.

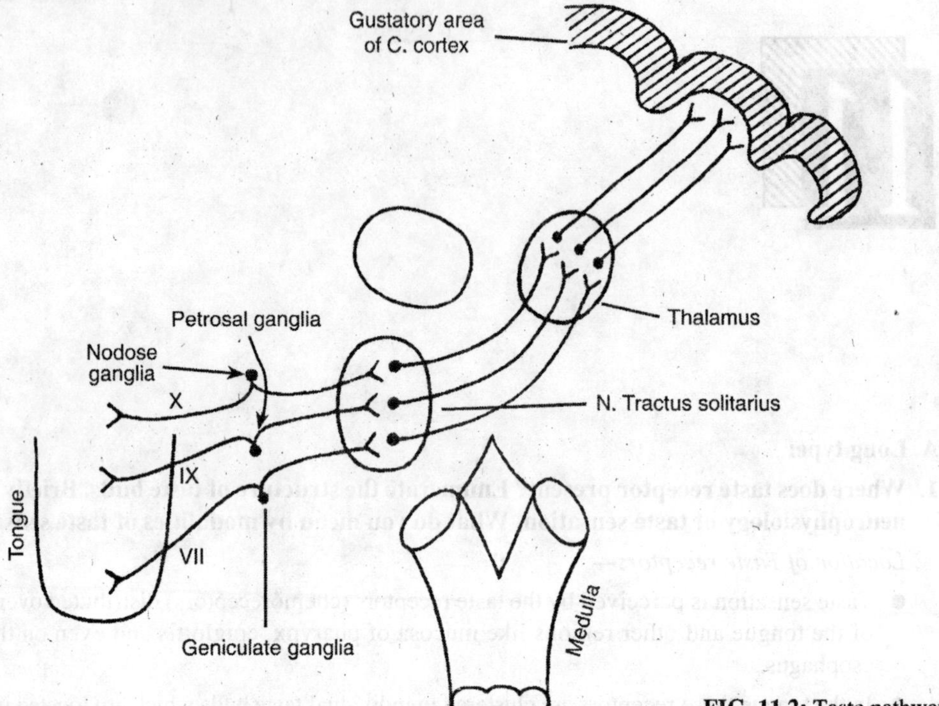

FIG. 11.2: Taste pathway

***Neural pathway responsible for taste sensation* (Fig. 11.2):**

- The taste buds are innervated by **3 cranial nerves**—
  - ***Corda tympani*** branch of facial nerve carries the sensation from anterior 2/3rd of tongue to the geniculate body from which the afferent fibers pass to the **nucleus tractus solitarius** (NTS) of medulla.
  - ***Glossopharyngeal nerve*** carries the sensation from posterior 1/3rd of tongue to the petrosal ganglia from which the afferent impulse goes to **NTS of medulla,**
  - ***Vagus*** nerve carries the sensations from larynx and proximal esophagus to the nodose ganglia which sends the afferent impulse to the **NTS of medulla.**
- The axons of post synaptic neurones enter the median lemniscus and thence enter the **ventropostero-medial nucleus of the thalamus** – to make another synapse.
- From the thalamus the sensation is carried to the post central gyrus in the **parietal cortex.**

***Modalities of taste sensation*:**

(a) *Types of primary taste sensation*: There are 4 types of primary taste sensation—Sweet, Sour, Salted and Bitter. Recently another type of taste sensation is added known as ***Umami*** which is pleasant and sweet but differs from standard sweet taste.

(b) Distribution of specific taste buds:

- taste buds highly sensitive to **sweet** is present **in the tip** of the tongue (Fig. 11.3).
- taste buds highly sensitive to **bitter** is present **in the back** of the tongue.
- taste buds highly sensitive to **sour** and **salty** are present **in the sides** of the tongue.

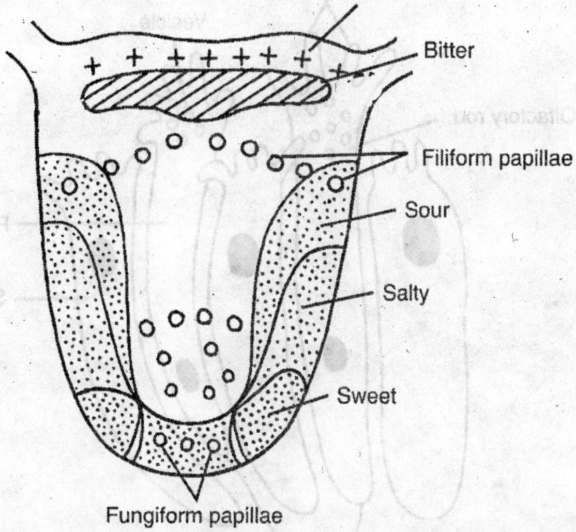

FIG. 11.3: Location of taste papillae including modalities of taste sensation

(c) *Stimulus of different taste sensation*:

- **Sweet taste**: Sweet taste is produced by—
  - mainly organic substances e.g. sugar, alcohol, aldehyde, ketone, saccharides etc.
  - inorganic substance like lead acetate.
- **Sour taste**: Sour taste is produced by acids (including organic acids) which is ionised to H^+ and stimulate taste receptor cells for sour sensation.
- **Salty taste**: It is produced by cations released from inorganic salts.
- **Bitter taste**: It is offered by long chain organic compounds that contain N_2 (e.g. quinine sulphate, urea, caffeine etc.) and also by alkaloids (nicotine, morphins etc.).

2. Enumerate the olfactory organ. With suitable diagram discuss the neural basis of olfaction. What do you mean by electroolfactogram?

Olfactory organ that lies in the olfactory epithelium on either side of nasal septum (superior part of each nostril) just inferior to the **cribriform plate** of ethmoid bone is known as ***olfactory neuro epithelium***.

Structure of olfactory neuro epithelium:

- It is composed of 3 types of cells and one gland known a ***Bowman's gland*** (interspaced among olfactory cells) that secretes mucous.
- The cells are:

(a) *Supporting cells*: These are columnar epithelial cells with large oval nuclei and ends in microvilli. It secretes mucous along with the golden brown pigment that gives the **golden yellow color of the nasal mucosa.**

(b) *Receptor cells*: These are bipolar neurone (known as ***olfactory rods*** which ends in fine cilia (0.3 μ in diameter). From each rods 6-12 cilia arise which lie in the mucous covering olfactory mucous membrane. These projecting olfactory hairs (cilia) are believed to react with odoriferous molecules present in the air and then stimulate the olfactory receptor cell.

(c) *Basal cells: They* are few in number and are parent cell of supporting cells.

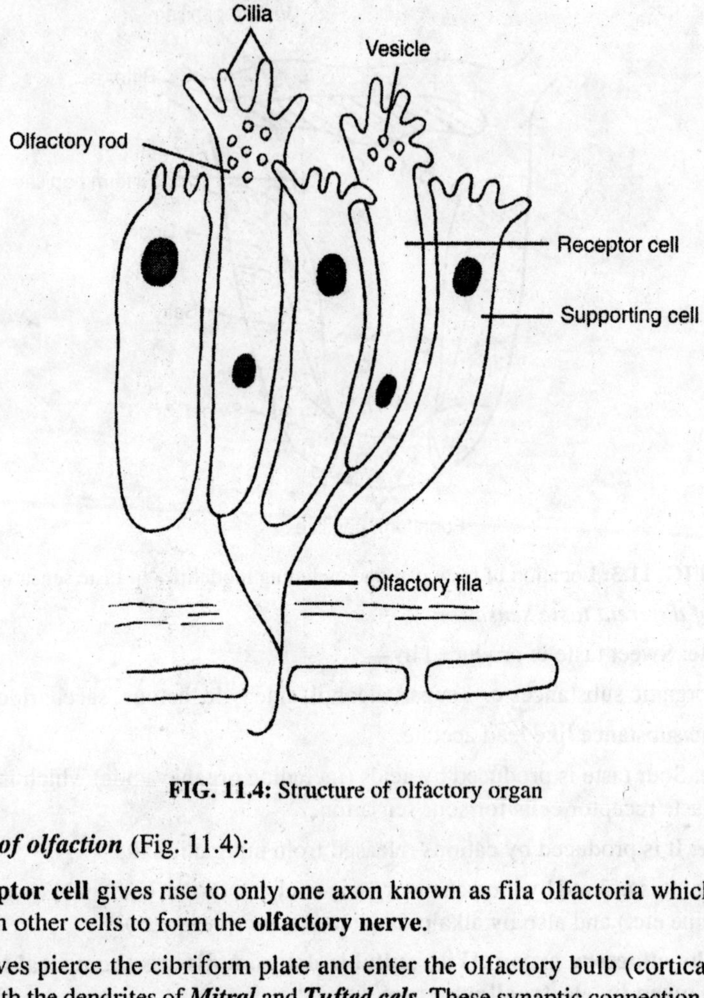

FIG. 11.4: Structure of olfactory organ

Neural basis of olfaction (Fig. 11.4):

- Each **receptor cell** gives rise to only one axon known as fila olfactoria which joins with other axons from other cells to form the **olfactory nerve**.
- These nerves pierce the cibriform plate and enter the olfactory bulb (cortical center) to make synapse with the dendrites of ***Mitral*** and ***Tufted cells.*** These synaptic connection between olfactory nerve fiber and dendrites of Mitral and Tufted cells is called as ***glomerulus.*** The axon of these Mitral and Tufted cells form olfactory tract.
- Olfactory tract originated from the Tufted cells run in the medial olfactory stria and cross the midline in the anterior commissure to form synapses with ***Granule cells*** in the opposite olfactory bulb. Some fibers of the medial olfactory stria originated from Tufted cell enters into medial olfactory area bilaterally.
- The olfactory nerve originated from the Mitral cells runs in the **lateral olfactory stria** and enters into **lateral olfactory area of brain**.

From these medial and lateral olfactory areas sensation is also relayed to secondary olfactory area of both sides of brain.

Electro-olfactogram—When an odorous molecule gets absorb in the olfactory mucosa a monophasic negative potential is recorded which lasts for 4-6 secs. This recorded electrical changes is known as ***electro-olfactogram.***

3. Draw a diagram of visual pathway and explain it. Indicate the effects of lesion at different levels of optic pathway.

General descriptions of visual pathway (Fig. 11.5):

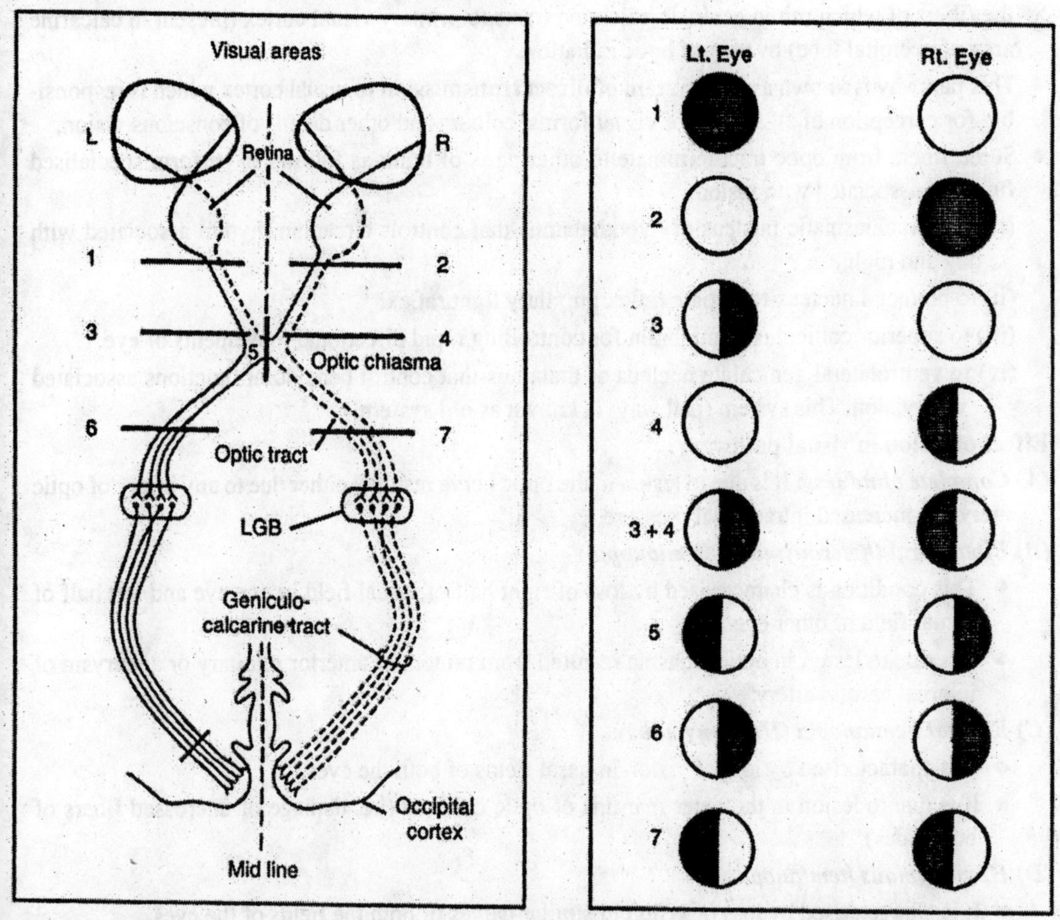

Fig. 11.5: Visual pathway (In left panel) along with conditions due to lesion in visual pathway (in right panel). 1 = lesion of left optic nerve that results total blindness of left eye, 2 = lesion of right optic nerve that results total blindness of right eye, 3 = lesion of lateral fibers of left side of optic chiasma that results left nasal hemianopia, 4 = lesion of lateral fibers of right side of optic chiasma that results right nasal hemianopia, 3 + 4 = lesion of lateral fibers of both side of optic chiasma that results binasal hemianopia, 5 = lesion of medial fibers of optic chiasma that results bitemporal hemianopia, 6 = lesion of left optic radiation that results right homonymous hemianopia and 7 = lesion of right optic radiation that results left homonymous hemianopia

- Rods and cones are the receptor cells for vision. Cones mainly function in bright light and are responsible for colour sensation whereas rods are excited during dim light and are responsible for perception of only shades of white and black.
- From rods and cones the 1st order neuron originates through which impulse passes to Bipolar cells present in the inner nuclear layer.

- 2nd order neuron from bipolar cell then sends the impulse to ganglion cell the axon of which forms the optic nerve.
- Optic nerve leaves the eye through optic disc. Some of the optic nerve fibers (nasal side) cross to opposite side and some (temporal side) remain uncrossed forming ***optic chiasma***. Thus at the optic chiasma all the fibers coming from nasal side of retina cross to the opposite side and join with fibers from the opposite temporal retina to form **optic tracts**.
- Each optic tract relays at dorsolateral geniculate nucleus from which 3rd order neuron originates the fibers of which run in geniculo-calcarine tracts to primary visual cortex (present in calcarine area of occipital lobe) by way of optic radiation.
- This pathway is known as **new system of direct transmission** to visual cortex which is responsible for perception of all aspects of visual forms, colours and other details of conscious vision.
- Some fibers from optic tract terminate to other parts of brain as follows to perform specialised function associated with vision.
  (i) to suprachiasmatic nucleus of hypothalamus-that controls circadian rhythm associated with day and night.
  (ii) to pretectal nucleus-to initiate reflex pupillary light reflex.
  (iii) to superior colliculus of midbrain for controlling rapid directional movements of eye.
  (iv) to ventrolateral geniculate nucleus of thalamus-that control behavioral functions associated with vision. This system (pathway) is known as **old system**.

Effect of lesion in visual pathway:

(A) Complete blindness: It is due to lesion in the optic nerve resulted either due to any injury of optic nerve or increased intracranial pressure.

(B) Bitemporal (heteronymous) hemianopia:

- This condition is characterised by loss of right half of visual field in one eye and left half of visual field of other eye.
- It is due to lesion in optic chiasma resulted from tumors of anterior pituitary or aneurysm of internal carotid artery.

(C) Binasal hemianopia (Heteronymous):

- It is characterised by loss of vision in nasal fields of both the eyes.
- It is due to lesion in the outer margins of optic chiasma (i.e. damage of uncrossed fibers of both sides).

(D) Homonymous hemianopia:

- It is characterised by loss of vision in similar halves of both the fields of the eyes.
- It is due to lesion in the optic chiasma (damage of uncross fiber of one side) and lateral geniculate body or optic radiations.

(E) Quadrantic hemianopia:

- Blindness in superior field of both the eyes are called quadrantic hemianopia.
- It may be of two types:
  - **Superior quandrantic bitemporal heminapia** (loss of vision in superior field of temporal side of both the eyes).
  - **Inferior quandrantic bitemporal hemianopia** (loss of vision in inferior field of temporal side of both the eyes.
- It is due to damage of crossed fibers of optic chiasma.

*(F) **Scotoma***: Presence of other blind spot than the normal blind spot is called as scotoma.

*(G) **Strabismus*** or ***squint***: Lack of fusion of eyes in one or more coordinates is called as squint or Strabismus.

4. Explain the auditory pathway. Add a note on auditory defects with special reference to tests of hearing. What is hearing aid?

Auditory pathway (Fig. 11.6):

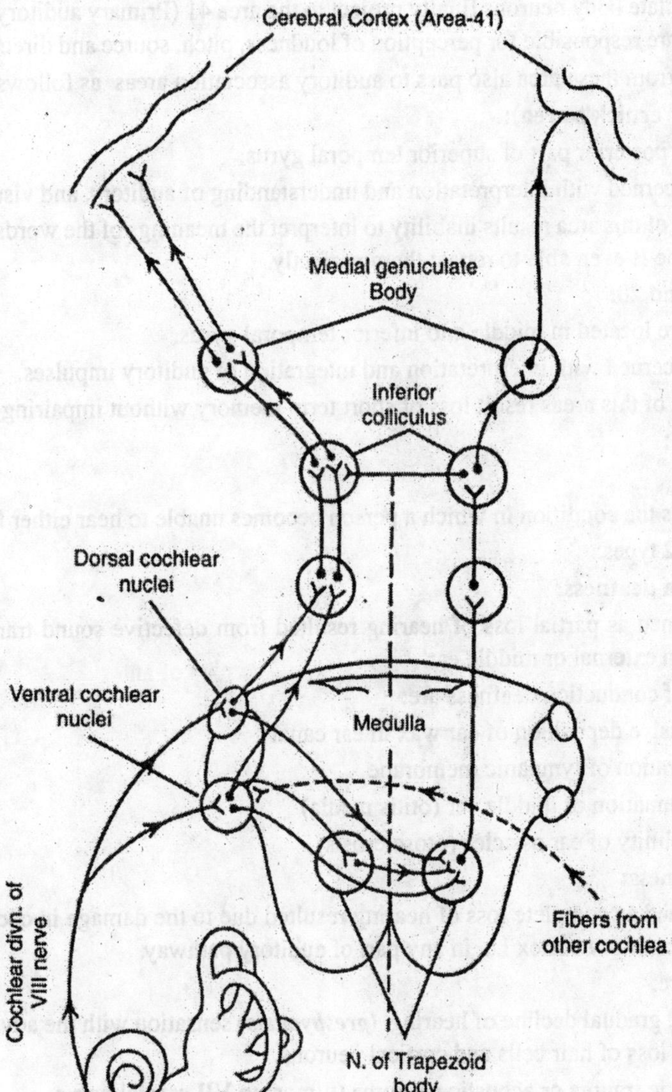

Fig. 11.6: Auditory pathway

- **Nerve fibers supplying hair cells of organ of corti go to spiral ganglia.**
- **The axons of spiral ganglia form the cochlear division of VIII cranial nerve (auditory nerve) which enter the medulla to terminate in ventral and dorsal cochlear nuclei.**

- From these nuclei second order neurons originate most of which terminate into superior olivary nucleus of opposite side by crossing through trapezoid body. Whereas some 2nd order neurons terminate to the ipsilateral superior olivary nucletus of same side.
- Third order neurons then pass to the inferior colliculus of both sides (center for auditory reflex) through the lateral lemniscus. Some of these fibers also send collaterals to the reticular formation and medial geniculate body.
- From the inferior colliculi the 4th order neuron arises which pass to the medial geniculate body.
- Median geniculate body neurons finally project to the area 41 (Primary auditory area) of cerebral cortex which are responsible for perception of loudness, pitch, source and direction of the sound.
- The impulses from these area also pass to auditory association areas as follows:

  (i) **Area 22 (Wernick's area):**
  - It lies in posterior part of superior temporal gyrus.
  - It is concerned with interpretation and understanding of auditory, and visual information.
  - Damage of this area results inability to interpret the meanings of the words the person hears though he is even able to repeat them perfectly.

  (ii) **Area 21 and 20:**
  - These are located in middle and inferior temporal gyrus.
  - It is concerned with interpretation and integration of auditory impulses.
  - Damage of this areas result loss of short term memory without impairing visual memory.

Auditory defects:

***A. Deafness*:**

- ***Definition*:** It is the condition in which a person becomes unable to hear either fully or partly.
- ***Types*:** It is of 2 types:

  (a) **Conduction deafness:**
  - It is defined as partial loss of hearing resulted from defective sound transmission due to defects in external or middle ear.
  - Causes of conduction deafness are:
    - ☐ Excessive deposition of ear wax in ear canal
    - ☐ Perforation of tympanic membrane
    - ☐ Inflammation of middle ear (otitis media)
    - ☐ Immobility of ear ossicles (otosclerosis)

  (b) **Nerve deafness:**
  - It is defined as complete loss of hearing resulted due to the damage in cochlea or cochlear nerve or auditory cortex i.e. in any part of auditory pathway.
  - Causes are:
    - ☐ Aging: gradual decline of hearing (***presbycusis***) sensation with the advancement of age due to loss of hair cells and cortical neurons.
    - ☐ Acoustic trauma or acoustic neuroma (tumor) to VII cranial nerve.
    - ☐ Prolonged exposure to high frequency noise.
    - ☐ Degeneration of VIII cranial nerve during meningitis, measles or due to streptomyosin injection.
- *Tests for detection of auditory defects*: There are three tests to differentiate between nerve and conduction deafness:

(a) **Rinne's Test**—See Table 11A.

(b) **Weber's Test**—See table 11A.

(c) **Audiometry**—This test is conducted in a sound proof room, and one ear at a time using audio meter.

Table 11A : Tuning fork tests to assess auditory function

Name of the test	Procedure	Observation	Inference
Rinne's test	1. The base of vibrating tuning fork is placed on the mastoid process of the subject.	1. If vibration in air is heard after bone conduction is over.	Normal
	2. The subject is asked whether he is listening the sound and instructed him to say "No" as soon as he stops listening the sound.	2. If vibration in air is not heard after bone conduction is over.	Conduction deafness
	3. The arm of the same vibrating fork is now brought near his ear.		
	4. The subject is asked whether he is listening the sound again or not.		
Weber's test	1. The base of the vibrating tuing fork is placed on the forehead of the subject.	1. If sound is louder (due to absence of masking effect of noise) in the diseased ear.	Conduction deafness
	2. The subject is asked whether he is listening the sound in both ear equally or not.	2. If sound is louder in the normal ear.	Nerve deafness (partial)

- *Hearing aids*: Hearing aids have been designed to help patients with impaired hearing-both conduction and nerve deafness provided the sense of hearing is not totally lost. It has 3 components:
  (i) Microphone—It converts sound signal to electrical signal.
  (ii) Amplifier—It amplifies the electrical signal.
  (iii) Ear phone—Transducer that converts amplified electrical signals to sound signal that is fed to the ear.

5. Explain the mechanism of hearing. Discuss in brief the theories regarding perception of pitch of the sound.

Mechanism of hearing:

Step I : Sound wave strikes Tympanic membrane (TM) that causes resonant vibration of TM.

Step II : Vibration of TM initiates movement of ear ossicles that lead inward pushing of Stapes to Oval window.

Step III : Generation of wave into cochlear fluid that travels toward Basilar membrane (BM).

Step IV : Upward and downward (***Rocking***) movement of BM.

Step V : Pulling and side bending of cilia of hair cells toward nodiolus.

Step VI : Depolarisation and hyperpolarisation of hair cells.

Step VII : Transmission of AP through cochlear nerve when hair cell gets depolarise.

Step VIII : When hair cell undergoes hyper polarisation due to downward movement of BM transmission of impulse through cochlear nerve is stopped.

Theories regarding perception of pitch of sound:

(a) *Telephonic theory of Rutherford*: It was postulated by scientist Rutherford which states that cochlea acts as a telephone transmitter responsible for transforming sounds into nerve impulse of same frequency which were then analysed by CNS.

(b) *Place Principle*: As per this theory the place (part) of BM discriminates the pitch of the sound. **For example**: If the frequency of sound wave is low there is maximum vibration of BM in its apical side (helicotremal side) whereas if the frequency is high there is the maximum vibration of BM in its basal side. Thus if the hair cells present near the helicotremal side are stimulated the pitch of the sound is perceived as lower frequency (low pitch), similarly if the hair cells, present at the basal side of cochlea are stimulated, it is perceived as high pitched sound.

(c) *Volley principle*: However, the place principle can not explain how the apical part of BM discriminates the low frequency sound of 200 cycles/Sec to 20 cycles/Sec. So there is postulation of another principle known as **Volley principle.** As per this principle each frequency of sound initiates different volley of impulse that leads generation of impulse of different intensity. So CNS interprets sounds of different frequency that activate different populations of afferent fibers.

(d) *Modern (Duplex) Theory*: It is the latest theory available, which states that both the Volley principle and Place principle together help in discrimination of pitch of sound.

6. Enumerate the retinal layers and cells present in them. Describe in brief the photo-chemistry of vision (phototransduction).

Retina contains **10 layers—**

(i) Layer of pigment layer
(ii) Layer of photoreceptors i.e. rods and cones
(iii) External limiting membrane
(iv) Outer nuclear layer
(v) Outer plexiform layer
(vi) Inner nuclear layer which contains Bipolar, Horizontal and amacrine cell
(vii) Inner plexiform layer
(viii) Ganglion cell layer
(ix) Layer of nerve fibers
(x) Internal limiting membrane

Photochemical basis of vision: When the image of any substance is focused on retina the light energy is converted to electrical energy which is fed to cerebral cortex and the sensation of vision is produced in cerebral cortex. Due to the differences of refractive index of different structures of eye the light rays from any object is refracted and brought to a focus on retina resulting inverted status of image. However, the cerebral cortex perceived it as upright position. The detail **process of image formation** is as follows:

(A) Photochemical basis:

- The photosensitive pigments present in rods and cones (receptor cells) are responsible for chemical basis of visual process. The chemical reactions that takes place in these pigments result generation of electrical impulse which are transmitted through optic nerve.

- When light strikes the retina it is passed to the inner sides of discs and this light energy is then absorbed by the ***rhodopsin*** or ***iodopsin*** (pigments). This results splitting of rhodopsin to ***retinine*** and ***opsin*** through various intermediate photochemical reaction (Fig. 11.7).

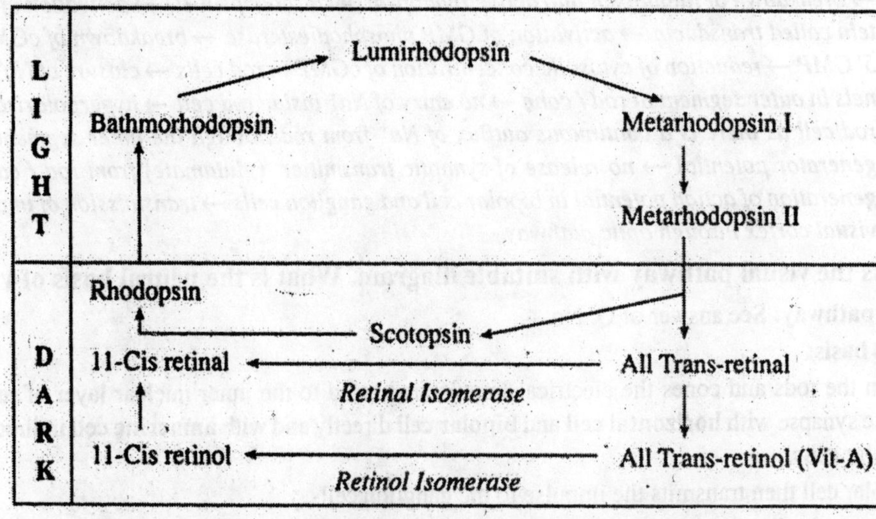

Fig. 11.7: Schematic diagram showing rhodopsin-retinine visual cycle

- The ***metarhodopsin II*** produced in this rhodopsin retinine visual cycle as intermediate product is responsible for genesis of receptor potential.
- The chemical changes that take place in cone are presumed to be same as rods.
- In this way in response to dim light rods are excited as rhodopsin is more sensitive and can react in presence of very small amount of light. This dim light vision by rod is known as **Scotopic vision.**
- Whereas vision in bright light is called as **Photopic vision** where cones are the receptors. The cone pigments have high threshold and help to analyze the details of the object seen. This is why the details including colours can only seen in bright light when cone pigments take parts. Hence the cones are responsible for acuity of vision.

***(B) Phototransduction*:**

- It is the process by which light energy is converted to receptor potential in visual receptors which are transmitted to visual cortex.
- In the dark the resting membrane potential of the visual receptors is slightly in depolarising state (– 40 mv). This is because normally in dark the Na^+ are pumped out of inner segments of rod cell to ECF which is leaked back into the rod cells through the membrane of outer segment and reduces the electronegativity inside the rod cell. This results continuous release of neurotransmitter during dark from the rod cells.
- The influx of Na^+ into the outer segment of rods is due to the constant opening of Na^+ leak channels by cGMP present in the cytoplasm of the rod cell.
- When light falls on retina the rhodopsin is splitted into metarhodopsin-II which activates a G-protein called **transducin** that activates the enzyme cGMP phosphodiesterase. This phosphodiesterase then converts the cGMP of cytoplasm to 5'-GMP, thereby reducing the concen-

tration of cGMP in cytoplasm of rod cells. This results closure of Na^+ leak channels in membrane of outer segment of rods preventing entry of Na^+ inside. This ultimately results hyperpolarisation of rod cell that leads reduction of release of synaptic transmitter. The whole sequence of events is illustrated with the help of following flow chart:

Light rays → absorption of light by photo pigments present in photo receptors (rod and cone) → breakdown of Rhodopsin into active rhodopsin (metarhodopsin-II) → activation of G protein called transducin → activation of GMP phosphodiesterase → breakdown of cGMP into 5' GMP → reduction of cytosolic concentration of cGMP in rod cells → closure of Na^+ channels in outer segment of rod / cone → no entry of Na^+ inside rod cell → hyperpolarisation of rod cell as there is a continuous outflux of Na^+ from rod through the inner segment → no generator potential → no release of synaptic transmitter (glutamate) from rod / cones → generation of action potential in bipolar cell and ganglion cells → transmission of impulse to visual cortex through optic pathway.

7. Discuss the visual pathway with suitable diagram. What is the neural basis of vision?

Visual pathway: See answer of Q. No. 4.

Neural basis:

- From the rods and cones the electrical impulse is passed to the inner nuclear layer of retina to make synapse with **horizontal cell** and **bipolar cell** directly and with **amacrine cell** indirectly via bipolar cells.
- Bipolar cell then transmits the impulse to the ganglion cells.
- Whereas the horizontal cells sends inhibitory signal horizontally i.e. laterally on either side of stimulated area resulting **lateral inhibition**. This lateral inhibition is responsible for neutralising spread of excitatory signals on either side, thus sharpening the boundary between dark and bright areas making contrast borders in visual image.
- Amacrine cells only send transient signals in response to change of light intensity.
- Ganglion cells are of 3 types—W cells, X cells and Y cells.
  - W cells are responsible for rod vision.
  - X cells are responsible for colour vision.
  - Y cells are responsible for rapid changes in the visual image.

  Ganglion cells inturn send the impulse to lateral geniculate body via optic nerve that ultimately is fed to the Primary and Associated visual areas.

8. Discuss the mechanism of Colour vision. Add a note on colour-blindness.

***Mechanism of colour vision*:** There are many theories to explain the mechanism of perception of colour vision. The most important and universally accepted theories are:

(i) Young Helmholz trichromatic theory

(ii) Granit's modulator and dominator theory.

(i) Young Helmholtz trichromatic theory:

- As per this theory there are 3 types of photosensitive pigments present in cone-***Iodopsin*** (Green sensitive photopigments), ***Porphyropsin*** (red sensitive pigments) and ***Cyanopsin*** (blue sensitive).
- Each of this photosensitive pigment is sensitive to a small range of light wavelength but maximally sensitive to only one wavelength (colour). For example: Iodopsin is maximally sensitive to green colour having wavelength 535 nm. Similarly porphyropsin is maximally

sensitive to red colour having wavelength 575 nm and cyanopsin is maximally sensitive to blue colour having wavelength 435 nm.

- As per this theory when the light having wavelength 535 nm falls on retina the iodopsin is excited resulting perception of light by the visual cortex. Similarly the light of wavelength 575 and 435 are responsible for excitation of porphyropsin and cyanopsin resulting perception of red and blue colour respectively.
- Whereas the different types of colour shades of visible spectrum can be obtained by **different combinations of these 3 basic colours** (Fig. 11.8). **For example** when monochromatic orange light with wavelength 580 nm falls on the retina then all these 3 cones are stimulated in

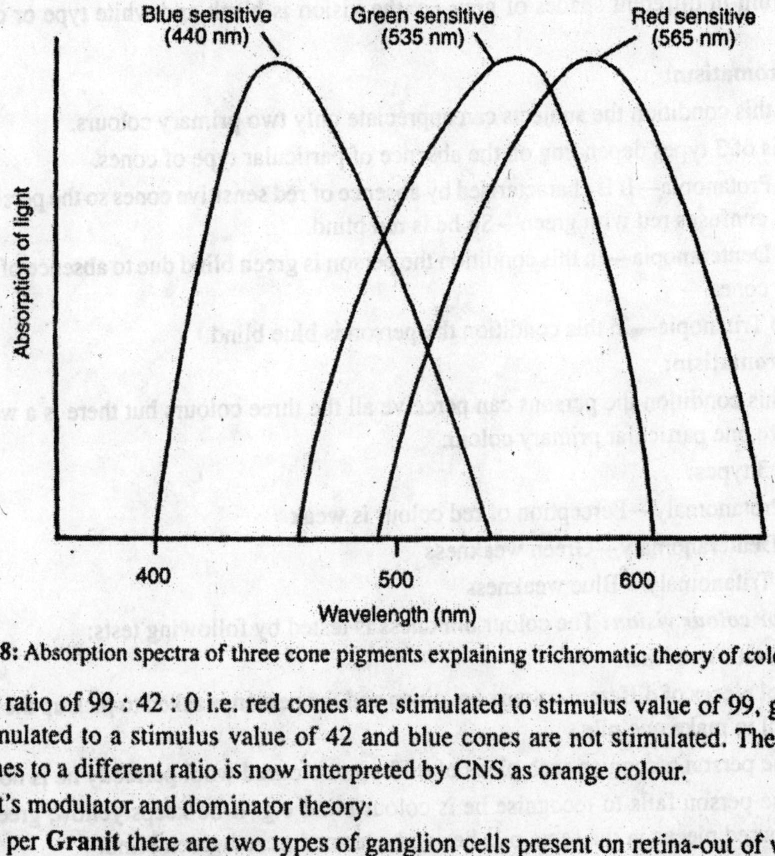

Fig. 11.8: Absorption spectra of three cone pigments explaining trichromatic theory of colour vision

the ratio of 99 : 42 : 0 i.e. red cones are stimulated to stimulus value of 99, green cones are stimulated to a stimulus value of 42 and blue cones are not stimulated. The stimulation of cones to a different ratio is now interpreted by CNS as orange colour.

(ii) Granit's modulator and dominator theory:

- As per **Granit** there are two types of ganglion cells present on retina-out of which **dominators are responsible for brightness** of light and **modulators are responsible for colour sensation.**
- Modulators are of 3 types—
  - *Modulators of blue*: stimulated by lights of wavelength 450-470 nm.
  - *Modulators of green*: stimulated by lights of wavelength of 520-540 nm.
  - *Modulators of red yellow*: stimulated by lights of wavelength of 580-600 nm.
- Light intensity of a particular wavelength when falls in the retina depending on the type of modulators stimulated, a particular colour of light is perceived by the brain. For example if green light falls on retina modulators of green are stimulated and other two are less affected. This is interpreted as green light by CNS.

Colour-blindness

- ***Definition***: Failure to differentiate some colours from the others is called colour-blindness. It is more common in males (8%) as this disease is inherited sex linked recessive disorder.
- ***Cause***: Absence of one group or more groups of cones in the retina.
- ***Classification***: On the basis of Young-Helmholtz's trichromatic theory it is of 3 types:
  (a) Monochromates
  (b) Dichromates
  (c) Trichromates

(a) Monochromatism: In this case subjects can not appreciate any colour but they see the whole spectrum in different shades of gray i.e. the vision is black and white type or complete colour blind.

(b) Dichromatism:

- In this condition the subjects can appreciate only two primary colours.
- It is of 3 types depending on the absence of particular type of cones.
  (i) Protanopia—It is characterised by absence of red sensitive cones so the person (protonopes) confuses red with green—So he is red blind.
  (ii) Deuteranopia—In this condition the person is green blind due to absence of green sensitive cones.
  (iii) Tritanopia—In this condition the person is blue blind.

(c) Trichromatism:

- In this condition the persons can perceive all the three colours but there is a weakness to perceive one particular primary colour.
- It is 3 types:
  (i) Protanomaly—Perception of red colour is weak
  (ii) Deuteranomaly—Green weakness
  (iii) Tritanomaly—Blue weakness

- ***Tests for colour vision***: The colour blindness is tested by following tests:

(a) *Holmgren's wool test*:

- Wool pieces of different colours are given and the person is asked to pick up the same coloured wool to make one pile.
- If the person recognise each piece of different coloured wool perfectly he is normal.
- If the person fails to recognise he is colour blind e.g. if he keeps yellow, green, orange, red coloured pieces in the same pile he can be termed as red-green blind.

(b) *Ishihara's chart*:

- This chart consists of a series of plate that has a background of coloured dots on which letter or number or line is written / drawn with different colours.
- The colours in the charts are arranged in such a way that only normal person can read all letters and numbers correctly or trace out the line correctly.
- The colour blind person is either not able to read or he reads wrongly. For example: Number '8' will be read as '8' by a normal person and as '3' by a subject with defective colour vision.

(c) *The Edridge—Green Lantern test*: In this test the subject has to identify the colour of the small illuminated area, size of which can be varied. This test is done during selection of engine or lorry drivers for detecting the colour defective vision.

B. Short Notes:

1. Cochlear microphonics:

- It is a type of dynamic electrical response seen in hair cells of cochlea when an auditory stimulus arrives at the cochlea.
- It is generated instantaneously due to the large current flow across the apical surface of hair cells along a favourable electrical gradient.
- It can be detected by placing electrodes on the round window or in areas near the cochlea by the process known as electrocochleography.
- The characteristics features of this electrical potential are:
  - Have no latency
  - Have no refractory period
  - Have no fatigue
  - Can not be masked
  - Occurs before the action potential.

2. Accommodation:

- To see an object clearly the object should be present at the focal point of the focusing apparatus by changing it's curvature of the anterior surface and this ability of eye to see the near object clearly is known as accommodation.
- Accommodation is achieved by contracting the ciliary muscles, pulling the ciliary body forwards and medially towards the lens, relaxing the suspensory ligaments and making the lens more convex.
- The accommodation is maximum at the near point i.e. the nearest point to the eye at which an object can be clearly seen.
- The maximum accommodation ability of the eye decreases with age so the near point recedes slowly. This gradual loss of accommodation is due to progressive loss of elasticity of the lens.
- Accommodation is an active process that is why watching television or reading book for long time results tiring of the ocular muscles and headache.
- *Abnormalities of accommodation*:

(i) Argyll Robertson pupil:

- Pupil that fails to respond to light but retained it's accommodation ability is known as **Argyll Robertson pupil.**
- It is a disease associated with lesions in or near the aqueduct of sylvius and superior colliculi interrupting the pathway for light reflex. It is the diagnostic sign of syphilis in CNS.

(ii) Reverse Argyll-Robertson pupil:

- In this case pupil retains light reflex but loss it's accommodation power.
- It is due to bilateral damage of frontal lobe or damage of it's descending fibers to III cranial nerve nucleus.

(iii) Horner's syndrome: It is characterised by—

(a) persistent constriction of pupil of affected side.

(b) persistent dilatation of blood vessels on the corresponding side of face and head.

(c) absence of sweating in face and head of affected side.

(d) drooping of superior eyelid on the corresponding side **(partial ptosis).**

It is due to damage of sympathetic nerves in cervical sympathetic chain.

- The range of accommodation is upto 10 diapters i.e. 59D to 69D.

3. Presbyopia:

- This is the physiological phenomenon seen in all persons at about age of 40 years in which the near point of vision recedes beyond the normal reading or working distance due to progressive loss of elasticity of the lens.
- As the near point recedes beyond the point which is about 28 cm from the eye, the person has difficulty in reading or writing and performing close work.
- It is usually corrected by a convex lens.

4. Electroretinogram:

- It is the record of electrical activity of retina in response to it's stimulation by a flash of light.

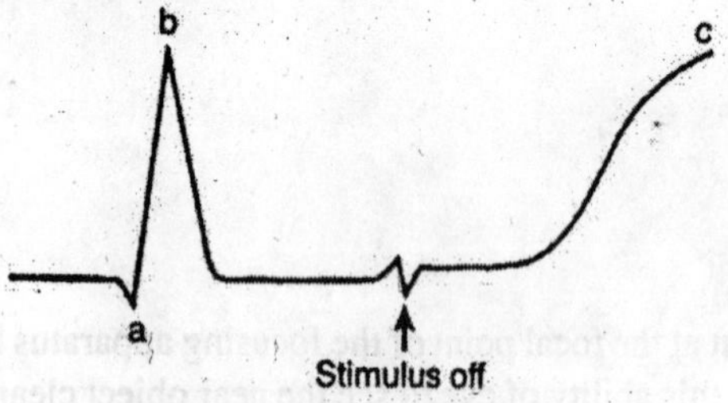

Fig. 11.9: Electroretinogram

- It has an initial rapid downward negative deflection i.e. 'a' wave followed by a bigger upward deflection i.e. 'b' wave of short duration followed by a prolonged small amplitude positive 'c' wave (Fig. 11.9). The 'a' wave originates from retinal photoreceptors, 'b' wave originates from bipolar cells and 'c' wave from the pigmented epithelium.
- It gives information about the rods located at the periphery of the retina and their connections.
- It is helpful in the diagnosis of retinal detachment, retinal dystrophy, vit-A deficiency.

5. Nystagmus:

- The involuntary rhythmical to and fro movement of the eyeball is known as nystagmus.
- It is of two types-physiological and pathological.
- When the gaze is fixed on a still object there is to and fro movement of the eyeball at a rate of 30-80 cycles per sec due to continuous contraction of few muscles fibers. This type of oscillatory movements of eye ball is known as *physiological nystagmus* which helps the eye to see the object clearly for a longer duration.
- Pathologically nystagmus results due to disorders of vestibular system or lesion of the neural pathways controlling the ocular movements.

6. Macular sparing:

- Lesion of geniculocalcarine tract damages ipsilateral temporal fibers and contralateral nasal fiber but the macular fibers that travel dorsal to the optic radiation are spared and thus escape the damage. This results homonymous hemianopia. This phenomenon is known as ***macular sparing***.
- Similarly lesion of occipital cortex also damages ipsilateral temporal fibers and contralateral nasal fibers with macular sparing.

7. Purkinjee shift:

- The colour perception depends not only on the wavelength of light but also illumination. When the spectral colours are seen in dim light the brightest part of the spectrum is green as the rods are most sensitive to the green light. On the other way when the same spectral colours are seen in high illumination e.g. in day light the brightest part of the spectrum is yellow as the cones have maximum sensitivity in the yellow region. Thus the brightest part of the spectrum shift to left during scotopic vision and shifts to right during photopic vision. This shift of the maximum sensitivity to the visible spectrum with change in illumination is known as purkinjee shift.

8. Glucoma:

- Increased intra-ocular pressure with characteristic degeneration of the retina is known as ***glucoma.***
- This is the abnormal condition in which vision is lost due to compression of optic nerve fibers at the optic disc.
- It is of two types-angle closure glaucoma and open-angle glaucoma.
- Medical treatment in both types of glucoma is common which is reduction of intra-ocular pressure by hyperosmotic drugs like mannitol, glycerol, sorbitrate or urea which causes shrinkage of vitreous humor and thus reduces the IOP. Besides this, intravenous acetazolamide, α-adrenergic blocker, cholinergic agonist, miotics (drugs causing constriction of pupil) are also useful.

9. Reduced eye:

- With light bending at multiple interfaces any mathematical treatment of visuocopic becomes very complicated. This is avoided by confining the mathematical approach to a simplified model of the eye is called as the reduced eye of Listing.
- In the reduced eye the multiple media i.e. cornea, aquous humor and vetrious humor are all replaced by a single media having refractive index 1.326. The edge of this hypothetical medium is located 1.4 cm behind the corneal surface. The edge is spherical with its radius of curvature being 5.6 mm. The nodal point of the medium is thus located 5.6 mm behind the air-medium interface.
- Rays of light passing through the nasal point does not undergo any refraction.

10. Organ of corti:

- The receptor organ for hearing is known as ***Organ of corti*** which are located on the basilar membrane present in the cochlea of internal ear. This is responsible for generation of nerve impulse in response to vibration of BM.
- The main features of organ of corti are the inner and outer rods of corti forming a single row, the upper ends of which coverage and join forming part of ***lamina reticularis*** (Fig. 11.10).
- The receptor cells in the organ of corti are of two types of hair cells—
  - **Single row of inner hair cells** (3500 in number and 12 μm in diameter).
  - **3-4 rows of outer hair cells** (12000 in number and 8 μm in diameter).

  The hairs coming out of upper end of these hair cells are covered by tectoral membrane. Basal and sides of the hair cells synapse with a network of cochlear nerve endings which lead to spiral ganglia of corti present in nodiolus and thence to cochlear nerve.

11. Tympanic reflex:

- The middle ear muscle ***Tensor tympani*** and ***Stapedius*** are responsible for initiation of this reflex.
- In response to loud sound these muscles contract → dampen the movement of ossicular system → decrease in sensitivity of acoustic apparatus (i.e. lowers the magnification of sound energy that strikes the cochlear fluid). Thus it helps to protect the structures of internal ear in response to very loud sound. This protective reflex is known as ***tympanic reflex*** or ***attenuation reflex.***

12. Cochlea:

- It is a coiled tube in the internal ear lying in the petrous part of temporal bone, which makes 2.5 to 2.75 turns.
- The lumen of the cochlea is divided throughout the length into **3 cavities** – ***Scala vestibule (SV), Scala media (SM), Scala tympani (ST)*** by two membrane ***Reissner's membrane (RM)*** and ***Basilar membrane (BM).***

- On the top of Reissner's membrane lies the scala vestibuli containing ***perilymph***. Between the RM and BM lies scala media containing ***endolymph***. Below BM there is scala tympani which contains also perilymph.
- Near the apex of cochlea, the scala vestibule communicates with the scala tympani via helicotrema.
- The RM is very **thin** and therefore do not cause any obstruction of sound. This is why so far as the conduction of sound wave, SV and SM are considered as a single chamber. However, the importance of **RM** is to **prevent the admixture of endolymph with perilymph as endolymph** is highly required for the normal function of the sound receptive hair cells.
- The **BM** is a fibrous membrane consisting of **20,000–30,000 basilar fibers** that project from the bony center of cochlea towards the outer wall.
- These basilar fibers are **stiff, elastic, reed like** structures that are fixed at their basal ends in the central bony structure of the cochlea but not fixed at their distal ends. As they are stiff and free at one end they can vibrate **like reeds of harmonica**, when sound wave strikes it.
- The **length** of basilar **fibers increases as the distance from bony ossicles** and diameter **decreases.** As a result stiff and short fibers are present near the oval window which vibrate best at higher frequency ad long limber fibers are present near the tip and vibrate best at a lower frequency sound.
- The receptor organ for hearing is known as ***Organ of corti*** which are located on the basilar membrane. This is responsible for generation of nerve impulse in response to vibration of BM.

13. Eustachian tube:

- It is 4-5 cm long tube that connects the middle ear cavity with the nasopharynx.
- Normally its pharyngeal opening remains close but opens during swallowing, chewing and yawning to allow air passage to middle ear cavity.
- When open it serves to equalize the pressure on the two sides of tympanic membrane to prevent inward or outward bulging of tympanic membrane that may lead the rupture of tympanic membrane.
- In **aeroplane journey** due to low atmospheric pressure there is outward bulging of tympanic membrane producing discomfort. To prevent it cotton plug is used or frequent acts of swallowing (by suckling lozenges) helps to equilibrate the pressure in two sides of tympanic membrane.

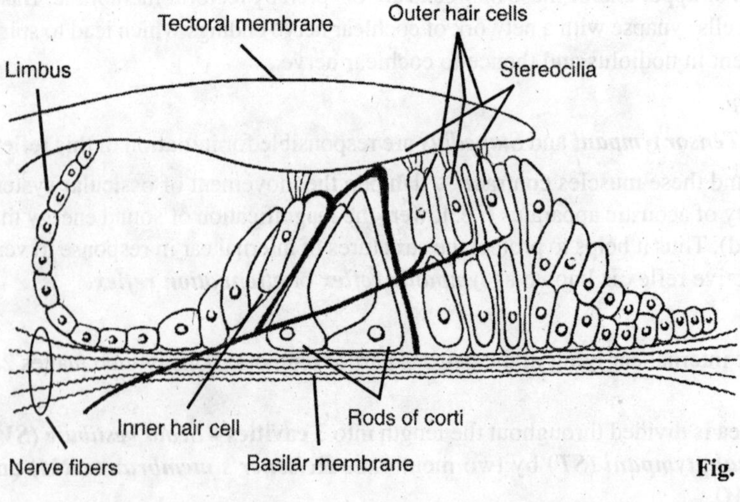

Fig. 11.10: Structure of organ of corti

14. Impedance matching device:

- This is a device by which tympanic membrane and ear ossicles magnifies the sound energy.
- Along with the tympanic membrane the ossicular system serves as a ***impedance matching device*** by two mechanism:
  - **High ratio of surface area** of tympanic membrane to oval window, which magnifies the pressure or force of sound wave, by 17 times.
  - **Mechanical advantage of lever system** of ear ossicles, which increases the force about **1.3 time.**

  Thus there is $17 \times 1.3 = 22$ times increase of energy of sound waves that is transmitted to the cochlear fluid.

15. Audiometry:

- This test is done to detect any abnormalities in hearing or not and is conducted in a sound proof room, and one ear at a time.
- Audio meter is an electronic oscillator to which earphone is connected. The audiometer is calibrated in such a way that zero intensity is the threshold intensity for all different frequencies.
- Now different frequencies of sound wave is presented to both of the ear one by one and by both routes (air and bone) in succession and the results are plotted graphically known as **audiogram.**
- In conduction deafness audiogram becomes normal when tested through bone conduction but hearing loss (especially for low frequency sound) is observed when tested through air conduction.
- In nerve deafness there will be hearing losses when tested by both air and bone conduction.

16. Ossicular system:

- It conducts the sound wave to the internal ear.
- It consists of 3 bones:
  - **Malleus**: The handle of malleus is attached to the inner side of tympanic membrane and head is firmly connected with incus by ligaments (Fig. 11.11).
  - **Incus**: It is attached to the head of malleus in one side and in other side articulates with the head of the Stapes.
  - **Stapes**: Whose foot plate is attached with the oval window by ligament.
- Ossicular system acts as a ***single lever.*** Every time the sound wave strikes the tympanic membrane → Malleus moves inward → Incus moves and causes the Stapes to push forward the cochlear fluid by striking inward at the oval window.
- Along with the tympanic membrane it also serves as a ***impedance matching device*** to protect the hair cells of the ear against loud sound.

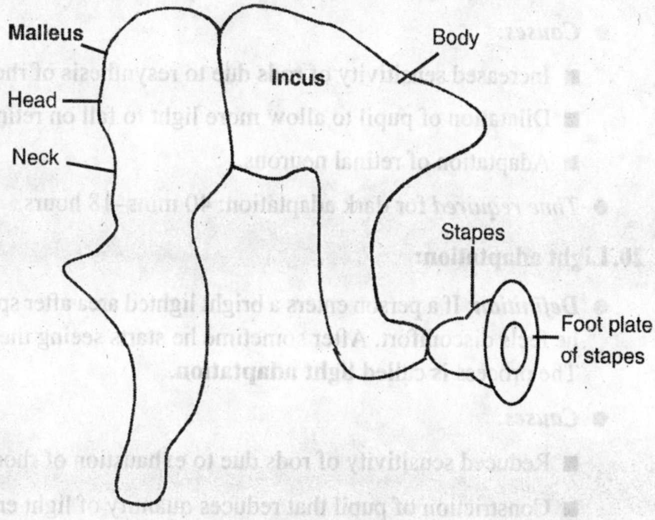

Fig. 11.11: Ear ossicles

17. Visual acuity:

- ***Definition*** — It is defined as the power of eye to recognise the separateness of two objects placed together i.e. the ability of the eye to determine the precise shape and details of any object.
- It is maximum in ***fovea centralis*** which contain densely packed cones.
- It is tested clinically with the help of **Snellen's chart** for distant vision and **Jeager's chart** for near vision.
- ***The factors affecting*** visual activity: These are:
  - (i) Type of stimulus.
  - (ii) Illumination of surface.
  - (iii) Site of retina.
  - (iv) Time of exposure.
  - (v) Brightness and contrast.
  - (vi) Errors of refraction.
- If there is any difficulty is seeing the distant or near object the defect is known as **refractive error** which can be corrected by using specific lens in spectacle.

18. Astigmatism:

- It is the defect in the refractive power of lens of the eye due to different refractive power of the lens in two planes.
- It is due to oblong shape of the lens or cornea resulting different curvature of lens in two plane.
- It is corrected by giving cylindrical lens in a defective axis (defective plane of lens which requires correction).

19. Dark adaptation:

- ***Definition***: If a person enters a dim lighted room after spending in bright light for prolonged time, initially he/she can not see the object. However, after sometime he/she can gradually see the object even in dim light. This process of vision in dim light is known as **dark adaptation**.
- ***Causes***:
  - ■ Increased sensitivity of rods due to resynthesis of rhodopsin.
  - ■ Dilatation of pupil to allow more light to fall on retina.
  - ■ Adaptation of retinal neurons.
- ***Time required*** for dark adaptation: 40 mins–18 hours.

20. Light adaptation:

- ***Definition***: If a person enters a bright lighted area after spending in dim light for long time initially he feels discomfort. After sometime he starts seeing the objects around without any discomfort. The process is called **light adaptation.**
- ***Causes***:
  - ■ Reduced sensitivity of rods due to exhaustion of rhodopsin.
  - ■ Constriction of pupil that reduces quantity of light entering the eye.
- ***Time requirement*** — 5 mins.

21. Rods:

Rod cells are cylindrical, 40-60 μ long and 2 μ in diameter (Fig. 11.12). Each rod cell has 4 parts namely — 1. Outer segment, 2. Inner segment, 3. Cell body, 4. Synaptic terminal.

The outer segment of rod cell is formed by the modified cilia and contains free floating flat membranous discs which contains the photosensitive pigment called ***Rhodopsin***. This outer segment is continuously renewed by formation of new discs at the inner edge and phagocytosis of old discs from the outer tip by cells of pigmented epithelium. The inner segment is rich in mitochondria.

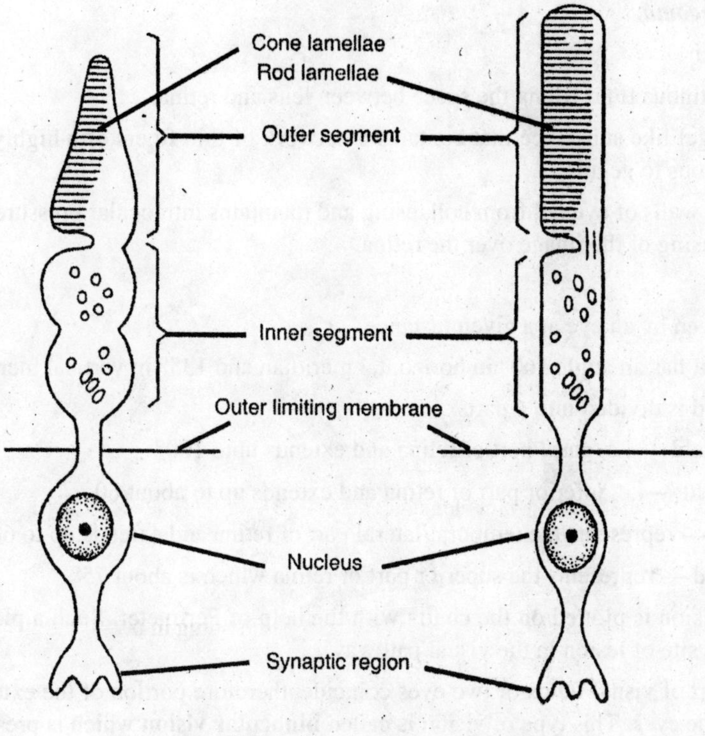

Fig. 11.12: Structure of rod and cone

22. Cones:

- These are generally flask shaped, 35-40 μ long and having a diameter of about 5 μ.
- Like rods it also have outer segment, inner segment, cell body, synaptic terminal (Fig. 11.12).
- The outer segment is small, conical and does not have discs like rods.
- Rather, in cone the cell membrane becomes folded to form saccules the surface of which contains pigment called ***Iodopsin*** (green sensitive). ***Porphyropsin*** (red sensitive) and ***Cyanopsin*** (blue sensitive).

23. Aqueous humor:

- It is thin and clear fluid present in the anterior and posterior chamber of the eye having following property:
  - Volume: 0.13 ml
  - pH: 7.5

- Viscosity: 1.029
- Sp. Gravity: 1.002 – 1.004
- Refractive index: 1.34

- It is formed from the capillaries of the ciliary process by active transport and diffusion and isotonic to plasma.
- It supplies nutrition to lens and cornea and maintains intraocular pressure to maintain the normal shape of the eyeball.
- Any obstruction of the outflow of aqueous humor results increased intraocular pressure which is known as ***glaucoma.***

24. Vitreous humor:

- It is clear gelatinous fluid filling the space between lens and retina.
- It consists of gel like substance that contains a network of thin fibers of a highly hygroscopic protein analogous to gelatin.
- It prevents the walls of eyeball from collapsing and maintains intraocular pressure. It also helps in normal focusing of the image over the retina.

25. Field of vision:

- It is the area seen by an eye at a given instance.
- In human eye it has an angle 160° in horizontal meridian and 135° in vertical meridian.
- The visual field is divided into 4 parts:
  - Temporal field — i.e. nasal part of retina and extends upto 100°
  - Superior field — i.e. inferior part of retina and extends up to about 60°
  - Nasal field — represents the temporal/lateral part of retina and extends up to 60°
  - Inferior field — represents the superior part of retina which is about 75°
- The field of vision is plotted on the charts with the help of Perimeter. Such a plot is useful in diagnosing the site of lesion in the visual pathway.
- The central part of visual fields of two eyes coincide, therefore portion of the external world is seen by both the eyes. This type of vision is called **binocular vision** which is present in human beings (In animals it is monocular vision).

26. Pupillary light reflex:

- *Definition*: When light is flashed into the eyes, pupil constricts. This is known as pupillary light reflex.
- *Types:* It is of 2 types:
  - Direct light reflex — When light is flashed into a particular eye there is constriction of pupil of that eye which is known as direct light reflex.
  - Indirect (consensual) light reflex — In response to flashing of light in one eye there is constriction of other eye also which is known as indirect light reflex which is due to crossing over of nerve fibers in the visual pathway mainly at optic chiasma.
- *Pathway of light reflex*: Receptors in retina → optic nerve → optic chiasma → optic tract → pretectal nucleus → Edinger — Westphal nucleus → oculomotor nerve → ciliary ganglion → ciliary nerves → sphincter pupillae muscle responsible for constriction of pupil.
- *Function*: It is to help the eye to adapt rapidly to changing light condition.

27. Refractory errors of eye:

(a) *Physiological refractive errors:*

(i) **Spherical aberration:** When parallel rays of light pass through the peripheral portions of the lens of the eye it does not exactly focus at the same point where rays, passing through central portion of the lens focus. This defect is physiological and known as ***spherical aberration*** which is minimised specially when pupil constricts as iris covers the peripheral portions of lens to prevent passing of light through peripheral portions of lens.

(ii) **Chromatic aberration:** The light rays of different colours get focused at different distances behind the lens. This type of physiological error is known as ***chromatic aberration.***

(iii) **Diffraction:** Bending of the light rays as they pass over the sharp borders of pupil is known as diffraction.

(b) *Pathological refractive errors*:

(i) **Myopia** (Short sightedness):

- It is the condition in which ciliary muscles completely relax resulting focusing of the parallel rays of light coming from the distant object in front of retina (Fig. 11.13). Therefore the person is unable to see the distant object.

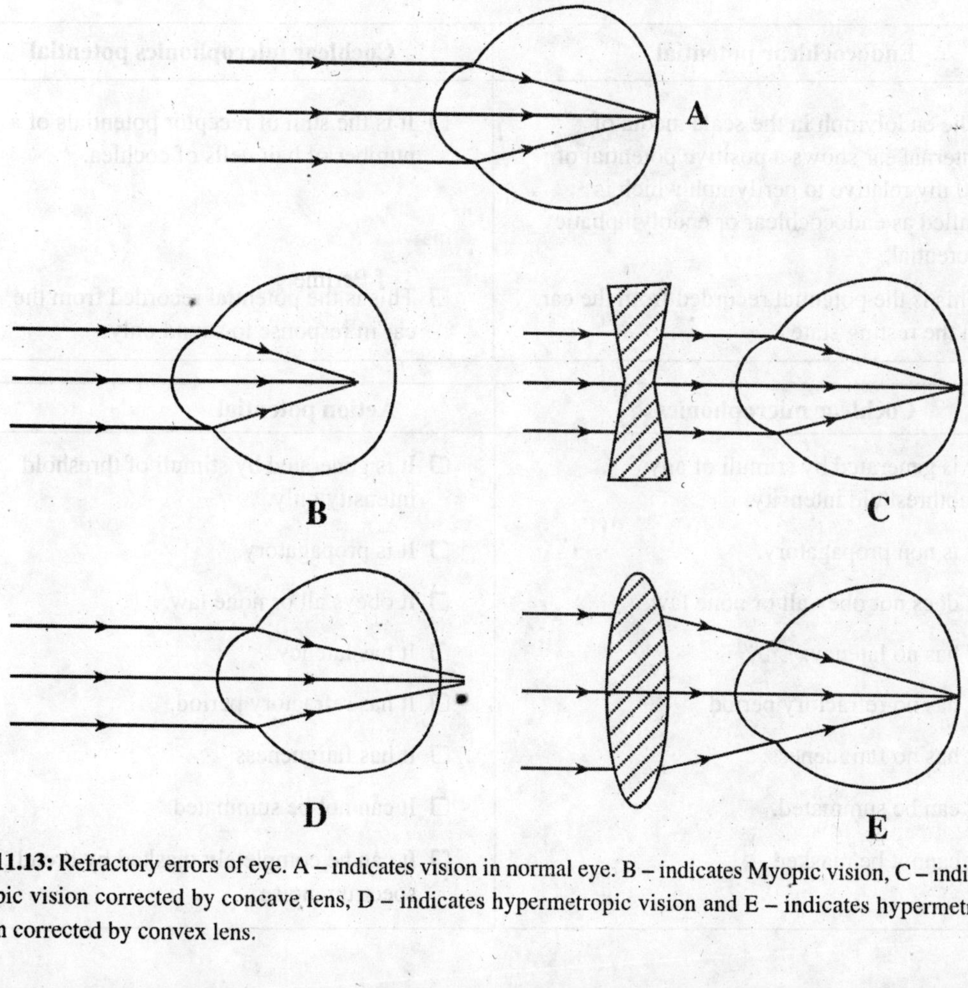

Fig. 11.13: Refractory errors of eye. A – indicates vision in normal eye. B – indicates Myopic vision, C – indicates Myopic vision corrected by concave lens, D – indicates hypermetropic vision and E – indicates hypermetropic vision corrected by convex lens.

- It is either due to long eyeball or increased refractive power of the lens.
- It is corrected by giving concave lens of appropriate refractive power (Fig. 11.13).

(ii) **Hypermetropia** (Far sightedness):

- It is the refractive error of the eye characterised by inability to see the near object due to focussing of parallel rays of light coming from distant object behind the retina (Fig. 11.13).
- It is either due to too short eyeball or decreased refractive power of the lens of eye.
- It is corrected by giving convex lens of appropriate refractive power.

(iii) **Astigmatism:**

- It is the defect in the refractive power of lens of the eye only in one place due to different refractive power of the lens in two planes.
- It is due to oblong shape of the lens or cornea resulting different curvature of lens in two plane.
- It is corrected by giving cylindrical lens in a defective axis (defective plane of lens which requires correction).

C. Differentiate between:

Endocochlear potential	Cochlear microphonics potential
❒ The endolymph in the scala media of internal ear shows a positive potential of 80 mv relative to perilymph which is called as endocochlear or endolymphatic potential.	❒ It is the sum of receptor potentials of a number of hair cells of cochlea.
❒ This is the potential recorded from the ear in the resting state.	❒ This is the potential recorded from the ear in response to sound only.

Cochlear microphonics	Action potential
❒ It is generated by stimuli of any subthreshold intensity.	❒ It is generated by stimuli of threshold intensity only.
❒ It is non propagatory.	❒ It is propagatory.
❒ It does not obey all or none law.	❒ It obeys all or none law.
❒ It has no latency.	❒ It has latency.
❒ It has no refractory period.	❒ It has refractory period.
❒ It has no fatigueness.	❒ It has fatigueness.
❒ It can be summated.	❒ It can not be summated.
❒ It cannot be masked.	❒ It can be completely masked by broad spectrum noise.

Perilymph	Endolymph
❒ Present in scala tympani and scala vestibuli.	❒ Present in scala media, utricle, saccule and semi circular canals.
❒ Contains high Na^+ and low K^+ and resembles ECF.	❒ Contains high K^+ and low Na^+ and resembles ICF.
❒ It is the ultrafiltrate of blood.	❒ It is the secretions from stria vascularis.
❒ It is required for passing of sound wave from oval window to scala media.	❒ It is required for activation of hair cells.

Inner hair cells	Outer hair cells
❒ Single row of hair cells present internal to the inner Rod's of corti.	❒ 3-4 rows of hair cells present external to the outer Rod's of corti.
❒ It is flask shaped.	❒ It is test tube shaped.
❒ It is responsible for initiation of auditory impulses and less in number (3500).	❒ It is responsible for modulation of the function of inner hair cells.

Vitreous humor	Aqueous humor
❒ It is present behind the retina in the space between lens and retina.	❒ It is present in front of the retina and fills the space between lens and cornea.
❒ It is a highly viscus and gelatinous substance formed by a fine fibriller network of proteo-glycan molecule.	❒ It is thin fluid containing mainly water.
❒ It is formed by diffusion from the blood.	❒ It is formed partly by active secretion and partly by ultrafiltration in the posterior chamber.
❒ It mainly helps in maintaining shape and pressure in eye ball.	❒ It mainly provides nutrition to the cornea and lens.
❒ It has negligible role in changing intraocular pressure.	❒ It has major role in changing intraocular pressure.

Direct light reflex	Indirect light reflex
❒ When light is flashed to a particular eye there is constriction of pupil of that eye which is known as direct light reflex.	❒ When light is flashed to a particular eye there is constriction of both the eyes which is known as indirect light reflex.

Argyll-Robertson pupil	Reverse Argyll-Robertson pupil
❒ Light reflexes are lost in this situation.	❒ Light reflexes are retained in this situation.
❒ Accommodation reflex is present.	❒ Accommodation reflex is absent.
❒ Pupils become small and irregular.	❒ Pupils become large.

Rods	Cons
❒ It is responsible for dim light vision	❒ It is responsible for day light vision.
❒ It can not direct colour	❒ It can detect colour.
❒ These are more in number (120 million).	❒ These are less in number (6 million).
❒ These are cylindrical and 40-60 μ long.	❒ These are flask shaped and 3.5-4.0 μ long.
❒ Present mainly in the peripheral retina.	❒ Present mainly in the central retina.
❒ More pigments per rod.	❒ Less pigments per cone.
❒ Present only type of pigment i.e. rhodopsin.	❒ Present 3 types of pigment.
❒ Receptive field is more.	❒ Receptive field is less.
❒ Resolution is less.	❒ Resolution is more.
❒ Loss of rod function leads to night blindness.	❒ Loss of cone function leads to functional blindness.

Myopia	Hypermetropia
❒ It is due to focusing of parallel rays of light from the distant object on the retina.	❒ It is due to focusing of parallel rays of light from the distant object behind the retina.
❒ The primary defect is increase in length of the eye ball or refractive power of the lens.	❒ The primary defect is decrease in length of the eye ball or refractive power of the lens.
❒ Far point of vision decreases below 6 mt.	❒ Far point of vision increases above 6 mt.
❒ Near point of vision remains close to eye.	❒ Near point of vision increases.
❒ Accommodation is not required for focusing distant objects.	❒ Accommodation is reqired for focusing distant objects.
❒ Range of accommodation decreases.	❒ Range of accommodation increases.
❒ Common in young adult.	❒ Rare in young adult.
❒ Refractive power of concave lens is expressed in negative diopter.	❒ Refractive power of convex lens is expressed in positive diopter.

Spherical aberration	Chromatic abberation
❒ When parallel rays of light pass through the peripheral portions of the lens of the eye it does not exactly focus at the same point where rays passing through central portion of the lens, focus. This defect is known as spherical aberration.	❒ When the light rays of different colours get focused at different distances behind the lens this type of error is known as chromatic aberration.

Binocular vision	Monocular vision
❒ Field of vision is more.	❒ Field of vision is less.
❒ Viewing of object as a single one with both eyes is called as a bionocular vision.	❒ Visual fields of both eyes overlap only to a small extent.

Bionocular vision	Monocula
❒ **Example:** Vision in human beings. ❒ It is due to presence of eye balls in front of the head.	❒ **Example:** Vision in animals like dog, rabbit etc. ❒ It is due to presence of eye balls at the side of the head.

Dark adaptation	Light adaptation
❒ If a person enters a dimlighted room after spending in bright light for prolonged time, initially he/she can not see the object even in dim-light. However after sometime he/she can see the object even in dim-light. This process of vision in dim-light is known as dark adaptation.	❒ If a person enters a bright lighted room after spending in dim-light for prolonged time, initially he/she feels discomfort but after sometime he/she can gradually see the object without any discomfort. This process of vision is known as light adaptation.
❒ Dark adapted retina is more sensitive (10,000 times).	❒ Dark adapted retina is less sensitive.
❒ Vit-A deficiency affects the dark adaptation.	❒ Vit-A deficiency does not affect the light adaptation.
❒ Vision changes from cones to rod (photopic to scotopic).	❒ Vision changes from rods to cones (scotopic to photopic).
❒ Concentration of photopigments increase.	❒ Concentration of photopigments decrease.
❒ Sensitivity of receptors to light increases.	❒ Sensitivity of receptors to light decreases.
❒ Visual acuity decreases.	❒ Visual acuity increases.
❒ Pupils dilate during this.	❒ Pupils constrict during this.

Rhodopsin	Iodopsin
❒ These are the photosensitive pigments in rods.	❒ These are the photosensitive pigments in cones.
❒ These are responsible for dim-light vision.	❒ These are responsible for colour vision.
❒ Vit-A deficiency affects rhodopsin formation.	❒ Vit-A deficiency does not affect iodopsin formation.

Primary colour	Complementary colour
❒ Three basic colours which when combined together in equal proportions can produce white colour is known as primary colour.	❒ Complimentary colours are those two colours which when are mixed or combined produce white colours.
❒ **Example**: red, green, blue.	❒ **Examples**: red and greenish blue, orange and cyan blue etc.

Photopic vision	Scotopic vision
❒ It is daylight vision.	❒ It is dimlight vision.
❒ It is due to activation of cone receptor.	❒ It is due to activation of rod receptor.
❒ It has higher threshold i.e. opertes at higher intensity of light.	❒ It has lower threshold i.e. operates at lower intensity of light.
❒ Its peak sensitivity is at 560 nm (green yellow).	❒ Its peak sensitivity is at 502 nm (blue green).

Conduction deafness	Nerve deafness
❒ It is defined as partial loss of hearing resulted from defective sound transmission due to defects in external or middle ear.	❒ It is defined as complete or partial loss of hearing resulted due to the complete or partial damage in cochlea or cochlear nerve or auditory cortex.
❒ In Rinne's test the vibration in air are not heard after bone conduction is over.	❒ It is Rinne's test insensitive.
❒ Can be corrected by hearing aids.	❒ Can not be corrected by hearing aids.
❒ Weber's test is lateralised to the affected side.	❒ Weber's test is lateralised to the normal side.
❒ Schwabach test shows better conduction than examiners.	❒ Schwabach test shows poorer conduction than examiners.

D. Short answer type:

1. Give physiological basis of decrease in olfaction in following cases.

(a) *If a person suffers from common cold*: In case of common cold mucous in the nasal passage prevent the odoriferous substances to transverse through → decrease of olfaction.

(b) *In old age*: In old age the olfactory thresold increases resulting loss of olfaction.

2. Why are organic acids more sour than mineral acids?

The degree of sour is directly related with the degree of dissociation of H^+ from an acid which is greater in organic acids.

3. What will happen and why to hearing?

(a) *If someone suffers from sore throat*: In sore throat → closure of pharyngotympanic tube due to inflammation in throat → ineffective swallowing → absorption of air present in middle ear → decrease in pressure in middle ear → inward bulging of tympanic membrane → decrease in vibration of tympanic membrane → loss of hearing.

(b) *If one auditory cortex is removed*: Hearing will remain unaffected with only slight decrease of the auditory acuity (sharpness). This is because that the fibers from either ear are projected to the both sides of cerebral cortex though the projection is more in contralateral side.

Index

Some exciting gifts are up for grabs with this book!!

PHYSIOLOGY : MADE EASY

Dr A K Basak

FREE Gifts Rs. 1000/-

Dear Readers

By now you must have gone through this book in the entirety. So we invite your assessment on this title with absolute impartiality and candid observations. After all, we publishers blindly depend on your benchmarking. Friends, please fill up the open spaces below with CAPITAL LETTERS. You may add some extra sheets of paper if the space provided is not sufficient for you.

i. What are the important topics of your syllabus which are not adequately covered in this book?

ii. In which chapters and on what topics the treatment of the subject-matter by the author is not satisfactory and why?

iii. Have you come across the typos, factual inaccuracies, inconsistencies, and other forms of mistakes in the book? If yes, then please specify the mistakes and page numbers.

iv. Name top three books on the same subject, which, in your consideration, are better than this book. Could you provide some reasons?

Your 1st Preference: ....

Your 2nd Preference: ....

Your 3rd Preference: ....

v. Any suggestion to improve the quality of illustrations, diagrams, etc.?

vi. How did you like the cover design? Any suggestion on colours?

vii. Suggestions for further improvement of production-standard:

viii. Who recommended you this book:

☐ Teacher ☐ Friend ☐ Parents ☐ Bookseller ☐ Librarian

ix. Name of the person who has recommended:

Designation: ....

Address: ....

Phone No.: ....

e-mail: ....